HANDBOOK OF EMOTION REGULATION

HANDBOOK OF EMOTION REGULATION

edited by James J. Gross

THE GUILFORD PRESS
New York   London

© 2007 The Guilford Press
A Division of Guilford Publications, Inc.
72 Spring Street, New York, NY 10012
www.guilford.com

Paperback edition 2009

Printed in the United States of America

This book is printed on acid-free paper.

Last digit is print number: 9 8 7 6 5 4 3

Library of Congress Cataloging-in-Publication Data
Handbook of emotion regulation / edited by James J. Gross.
    p. cm.
  Includes bibliographical references and index.
  ISBN 978-1-59385-148-4 (hardcover: alk. paper)
  ISBN 978-1-60623-354-2 (paperback: alk. paper)
  1. Emotions. I. Gross, James J., Ph.D.
  [DNLM: 1. Emotions—physiology. 2. Brain—physiology. 3. Cog-
nition. 4. Human Development. 5. Mental Disorders—etiology.
6. Mental Disorders—therapy. WL 103 H23565 2007]
  BF531.H324 2007
  152.4—dc22
                                            2006028625

To my parents

About the Editor

James J. Gross, PhD, is an Associate Professor in the Department of Psychology, a faculty member in the Neurosciences Program, and the Director of the Stanford Psychophysiology Laboratory at Stanford University. He is a leading researcher in the areas of emotion and emotion regulation, and is well known for his innovative theoretical and experimental analyses of emotion regulation processes. He is also an award-winning teacher, a Bass University Fellow in Undergraduate Education, and the Director of the Stanford Psychology One Teaching Program. Dr. Gross earned his BA in philosophy from Yale University and his PhD in clinical psychology from the University of California, Berkeley. He has received early career awards from the American Psychological Association, the Western Psychological Association, and the Society for Psychophysiological Research. Dr. Gross has an extensive program of investigator-initiated research, with grants from both the National Science Foundation and the National Institutes of Health. His publications include *Psychology* (with Henry Gleitman and Daniel Reisberg), and his current research examines emotion regulation processes in healthy and clinical populations using behavioral, autonomic, and functional magnetic resonance imaging measures.

Contributors

Dustin Albert, MA, Department of Psychology, Wake Forest University, Winston–Salem, North Carolina

John A. Bargh, PhD, Department of Psychology, Yale University, New Haven, Connecticut

David H. Barlow, PhD, Department of Psychology, Boston University, Boston, Massachusetts

Lisa Feldman Barrett, PhD, Department of Psychology, Boston College, Chestnut Hill, Massachusetts

Roy F. Baumeister, PhD, Department of Psychology, Florida State University, Tallahassee, Florida

Jennifer S. Beer, PhD, Department of Psychology and the Center for Mind and Brain, University of California at Davis, Davis, California

Pavel S. Blagov, MA, Department of Psychology, Emory University, Atlanta, Georgia

Martin Bohus, MD, The Medical Faculty of Mannheim, University of Heidelberg, Heidelberg, Germany

Matthew M. Botvinick, MD, PhD, Department of Psychiatry and Center for Cognitive Neuroscience, University of Pennsylvania, Philadelphia, Pennsylvania

Susan D. Calkins, PhD, Department of Psychology, University of North Carolina, Greensboro, North Carolina

Laura Campbell-Sills, PhD, Department of Psychiatry, University of California at San Diego, La Jolla, California

Laura L. Carstensen, PhD, Department of Psychology, Stanford University, Stanford, California

Susan Turk Charles, PhD, Department of Psychology and Social Behavior, University of California at Irvine, Irvine, California

Jonathan D. Cohen, PhD, Department of Psychology and Center for the Study of Brain, Mind, and Behavior, Princeton University, Princeton, New Jersey

William A. Cunningham, PhD, Department of Psychology, The Ohio State University, Columbus, Ohio

Richard J. Davidson, PhD, Department of Psychology, University of Wisconsin–Madison, Madison, Wisconsin

Nancy Eisenberg, PhD, Department of Psychology, Arizona State University, Tempe, Arizona

Erika E. Forbes, PhD, Department of Psychiatry, University of Pittsburgh, Pittsburgh, Pennsylvania

Andrew Fox, BA, Waisman Center for Brain Imaging and Behavior, University of Wisconsin–Madison, Madison, Wisconsin

Joshua D. Greene, PhD, Department of Psychology, Princeton University, Princeton, New Jersey

Emily R. Grekin, PhD, Department of Psychological Sciences, University of Missouri–Columbia, Columbia, Missouri

James J. Gross, PhD, Department of Psychology, Stanford University, Stanford, California

Ahmad R. Hariri, PhD, Department of Psychiatry, University of Pittsburgh, Pittsburgh, Pennsylvania

Ashley Hill, PhD, Center for Developmental Science, University of North Carolina, Chapel Hill, North Carolina

Stephen P. Hinshaw, PhD, Department of Psychology, University of California at Berkeley, Berkeley, California

Claire Hofer, PhD, Department of Psychology, Arizona State University, Tempe, Arizona

Oliver P. John, PhD, Department of Psychology, University of California at Berkeley, Berkeley, California

Ned H. Kalin, MD, Department of Psychiatry, University of Wisconsin–Madison, Madison, Wisconsin

Marsha M. Linehan, PhD, Behavioral Research and Therapy Clinics, University of Washington, Seattle, Washington

George Loewenstein, PhD, Social and Decision Sciences, Carnegie Mellon University, Pittsburgh, Pennsylvania

Michael V. Lombardo, BA, Department of Psychology and the Center for Mind and Brain, University of California at Davis, Davis, California

Thomas R. Lynch, PhD, Department of Psychology and Neuroscience, Duke University, Durham, North Carolina

Samuel M. McClure, PhD, Department of Psychology and Center for the Study of Brain, Mind, and Behavior, Princeton University, Princeton, New Jersey

Mark Meerum Terwogt, PhD, Department of Developmental Psychology, Vrije Universiteit Amsterdam, Amsterdam, Holland

Batja Mesquita, PhD, Department of Psychology, Wake Forest University, Winston–Salem, North Carolina

Sara Meyer, MA, Department of Psychology, University of California at Davis, Davis, California

Mario Mikulincer, PhD, Department of Psychology, Bar-Ilan University, Ramat-Gan, Israel

Benjamin C. Mullin, BA, Department of Psychology, University of California at Berkeley, Berkeley, California

Kevin N. Ochsner, PhD, Department of Psychology, Columbia University, New York, New York

Nansook Park, PhD, Department of Psychology, University of Rhode Island, Kingston, Rhode Island

Christopher Peterson, PhD, Department of Psychology, University of Michigan, Ann Arbor, Michigan

Gregory J. Quirk, PhD, Department of Psychology, Ponce School of Medicine, Ponce, Puerto Rico

Bernard Rimé, PhD, Department of Psychology, Université Catholique de Louvain, Louvain-la-Neuve, Belgium

Mary K. Rothbart, PhD, Department of Psychology, University of Oregon, Eugene, Oregon

Peter Salovey, PhD, Department of Psychology, Yale University, New Haven, Connecticut

Robert M. Sapolsky, PhD, Department of Biological Sciences, Stanford University, Stanford, California

Phillip R. Shaver, PhD, Department of Psychology, University of California at Davis, Davis, California

Brad E. Sheese, PhD, Department of Psychology, University of Oregon, Eugene, Oregon

Kenneth J. Sher, PhD, Department of Psychology, University of Missouri–Columbia, Columbia, Missouri

Hedy Stegge, PhD, Department of Developmental Psychology, Vrije Universiteit Amsterdam, Amsterdam, Holland

Ross A. Thompson, PhD, Department of Psychology, University of California at Davis, Davis, California

Dianne M. Tice, PhD, Department of Psychology, Florida State University, Tallahassee, Florida

Julie Vaughan, BA, Department of Psychology, Arizona State University, Tempe, Arizona

Fraser Watts, PhD, Faculty of Divinity, University of Cambridge, Cambridge, United Kingdom

Drew Westen, PhD, Department of Psychology, Emory University, Atlanta, Georgia

Lawrence E. Williams, MS, Department of Psychology, Yale University, New Haven, Connecticut

Tanja Wranik, PhD, Department of Psychology, University of Geneva, Geneva, Switzerland

Nick Yeung, PhD, Department of Psychology, Carnegie Mellon University, Pittsburgh, Pennsylvania

Philip David Zelazo, PhD, Department of Psychology, University of Toronto, Toronto, Canada

Anne L. Zell, MA, Department of Psychology, Florida State University, Tallahassee, Florida

Preface

The topic of emotion regulation has now come into its own. Books, articles, and conferences related to emotion regulation seem to be everywhere. This growing interest is reflected in citation trends. As shown in Figure P.1, until the early 1990s, there were just a few citations a year containing the phrase "emotion regulation." Since this time, there has been an approximately fivefold increase in citations each 5-year period.

Popularity is a wonderful thing, but there remains an unfortunate degree of confusion about what emotion regulation is (and isn't), how it changes over time, and what effects—if any—emotion regulation has on important life outcomes. In part, this confusion stems from the fact that theoretical discussions and empirical studies related to emotion regulation are so widely dispersed across a number of disciplines. I hope, in this volume, to bring some clarity to the topic.

The goals of this handbook are (1) to facilitate cumulative science by integrating developmental and adult literatures on emotion regulation, and by bridging the gap between research on basic processes and clinical applications; (2) to provide an authoritative and up-to-date account of the findings in this field in a format that will be useful to educators and health care professionals who regularly face emotion regulation challenges in school and therapeutic contexts; and (3) to encourage cross-disciplinary dialogue about one of the most fascinating puzzles regarding the human condition, namely, that we are at once governed by—and governors of—our emotions.

The primary audience for this handbook consists of social scientists interested in emotion and self-regulation who study infants, children, or adults, as well as educators, clinicians, and other health professionals whose work with patients centers around emotion and emotion regulation. I also hope this handbook will be of interest to scholars in other fields, including (among others) philosophy, economics, law, history, sociology, anthropology, religious studies, linguistics, and literature.

The organization of this handbook is straightforward. Nearly a decade ago, I noted that the (at that time) emerging field of emotion regulation cuts across traditional subdisciplinary boundaries (Gross, 1998). In particular, I suggested that emotion regulation may be seen as drawing upon insights and findings from biological, cognitive,

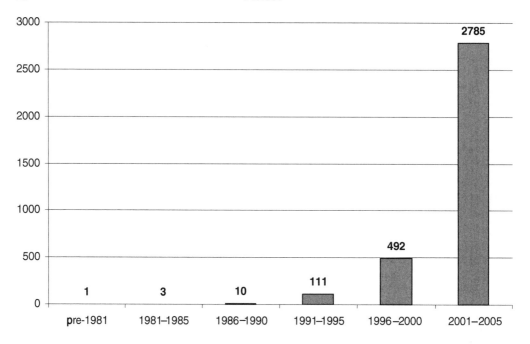

FIGURE P.1. Citations for "emotion regulation" in PsycLIT. A similar citation trend is apparent when using a broader bandwidth search tool such as Google Scholar.

developmental, personality, social, and clinical/health domains. As shown in Figure P.2, this is the organizational scheme I have used to structure this handbook.

The handbook begins with a foundations section in which Ross Thompson and I provide a conceptual foundation for the field. To this end, we first set emotion in the context of other affective processes. Next, we relate emotion regulation to other forms of self-regulation. We then present a process model of emotion regulation that distinguishes five points in the emotion-generative process at which emotions may be regulated. Using this model as our framework, we review research drawn from developmental and adult literatures related to each of five major families of emotion-regulatory processes.

The second section considers biological bases of emotion regulation, with chapters that draw on lesion and activation studies in rats and primates, neuropsychological studies, brain imaging studies, and imaging genetics. Gregory Quirk considers the animal literature concerning the nature of prefrontal–amygdala interactions in the regulation of fear, and suggests that deficits in prefrontal–amygdala extinction circuits may underlie emotion dysregulation. Richard Davidson and colleagues draw on studies of nonhuman primates and humans to elucidate the neural bases of emotion regulation. Jennifer Beer and Michael Lombardo examine the neuropsychological literature, finding that common control systems underlie the regulation of emotional and nonemotional behavior. Kevin Ochsner and I review the neuroimaging literature of emotion regulation, with a particular focus on two types of regulation: attentional deployment and cognitive change. Finally, Ahmad Hariri and Erika Forbes synthesize the literature on imaging genetics and present evidence that the serotonin system is crucially involved in emotion regulation.

The third section considers cognitive aspects of emotion regulation. Based on the literature on executive function, Philip Zelazo and William Cunningham propose a model that highlights the role of reflection and rule use in the regulation of emotion. Christopher Peterson and Nansook Park summarize the literature on explanatory style and argue that differences in how people habitually explain the causes of events shed light on how they regulate emotions. George Loewenstein considers the intersection of affect regulation and affective forecasting, demonstrating that the way people regulate their emotions depends on their beliefs. Finally, Samuel McClure and colleagues draw on findings in the areas of economic decision making, social exchange, and moral judgment to examine how competition between emotional and cognitive processes is adjudicated.

The fourth section focuses on developmental considerations, ranging from infancy through old age. Susan Calkins and Ashley Hill consider how biological and environmental transactions in early development shape emerging emotion regulation capabilities, with a particular focus on caregiver–child relationships. Ross Thompson and Sara Meyer consider family socialization of emotion regulation in the context of both typical and atypical development. Continuing this theme, Hedy Stegge and Mark Meerum Terwogt consider how children learn to regulate their emotions (or fail to do so), with particular emphasis on the role of self-awareness and self-reflection. Nancy Eisenberg and colleagues examine the impact of effortful control in childhood on social cognition, adjustment, social competence, and moral/prosocial development. Finally, Susan Turk Charles and Laura Carstensen take a lifespan perspective, and show how biological and motivational changes interact to shape the trajectory of emotion regulation through adulthood and into older age.

The fifth section considers personality processes and individual differences. Mary Rothbart and Brad Sheese present a temperament systems approach, which provides a context for understanding individual differences and the development of emotion regulation. Oliver John and I use the conceptual framework from the first chapter of this handbook to consider personality trait (Big Five domains), dynamic (coping styles and attachment), and social–cognitive (optimism, meta-mood processes, and implicit theories) paradigms. Drew Westen and Pavel Blagov consider links among psychological defense, motivated reasoning, and emotion regulation. Tanja Wranik and colleagues use an emotional intelligence framework to consider how emotion-related skills help individuals adapt to life challenges. Finally, Roy Baumeister and colleagues consider how emotions facilitate and impair self-regulation.

The sixth section considers social-psychological approaches to emotion regulation. John Bargh and Lawrence Williams review the mechanisms that underlie nonconscious self-regulation and suggest that emotions might be nonconsciously managed in a similar fashion. Phillip Shaver and Mario Mikulincer present a model of attachment and emo-

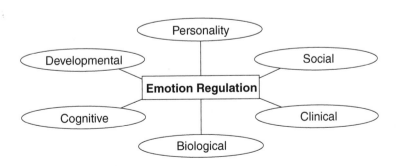

FIGURE P.2. Emotion regulation and six subfields of psychology. These—along with the conceptual foundations section—make up the seven sections of this handbook.

tion regulation that helps to explain the emotional correlates and consequences of individual differences in attachment-system functioning. Bernard Rimé investigates how emotions are regulated interpersonally, addressing the question of why people so often seek to share their emotions with others. Batja Mesquita and Dustin Albert offer a cultural perspective on emotion regulation, arguing that emotion regulation is necessarily embedded in cultural models of self and other. Finally, Fraser Watts explores links between emotion regulation and religious beliefs and practices, with a particular focus on anger.

The seventh section considers clinical applications of emotion regulation. Benjamin Mullin and Stephen Hinshaw explore the role of emotional reactivity and regulation in externalizing disorders in children and adults. Laura Campbell-Sills and David Barlow argue that counterproductive efforts to regulate emotions are a major feature of anxiety and mood disorders, and present a treatment protocol that is grounded in basic research on emotion and emotion regulation. Kenneth Sher and Emily Grekin review literature concerning both the effects of alcohol use on affect and the effects of affect on alcohol use. Marsha Linehan and colleagues describe the application and theoretical rationale of a set of emotion regulation skills developed within the context of dialectical behavior therapy, a treatment developed for individuals with severe and pervasive disorders of emotion regulation. Finally, in the last chapter, Robert Sapolsky reviews links among stress, stress-related disease, and emotion regulation.

It bears noting that although this handbook is divided into sections, one of its major goals is breaking down barriers to cross-area communication. For this reason, there are considerably more cross-chapter links and citations than is typical in a handbook. There are also many points at which an author in one section will present material that makes contact with ideas, methods, and evidence from another section (e.g., developmental considerations in the clinical applications section; neuroscience in the cognitive section; analyses of individual differences in the social section). My hope is that these carefully assembled chapters—which are written by leading scholars in the field—will bring the field of emotion regulation together in a way that will be productive and new.

A large number of wonderful people helped to bring this handbook into being. I am grateful to Seymour Weingarten, Editor-in-Chief at The Guilford Press, for convincing me that the time had come for this handbook, and to Robert Levenson, with whom my work on emotion regulation began. I am also grateful to the many friends and colleagues who provided crucial guidance as I laid the plan for this handbook, including Ross Thompson, Oliver John, Richard Davidson, Lisa Feldman Barrett, and Kevin Ochsner. I would also like to thank the many generous reviewers who provided helpful feedback on each of these chapters. Finally, I would like to acknowledge the contributions of the members of the Stanford Psychophysiology Laboratory, who help make Stanford such a fun place to be.

REFERENCE

Gross, J. J. (1998). The emerging field of emotion regulation: An integrative review. *Review of General Psychology, 2*, 271–299.

Contents

VII. CLINICAL APPLICATIONS

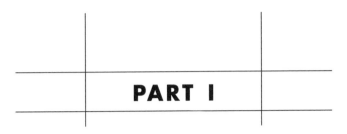

PART I

FOUNDATIONS

CHAPTER 1

Emotion Regulation
CONCEPTUAL FOUNDATIONS

JAMES J. GROSS
ROSS A. THOMPSON

Standing in a long line at the supermarket check-out counter probably isn't anyone's idea of a good time. But when the line's glacial pace is further slowed by a gossipy clerk, annoyance turns to anger, and changes become apparent in our thoughts, feelings, behavior, and indeed, throughout our body. Our blood pressure rises, our fingers grip the cart more tightly, and we prepare a scathing remark for the clerk. But, at the last moment, the thought crosses our mind that a cutting comment will make a bad situation worse. And so we opt to bite our tongue and keep our mouth shut as the dual decisions of credit or debit, paper or plastic are made.

Quotidian acts of emotion regulation such as this constitute one important thread in the fabric of civilization. After all, civilization is defined by coordinated social interchanges that require us to regulate how emotions are experienced and expressed. But what do people do to regulate their emotions? Are some ways of regulating emotions more successful than others? How do temperament and learning interact to shape an individual's unique style of emotion regulation? In this chapter, we provide a conceptual foundation for answering such questions as they arise in developmental and adult literatures relevant to emotion regulation.

Because a discussion of emotion regulation presupposes an understanding of what emotion is, we first consider emotion in the context of the larger family of affective processes to which it belongs. Next, we distinguish emotion regulation from other major forms of self-regulation. This prepares the way for our presentation of the framework we use to organize the many different types of emotion regulation. Using this framework, we review findings from developmental and adult literatures. In the last section, we highlight some of the biggest challenges—and opportunities—for those interested in emotion and emotion regulation.

EMOTIONS AND RELATED PROCESSES

Contemporary functionalist perspectives emphasize the important roles emotions play as they ready necessary behavioral responses, tune decision making, enhance memory for important events, and facilitate interpersonal interactions. However, emotions can hurt as well as help. They do so when they occur at the wrong time or at the wrong intensity level. Inappropriate emotional responses are implicated in many forms of psychopathology (Campbell-Sills & Barlow, this volume; Mullin & Hinshaw, this volume; Linehan & Bohus, this volume; Sher & Grekin, this volume), in social difficulties (Wranik, Barrett, & Salovey, this volume; Eisenberg, Hofer, & Vaughan, this volume; Shaver & Mikulincer, this volume), and even in physical illness (Sapolsky, this volume). Clearly, a great deal hinges on our ability to successfully regulate emotions.

To understand emotion regulation, we first need to know what is being regulated. This sounds simple, but emotion has proven famously difficult to pin down. Part of the problem is that what people seem to want when they try to "pin down" emotion is the list of necessary and sufficient conditions for something to qualify as an emotion. What is it that we must have for something to be an emotion (necessary conditions)? What is it that—if present—guarantees that something is an emotion (sufficient conditions)? Efforts to derive this sort of tidy classical definition run athwart the fact that "emotion" is a term that was lifted from common language, and refers to an astonishing array of happenings, from the mild to the intense, the brief to the extended, the simple to the complex, and the private to the public. Irritation with a gossipy clerk counts. So does amusement at a cartoon, anger at economic disparities around the world, surprise at a friend's new tatoo, grief at the death of a loved one, and embarrassment at a child's misbehavior.

A growing appreciation of the mismatch between the wished for definitional precision and the ill-bounded subject matter has led to an increasing reliance on prototype conceptions of emotion. Unlike classical conceptions, prototype conceptions emphasize typical features, which may or may not be evident in any given case, but whose presence makes it more likely that something is an emotion. In the next section, we focus on three core features of the emotion prototype that relate to emotion antecedents, emotion responses, and the link between emotion antecedents and responses.

Core Features of Emotion

First, emotions arise when an individual attends to a situation and sees it as relevant to his or her goals. The goals that support this evaluation may be enduring (staying alive) or transient (seeing our team win the game). They may be central to our sense of self (being a good student) or peripheral (opening a cereal box). Goals may be conscious and complicated (plotting revenge on a classroom bully) or unconscious and simple (ducking a punch). They may be widely shared and understood (having friends) or highly idiosyncratic (finding a new beetle for our collection). Whatever the goal, and whatever the source of the situational meaning for the individual, it is this meaning that gives rise to emotion. As this meaning changes over time (due either to changes in the situation itself or to changes in the meaning the situation holds), the emotion will also change.

Second, emotions are multifaceted, whole-body phenomena that involve loosely-coupled changes in the domains of *subjective experience*, *behavior*, and *central and peripheral physiology* (Mauss, Levenson, McCarter, Wilhelm, & Gross, 2005). The subjective aspect of emotion is, of course, so tightly bound up with what we mean by emotion that in everyday usage the terms "emotion" and "feeling" often are used interchangeably. But emotions not only make us feel something, they make us feel like *doing* something (Frijda, 1986). This is reflected in the language we use to describe emotions: We say we were "hopping mad," "moved to tears," or "frozen with fear." These impulses to act in certain ways (and not act in others) are associated with autonomic and neuroendocrine changes that both anticipate the associated behavioral response (thereby providing metabolic support for the action) and follow it, often as a consequence of the motor activity associated with the emotional response. Maturational changes in behavioral and physiological response systems involved in emotion play a fundamental role in the development of emotion, particularly in infancy and early childhood.

Third, the multisystem changes associated with emotion are rarely obligatory. Emotions do possess an imperative quality—which Frijda (1986) has termed "control precedence"—meaning that they can interrupt what we are doing and force themselves on our awareness. However, emotions often must compete with other responses that are also occasioned by the social matrix within which our emotions typically play out. The malleability of emotion has been emphasized since William James (1884), who viewed emotions as response tendencies that may be modulated in a large number of ways. It is this third aspect of emotion that is most crucial for an analysis of emotion regulation, because it is this feature that makes such regulation possible.

The Modal Model of Emotion

Together, these three core features of emotion constitute what we refer to as the "modal model" of emotion: a person–situation transaction that compels attention, has particular meaning to an individual, and gives rise to a coordinated yet flexible multisystem response to the ongoing person–situation transaction. We believe that this modal model underlies lay intuitions about emotion (Barrett, Ochsner, & Gross, in press) and also—not coincidentally—represents major points of convergence among researchers and theoreticians concerned with emotion.

In Figure 1.1, we present the highly abstracted and simplified situation–attention–appraisal–response sequence specified by the modal model of emotion (with the organismal "black box" interposed between situation and response). This sequence begins with a psychologically relevant situation, which is often external, and hence physically specifiable, such as the checkout line in the opening example. However, psychologically relevant "situations" also can be internal, and based on mental representations. Whether external or internal, situations are attended to in various ways, giving rise to appraisals that constitute the individual's assessment of—among other things—the situation's familiarity, valence, and value relevance (Ellsworth & Scherer, 2003). Different theorists have postulated different appraisal steps or dimensions, and these appraisal processes change developmentally, but there is broad agreement that it is these appraisals that give rise to emotional responses. As noted previously, the emotional responses generated by appraisals are thought to involve changes in experiential, behavioral, and neurobiological response systems.

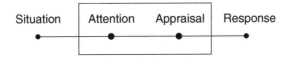

FIGURE 1.1. The "modal model" of emotion.

Like many other responses, an emotional response often changes the situation that gave rise to the response in the first place. One way to depict this recursive aspect of emotion is shown in Figure 1.2A, which has the response feeding back to (and modifying) the situation. A second way of depicting recursion is shown in Figure 1.2B. Here, time is on the X-axis, and three miniature versions of Figure 1.2A are drawn back to back. To make this idea of recursion more concrete, imagine two colleagues (or a parent and child) who are in situation S (disagreeing heatedly) when one emits response R (starts to cry). This emotional response substantially alters the interpersonal situation, transforming it into situation S' (interacting with someone you have just made cry). This situation now gives rise to a new response R' (an apology), which further transforms the situation, into situation S'' (responding to someone who has just apologized). This situation, in turn, provokes still another response, R'' (embarrassment), and so on. The key idea in Figures 1.2A and 1.2B is that emotions have a recursive aspect, in that they can lead to changes to the environment which have the effect of altering the probability of subsequent instances of that (and other) emotions.

Emotions and Other Affective Processes

Dozens of terms swirl about in the emotion literature (affect, reflex, mood, impulse, feeling, etc.), making communication difficult. Following Scherer (1984), we use *affect* as the superordinate category for various kinds of states that involve relatively quick good–bad discriminations (and thus have in common certain attentional processes and valence appraisals). These affective states include (1) general *stress responses* to taxing circumstances, (2) *emotions* such as anger and sadness, (3) *moods* such as depression and euphoria, and (4) *other motivational impulses* such as those related to eating, sex, aggression, or pain. Although these terms overlap in complex ways (see later in chapter), a simple depiction of these key terms is given as Figure 1.3.

How are these various affective processes distinguished? While both stress and emotion involve whole-body responses to significant events, stress typically refers to negative (but otherwise unspecified) affective responses, whereas emotion refers to both negative and positive affective states (Lazarus, 1993). Emotions also may be distinguished from moods (Parkinson, Totterdell, Briner, & Reynolds, 1996). Moods often last longer than emotions, and compared to moods, emotions typically have specific

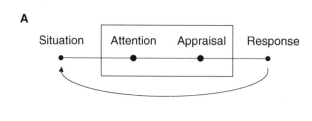

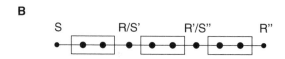

FIGURE 1.2. Recursion in emotion shown using a feedback loop in the modal model (Figure 1.2A), or, equivalently, using three iterations of the modal model (Figure 1.2B).

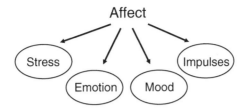

FIGURE 1.3. Emotion and related affective processes.

objects and give rise to behavioral response tendencies relevant to these objects. By contrast, moods are more diffuse, and although they may give rise to broad action tendencies such as approach or withdrawal (Lang, 1995), moods bias cognition more than they bias action (Clore, Schwarz, & Conway, 1994; Davidson, 1994; Fiedler, 1988). Emotions also may be distinguished from other motivational impulses (e.g., hunger, thirst, sex, and pain). Like emotions, each of these motivational impulses has a valence and motive force, directing and energizing behavior (Ferguson, 2000). Emotions are different from other motivational impulses, however, because of the flexibility with which they are deployed and the much broader range of potential targets. Thus, we can distinguish approach from withdrawal emotions, but it is difficult to more precisely specify the nature of an emotion's action tendency without referring to the context within which the emotion is taking place.

Lest these distinctions seem overly academic, consider the term "affect." We place affect at the "top" of the hierarchy. Others use the terms "affect" and "emotion" interchangeably. For still others, affect is used to refer to the experiential (Buck, 1993; MacLean, 1990) or behavioral (American Psychiatric Association, 1994; Kaplan & Sadock, 1991) components of emotion. Clearly, there is no reason to expect neat distinctions among the many types of motivationally relevant affective processes with which we have been endowed. However, clarity regarding these constructs is a prerequisite for an analysis of how these various processes are (or are not) regulated.

EMOTION REGULATION AND RELATED PROCESSES

Contemporary research on emotion regulation has its roots in the study of psychological defenses (Freud, 1926/1959), psychological stress and coping (Lazarus, 1966), attachment theory (Bowlby, 1969), and, of course, emotion theory (Frijda, 1986). Emotion regulation first gained currency as a distinct construct in the developmental literature (Campos, Campos, & Barrett, 1989; Thompson, 1990, 1991), and then subsequently in the adult literature (e.g., Izard, 1990; Gross & Levenson, 1993). Despite richly overlapping concerns, to date there has been a surprising lack of integration across developmental and adult literatures on emotion regulation.

On its own, the phrase "emotion regulation" is crucially ambiguous, as it might refer equally well to how emotions regulate something else, such as thoughts, physiology, or behavior (regulation *by* emotions) or to how emotions are themselves regulated (regulation *of* emotions). However, if a primary function of emotions is to coordinate response systems (Levenson, 1999), the first sense of emotion regulation is coextensive with emotion. For this reason, we prefer the second usage, in which emotion regulation refers to the heterogeneous set of processes by which emotions are themselves regulated.

Emotion regulatory processes may be automatic or controlled, conscious or unconscious, and may have their effects at one or more points in the emotion generative process (we return to this idea in a later section). Because emotions are multicomponential processes that unfold over time, emotion regulation involves changes in "emotion dynamics" (Thompson, 1990), or the latency, rise time, magnitude, duration, and offset of responses in behavioral, experiential, or physiological domains. Emotion regulation may dampen, intensify, or simply maintain emotion, depending on an individual's goals. Emotion regulation also may change the degree to which emotion response components cohere as the emotion unfolds, such as when large changes in emotion experience and physiological responding occur in the absence of facial behavior.

One as-yet-unresolved issue is whether emotion regulation refers to intrinsic processes (Fred regulates his own emotions: emotion regulation *in self*), to extrinsic processes (Sally regulates Bob's emotions: emotion regulation *in other*), or to both. In general, researchers in the adult literature typically focus on intrinsic processes (Gross, 1998b). By contrast, researchers in the developmental literature focus more on extrinsic processes, perhaps because extrinsic processes are so salient in infancy and early childhood (e.g., Cole, Martin, & Dennis, 2004). We believe that both intrinsic and extrinsic regulatory processes are essential, and recommend using the qualifiers "intrinsic" and "extrinsic" whenever clarification is needed, such as when Sally regulates Bob's emotions in order to calm herself down.

Core Features of Emotion Regulation

Three aspects of this conception of emotion regulation warrant particular comment. First, we explicitly include the possibility that people may regulate either negative or positive emotions, either by decreasing them or by increasing them. Little is known about whether the emotions people try to change differ depending on their developmental stage. However, in an interview study, young adults predominantly reported trying to downregulate negative emotions (especially anger, sadness, and anxiety), with a focus on regulating experiential and behavioral aspects of emotion (Gross, Richards, & John, 2006). These emotion regulation episodes were nearly always social in nature, and although participants did regulate positive emotions (e.g., decreasing happiness to fit in socially), they did so far less frequently than negative emotions.

Second, although prototypical examples of emotion regulation are conscious, such as our opening example of the supermarket checkout line, we can imagine emotion regulatory activity that is initially deliberate but later occurs without conscious awareness. Examples include hiding the anger we feel when we are rejected by a peer or quickly turning our attention away from potentially upsetting material. Previous discussions have distinguished categorically between conscious and unconscious processes (Masters, 1991). However, we prefer to think of a continuum from conscious, effortful, and controlled regulation to unconscious, effortless, and automatic regulation. It is difficult to adequately assess automatic emotion regulation processes. However, there are behavioral (Bargh & Williams, this volume; Mauss, Evers, Wilhelm, & Gross, 2006) and physiological approaches (Davidson, Fox, & Kalin, this volume; Hariri & Forbes, this volume; Ochsner & Gross, this volume) that show promise in elucidating automatic emotion regulation processes.

Third, we make no a priori assumptions as to whether any particular form of emotion regulation is necessarily good or bad (Thompson & Calkins, 1996). This is important, as it avoids the confusion that was created in the stress and coping literature, where defenses were predefined as maladaptive and contrasted with coping strategies, which were predefined as adaptive (Parker & Endler, 1996). These predefinitions made it difficult to consider the costs and benefits of defensive processes (Lazarus, 1985). In our view, emotion regulation processes may be used to make things either better or worse, depending on the context. For example, cognitive strategies that dampen negative emotions may help a medical professional operate efficiently in stressful circumstances, but also may neutralize negative emotions associated with empathy, thereby decreasing helping. Moreover, consistent with our functionalist orientation, regulatory strategies may accomplish a person's own goals but nonetheless be perceived by others as maladaptive, such as when a child cries loudly in order to get attention.

Emotion Regulation and Related Constructs

Paralleling the distinctions drawn among members of the affective family in Figure 1.3, we see emotion regulation as subordinate to the broader construct of *affect regulation*. Under this broad heading fall all manner of efforts to influence our valenced responses (Westen, 1994).

As depicted in Figure 1.4, affect regulation includes (among other things) four overlapping constructs: (1) *coping*, (2) *emotion regulation*, (3) *mood regulation*, and (4) *psychological defenses*. Because virtually all goal-directed behavior can be construed as maximizing pleasure or minimizing pain—and is thus affect regulatory in a broad sense—we believe it is important to narrow the focus by examining the four second-level families of processes shown here.

Coping is distinguished from emotion regulation both by its predominant focus on decreasing negative affect, and by its emphasis on much larger periods of time (e.g., coping with bereavement). As noted earlier, moods are typically of longer duration and are less likely to involve responses to specific "objects" than emotions (Parkinson et al., 1996). In part due to their less well defined behavioral response tendencies, in comparison with emotion regulation, mood regulation and mood repair are more concerned with altering emotion experience than emotion behavior (Larsen, 2000). Like coping, defenses typically have as their focus the regulation of aggressive or sexual impulses and their associated negative emotion experience, particularly anxiety. Defenses usually are unconscious and automatic (Westen & Blagov, this volume) and are usually studied as stable individual differences (Cramer, 2000).

EMOTION REGULATION STRATEGIES

To set the stage for our discussion of specific emotion regulation strategies, imagine a father who decides to take his child for the child's first proper (i.e., nonparental) haircut. Before mentioning the idea to his child, the father scouts out a few places. Some

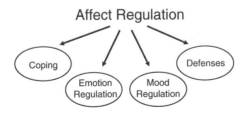

FIGURE 1.4. Emotion regulation and related processes.

are generic adult-only barber shops. Others look more kid friendly, with brightly colored walls and racks of toys. Once his child is planted in a chair at Cuts 'R' Us, the father waits nervously. The first barber that comes over is the least promising of the lot, with a huge beard and a terrifying demeanor. As he approaches—scissors in hand—the child screams bloody murder. The father asks to wait for the next available barber. When a second barber finally becomes free, the haircut begins. At first, the child watches the flurry of falling hair with great interest. After a few minutes of calm, the child loses interest and wants to leave. The father says they will certainly leave, but first asks what the child would like for his birthday. This distracts the child until the barber turns on a noisy shaver. The child bursts into tears, terrified by the "monster's roar." The father says the noise is the machine purring, just like their cat. This yields a few more minutes of tranquility until the child notices the pile of hair trimmings around the chair, which again provokes an emotional outburst. In desperation, the father says that big kids shouldn't cry and tells the child to stop it right now.

As this barbershop story suggests, one of the challenges in thinking about emotion regulation is finding a conceptual framework that can help to organize the myriad forms of emotion regulation that are encountered in everyday life. The modal model of emotion (Figure 1.1) suggests one approach, in that it specifies a sequence of processes involved in emotion generation, each of which is a potential target for regulation. In Figure 1.5, we have redrawn the modal model, highlighting five points at which individuals can regulate their emotions.

These five points represent five families of emotion regulation processes: situation selection, situation modification, attentional deployment, cognitive change, and response modulation (Gross, 1998b). These families are distinguished by the point in the emotion-generative process at which they have their primary impact. We emphasize the notion of families, which harkens back to the prototype conception of emotion emphasized earlier, and we regard these families as loose-knit constellations of processes.

For purposes of presentation, we focus on between-family differences (e.g., the difference between cognitive change and response modulation). However, there are also higher-order commonalities. For example, the first four emotion regulation families may be considered *antecedent-focused*, in that they occur before appraisals give rise to full-blown emotional response tendencies, and may be contrasted with *response-focused* emotion regulation, which occurs after the responses are generated (Gross & Munoz, 1995). As we describe later, there are also considerable within-family differences. In the

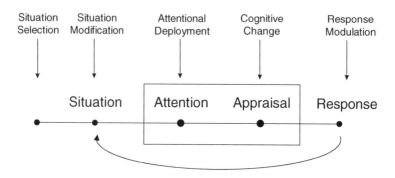

FIGURE 1.5. A process model of emotion regulation that highlights five families of emotion regulation strategies.

following sections, we review adult and developmental literatures related to each of the five families of emotion regulation processes.

Situation Selection

The most forward-looking approach to emotion regulation is *situation selection*. This type of emotion regulation involves taking actions that make it more (or less) likely that we will end up in a situation we expect will give rise to desirable (or undesirable) emotions. In the example of the father taking his child for a haircut, situation selection is illustrated by the father choosing the barbershop that he thinks is likely to maximize the chances that the child will tolerate the haircut. Other examples include avoiding an offensive coworker, renting a funny movie after a bad day, or seeking out a friend with whom we can have a good cry.

Situation selection requires an understanding of likely features of remote situations, and of expectable emotional responses to these features. There is a growing appreciation of just how difficult it is to gain such an understanding. Looking backward in time, there is a profound gap between the "experiencing self" and the "remembering self" (Kahneman, 2000). In particular, real-time ratings of emotion experience (e.g., how I'm feeling at each moment throughout an emotional film) diverge from retrospective summary reports (e.g., how I felt during the film) in that retrospective reports are predicted by peak and end feelings but are curiously insensitive to duration. Looking forward in time, people profoundly misestimate their emotional responses to future scenarios (Gilbert, Pinel, Wilson, Blumberg, & Wheatley, 1998; Loewenstein, this volume). In particular, people overestimate how long their negative responses to various outcomes (e.g., being denied tenure and breaking up with a partner) will last. These backward- and forward-looking biases make it difficult to appropriately represent past or future situations for the purposes of situation selection.

Another barrier to effective situation selection is appropriately weighing short-term benefits of emotion regulation versus longer-term costs. For example, a shy person may feel much better in the short term if she avoids social situations. However, this short-term relief may come at the cost of longer-term social isolation. Because of the complexity of these trade-offs, situation selection often requires the perspective of others, ranging from parents to therapists.

Indeed, people commonly intervene in this way to manage the feelings of a child, spouse, friend, or acquaintance, whether by dissuading them from going to events that may be stressful, joining them for activities that are likely to be emotionally satisfying, or offering warm conversation and a sympathetic ear. This form of extrinsic emotion regulation is important throughout life, but is most evident in infancy and early childhood when parents strive to create daily routines with manageable emotional demands for their offspring. This can involve careful selection of child care arrangements, predictable routines, scheduling naps and breaks to assist young children's coping, and managing the broader emotional climate of family life. Early emotional life is strongly influenced by situation selection because infants and young children are less capable of choosing their circumstances for themselves.

Using situation selection to manage another's emotions requires the same kinds of predictive judgments that are involved in managing our own feelings in this way, with the additional complication that we must estimate the emotional consequences for another. In this regard, extrinsic emotion regulation using situation selection occurs in concert with estimations of the recipient's self-regulatory capacities. Parents thus must arrange the schedule of their offspring with due regard, for example, to their particular child's temperamental qualities, activity level, interests, and capacities for managing arousal (Fox & Calkins, 2003).

Situation Modification

Potentially emotion-eliciting situations—such as the approach of the terrifying barber in the earlier example—do not inevitably lead to emotional responses. After all, we can always ask to wait until a less frightening barber is free. Such efforts to directly modify the situation so as to alter its emotional impact constitute a potent form of emotion regulation.

When conservative in-laws visit, situation modification may take the form of hiding politically incindiary artwork. Situation modification is also a mainstay of parenting, where it takes the form of helping with a frustrating puzzle or setting up for an elaborate doll tea party. With older children and adults, situation modification can include verbal prompts to assist in problem solving, or to confirm the legitimacy of an emotion response. It is important to recognize that in these situations, situation modification is created both by the supportive presence of a partner and by that partner's specific interventions. A study by Nachmias, Gunnar, Mangelsdorf, Parritz, and Buss (1996) found, for example, that toddlers' emotional coping in a stressful situation was aided both by the specific interventions of their mothers and the existence of a secure attachment between them.

Given the vagueness of the term "situation," it is sometimes difficult to draw the line between situation selection and situation modification. This is because efforts to modify a situation may effectively call a new situation into being. Also, although we have previously emphasized that situations can be external or internal, situation modification—as we mean it here—has to do with modifying external, physical environments. We consider efforts at modifying "internal" environments (i.e. cognitions) under the section on "Cognitive Change."

Another boundary issue arises when considering the social consequences of emotion expression. As we noted earlier, emotional expressions have important social consequences and can dramatically alter ongoing interactions (Keltner & Kring, 1998). If our partner suddenly looks sad, this can shift the trajectory of an angry interaction, as we pause to express concern, backpedal, or offer support. In this sense, emotion expressions can be powerful extrinsic forms of emotion regulation, changing the nature of the situation (Rimé, this volume).

One context in which the emotion regulatory effects of emotion expression has been examined is parents' emotional responses to their children's emotions. A considerable body of research indicates that when parents respond supportively and sympathetically to the emotional expressions of offspring, children cope more adaptively with their emotions in the immediate situation and acquire more positive emotion regulatory capacities in the long run. By contrast, when parents respond to their children's emotions in ways that are denigrating, punitive, or dismissive, more negative outcomes are likely (Denham, 1998; Eisenberg, Cumberland, & Spinrad, 1998, for reviews; see also Thompson & Meyer, this volume). The latter is a reminder that emotional expressions can elicit social responses that modify the situation in ways that undermine effective emotion regulation rather than facilitate it. More generally, these developmental studies alert us to how emotional expressions inaugurate social processes that progressively modify the situation that initially elicited emotion—sometimes aiding emotion regulation while on other occasions impairing it. This is one way that the broader emotional climate of the family influences the development of emotion regulatory capacities in children.

Attentional Deployment

Situation selection and situation modification help shape the individual's situation. However, it also is possible to regulate emotions without actually changing the environment. Situations have many aspects, and *attentional deployment* refers to how individuals direct their attention within a given situation in order to influence their emotions.

Attentional deployment is one of the first emotion regulatory processes to appear in development (Rothbart, Ziaie, & O'Boyle, 1992) and appears to be used from infancy through adulthood, particularly when it is not possible to change or modify our situation. Not only do infants and young children spontaneously look away from aversive events (and toward pleasant ones) but their attentional processes can also be guided by others for purposes of emotion management. In the example given earlier, emotion regulation involved facilitating an attentional shift in the child by getting the child to focus on birthday wishes. Attentional deployment might be considered an internal version of situation selection. Two major attentional strategies are distraction and concentration.

Distraction focuses attention on different aspects of the situation, or moves attention away from the situation altogether, such as when an infant shifts its gaze from the emotion-eliciting stimulus to decrease stimulation (Rothbart & Sheese, this volume; Stifter & Moyer, 1991). Distraction also may involve changing internal focus, such as when individuals invoke thoughts or memories that are inconsistent with the undesirable emotional state (Watts, this volume), or when an actor calls to mind an emotional incident in order to portray that emotion convincingly.

Concentration draws attention to emotional features of a situation. Wegner and Bargh (1998) have termed this "controlled starting" of emotion. When attention is repetitively directed to our feelings and their consequences, it is referred to as rumination. Ruminating on sad events leads to longer and more severe depressive symptoms (Just & Alloy, 1997; Nolen-Hoeksema, 1993). However, Borkovec, Roemer, and Kinyon (1995) have argued that when attention is focused on possible future threats, it may have the effect of increasing low-grade anxiety but decreasing the strength of the negative emotional responses.

Attentional deployment thus may take many forms, including physical withdrawal of attention (such as covering the eyes or ears), internal redirection of attention (such as through distraction or concentration), and responding to others' redirection of our attention (such as the father and the haircut). As children become more aware of the internal determinants of emotional experience, their reliance on attentional deployment to manage emotions increases. Attentional deployment is enlisted beginning in early childhood, for example by children who are waiting for delayed rewards (Mischel & Ayduk, 2004). By grade school, children are well aware of how the intensity of emotion wanes over time as they think less of emotionally arousing situations (Harris, Guz, Lipian, & Man-Shu, 1985; Harris & Lipian, 1989).

Cognitive Change

Even after a situation has been selected, modified, and attended to, an emotional response is by no means a foregone conclusion. Emotion requires that percepts be imbued with meaning and that individuals evaluate their capacity to manage the situation. As described previously, appraisal theorists have described the cognitive steps needed to transform a percept into something that elicits emotion. *Cognitive change* refers to changing how we appraise the situation we are in to alter its emotional significance, either by changing how we think about the situation or about our capacity to manage the demands it poses.

In the earlier example, cognitive change is exemplified by the father's comment that the barber's buzzer sounded like a cat purring (rather than a monster roaring). One common application of cognitive change in the social domain is downward social comparison, which involves comparing our situation with that of a less fortunate person, thereby altering our construal and decreasing negative emotion (Taylor & Lobel, 1989; Wills, 1981). Because psychologically relevant events or situations can be internal as well as external, cognitive change also can be applied to our internal experience of the event. It is likely that individuals who interpret their physiological arousal prior to a stressful athletic or musical performance as competence enhancing ("getting pumping up") rather than debilitating ("stage fright") are more capable of managing emotion, although little is known of how individuals interpret or reconstrue their physiological signs of emotional arousal.

One form of cognitive change that has received particular attention is reappraisal (Gross, 2002; John & Gross, this volume; Ochsner & Gross, this volume). This type of cognitive change involves changing a situation's meaning in a way that alters its emotional impact. Leading subjects to reappraise negatively valenced films has been shown to result in decreased negative emotion experience. Decreases in physiological responding are not always evident (Gross, 1998a; Steptoe & Vogele, 1986), however, perhaps because so little cognitive processing is needed in order to translate the potent images that have been used in these studies into physiological responses.

For children, cognitive appraisals related to emotion are significantly influenced by their developing representations of emotions, including the causes and consequences of these emotions (Stegge & Meerum Terwogt, this volume). This development has implications for children's efforts to manage emotion. Not surprisingly, parents, and later peers and other caregivers, are highly influential in children's developing emotion-related appraisals. Parents influence how children appraise emotion-relevant situations by (1) the information they provide about these circumstances (describing a camping trip as fun outdoors, but not mentioning mosquitoes or bears), (2) explaining the causes of the emotions the child feels or observes in others ("Your brother is scared of the dog because another dog barked at him yesterday"), and (3) enlisting feeling rules or emotion scripts ("big kids don't fuss and cry when they're at someone's home"). Parents also coach emotion regulatory strategies involving cognitive change (such as thinking happy thoughts in the dark at bedtime), and directly provoke cognitive change by reinterpreting the situation for the child ("We don't laugh at people who fall down—how do you think they feel?") (Denham, 1998; Eisenberg et al., 1998; Thompson, 1994). In these and other ways, socialized representations of emotion shape children's evaluations of emotion-relevant situations and their emotion-regulatory reappraisals (Mesquita & Albert, this volume). Over time, these experiences shape how an individual construes both the self and the environment (Peterson & Park, this volume).

The importance of these developmental influences is reflected in culturally comparative studies of children's representations of emotion and emotion regulation. As early as age 6, for example, Nepalese children differ significantly from American children in their appraisals of interpersonal conflict (as eliciting shame or guilt) and their beliefs about whether negative emotion of any kind should be expressed (Cole, Bruschi, & Tamang, 2002; Cole & Tamang, 1998). Studies such as these suggest how much the development of children's emotion-related appraisals is culturally constructed through socialization processes that begin at home.

Response Modulation

In contrast with other emotion regulatory processes, *response modulation* occurs late in the emotion-generative process, after response tendencies have been initiated. Response modulation refers to influencing physiological, experiential, or behavioral responding as directly as possible. Attempts at regulating the physiological and experiential aspects of emotion are common. Drugs may be used to target physiological responses such as muscle tension (anxiolytics) or sympathetic hyperreactivity (beta blockers). Exercise and relaxation also can be used to decrease physiological and experiential aspects of negative emotions, and, alcohol, cigarettes, drugs, and even food also may be used to modify emotion experience.

Another common form of response modulation involves regulating emotion-expressive behavior (Gross, Richards, & John, 2006). We may wish to regulate expressive behavior for many reasons, ranging from an assessment that it would be best to hide our true feelings from another person (e.g., hiding our fear when standing up to a bully) to direct prompts from a parent (e.g., in the barbershop example). By and large, studies have shown that initiating emotion-expressive behavior slightly increases the feeling of that emotion (Izard, 1990; Matsumoto, 1987). Interestingly, decreasing emotion-expressive behavior seems to have mixed effects on emotion experience (decreasing positive but not negative emotion experience) and actually increasing sympathetic activation (Gross, 1998a; Gross & Levenson, 1993, 1997).

In general terms, children and adults seem to be more capable of regulating emotions if they can find ways of expressing them in adaptive rather than maladaptive ways (Thompson, 1994). The parental maxim to toddlers—"use words to say how you feel"—reflects the psychological reality that developing language ability significantly facilitates young children's capacities to understand, convey, reflect on, and manage their emotions (Kopp, 1992). At older ages, the extent to which emotions can be successfully managed is based, in part, on the availability of adaptive response alternatives for expressing emotion, such as to provoke problem solving or interpersonal understanding rather than simply venting.

This conclusion has several implications, all consistent with functionalist emotions theory. First, "adaptive response alternatives" may vary significantly in different situations. For example, crying is likely to be maladaptive for toddlers in some situations (e.g., when resisting mother's request) but to accomplish valuable goals in others (e.g., calling attention to sudden danger or an older sibling's aggression). Thus it is not the emotional response *per se* that is adaptive or maladaptive but the response in its immediate context. Second, evaluating broader individual differences in emotion regulatory capacities must likewise incorporate attention to the contexts in which the individual's emotions are expressed and the potentially adaptive consequences of these emotions. Sometimes examples of "emotional dysregulation" by children or adults can be viewed as the only adaptive response options in the circumstances in which these individuals are expressing emotion, such as in the context of an emotionally abusive family. Third, cultural values are significant in determining what constitutes "adaptive response alternatives" for expressing emotion for persons of any age. As indicated in Cole's studies of

Nepalese children profiled earlier, expressing negative emotion may be viewed by American adults as appropriately assertive but by Nepalese adults as woefully inappropriate. This indicates how response modulation must be considered within the broader cultural context in which emotion is experienced, expressed, and regulated.

ELABORATIONS AND COMPLICATIONS

Our process model provides an integrative framework for organizing the dizzying array of emotion regulatory processes. Like any model, however, it makes a number of simplifying assumptions. As our understanding of emotion grows, we will naturally outgrow the modal model of emotion in the sense that we will be able to better specify constituent processes, and thus will be able to describe the emotion-generative processes in greater detail. This will in turn permit us to refine our conception of emotion regulation processes. In the following section, we consider three specific aspects of our model of emotion regulation that bear particular comment.

Time and Feedback

In discussing the model presented in Figure 1.5, we have focused on just one cycle of the emotion-generative process. Movement from left to right in this figure captures movement through time: a particular situation is selected, modified (or not), attended to, appraised in a certain way, and yields a particular set of emotional responses. However, as we have emphasized in Figure 1.2, emotion generation is an ongoing process, not a one-shot deal. This dynamic aspect of emotion and emotion regulation is signaled by the feedback arrow in Figure 1.5 from the emotional response back to the situation. This arrow is meant to suggest the dynamic and reciprocally determined nature of emotion regulation as it occurs in the context of an ongoing stream of emotional stimulation and behavioral responding. Similar feedback arrows might also be drawn from the emotional response to each of the other steps in the emotion-generative process. Each of these in turn influences subsequent emotional responses. On the antecedent side, for example, which emotions we have and how we express them are potent inputs into a new emotion cycle (e.g., feeling embarrassment about an angry outburst: see Ekman, 1993). On the response side, too, it seems likely that our current emotional state (which is the result of previous emotion regulatory efforts) may influence how we decide to modulate the current emotional response tendencies (e.g., deciding to "really let someone have it" when we are angry). Furthermore, as we have noted, the reactions of other people to our emotions constitute significant changes in the situation that further influence emotional responding. Modeling these real-time influences is a significant conceptual and empirical challenge.

Antecedent-Focused versus Response-Focused Regulation

This recursive aspect of emotion generation is essential for understanding the broad distinction between antecedent-focused and response-focused emotion regulation. In view of the cyclic nature of emotion (see Figures 1.2A and 1.2B), a given instance of emotion regulation is antecedent-focused or response-focused *with respect to a given cycle through the emotion-generative process.* Consider the use of cognitive change to help regulate the anxiety we feel about an upcoming exam. The night before the exam, in an effort to decrease our anxiety, we might try to think in a way that decreases the significance the exam has for our long-term goals (we might focus on how well we have done with the other aspects of the course so far, or remind ourselves that there are more important things in life than grades, etc.).

It is true that this instance of emotion regulation occurs before the exam, but this is not what makes this regulatory strategy antecedent-focused. Indeed, we could mount the same effort at cognitive change during the exam, and it would still be antecedent-focused in our sense. What sense is that? As we have described, emotions unfold over time, and in each cycle of emotion generation, our responses in that cycle influence our subsequent responses. When a person uses cognitive regulation either before or during an exam, we regard these efforts as antecedent-focused in the sense that they take place early in a given emotion-generative cycle. At the heart of this distinction between antecedent- and response-focused emotion regulation, then, is the notion of a fast cycling system that gives rise to an emotional "pulse" in each iteration. Emotion regulation efforts that target prepulse processes (in any given cycle of the emotion-generative process shown in Figure 1.5) are antecedent-focused, whereas emotion regulation efforts that target postpulse processes are response-focused.

From One Process to Many

For clarity of presentation, our examples have been cases in which an individual has used one type of emotion regulation at a time. Thus, in the previous section, we considered using cognitive change to decrease feelings of exam-related anxiety. However, emotion regulation can also occur in parallel at multiple points in the emotion generative process. Using many forms of emotion regulation might in fact be the modal case. This approach of "throwing everything you've got at it" makes sense. There are many different ways of influencing the emotion-generative process, and if we want to make a big change in a hurry, it may be useful to try several things at once. Thus, what we do to regulate our emotions—such as going out to a bar with friends in order to get our mind off a bad day at work—often involves multiple regulatory processes.

One important and as yet unanswered question is how different forms of emotion regulation typically co-occur. We believe that this question may be profitably addressed both by considering particular contexts (e.g., exam taking) and by considering particular individuals (e.g., does a person who uses a particular type of cognitive change also typically use a particular type of response modulation: see John & Gross, this volume). Even if regulatory processes are often coactive and adjusted dynamically, we believe that a process-oriented approach will bring us closer to understanding the causes, consequences, and underlying mechanisms. Moreover, such a process-oriented approach is well suited to the study of developmental changes in emotion regulation, and encourages investigators to examine the interaction of external and intrinsic influences.

FUNDAMENTAL QUESTIONS AND DIRECTIONS FOR FUTURE INQUIRY

As is the case with any new and vital area of science, the study of emotion regulation has generated many more questions than answers. In the following sections, we consider three such questions that we believe are particularly important to the field of emotion regulation.

How Separable Are Emotion and Emotion Regulation?

The notion of emotion regulation presupposes that it is possible (and sensible) to separate emotion generation from emotion regulation. However, emotion regulation is so tightly intertwined with emotion generation that some theorists view emotion regulation as part and parcel of emotion (Campos, Frankel, & Camras, 2004; Frijda, 1986). On the one hand, this perspective is consistent with the observation that adult emotions are almost always regulated (Tomkins, 1984), and that emotion-generative brain centers are tonically restrained by the prefrontal cortex (Stuss & Benson, 1986). On the other hand, both common sense and its academic counterpart—the modal model—suggest the need to distinguish between emotion and emotion regulation.

Admittedly, making this distinction is difficult, because emotion regulation often must be inferred when an emotional response would have proceeded in one fashion but instead is observed to proceed in another. For example, a still face in someone who typically expresses lots of emotion may be rich with meaning, but the same lack of expression in someone who rarely shows any sign of emotion is less strongly suggestive of emotion regulation. However, recent advances in neuroimaging have made it possible to begin to assess whether (particularly in the context of explicit manipulations of emotion regulation) there are differences either in the magnitude or regional locus of brain activation associated with emotion alone versus emotion in addition to emotion regulation (Ochsner et al., 2004). Emotion regulation also may be inferred from changes in how response components are interrelated as the emotion unfolds over time (e.g., a dissociation between facial expression and physiology, suggestive of suppression).

At the highest level, emotion and emotion regulation processes (and all other psychological processes for that matter) co-occur in the same brain, often at the same time. The question of whether two sets of processes are separable (e.g., emotion and memory; emotion and emotion regulation) is therefore a question about the value of distinguishing processes for a particular purpose. We believe that a two-factor approach that distinguishes emotion from emotion regulation is a useful approach for analyzing basic processes, individual differences, and fashioning clinical interventions. That said, we also believe that it is crucial to be as explicit as possible about the grounds for inferring the existence of emotion regulation in any given context.

One particular challenge in this regard is understanding the *bidirectional* links between limbic centers that generate emotion and cortical centers that regulate emotion (Beer & Lombardo, this volume; Davidson, Fox, & Kalin, this volume; Ochsner & Gross, this volume; Quirk, this volume). At present, we would hypothesize that (1) emotion regulation often co-occurs with emotion, whether or not emotion regulation is explicitly manipulated; and (2) emotion regulation engages some (and perhaps many) of the same brain regions that are implicated in emotion generation. Given our nascent understanding of both emotion and emotion regulation processes, we believe it is appropriate to be very cautious indeed when inferring whether emotion regulation processes are operative in a particular context. At the same time, however, we would argue that the question "Is emotion ever *not* regulated?" is misleading in that it suggests an all-or-none affair. A conception of varying amounts and types of emotion regulation seems more appropriate.

What Are the Developmental Trajectories of Emotion Regulation?

One powerful tool for understanding emotion regulation is to chart the development of emotion regulation. Much of the developmental literature on emotion regulation has focused on the period from infancy through adolescence (e.g., Thompson, 1990, 1994). This is a crucial period because it is a time when temperamental, neurobiological (e.g., the development of the frontal lobes), conceptual (e.g., understanding of emotional processes), and social (e.g., family, teachers, and peers) forces come together to lay the foundation for the individual differences in emotion regulation we observe in adulthood (Calkins & Hill, this volume; Rothbart & Sheese, this volume; Thompson & Meyer, this volume).

Because the developmental study of emotion regulation has been influenced by constructivist and relational approaches to emotional development, it has emphasized the person-in-context (Thompson & Lagattuta, 2006). Contextual factors considered pivotal in the development of emotion regulation include the varieties of caregiving influences on which infants and young children rely for managing their emotions; the growth of language by which emotions are understood, conveyed, and managed; the settings in which the expression of emotion may have adaptive or maladaptive outcomes; and cultural values that define how the emotions of men and women should be regulated in social contexts. In later childhood and adolescence, as emotions themselves are understood in more complex terms, children begin to appreciate the diverse internal constituents of emotional experience that can be targets of regulatory efforts (such as our thoughts, expectations, attitudes, personal history, and other facets of cognitive appraisal processes). Over time, individual differences in emotional regulatory capacities develop in concert with personality, so that children manage their feelings in a way that is consistent with their temperament-based tolerances, needs for security or stimulation, capacities for self-control, and other personality processes (Thompson, 2006). Understanding how these developmental processes emerge and are integrated in the growth of emotion regulation skills is a conceptual challenge, and developmental research on emotion regulation faces unique difficulties in empirically operationalizing these processes (Cole et al., 2004).

There is also reason to believe that emotion regulation processes continue to change and develop throughout the adult years (see Charles & Carstensen, this volume). In part, age-related shifts in emotion regulation should be expected due to changes in contextual factors: There may be more situations that require suppression in early adulthood than later adulthood (e.g., in the work setting). Increasing life experience and wisdom regarding the relative costs and benefits of different forms of emotion regulation also suggest that changes will take place with age (Gross & John, 2002). For example, if cognitive reappraisal has a healthier profile of consequences than expressive suppression, as individuals mature and gain in life experience, they might increasingly learn to make greater use of healthy emotion regulation strategies (such as reappraisal) and lesser use of less healthy emotion regulation strategies (such as suppression). Evidence now exists that just such an age-related change does occur (John & Gross, 2004). More broadly, later-life developmental changes in emotion regulation likely occur in concert with broader life goals for older individuals, such as conserving physical energy, ensuring consistent emotional demands, and heightening positive emotional experience (Carstensen et al., 1999).

How Does Emotion Regulation Relate to Other Forms of Self-Regulation?

Emotional impulses are far from the only psychological processes we must regulate. How does emotion regulation relate to the regulation of stress, moods, thoughts, attention, and impulses such as hunger, aggression, and sexual arousal? Are impulses to respond—and the processes by which they are modulated—crucially similar, as suggested by Block and Block (1980) and by recent discussions of ego depletion (Baumeister, Geyer, & Tice, this volume)? Or is it necessary to maintain distinctions among various forms of self-regulation?

There is certainly reason to see continuity among regulatory processes across response domains. For example, Mischel's (1996) famous "marshmallow studies" of young children's ability to delay gratification highlight the role of attentional processes such as distraction and reframing that are closely related to those implicated in emotion regulation. Similarly, the neural bases of emotion regulation seem to overlap considerably with those associated with pain regulation (Ochsner & Gross, 2005). Nonetheless, in our discussion of emotion and emotion regulation processes above, we have emphasized our preference for making distinctions among various loosely defined types of affective processes and, hence, similar distinctions among various equally loosely defined types of self-regulation.

In part, our emphasis on distinctions among affective processes reflects our abiding respect for the complexity of both the affective processes themselves and the regulatory processes involved. We are entirely comfortable with the proposition that there may be domain-general aspects of executive control (e.g., set switching, updating, and response inhibition; Botvinick, Young, Greene, & Cohen, this volume; Miyake et al., 2000; Zelazo & Cunningham, this volume) but believe it is currently an open question as to whether either (1) different regulatory processes are engaged in the context of different affective processes such as moods, emotions, and other impulses, and/or (2) the same regulatory processes have different consequences in the context of different affective processes. By drawing as explicit distinctions as we can now, we will be able to discern whether these differences matter. If so, we have learned something important about the regulatory processes in question. If not, so much the better—we will then have context-general principles by which to understand self-regulation. For the moment, we recommend a dual strategy of making as explicit distinctions as possible in each study, and then paying careful attention across studies to the points of difference and similarity.

ACKNOWLEDGMENTS

We would like to thank Sara Meyer and members of the Stanford Psychophysiology Laboratory for comments on a prior version of this chapter. Preparation of this chapter was supported by Grant No. MH58147 and MH66957 from the National Institute of Mental Health to James J. Gross.

REFERENCES

American Psychiatric Association (1994). *Diagnostic and statistical manual of mental disorders* (4th ed.). Washington, DC: Author.

Bargh, J. A., & Williams, L. E. (2007). The nonconscious regulation of emotion. In J. J. Gross (Ed.), *Handbook of emotion regulation* (pp. 429–445). New York: Guilford Press.

Barrett, L. F., Ochsner, K. N., & Gross, J. J. (in press). Automaticity and emotion. In J. Bargh (Ed.), *Automatic processes in social thinking and behavior*. New York: Psychology Press.

Baumeister, R. F., Zell, A. L., & Tice, D. M. (2007). How emotions facilitate and impair self-regulation. In J. J. Gross (Ed.), *Handbook of emotion regulation* (pp. 408–426). New York: Guilford Press.

Beer, J. S., & Lombardo, M. V. (2007). Insights into emotion regulation from neuropsychology. In J. J. Gross (Ed.), *Handbook of emotion regulation* (pp. 69–86). New York: Guilford Press.

Block, J. H., & Block, J. (1980). The role of ego-control and ego-resiliency in the organization of behavior. In W. A. Collins (Ed.), *The Minnesota symposia on child psychology: Vol. 13. Development of cognition, affect, and social relations* (pp. 39–51). Hillsdale, NJ: Erlbaum.

Borkovec, T. D., Roemer, L., & Kinyon, J. (1995). Disclosure and worry: Opposite sides of the emotional processing coin. In J. W. Pennebaker (Ed.), *Emotion, disclosure, and health* (pp. 47–70). Washington, DC: American Psychological Association.

Botvinick, M. M., Yeung, N., Greene, J. D., & Cohen, J. D. (2007). Conflict monitoring in cognition–emotion competition. In J. J. Gross (Ed.), *Handbook of emotion regulation* (pp. 204–226). New York: Guilford Press.

Bowlby, J. (1969). *Attachment and loss: Attachment.* New York: Basic Books.

Buck, R. (1993). What is this thing called subjective experience? Reflections on the neuropsychology of qualia. *Neuropsychology, 7,* 490–499.

Calkins, S. D., & Hill, A. (2007). Caregiver influences on emerging emotion regulation: Biological and environmental transactions in early development. In J. J. Gross (Ed.), *Handbook of emotion regulation* (pp. 229–248). New York: Guilford Press.

Campbell-Sills, L., & Barlow, D. H. (2007). Incorporating emotion regulation into conceptualizations and treatments of anxiety and mood disorders. In J. J. Gross (Ed.), *Handbook of emotion regulation* (pp. 542–559). New York: Guilford Press.

Campos, J. J., Campos, R. G., & Barrett, K. C. (1989). Emergent themes in the study of emotional development and emotion regulation. *Developmental Psychology, 25,* 394–402.

Campos, J. J., Frankel, C. B., & Camras, L. (2004). On the nature of emotion regulation. *Child Development, 75,* 377–394.

Carstensen, L. L., Isaacowitz, D. M., & Charles, S. T. (1999). Taking time seriously. *American Psychologist, 154,* 165–181.

Charles, S. T., & Carstensen, L. L. (2007). Emotion regulation and aging. In J. J. Gross (Ed.), *Handbook of emotion regulation* (pp. 307–327). New York: Guilford Press.

Clore, G. L., Schwarz, N., & Conway, M. (1994). Affective causes and consequences of social information processing. In R. S. Wyer & T. K. Srull (Eds.), *Handbook of social cognition* (pp. 323–417). Hillsdale, NJ: Erlbaum.

Cole, P. M., Bruschi, C. J., & Tamang, B. L. (2002). Cultural differences in children's emotional reactions to difficult situation. *Child Development, 73,* 983–996.

Cole, P., Martin, S., & Dennis, T. (2004). Emotion regulation as a scientific construct: Methodological challenges and directions for child development research. *Child Development, 75,* 317–333.

Cole, P. M., & Tamang, B. L. (1998). Nepali children's ideas about emotional displays in hypothetical challenges. *Developmental Psychology, 34,* 640–646.

Cramer, P. (2000). Defense mechanisms in psychology today. *American Psychologist, 55,* 637–646.

Davidson, R. J. (1994). On emotion, mood, and related affective constructs. In P. Ekman & R. J. Davidson (Eds.), *The nature of emotion: Fundamental questions* (pp. 51–55). New York: Oxford University Press.

Davidson, R. J., Fox, A., & Kalin, N. H. (2007). Neural bases of emotion regulation in nonhuman primates and humans. In J. J. Gross (Ed.), *Handbook of emotion regulation* (pp. 47–68). New York: Guilford Press.

Denham, S. (1998). *Emotional development in young children.* New York: Guilford Press.

Eisenberg, N., Cumberland, A., & Spinrad, T. L. (1998). Parental socialization of emotion. *Psychological Inquiry, 9,* 241–273.

Eisenberg, N., Hofer, C., & Vaughan, J. (2007). Effortful control and its socioemotional consequences. In J. J. Gross (Ed.), *Handbook of emotion regulation* (pp. 287–306). New York: Guilford Press.

Ekman, P. (1993). Facial expression and emotion. *American Psychologist, 48,* 384–392.

Ellsworth, P. C., & Scherer, K. R. (2003). Appraisal processes in emotion. In R. J. Davidson, K. R. Scherer, & H. H. Goldsmith (Eds.), *Handbook of affective sciences* (pp. 572–595). New York: Oxford University Press.

Ferguson, E. D. (2000). *Motivation: A biosocial and cognitive integration of motivation and emotion.* New York: Oxford University Press.

Fiedler, K. (1988). Emotional mood, cognitive style, and behavior regulation. In K. Fiedler & J. Forgas (Eds.), *Affect, cognition and social behavior: New evidence and integrative attempts* (pp. 100–119). Toronto: Hogrefe.

Fox, N. A., & Calkins, S. D. (2003). The development of self-control of emotion: Intrinsic and extrinsic influences. *Motivation and Emotion, 27,* 7–26.

Freud, S. (1959). *Inhibitions, symptoms, anxiety* (A. Strachey, Trans., & J. Strachey, Ed.). New York: Norton. (Original work published 1926)

Frijda, N. H. (1986). *The emotions.* Cambridge, UK: Cambridge University Press.

Gilbert, D. T., Pinel, E. C., Wilson, T. D., Blumberg, S. J., & Wheatley, T. P. (1998). Immune neglect: A source of durability bias in affective forecasting. *Journal of Personality and Social Psychology, 75,* 617–638.

Gross, J. J. (1998a). Antecedent- and response-focused emotion regulation: Divergent consequences for experience, expression, and physiology. *Journal of Personality and Social Psychology, 74,* 224–237

Gross, J. J. (1998b). The emerging field of emotion regulation: An integrative review. *Review of General Psychology, 2,* 271–299.

Gross, J. J. (2002). Emotion regulation: Affective, cognitive, and social consequences. *Psychophysiology, 39,* 281–291.

Gross, J. J., & John, O. P. (2002). Wise emotion regulation. In L. F. Barrett & P. Salovey (Eds.), *The wisdom of feelings: Psychological processes in emotional intelligence* (pp. 297–318). New York: Guilford Press.

Gross, J. J., & Levenson, R. W. (1993). Emotional suppression: Physiology, self-report, and expressive behavior. *Journal of Personality and Social Psychology, 64,* 970–986.

Gross, J. J., & Levenson, R. W. (1997). Hiding feelings: The acute effects of inhibiting positive and negative emotions. *Journal of Abnormal Psychology, 106,* 95–103.

Gross, J. J., & Munoz, R. F. (1995). Emotion regulation and mental health. *Clinical Psychology: Science and Practice, 2,* 151–164.

Gross, J. J., Richards, J. M., & John, O. P. (2006). Emotion regulation in everyday life. In D. K. Snyder, J. A. Simpson, & J. N. Hughes (Eds.), *Emotion regulation in couples and families: Pathways to dysfunction and health* (pp. 13–35). Washington, DC: American Psychological Association.

Hariri, A. R., & Forbes, E. E. (2007). Genetics of emotion regulation. In J. J. Gross (Ed.), *Handbook of emotion regulation* (pp. 110–132). New York: Guilford Press.

Harris, P. L., Guz, G. R., Lipian, M. S., & Man-Shu, Z. (1985). Insight into the time course of emotion among Western and Chinese children. *Child Development, 56,* 972–988.

Harris, P. L., & Lipian, M. S. (1989). Understanding emotion and experiencing emotion. In C. Saarni & P. L. Harris (Eds.), *Children's understanding of emotion* (pp. 241–258). New York: Cambridge University Press.

Izard, C. E. (1990). Facial expressions and the regulation of emotions. *Journal of Personality and Social Psychology, 58,* 487–498.

James, W. (1884). What is an emotion? *Mind, 9,* 188–205.

John, O. P., & Gross, J. J. (2007). Individual differences in emotion regulation. In J. J. Gross (Ed.), *Handbook of emotion regulation* (pp. 351–372). New York: Guilford Press.

John, O. P., & Gross, J. J. (2004). Healthy and unhealthy emotion regulation: Personality processes, individual differences, and lifespan development. *Journal of Personality, 72,* 1301–1334.

Just, N., & Alloy, L. B. (1997). The response styles theory of depression: Tests and an extension of the theory. *Journal of Abnormal Psychology, 106,* 221–229.

Kahneman, D. (2000). Experienced utility and objective happiness: A moment-based approach. In D. Kahnemannm & A. Tversky (Ed.), *Choices, values, and frames* (pp. 673–692). Cambridge, UK: Cambridge University Press.

Kaplan, H. I., & Sadock, B. J. (1991). *Synopsis of psychiatry* (6th ed.). Baltimore: Williams & Wilkins.

Keltner, D., & Kring, A. M. (1998). Emotion, social function, and psychopathology. *Review of General Psychology, 2,* 320–342.

Kopp, C. B. (1992). Emotional distress and control in young children. In N. Eisenberg & R. A. Fabes (Eds.), *Emotion and its regulation in early development* (pp. 41–56). San Francisco: Jossey-Bass.

Lang, P. J. (1995). The emotion probe: Studies of motivation and attention. *American Psychologist, 50,* 372–385.

Larsen, R. J. (2000). Toward a science of mood regulation. *Psychological Inquiry, 11,* 129–141.

Lazarus, R. S. (1966). *Psychological stress and the coping process.* New York: McGraw Hill.

Lazarus, R. S. (1985). The costs and benefits of denial. In A. Monat & R. S. Lazarus (Eds.), *Stress and coping: An anthology* (2nd ed., pp. 154–173). New York: Columbia University Press.

Lazarus, R. S. (1993). From psychological stress to the emotions: A history of changing outlooks. *Annual Review of Psychology, 44,* 1–21.

Levenson, R. W. (1999). The intrapersonal functions of emotion. *Cognition and Emotion, 13,* 481–504.

Linehan, M. M., Bohus, M., & Lynch, T. R. (2007). Dialectical behavior therapy for pervasive emotion dysregulation: Theoretical and practical underpinnings. In J. J. Gross (Ed.), *Handbook of emotion regulation* (pp. 581–605). New York: Guilford Press.

Loewenstein, G. (2007). Affective regulation and affective forecasting. In J. J. Gross (Ed.), *Handbook of emotion regulation* (pp. 180–203). New York: Guilford Press.

MacLean, P. D. (1990). *The triune brain in evolution: Role in paleocerebral functions.* New York: Plenum Press.

Masters, J. C. (1991). Strategies and mechanisms for the personal and social control of emotion. In J. Garber & K. A. Dodge (Eds.), *The development of emotion regulation and dysregulation* (pp. 182–207). Cambridge, UK: Cambridge University Press.

Matsumoto, D. (1987). The role of facial response in the experience of emotion: More methodological problems and a meta-analysis. *Journal of Personality and Social Psychology, 52,* 769–774.

Mauss, I. B., Evers, C., Wilhelm, F. H., & Gross, J. J. (2006). How to bite your tongue without blowing your top: Implicit evaluation of emotion regulation predicts affective responding to anger provocation. *Personality and Social Psychology Bulletin, 32,* 589–602.

Mauss, I. B., Levenson, R. W., McCarter, L., Wilhelm, F. H., & Gross, J. J. (2005). The tie that binds?: Coherence among emotion experience, behavior, and physiology. *Emotion, 5,* 175–190.

Mesquita, B., & Albert, D. (2007). The cultural regulation of emotions. In J. J. Gross (Ed.), *Handbook of emotion regulation* (pp. 486–503). New York: Guilford Press.

Mischel, W. (1996). From good intentions to willpower. In P. Gollwitzer & J. Bargh (Eds.), *The psychology of action* (pp. 197–218). New York: Guilford Press.

Mischel, W., & Ayduk, O. (2004). Willpower in a cognitive–affective–processing system: The dynamics of delay of gratification. In R. F. Baumeister & K. D. Vohs (Eds.), *Handbook of self regulation: Research, theory, and applications* (pp. 99–129). New York: Guilford Press.

Miyake, A., Friedman, N. P., Emerson, M. J., Witzki, A. H., Howerter, A., & Wager, T. D. (2000). The unity and diversity of executive functions and their contributions to complex "frontal lobe" tasks: A latent variable analysis. *Cognitive Psychology, 41,* 49–100.

Mullin, B. C., & Hinshaw, S. P. (2007). Emotion regulation and externalizing disorders in children and adolescents. In J. J. Gross (Ed.), *Handbook of emotion regulation* (pp. 523–541). New York: Guilford Press.

Nachmias, M., Gunnar, M., Mangelsdorf, S., Parritz, R., & Buss, K. (1996). Behavioral inhibition and stress reactivity: The moderating role of attachment security. *Child Development, 67,* 508–522.

Nolen-Hoeksema, S. (1993). Sex differences in control of depression. In D. M. Wegner & J. W. Pennebaker (Eds.), *Handbook of mental control* (pp. 306–324). Englewood Cliffs, NJ: Prentice Hall.

Ochsner, K. N., & Gross, J. J. (2007). The neural architecture of emotion regulation. In J. J. Gross (Ed.), *Handbook of emotion regulation* (pp. 87–109). New York: Guilford Press.

Ochsner, K. N., & Gross, J. J. (2005). The cognitive control of emotion. *Trends in Cognitive Sciences, 9,* 242–249.

Ochsner, K. N., Ray, R. R., Cooper, J. C., Robertson, E. R., Chopra, S., Gabrieli, J. D. E., & Gross, J. J. (2004). For better or for worse: Neural systems supporting the cognitive down- and up-regulation of negative emotion. *NeuroImage, 23,* 483–499.

Parker, J. D. A., & Endler, N. S. (1996). Coping and defense: A historical overview. In M. Zeidner & N. S. Endler (Eds.), *Handbook of coping: Theory, research, applications* (pp. 3–23). New York: Wiley.

Parkinson, B., Totterdell, P., Briner, R. B., & Reynolds, S. (1996). *Changing moods: The psychology of mood and mood regulation.* London: Longman.

Peterson, C., & Park, N. (2007). Explanatory style and emotion regulation. In J. J. Gross (Ed.), *Handbook of emotion regulation* (pp. 159–179). New York: Guilford Press.

Quirk, G. J. (2007). Prefrontal–amygdala interactions in the regulation of fear. In J. J. Gross (Ed.), *Handbook of emotion regulation* (pp. 27–46). New York: Guilford Press.

Rimé, B. (2007). Interpersonal emotion regulation. In J. J. Gross (Ed.), *Handbook of emotion regulation* (pp. 466–485). New York: Guilford Press.

Rothbart, M. K., & Sheese, B. E. (2007). Temperament and emotion regulation. In J. J. Gross (Ed.), *Handbook of emotion regulation* (pp. 331–350). New York: Guilford Press.

Rothbart, M. K., Ziaie, H., & O'Boyle, C. G. (1992). Self-regulation and emotion in infancy. In N. Eisenberg & R. A. Fabes (Eds.), *Emotion and its regulation in early development* (pp. 7–23). San Francisco: Jossey-Bass.

Sapolsky, R. M. (2007). Stress, stress-related disease, and emotion regulation. In J. J. Gross (Ed.), *Handbook of emotion regulation* (pp. 606–615). New York: Guilford Press.

Scherer, K. R. (1984). On the nature and function of emotion: A component process approach. In K. R. Scherer & P. E. Ekman (Eds.), *Approaches to emotion* (pp. 293–317). Hillsdale, NJ: Erlbaum.

Shaver, P. R., & Mikulincer, M. (2007). Adult attachment strategies and the regulation of emotion. In J. J. Gross (Ed.), *Handbook of emotion regulation* (pp. 446–465). New York: Guilford Press.

Sher, K. J., & Grekin, E. R. (2007). Alcohol and affect regulation. In J. J. Gross (Ed.), *Handbook of emotion regulation* (pp. 560–580). New York: Guilford Press.

Stegge, H., & Meerum Terwogt, M. (2007). Awareness and regulation of emotion in typical and atypical development. In J. J. Gross (Ed.), *Handbook of emotion regulation* (pp. 269–286). New York: Guilford Press.

Steptoe, A., & Vogele, C. (1986). Are stress responses influenced by cognitive appraisal?: An experimental comparison of coping strategies. *British Journal of Psychology, 77,* 243–255.

Stifter, C. A., & Moyer, D. (1991). The regulation of positive affect: Gaze aversion activity during mother–infant interaction. *Infant Behaviors and Development, 14,* 111–123.

Stuss, D., & Benson, D. (1986). *The frontal lobes.* New York: Raven Press.

Taylor, S. E., & Lobel, M. (1989). Social comparison activity under threat: Downward evaluation and upward contacts. *Psychological Review, 96,* 569–575.

Thompson, R. A. (1990). Emotion and self-regulation. In R. A. Thompson (Ed.), *Socioemotional development. Nebraska Symposium on Motivation* (Vol. 36, pp. 367–467). Lincoln: University of Nebraska Press.

Thompson, R. A. (1991). Emotional regulation and emotional development. *Educational Psychology Review, 3,* 269–307.

Thompson, R. A. (1994). Emotion regulation: A theme in search of definition. The development of emotion regulation: Biological and behavioral considerations. *Monographs of the Society for Research in Child Development, 59,* 25–52.

Thompson, R. A. (2006). The development of the person: Social understanding, relationships, self, conscience. In W. Damon & R. M. Lerner (Eds.), *Handbook of child psychology. Social, emotional, and personality development* (N. Eisenberg, Vol. ed., 6th ed., pp. 24–98). New York: Wiley.

Thompson, R. A., & Calkins, S. D. (1996). The double-edged sword: Emotional regulation for children at risk. *Development and Psychopathology, 8,* 163–182.

Thompson, R. A., & Lagatutta, K. (2006). Feeling and understanding: Early emotional development. In K. McCartney & D. Phillips (Ed.), *The Blackwell handbook of early childhood development* (pp. 317–337). Oxford, UK: Blackwell.

Thompson, R. A., & Meyer, S. (2007). Socialization of emotion regulation in the family. In J. J. Gross (Ed.), *Handbook of emotion regulation* (pp. 249–268). New York: Guilford Press.

Tomkins, S. S. (1984). Affect theory. In P. Ekman (Ed.), *Emotion in the human face* (2nd ed., pp. 353–395). New York: Cambridge University Press.

Watts, F. (2007). Emotion regulation and religion. In J. J. Gross (Ed.), *Handbook of emotion regulation* (pp. 504–520). New York: Guilford Press.

Wegner, D. M., & Bargh, J. A. (1998). Control and automaticity in social life. In D. Gilbert, S. T. Fiske, & G. Lindzey (Eds.), *Handbook of social psychology* (4th ed., Vol. 1, pp. 446–496). New York: McGraw-Hill.

Westen, D. (1994). Toward an integrative model of affect regulation: Applications to social–psychological research. *Journal of Personality, 62,* 641–667.

Westen, D., & Blagov, P. S. (2007). A clinical–empirical model of emotion regulation: From defense and motivated reasoning to emotional constraint satisfaction. In J. J. Gross (Ed.), *Handbook of emotion regulation* (pp. 373–392). New York: Guilford Press.

Wills, T. A. (1981). Downward social comparison principles in social psychology. *Psychological Bulletin, 90,* 245–271.

Wranik, T., Barrett, L. F., & Salovey, P. (2007). Intelligent emotion regulation: Is knowledge power? In J. J. Gross (Ed.), *Handbook of emotion regulation* (pp. 393–407). New York: Guilford Press.

Zelazo, P. D., & Cunningham, W. A. (2007). Executive function: Mechanisms underlying emotion regulation. In J. J. Gross (Ed.), *Handbook of emotion regulation* (pp. 135–158). New York: Guilford Press.

PART II

BIOLOGICAL BASES

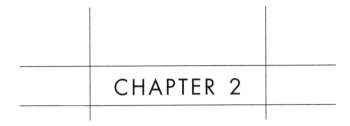

CHAPTER 2

Prefrontal–Amygdala Interactions in the Regulation of Fear

GREGORY J. QUIRK

The nervous system of every living thing is but a bundle of predispositions to react in particular ways upon the contact of particular features of the environment.

—JAMES (1884, p. 190)

The idea that we are "predisposed" to react in certain ways to environmental stimuli has a long history. While some predispositions may be hardwired in the brain, many more are learned through experience, such as classical conditioning. This is particularly true in the emotional domain, where associations can be rapidly acquired sometimes in the absence of conscious awareness. From the point of view of emotional health, there must be systems capable of regulating the expression of these associations, determining when and where their expression is appropriate and advantageous. The study of emotion regulation therefore is intimately associated with the concept of inhibition, namely, that higher cortical areas are responsible for inhibiting subcortical areas that generate prepotent responses to conditioned stimuli. For this reason, understanding the neural mechanisms of inhibition within limbic emotion networks is critical for understanding emotion regulation.

EARLY STUDIES OF INHIBITION

The physiological basis of inhibition originated in the 1840s with the observation that electrical stimulation of the vagus nerve in the frog *decreased* heart rate (Weber & Weber, 1846). This finding conflicted with the prevailing view that excitation of nerves always provoked increases in activity, and it was not fully accepted until acetylcholine was isolated from the vagus nerve many years later (Loewi, 1921). The idea that the brain was capable of generating inhibition was first introduced by Russian physiologist Ivan Sechenov, who demonstrated that the withdrawal reflex in frogs' legs was quickened by transecting the brain at the level of the midbrain (Sechenov, 1866). This provided evidence that descending projections from the brain were responsible for inhibiting spinal reflexes. Sechenov's suggestion that psychological concepts could be explained by physiological processes was met with strong opposition but laid the groundwork for fellow Russian Ivan Pavlov's subsequent work with conditioned reflexes in dogs.

Within the context of emotion, inhibitory theories of cortical function date back to the middle of the 19th century with the famous case of Phineas Gage, who suffered a large frontal lobe lesion in a railroad construction site accident. Following his recovery, Gage exhibited personality changes, becoming childlike, impulsive, and capricious (Harlow, 1868). Similar such patients were described soon afterward (Starr, 1884) laying the groundwork for the notion that pathology arises from "over-action of lower centers as a consequence of loss of control from inaction of higher centers" (Jackson, 1884). Experimenting with dogs, the Italian psychiatrist Leonardo Bianchi noted that prefrontal lesions tended to exaggerate emotional traits, so that timid dogs became more withdrawn and affectionate dogs more likely to seek affection (Bianchi, 1895). Later work in humans (Milner, 1964) and monkeys (Butter, Mishkin, & Rosvold, 1963) revealed a perseverative effect of prefrontal lesions, such that subjects would continue responding to previously rewarded cues that no longer predicted reward. These observations laid the groundwork for the idea that the prefrontal cortex is necessary for inhibiting conditioned responses, thereby permitting behavioral flexibility.

FEAR CONDITIONING AND THE AMYGDALA

Modern investigations of emotion regulation have increasingly used classical fear conditioning procedures in which animals associate sensory stimuli with aversive outcomes. In fear conditioning, rats are exposed to a simple sensory or contextual conditioned stimulus (CS) paired with footshock unconditioned stimulus (US). A single pairing is sufficient for the CS alone to elicit species-specific fear responses such as freezing, hypertension, analgesia, and potentiation of somatic reflexes (Blanchard & Blanchard, 1972; Davis, 1997; De Oca, DeCola, Maren, & Fanselow, 1998; LeDoux, 2000). Freezing is the most commonly used measure of conditioned fear in rodents and is employed in most of the studies cited here. Fear conditioning offers several important advantages for the study of emotional regulation: (1) fear responses to the CS are easily measured and quantified, (2) the neural circuits of fear conditioning have been extensively studied, and (3) psychological theories regarding control of fear expression make specific predictions as to how neural structures might signal conditioned stimuli.

In humans, the pairing of a tone and a shock is thought to generate two types of fear memory: a declarative form of memory in which the subject can consciously describe the link between the CS and US and a nondeclarative form responsible for the body's autonomic and reflexive behavioral responses to the fear stimulus (Bechara et al., 1995; LeDoux, 1996). While declarative memory depends on the hippocampus, nondeclarative fear memory depends on the amygdala, and is the focus of this chapter. The hypothesis that the amygdala stores fear associations was originally based on lesion evidence (Blanchard & Blanchard, 1972; Iwata, LeDoux, Meeley, Arneric, & Reis, 1986; LeDoux, Cicchetti, Xagoraris, & Romanski, 1990), but more recent studies have employed temporary inactivation (Helmstetter & Bellgowan, 1994; Wilensky, Schafe, & LeDoux, 1999), single-unit recording (Quirk, Repa, & LeDoux, 1995; Collins, & Pare,

2000; Repa et al., 2001), field potentials (Rogan, Leon, Perez, & Kandel, 2005), local infusion of antagonists (Miserendino, Sananes, Melia, & Davis, 1990; Fanselow & Kim, 1994; Schafe & LeDoux, 2000), and transgenic approaches (Kida et al., 2002; Shumyatsky et al., 2002).

These studies converge on the idea that the lateral amygdala (LA) is a critical storage site for the tone–shock association (see Figure 2.1). The LA receives tone and shock input from the thalamus and cortex and is the first site in the ascending sensory steam to show massive convergence of tone and shock inputs (LeDoux et al., 1990). LA projects to the central nucleus of the amygdala (Ce) directly and via the basal amygdala nuclei (Pare, Smith, & Pare, 1995; Pitkanen, Savander, & LeDoux, 1997). The Ce is the origin of amygdala outputs to fear generating structures in the hypothalamus and brainstem (LeDoux, Iwata, Cicchetti, & Reis, 1988; De Oca et al., 1998; Davis, 2000). Thus, LA is seen as the site of fear memory, while Ce is seen as the site of fear expression (LeDoux, 2000; Davis, 2000; Maren, 2001). Pretraining lesions of cortical areas do not prevent acquisition of fear conditioning (Romanski & LeDoux, 1992; Morgan, Romanski, & LeDoux, 1993; Campeau & Davis, 1995), indicating that subcortical amygdala circuits are sufficient for simple fear learning.

More recent findings, however, have modified this view of amygdala function. Posttraining lesion or inactivation of cortical areas impairs expression of conditioned fear (Corodimas & LeDoux, 1995; Campeau & Davis, 1995; Sacchetti, Lorenzini, Baldi, Tassoni, & Bucherelli, 1999; Sierra-Mercado, Corcoran, Lebron, & Quirk, 2006), indicating that cortical sites are more important than previously thought. Similarly, the basal nuclei of the amygdala were excluded from the circuit because pre-training lesions had no effect (Nader, Majidishad, Amorapanth, & LeDoux, 2001). It has been recently observed, however, that posttraining lesions of basal amygdala completely block the expression of conditioned fear (Anglada-Figueroa & Quirk, 2005), suggesting that the basal amygdala is a critical site of fear-related plasticity in the intact brain. Finally, recent evidence suggests that Ce is not simply a relay for fear expression, but is itself an

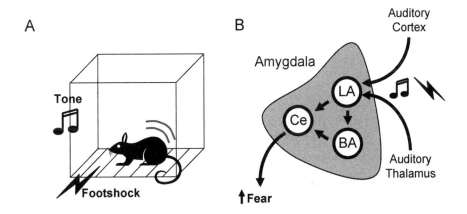

FIGURE 2.1. Fear conditioning depends on the amygdala. (A) Rats are exposed to a tone CS paired with a footshock US, and develop conditioned freezing responses to the tone. (B) Tone and shock information enter the lateral amygdala (LA) via thalamic and cortical inputs. The LA projects to the central nucleus (Ce) directly and indirectly via the basal amygdala (BA). The Ce projects to fear-generating structures in the hypothalamus and brainstem. All three amygdala regions (LA, BA, Ce) store the tone–shock association.

important site of plasticity (reviewed in Pare, Quirk, & LeDoux, 2004). Thus, fear learning is not limited to the LA but appears to be distributed throughout the amygdala, as well as in parts of cortex and even the brainstem (Heldt & Falls, 2003). The large number of critical sites of plasticity in fear conditioning increases the possibilities for modulation of fear expression by descending projections from the cortex.

INHIBITION OF FEAR EXPRESSION: EXTINCTION

Once acquired, fear associations are not always expressed (Rescorla, 2004). In situations in which danger is unlikely, conditioned fear stimuli do not elicit fear. This is most easily observed during extinction, where repeated presentations of the CS in the absence of the US leads to a diminution of fear responses. In his early investigations of appetitive conditioning in dogs, Pavlov observed that extinguished responses spontaneously recovered with the passage of time (Pavlov, 1927). This important observation indicated that extinction inhibited the conditioned response rather than erasing the conditioning memory. More recent behavioral studies have confirmed and extended this finding for conditioned fear (Quirk, 2002; Myers, & Davis, 2002; Rescorla, 2002). For example, extinguished fear responses can be reinstated by exposure to a single US (Rescorla & Heth, 1975), or renewed by delivering the CS in a context other than where extinction occurred (Bouton, 2002). Thus, fear memories are continually present in the brain and can be expressed any time that inhibition is reduced.

If extinction is not erasure, it must involve the formation of a new memory (Figure 2.2). The "extinction as new memory" hypothesis gained support from the observation that memory for extinction required activation of N-methyl-D-aspartate (NMDA) receptors (Falls, Miserendino, & Davis, 1992; Baker & Azorlosa, 1996; Santini, Muller, & Quirk, 2001). NMDA receptors are glutamate-gated ion channels that permit the influx of calcium ions, which trigger molecular cascades involved in memory consolidation (Collingridge & Bliss, 1995). Along the same lines, inhibitors of protein synthesis also block the formation of extinction memory (Vianna, Szapiro, McGaugh, Medina, & Izquierdo, 2001; Eisenberg, Kobilo, Berman, & Dudai, 2003; Santini, Ge, Ren, Pena, & Quirk, 2004). The involvement of a molecular cascade that has been repeatedly implicated in memory formation strongly suggests that extinction forms a "safety memory"

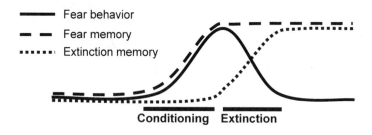

FIGURE 2.2. Memory for extinction and conditioning coexist in the extinguished brain. During the conditioning phase, rats learn the tone–shock association and display fear to the tone. During extinction, fear responses decline but fear memory remains intact, because extinction (safety) memory accumulates. This schema predicts that some structure or structures in the brain increase their activity following extinction, so as to inhibit the expression of fear behavior. Adapted from Milad, Rauch, and Quirk (2006). Copyright 2006 by Elsevier. Adapted by permission.

which competes with the fear memory for control of behavior. It has been suggested that anxiety disorders may result from a lack of balance between fear and safety memories (Quirk & Gehlert, 2003; Charney, 2004; Rogan et al., 2005; Milad et al., 2006), indicating that extinction of fear is a clinically relevant example of emotion regulation.

INHIBITION WITHIN THE AMYGDALA

Given the amygdala's well established plasticity mechanisms and projections to multiple fear-generating sites (Davis, 2000), it has been called a "hub" of fear learning and expression (LeDoux, 2000). Therefore, modulation of amygdala plasticity and/or output would be an efficient way of regulating fear expression. Recent work has focused on inhibitory circuits within the amygdala. Neurons in the basolateral complex (BLA) and central nucleus tend to fire at very low rates in vivo (Quirk et al., 1995; Collins & Pare, 1999), consistent with high levels of tonic inhibition. In fact, long-term potentiation of thalamic inputs to LA is accompanied by a reduction in inhibition (Bissiere, Humeau, & Luthi, 2003), suggesting that amygdala inhibition must be reduced in order to acquire fear memories (Rosenkranz, Moore, & Grace, 2003).

In addition to LA, there is also powerful inhibition of the Ce output neurons of the amygdala. Situated between the BLA and Ce are islands of GABA(gamma-amnobutyric acid)-ergic "intercalated" (ITC) cells (Nitecka & Ben Ari, 1987). These cells receive input from BLA and project to Ce output neurons, thereby acting as an inhibitory interface between centers of fear learning and fear expression (Pare & Smith, 1993; Royer, Martina, & Pare, 1999). Interestingly, these inhibitory circuits exhibit plasticity, as evidenced by long-term potentiation. High-frequency stimulation of thalamic inputs potentiated inhibitory interneurons in LA (Mahanty & Sah, 1998; Bauer & LeDoux, 2004), and high-frequency stimulation of BLA potentiated GABA-ergic ITC cells (Royer & Pare, 2002). Thus, in addition to learning fear associations, the amygdala is also capable of learning fear inhibition.

NEURAL CIRCUITS OF EXTINCTION LEARNING

Prefrontal Cortex and Amygdala

If extinction is new learning, some structure or structures must be activated by extinction in order to trigger inhibitory circuits responsible for reducing fear expression. Despite early theoretical formulations of extinction-related inhibition (Pavlov, 1927; Konorski, 1967), the search for inhibitory circuits has been largely unsuccessful (Kimble & Kimble, 1970; Chan, Morell, Jarrard, & Davidson, 2001). Recent studies, however, point to the medial prefrontal cortex (mPFC) as a possible inhibitor of fear in extinction (Quirk, Garcia, & Gonzalez-Lima, 2006). Early studies implicated the primate ventromedial prefrontal cortex (vmPFC) in extinction of appetitive conditioning (Butter et al., 1963; Fuster, 1997). Following this, LeDoux and colleagues demonstrated that lesions of a homologous area in rats impaired extinction of conditioned fear (Morgan et al., 1993). Rats with vmPFC lesions could acquire conditioned fear normally but had difficulty extinguishing fear responses across several days of extinction testing. The rat vmPFC is composed of infralimbic (IL) and prelimbic (PL) subregions. IL and PL do not have the same targets in the amygdala. PL targets mostly the basolateral and accessory basal nuclei, whereas the IL targets areas that inhibit amygdala output such as the capsular and lateral divisions of the central nucleus (McDonald, Mascagni, & Guo,

1996; Vertes, 2004). IL also projects to subcortical targets of the amygdala in the hypothalamus, midbrain, and brainstem (McDonald et al., 1996; Floyd, Price, Ferry, Keay, & Bandler, 2000; Vertes, R. P., 2004). IL is therefore well situated to inhibit the expression of fear, either via the amygdala or by acting directly on lower centers (see Figure 2.3).

More recent work has extended our understanding of the role of vmPFC in extinction (see Figure 2.4A). Rats with pretraining lesions of vmPFC can acquire conditioned fear responses normally, and can extinguish those responses during an extinction training session. The next day, however, fear responses to the tone spontaneously recover in lesioned rats (Quirk, Russo, Barron, & Lebron, 2000; Lebron, Milad, & Quirk, 2004). Thus, vmPFC-lesioned rats can learn extinction, but have difficulty recalling extinction after a long delay, suggesting that vmPFC is necessary for long-term retention of extinction. However, extending extinction training over consecutive days does eventually lead to recall of extinction in lesioned rats (Lebron et al., 2004), suggesting that vmPFC lesions delay but do not prevent access to extinction information. Paralleling these lesion findings, single neurons in IL do not signal the tone during conditioning or extinction training but do show tone responses the day after conditioning when rats are recalling extinction (Milad & Quirk, 2002) (see Figure 2.4B). This "extinction signal" is largest in rats showing the lowest levels of conditioned fear, consistent with an inhibitory role.

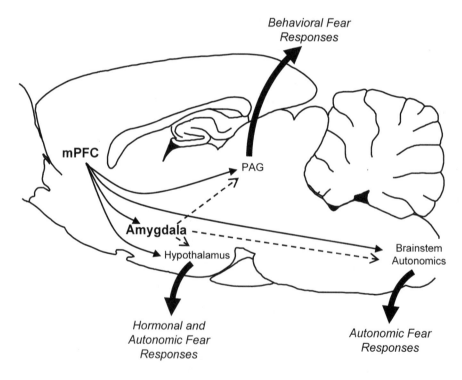

FIGURE 2.3. Descending projections of the infralimbic (IL) mPFC. IL projects to the amygdala, as well as to the amygdala's targets in the hypothalamus, periaqueductal gray (PAG), and brainstem, structures which mediate the expression of fear responses. Thus, IL is in a good position to modulate the expression of fear after extinction. Adapted from Paxinos and Watson (1998). Copyright 1998 by Elsevier. Adapted by permission.

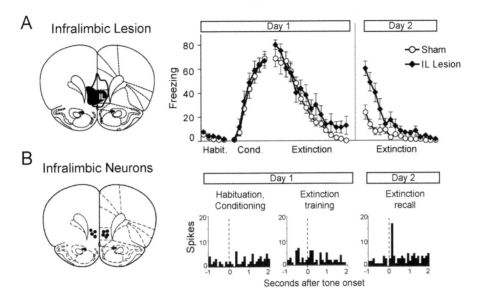

FIGURE 2.4. Infralimbic prefrontal cortex (IL) is necessary for recall of extinction. (A) Rats with lesions of IL can acquire and extinguish conditioned fear normally on Day 1, but have difficulty recalling extinction the following day. Adapted from Quirk et al. (2000). Copyright 2000 by the Society for Neuroscience. Adapted by permission. (B) Paralleling this, IL neurons signal the tone CS only during recall of extinction on Day 2. Dotted line indicates tone onset. These and other data suggest that extinction-induced potentiation of IL is necessary for suppression of fear after extinction. Adapted from Milad and Quirk (2002). Copyright 2002 by Milad and Quirk. Adapted by permission.

Potentiation of IL activity during recall of extinction has been demonstrated with other techniques such as evoked potentials (increased IL response to thalamic stimulation) (Herry & Garcia, 2002), glucose metabolism (increased uptake of labeled glucose in IL) (Barrett, Shumake, Jones, & Gonzalez-Lima, 2003), and induction of *c-Fos* (an immediate early gene associated with neural activation) (Santini et al., 2004; Herry & Mons, 2004). Infusion of drugs into the vmPFC that interfere with molecular cascades necessary for plasticity prevent long-term extinction memory (see Figure 2.5). These include NMDA receptor antagonist (3-((+/–)20carboxypiperazin-4yl) propel-1-phosphate, CPP) (Burgos-Robles, Santini, & Quirk, 2004), MAP (mitrogen-activated protein kinase) kinase inhibitor PD098059 (Hugues, Deschaux, & Garcia, 2004), and protein synthesis inhibitor anisomycin (Santini et al., 2004). Interestingly, all of these manipulations yield the same pattern of effects, namely, intact extinction learning but deficient recall of extinction the following day. Thus, multiple lines of evidence support the hypothesis that extinction forms a new memory of safety, and that memory exists, at least partially, in the vmPFC.

There is also a parallel line of evidence indicating that extinction memory is formed and stored in the amygdala (Myers & Davis, 2002). Inhibition of NMDA receptors (Walker & Davis, 2002), MAP kinase (Lu, Walker, & Davis, 2001), or protein synthesis (Lin, Yeh, Lu, & Gean, 2003) in the amygdala prevent extinction of conditioned fear. Cannabinoid receptors in the amygdala, which modulate the activity of inhibitory interneurons, have also been implicated in fear extinction (Marsicano et al., 2002; Chhatwal, Davis, Maguschak, & Ressler, 2005). As stated earlier, interfering with vmPFC does not prevent

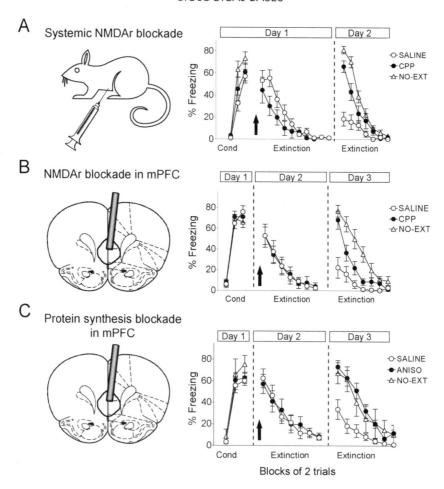

FIGURE 2.5. NMDA receptors and protein synthesis in mPFC are important for long-term, but not short-term, extinction memory. (A) Rats given the NMDA receptor antagonist CPP systemically could extinguish fear, but could not recall extinction the following day. Thus, long-term extinction memory is NMDA-dependent. A similar effect was seen when CPP was infused directly into the mPFC (B) or when protein synthesis inhibitor anisomycin was infused directly into the mPFC (C). Arrows indicate the time of infusion. Adapted from Santini et al. (2001, 2004). Copyright 2001 and copyright 2004 by the Society for Neuroscience. Adapted by permission.

extinction learning per se but prevents recall of extinction after a long delay. The fact that vmPFC-lesioned rats can eventually recall extinction with overtraining suggests that other structures such as the amygdala are capable of learning and expressing extinction. It has been suggested that the amygdala is necessary for short-term extinction learning, whereas the vmPFC is necessary for expression of extinction after a delay, when intervening temporal and contextual changes render the CS ambiguous (Lin et al., 2003; Quirk, Garcia, & Gonzalez-Lima, 2006; Santini et al., 2004).

Hippocampus

As already mentioned, the major factor in determining the response to an extinguished CS is context; recall of extinction only occurs in the context in which extinction training occurred. This suggests that contextual machinery located in the hippocampus plays a key role in the expression of extinction. In support of this, contextual renewal of fear responses after extinction is prevented when the hippocampus is pharmacologically inactivated at test (Corcoran & Maren, 2001). Interestingly, inactivation of the hippocampus prior to extinction training leads to impaired recall of extinction (high fear) the following day (Corcoran, Desmond, Frey, & Maren, 2005). This is similar to the effects of vmPFC lesions (Quirk et al., 2000) and inactivation (Sierra-Mercado et al., 2006), suggesting that the hippocampus and vmPFC act together to regulate the expression of fear responses to a CS following extinction (Maren & Quirk, 2004). Projections from the hippocampus to the mPFC show long-term potentiation (Jay, Burette, & Laroche, 1995) as well as long-term depression (Takita, Izaki, Jay, M., Kaneko, & Suzuki, 1999), consistent with extinction-related plasticity in this pathway. The hippocampus also has direct projections to the BLA, which exhibit long-term potentiation (Maren & Fanselow, 1995) and could mediate contextual modulation of fear independently of the mPFC (Hobin, Goosens, & Maren, 2003).

In addition to contextual gating of fear responses to extinguished stimuli, the hippocampus is also necessary for extinction of contextual fear learning, in which a shock is paired not with a tone but with a unique context. Extinction of contextual fear is prevented by intrahippocampal infusion of antagonists of NMDA receptors and MAP kinase (Szapiro, Vianna, McGaugh, Medina, & Izquierdo, 2003). Interestingly, the extinction of contextual fear is not impaired by lesions of the vmPFC (Morgan et al., 1993), suggesting that direct projections from the hippocampus to the amygdala are sufficient for contextual extinction. Thus, the hippocampal–prefrontal system may be particularly important in using contextual information to disambiguate the response to an extinguished tone CS.

PREFRONTAL–AMYGDALA INTERACTIONS IN THE REGULATION OF FEAR EXPRESSION

The increased activity in IL following extinction is consistent with Pavlov's suggestion that extinction activates a cortical inhibitor responsible for reducing fear (Pavlov, 1927). But is there any evidence that IL neurons act to inhibit fear? Using chronically implanted stimulating electrodes, it was shown that a single brief train of electrical impulses delivered to IL reduces conditioned freezing to a tone CS (Milad & Quirk, 2002). To reduce fear, the stimulation had to be delivered with the same timing and duration as actual IL tone responses (Milad, Vidal-Gonzalez, & Quirk, 2004). This suggests that stimulation of IL was able to mimic the extinction safety signal in rats that had not received extinction training.

IL sends a robust projection to the amygdala ITC cells and the lateral subdivision of Ce (Sesack, Deutch, Roth, & Bunney, 1989; McDonald et al., 1996; Vertes, 2004), both of which inhibit Ce output neurons. Following extinction, IL can exert feed-forward inhibition of the amygdala via the ITC cells (see Figure 2.6). In support of this idea, electrical stimulation of IL reduced the responsiveness of Ce output neurons to basolateral amygdala stimulation in both rats and cats (Quirk, Likhtik, Pelletier, & Pare, 2003). The source of Ce inhibition is likely the ITC cells, in light of recent evidence that IL stimulation activates c-Fos expression in ITC cells (Berretta, Pantazopoulos, Caldera, Pantazopoulos, & Pare, 2005). Thus, the IL has access to a powerful "off switch" for fear in the form of the ITC cells. It has also been suggested that vmPFC inhibits BLA neurons and thereby prevents the acquisition of fear conditioning (Rosenkranz & Grace,

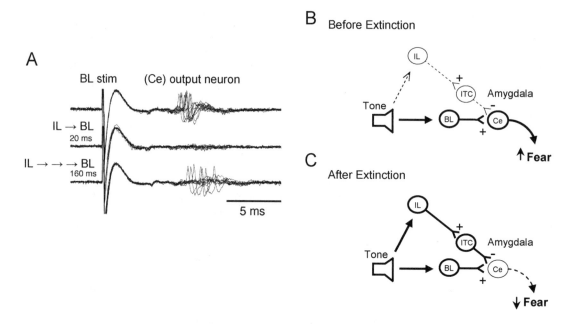

FIGURE 2.6. IL stimulation reduces amygdala output. (A) Recordings from a central nucleus (Ce) output neuron in an anesthetized cat. Stimulation of the amygdala basolateral nucleus (BL) alone activated Ce, but stimulating IL 20 msec prior to BL prevented Ce from being activated. Increasing the IL–BL stimulation interval to 160 msec eliminated the inhibitory effect of IL stimulation presumably because the inhibitory effect of ITC activation dissipated before BL was activated. These data suggest that IL can gate the excitability of Ce neurons, over a brief time window. Adapted from Quirk et al. (2003). Copyright 2003 by the Society for Neuroscience. Adapted by permission. (B) Suggested schema of how this circuit might function in conditioning and extinction. When recalling conditioning memory, the tone strongly activates BL, which strongly activates Ce resulting in high levels of fear. When recalling extinction, the tone also activates IL, which in turn activates GABA-ergic intercalated (ITC) cells in the amygdala. ITC inhibition of Ce cancels BL's excitatory effect, resulting in lower freezing. Adapted from Milad et al. (2004). Copyright 2004 by the American Psychological Association. Adapted by permission.

2001; Rosenkranz, Moore, & Grace, 2003; but see Likhtik, Pelletier, Paz, & Pare, 2005). Indeed, the conditioned tone responses of LA neurons are smaller in extinction contexts compared to no-extinction contexts (Hobin et al., 2003), suggesting that some extinction-related inhibition of the amygdala occurs prior to the ITC cells.

In addition to inhibiting the amygdala, there is growing evidence that some parts of the mPFC can excite the amygdala and increase fear. Acquisition of certain types of fear conditioning can be blocked by lesioning the vmPFC (Frysztak & Neafsey, 1994; McLaughlin, Skaggs, Churchwell, & Powell, 2002) or by locally inhibiting MAP kinase (Runyan, Moore, & Dash, 2004) or dopamine receptors (Laviolette, Lipski, & Grace, 2005) in the mPFC. Consistent with projections from PL to the basal nuclei of the amygdala (McDonald et al., 1996; Vertes, 2004), cross-correlation analysis has shown that BLA neurons tend to fire 20 msec after PL neurons (Likhtik et al., 2005), consistent with PL driving of BLA. We have ovserved that inactivation of vmPFC reduces the expression of conditioned fear (Sierra-Mercado et al., 2006). Therefore, prefrontal regulation of fear expression may work through separate modules for inhibiting (IL) and exciting (PL) fear responses.

In addition to descending projections to the amygdala, the vmPFC receives extensive return projections from the amygdala, particularly the basal nuclei (McDonald, 1991; Conde, Maire-Lepoivre, Audinat, & Crepel, 1995). There is still no consensus as to the role of these ascending projections for conditioned fear. CS-responsive inputs from the basal nuclei might be a major source of CS excitation (Laviolette et al., 2005) or inhibition (Garcia, Vouimba, Baudry, & Thompson, 1999) of vmPFC neurons during fear conditioning. Physiological studies show that stimulation of the BLA excites IL neurons (Ishikawa & Nakamura, 2003), and long-term potentiation has been observed in the BLA–IL pathway (Maroun & Richter-Levin, 2003). It has been suggested that short-term extinction memory learned by the amygdala is subsequently transferred to vmPFC for long-term storage (Milad & Quirk, 2002; Santini et al., 2004); however, lesions of the main source of amygdala afferents to the vmPFC (basal nuclei) do not prevent extinction (Sotres-Bayon, Bush, & LeDoux, 2004; Anglada-Figueroa & Quirk, 2005). Nevertheless, the projections from the BLA to both PL and IL are extensive. Given IL's return projections to inhibitory centers within the amygdala, the ascending projections from BLA may provide a route by which the amygdala inhibits its own output via the cortex. This would allow for integration of conditioned fear signals with cortical-level contextual and mnemonic factors capable of gating emotional responses. In support of this idea, hippocampal stimulation has been shown to gate the responsiveness of IL neurons to BL input (Ishikawa & Nakamura, 2003).

RELATION OF EXTINCTION TO OTHER PREFRONTAL FUNCTIONS

Extinction processes may be important to other functions of the mPFC such as reversal learning, valuation, and attentional set shifting. During discriminative instrumental conditioning, rats and monkeys learn to respond to a stimulus that predicts reward and withhold responding to a stimulus that does not predict reward. Lesions of PFC do not prevent learning or expression of such discriminations but impair the ability of the animal to modify its behavior following some change in the reward contingencies (Dalley, Cardinal, & Robbins, 2004; Schoenbaum & Roesch, 2005). For example, prefrontal-lesioned animals have difficulty reversing their responses with reversal of the reward contingency (Rolls, Critchley, Mason, & Wakeman, 1996), or altering their response appropriately when the discrimination requires a shift from one set of stimuli to another (Dias, Robbins, & Roberts, 1996). Similarly, when a rewarding US is subsequently "devalued" by pairing it with an aversive experience, prefrontal-lesioned rats maintain high rates of responding despite the devaluation (Pickens, Saddoris, Gallagher, & Holland, 2005). In each of these situations, the animal must extinguish responding to the original contingency in order to adjust to the new contingency. vmPFC lesions have been shown to interfere with recall of extinction in appetitive Pavlovian conditioning (Rhodes & Killcross, 2004), suggesting that prefrontal extinction mechanisms may underlie behavioral flexibility in various forms of appetitive learning.

DYSREGULATION OF THE PREFRONTAL–AMYGDALA SYSTEM

A window into the normal functioning of emotion regulation systems is provided by emotional pathologies. With respect to fear, this can take the form of phobias and post-traumatic stress disorder (PTSD). Both of these conditions are characterized by fear responses to stimuli which at some point appeared dangerous or life-threatening. In a sense, they are normal reactions to potentially dangerous stimuli. Long after the probability of danger has decreased, however, the person is unable to inhibit the expression of the latent fear associations.

Substantial evidence suggests that these disorders of emotional regulation are associated with pathology in the prefrontal–amygdala system. Specifically, loss of top-down inhibition of the amygdala by the vmPFC has been associated with anxiety and mood disorders (Drevets, 2001; Cannistraro & Rauch, 2003). People suffering from PTSD show impairments in a functional network involving the amygdala and anterior cingulate cortex (ACC) (Shin et al., 2001; Gilboa et al., 2004). Brain imaging studies of PTSD patients show reduced activity (Bremner, 2002; Shin et al., 2004; Britton, Phan, Taylor, Fig, & Liberzon, 2005) and reduced volume (Rauch et al., 2003) in the perigenual PFC, an area thought to be homologous with extinction-related regions of rodent mPFC (Ongur & Price, 2000) (see Figure 2.7). When exposed to reminders of traumatic events, patients with PTSD show a negative correlation between vmPFC activity (underactive) and amygdala activity (overactive) (Shin et al., 2004), consistent with a loss of prefrontal inhibition. Recent functional imaging and volumetric studies demonstrate that extinction of conditioned fear activates the same parts of vmPFC compro-

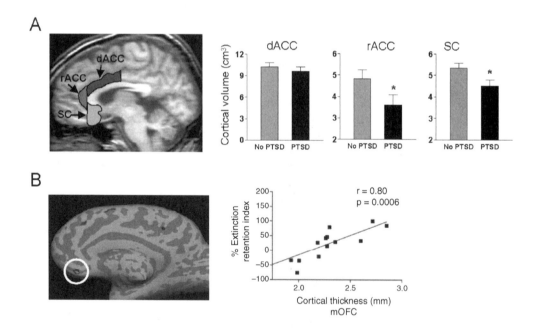

FIGURE 2.7. Human pericallosal mPFC is associated with posttraumatic stress disorder (PTSD) and extinction of fear. (A) The size of different subregions of the anterior cingulate cortex (ACC) in PTSD subjects and non-PTSD subjects. The rostral anterior cingulate (rACC) and subcallosal (SC) areas were significantly smaller in PTSD subjects. $*p < .05$. Adapted from Rauch et al. (2003). Copyright 2003 by Lippincott Williams & Wilkins. Adapted by permission. (B) The thickness of a similar region of vmPFC (circle) was correlated with retention of extinction memory in a fear conditioning task in humans. This suggests that a predisposing factor for developing PTSD is a deficient prefrontal regulatory network controlling extinction. Adapted from Milad et al. (2005). Copyright 2005 by the National Academy of Sciences, U.S.A.. Adapted by permission.

mised in PTSD (Phelps, Delgado, Nearing, & LeDoux, 2004; Milad et al., 2005) (see Figure 2.7). These same ventral prefrontal areas are also compromised in major depression (Mayberg, 2003), individuals at risk for depression (Pezawas et al., 2005), and normals showing introverted personality traits (Rauch et al., 2005). Thus, deficits in prefrontal inhibition of the amygdala may underlie several related pathologies.

A clue to how the prefrontal–amygdala system becomes compromised comes from recent experiments on the effects of chronic stressors on neuronal structure and function. Rats exposed to an early life stressor related to maternal care develop permanent alterations in GABA-ergic function in vmPFC and amygdala (Caldji, Diorio, & Meaney, 2003). Daily chronic restraint decreases dendritic branching and reduces the density of synaptic spines in vmPFC (Radley et al., 2004; Radley et al., 2006). In the amygdala, chronic restraint has the opposite effect, causing increased dendritic branching and increased spines (Vyas, Mitra, Shankaranarayana Rao, & Chattarji, 2002; Mitra, Jadhav, McEwen, Vyas, & Chattarji, 2005). Together, these findings suggest that chronic stress increases the ability of the amygdala to learn and express fear associations, while at the same time reducing the ability of the prefrontal cortex to control fear. This can create a vicious cycle in which increased fear and anxiety leads to more stress, which leads to further dysregulation. This situation has been termed "allostatic load" (McEwen, 2003) and could explain why stressful situations sometimes spiral into pathological states. Recent behavioral data support the idea that chronic stress impairs extinction learning (Miracle, Brace, Huyck, Singler, & Wellman, 2006). Following the cessation of stress, prefrontal changes are reversible (Radley et al., 2005), but amygdala changes are not (Vyas, Pillai, & Chattarji, 2004), suggesting that chronic stress can induce permanent alterations in fear circuits. It is well documented that chronic stress induces pathology in the hippocampus (McEwen, 2003), which is another structure compromised in PTSD (Gilbertson et al., 2002; Kitayama, Vaccarino, Kutner, Weiss, & Bremner, 2005). Deficient hippocampal function could deprive the subject of the contextual information needed to recognize an environment as safe.

ENHANCING EXTINCTION OF FEAR

If pathology results from deficient prefrontal–amygdala extinction circuits, an obvious clinical approach would be to restore the balance between prefrontal inhibition and amygdala excitation of fear. Behavioral therapy for PTSD, termed "exposure therapy," is based mainly on the process of extinction (Rothbaum & Schwartz, 2002; Hermans et al., 2005). Patients are repeatedly exposed to traumatic reminders within the safety of the therapist's office in an attempt to extinguish traumatic associations. A recent meta-analysis has shown that 68% of individuals completing exposure therapy for PTSD no longer met the criteria for PTSD (Bradley, Greene, Russ, Dutra, & Westen, 2005). While encouraging, such statistics might be improved by facilitating extinction learning during exposure therapy.

Recent rodent studies have used a variety of approaches to augment prefrontal function in order to strengthen extinction of fear (Quirk et al., 2006). High-frequency stimulation of the IL directly (Milad & Quirk, 2002), or indirectly via its thalamic afferent (Herry & Garcia, 2002), improves long-term retention of extinction. Systemic administration of the metabolic enhancer methylene blue, which increases metabolism in the vmPFC during extinction, strengthens extinction memory (Gonzalez-Lima & Bruchey, 2004). Extinction learning can also be augmented with systemic drugs including dopamine antagonists (Ponnusamy, Nissim, & Barad, 2005), noradrenergic agonists (Cain, Blouin, & Barad, 2004), and cannabinoid agonists (Chhatwal et al., 2005). The locus and mechanism of these treatments remains to be determined, although D-cycloserine, a partial agonist of the NMDA receptor, augments extinction when infused into the amygdala (Walker, Ressler, Lu, & Davis, 2002; Ledgerwood, Richardson, & Cranney, 2003). Additional approaches to activating the prefrontal cortex include repetitive transcranial magnetic stimulation (Cohen et al., 2004), deep brain stimulation (Abelson et al., 2005), or even meditation (Lazar et al., 2000). Thus, augmenting prefrontal activity pharmacologically, physiologically, or psychologically could restore balance to emotional regulatory mechanisms that have become compromised through repeated stress and trauma. Functional imaging studies are needed to evaluate the effect of extinction and extinction-related treatments on emotion circuits in humans, and to more fully understand cortical regulation of emotion in health and disease.

ACKNOWLEDGMENTS

This work was supported by Grants Nos. MH058883, MH072156, and GM008239 from the National Institutes of Health. I thank Dr. Kevin A. Corcoran for comments on the manuscript.

REFERENCES

Abelson, J. L., Curtis, G. C., Sagher, O., Albucher, R. C., Harrigan, M., Taylor, S. F., et al. (2005). Deep brain stimulation for refractory obsessive–compulsive disorder. *Biological Psychiatry, 57,* 510–516.

Anglada-Figueroa, D., & Quirk, G. J. (2005). Lesions of the basal amygdala block expression of conditioned fear but not extinction. *Journal of Neuroscience, 25,* 9680–9685.

Baker, J. D., & Azorlosa, J. L. (1996). The NMDA antagonist MK-801 blocks the extinction of Pavlovian fear conditioning. *Behavioral Neuroscience, 110,* 618–620.

Barrett, D., Shumake, J., Jones, D., & Gonzalez-Lima, F. (2003). Metabolic mapping of mouse brain activity after extinction of a conditioned emotional response. *Journal of Neuroscience, 23,* 5740–5749.

Bauer, E. P., & LeDoux, J. E. (2004). Heterosynaptic long-term potentiation of inhibitory interneurons in the lateral amygdala. *Journal of Neuroscience, 24,* 9507–9512.

Bechara, A., Tranel, D., Damasio, H., Adolphs, R., Rockland, C., & Damasio, A. R. (1995). Double dissociation of conditioning and declarative knowledge relative to the amygdala and hippocampus in humans. *Science, 269,* 1115–1118.

Berretta, S., Pantazopoulos, H., Caldera, M., Pantazopoulos, P., & Pare, D. (2005). Infralimbic cortex activation increases c-Fos expression in intercalated neurons of the amygdala. *Neuroscience, 132,* 943–953.

Bianchi, L. (1895). The functions of the frontal lobes. *Brain, 18,* 497–530.

Bissiere, S., Humeau, Y., & Luthi, A. (2003). Dopamine gates LTP induction in lateral amygdala by suppressing feedforward inhibition. *Nature Neuroscience, 6,* 587–592.

Blanchard, D. C., & Blanchard, R. J. (1972). Innate and conditioned reactions to threat in rats with amygdaloid lesions. *Journal of Comparative Physiology and Psychology, 81,* 281–290.

Bouton, M. E. (2002). Context, ambiguity, and unlearning: Sources of relapse after behavioral extinction. *Biological Psychiatry, 52,* 976–986.

Bradley, R., Greene, J., Russ, E., Dutra, L., & Westen, D. (2005). A multidimensional meta-analysis of psychotherapy for PTSD. *American Journal of Psychiatry, 162,* 214–227.

Bremner, J. D. (2002). Neuroimaging studies in post-traumatic stress disorder. *Current Psychiatry Report, 4,* 254–263.

Britton, J. C., Phan, K. L., Taylor, S. F., Fig, L. M., & Liberzon, I. (2005). Corticolimbic blood flow in posttraumatic stress disorder during script-driven imagery. *Biological Psychiatry, 57,* 832–840.

Burgos-Robles, A., Santini, E., & Quirk, G. J. (2004). Blockade of NMDA receptors in the medial prefrontal cortex impairs consolidation of fear extinction. *Society of Neuroscience Abstracts, Program No. 328.14.*

Butter, C. M., Mishkin, M., & Rosvold, H. E. (1963). Conditioning and extinction of a food-rewarded response after selective ablation of frontal cortex in Rhesus monkeys. *Experimental Neurology, 7,* 65–75.

Cain, C. K., Blouin, A. M., & Barad, M. (2004). Adrenergic transmission facilitates extinction of conditional fear in mice. *Learning and Memory, 11,* 179–187.

Caldji, C., Diorio, J., & Meaney, M. J. (2003). Variations in maternal care alter GABA(A) receptor subunit expression in brain regions associated with fear. *Neuropsychopharmacology, 28,* 1950–1959.

Campeau, S., & Davis, M. (1995). Involvement of subcortical and cortical afferents to the lateral nucleus of the amygdala in fear conditioning measured with fear-potentiated startle in rats trained concurrently with auditory and visual conditioned stimuli. *Journal of Neuroscience, 15,* 2312–2327.

Cannistraro, P. A., & Rauch, S. L. (2003). Neural circuitry of anxiety: Evidence from structural and functional neuroimaging studies. *Psychopharmacological Bulletin, 37,* 8–25.

Chan, K. H., Morell, J. R., Jarrard, L. E., & Davidson, T. L. (2001). Reconsideration of the role of the hippocampus in learned inhibition. *Behavioral Brain Research, 119,* 111–130.

Charney, D. S. (2004). Psychobiological mechanisms of resilience and vulnerability: Implications for successful adaptation to extreme stress. *American Journal of Psychiatry, 161,* 195–216.

Chhatwal, J. P., Davis, M., Maguschak, K. A., & Ressler, K. J. (2005). Enhancing cannabinoid neurotransmission augments the extinction of conditioned fear. *Neuropsychopharmacology, 30,* 516–524.

Cohen, H., Kaplan, Z., Kotler, M., Kouperman, I., Moisa, R., & Grisaru, N. (2004). Repetitive transcranial magnetic stimulation of the right dorsolateral prefrontal cortex in posttraumatic stress disorder: A double-blind, placebo-controlled study. *American Journal of Psychiatry, 161,* 515–524.

Collingridge, G. L., & Bliss, T. V. (1995). Memories of NMDA receptors and LTP. *Trends in Neuroscience, 18,* 54–56.

Collins, D. R., & Pare, D. (1999). Reciprocal changes in the firing probability of lateral and central medial amygdala neurons. *Journal of Neuroscience, 19,* 836–844.

Collins, D. R., & Pare, D. (2000). Differential fear conditioning induces reciprocal changes in the sensory responses of lateral amygdala neurons to the CS(+) and CS(−). *Learning and Memory, 7,* 97–103.

Conde, F., Maire-Lepoivre, E., Audinat, E., & Crepel, F. (1995). Afferent connections of the medial frontal cortex of the rat. II. Cortical and subcortical afferents. *Journal of Comparative Neurology, 352,* 567–593.

Corcoran, K. A., Desmond, T. J., Frey, K. A., & Maren, S. (2005). Hippocampal inactivation disrupts the acquisition and contextual encoding of fear extinction. *Journal of Neuroscience, 25,* 8978–8987.

Corcoran, K. A., & Maren, S. (2001). Hippocampal inactivation disrupts contextual retrieval of fear memory after extinction. *Journal of Neuroscience, 21,* 1720–1726.

Corodimas, K. P., & LeDoux, J. E. (1995). Disruptive effects of posttraining perirhinal cortex lesions on conditioned fear: Contributions of contextual cues. *Behavioral Neuroscience, 109,* 613–619.

Dalley, J. W., Cardinal, R. N., & Robbins, T. W. (2004). Prefrontal executive and cognitive functions in rodents: Neural and neurochemical substrates. *Neuroscience and Biobehavioral Review, 28,* 771–784.

Davis, M. (1997). Neurobiology of fear responses: The role of the amygdala. *Journal of Neuropsychiatry and Clinical Neuroscience, 9,* 382–402.

Davis, M. (2000). The role of the amygdala in conditioned and unconditioned fear and anxiety. In J. P. Aggleton (Ed.), *The amygdala* (pp. 213–288). Oxford, UK: Oxford University Press.

De Oca, B. M., DeCola, J. P., Maren, S., & Fanselow, M. S. (1998). Distinct regions of the periaqueductal gray are involved in the acquisition and expression of defensive responses. *Journal of Neuroscience, 18,* 3426–3432.

Dias, R., Robbins, T. W., & Roberts, A. C. (1996). Dissociation in prefrontal cortex of affective and attentional shifts. *Nature, 380,* 69–72.

Drevets, W. C. (2001). Neuroimaging and neuropathological studies of depression: implications for the cognitive-emotional features of mood disorders. *Current Opinion in Neurobiology, 11,* 240–249.

Eisenberg, M., Kobilo, T., Berman, D. E., & Dudai, Y. (2003). Stability of retrieved memory: Inverse correlation with trace dominance. *Science, 301,* 1102–1104.

Falls, W. A., Miserendino, M. J., & Davis, M. (1992). Extinction of fear-potentiated startle: blockade by infusion of an NMDA antagonist into the amygdala. *Journal of Neuroscience, 12,* 854–863.

Fanselow, M. S., & Kim, J. J. (1994). Acquisition of contextual Pavlovian fear conditioning is blocked by application of an NMDA receptor antagonist D,L-2-amino-5-phosphonovaleric acid to the basolateral amygdala. *Behavioral Neuroscience, 108,* 210–212.

Floyd, N. S., Price, J. L., Ferry, A. T., Keay, K. A., & Bandler, R. (2000). Orbitomedial prefrontal cortical projections to distinct longitudinal columns of the periaqueductal gray in the rat. *Journal of Comparative Neurology, 422,* 556–578.

Frysztak, R. J., & Neafsey, E. J. (1994). The effect of medial frontal cortex lesions on cardiovascular conditioned emotional responses in the rat. *Brain Research, 643,* 181–193.

Fuster, J. (1997). *The prefrontal cortex: Anatomy, physiology, and neuropsychology of the frontal lobe.* Baltimore: Lippincott Williams & Wilkins.

Garcia, R., Vouimba, R. M., Baudry, M., & Thompson, R. F. (1999). The amygdala modulates prefrontal cortex activity relative to conditioned fear. *Nature, 402,* 294–296.

Gilbertson, M. W., Shenton, M. E., Ciszewski, A., Kasai, K., Lasko, N. B., Orr, S. P., et al. (2002). Smaller hippocampal volume predicts pathologic vulnerability to psychological trauma. *Nature Neuroscience, 5,* 1242–1247.

Gilboa, A., Shalev, A. Y., Laor, L., Lester, H., Louzoun, Y., Chisin, R., et al. (2004). Functional connectivity of the prefrontal cortex and the amygdala in posttraumatic stress disorder. *Biological Psychiatry, 55,* 263–272.

Gonzalez-Lima, F., & Bruchey, A. K. (2004). Extinction memory improvement by the metabolic enhancer methylene blue. *Learning and Memory, 11,* 633–640.

Harlow, J. M. (1868). Recovery from the passage of an iron bar through the head. *Publications of the Massachusetts Medical Society, 2,* 327–347.

Heldt, S. A., & Falls, W. A. (2003). Destruction of the inferior colliculus disrupts the production and inhibition of fear conditioned to an acoustic stimulus. *Behavior Brain Research, 144,* 175–185.

Helmstetter, F. J., & Bellgowan, P. S. (1994). Effects of muscimol applied to the basolateral amygdala on acquisition and expression of contextual fear conditioning in rats. *Behavioral Neuroscience, 108,* 1005–1009.

Hermans, D., Dirikx, T., Vansteenwegenin, D., Baeyens, F., Van den, B. O., & Eelen, P. (2005). Reinstatement of fear responses in human aversive conditioning. *Behavior Research and Therapy, 43,* 533–551.

Herry, C., & Garcia, R. (2002). Prefrontal cortex long-term potentiation, but not long-term depression, is associated with the maintenance of extinction of learned fear in mice. *Journal of Neuroscience, 22,* 577–583.

Herry, C., & Mons, N. (2004). Resistance to extinction is associated with impaired immediate early gene induction in medial prefrontal cortex and amygdala. *European Journal of Neuroscience, 20,* 781–790.

Hobin, J. A., Goosens, K. A., & Maren, S. (2003). Context-dependent neuronal activity in the lateral amygdala represents fear memories after extinction. *Journal of Neuroscience, 23,* 8410–8416.

Hugues, S., Deschaux, O., & Garcia, R. (2004). Postextinction infusion of a mitogen-activated protein kinase inhibitor into the medial prefrontal cortex impairs memory of the extinction of conditioned fear. *Learning and Memory, 11,* 540–543.

Ishikawa, A., & Nakamura, S. (2003). Convergence and interaction of hippocampal and amygdalar projections within the prefrontal cortex in the rat. *Journal of Neuroscience, 23,* 9987–9995.

Iwata, J., LeDoux, J. E., Meeley, M. P., Arneric, S., & Reis, D. J. (1986). Intrinsic neurons in the amygdaloid field projected to by the medial geniculate body mediate emotional responses conditioned to acoustic stimuli. *Brain Research, 383,* 195–214.

Jackson, J. H. (1884). Croonian Lectures on evolution and dissolution of the nervous system. *Lancet, i,* 555–558.

James, W. (1884). What is an emotion? *Mind, 9,* 188–205.

Jay, T. M., Burette, F., & Laroche, S. (1995). NMDA receptor-dependent long-term potentiation in the hippocampal afferent fibre system to the prefrontal cortex in the rat. *European Journal of Neuroscience, 7,* 247–250.

Kida, S., Josselyn, S. A., de Ortiz, S. P., Kogan, J. H., Chevere, I., Masushige, S., et al. (2002). CREB required for the stability of new and reactivated fear memories. *Nature Neuroscience, 5,* 348–355.

Kimble, D. P., & Kimble, R. J. (1970). The effect of hippocampal lesions on extinction and "hypothesis" behavior in rats. *Physiology and Behavior, 5,* 735–738.

Kitayama, N., Vaccarino, V., Kutner, M., Weiss, P., & Bremner, J. D. (2005). Magnetic resonance imaging (MRI) measurement of hippocampal volume in posttraumatic stress disorder: A meta-analysis. *Journal of Affective Disorders, 88,* 79–86.

Konorski, J. (1967). *Integrative activity of the brain.* Chicago: University of Chicago Press.

Laviolette, S. R., Lipski, W. J., & Grace, A. A. (2005). A subpopulation of neurons in the medial prefrontal cortex encodes emotional learning with burst and frequency codes through a dopamine D4 receptor-dependent basolateral amygdala input. *Journal of Neuroscience, 25,* 6066–6075.

Lazar, S. W., Bush, G., Gollub, R. L., Fricchione, G. L., Khalsa, G., & Benson, H. (2000). Functional brain mapping of the relaxation response and meditation. *Neuroreport, 11,* 1581–1585.

Lebron, K., Milad, M. R., & Quirk, G. J. (2004). Delayed recall of fear extinction in rats with lesions of ventral medial prefrontal cortex. *Learning and Memory, 11,* 544–548.

Ledgerwood, L., Richardson, R., & Cranney, J. (2003). Effects of D-cycloserine on extinction of conditioned freezing. *Behavioral Neuroscience, 117,* 341–349.

LeDoux, J. E. (1996). *The emotional brain.* New York: Simon & Schuster.

LeDoux, J. E. (2000). Emotion circuits in the brain. *Annual Review of Neuroscience, 23,* 155–184.

LeDoux, J. E., Cicchetti, P., Xagoraris, A., & Romanski, L. M. (1990). The lateral amygdaloid nucleus: Sensory interface of the amygdala in fear conditioning. *Journal of Neuroscience, 10,* 1062–1069.

LeDoux, J. E., Iwata, J., Cicchetti, P., & Reis, D. J. (1988). Different projections of the central amygdaloid nucleus mediate autonomic and behavioral correlates of conditioned fear. *Journal of Neuroscience, 8,* 2517–2529.

Likhtik, E., Pelletier, J. G., Paz, R., & Pare, D. (2005). Prefrontal control of the amygdala. *Journal of Neuroscience, 25,* 7429–7437.

Lin, C. H., Yeh, S. H., Lu, H. Y., & Gean, P. W. (2003). The similarities and diversities of signal pathways leading to consolidation of conditioning and consolidation of extinction of fear memory. *Journal of Neuroscience, 23,* 8310–8317.

Loewi, O. (1921). Uber humorale Ubertragbarkeit der Herznervenwirkung. *Pfluger's Archiv fir die gesamte Physiologie, 189,* 201–213.

Lu, K. T., Walker, D. L., & Davis, M. (2001). Mitogen-activated protein kinase cascade in the basolateral nucleus of amygdala is involved in extinction of fear-potentiated startle. *Journal of Neuroscience, 21,* RC162.

Mahanty, N. K., & Sah, P. (1998). Calcium-permeable AMPA receptors mediate long-term potentiation in interneurons in the amygdala. *Nature, 394,* 683–687.

Maren, S. (2001). Neurobiology of Pavlovian fear conditioning. *Annual Review of Neuroscience, 24,* 897–931.

Maren, S., & Fanselow, M. S. (1995). Synaptic plasticity in the basolateral amygdala induced by hippocampal formation stimulation *in vivo. Journal of Neuroscience, 15,* 7548–7564.

Maren, S., & Quirk, G. J. (2004). Neuronal signalling of fear memory. *Nature Review of Neuroscience, 5,* 844–852.

Maroun, M., & Richter-Levin, G. (2003). Exposure to acute stress blocks the induction of long-term potentiation of the amygdala-prefrontal cortex pathway *in vivo. Journal of Neuroscience, 23,* 4406–4409.

Marsicano, G., Wotjak, C. T., Azad, S. C., Bisogno, T., Rammes, G., Cascio, M. G., et al. (2002). The endogenous cannabinoid system controls extinction of aversive memories. *Nature, 418,* 530–534.

Mayberg, H. S. (2003). Modulating dysfunctional limbic-cortical circuits in depression: towards development of brain-based algorithms for diagnosis and optimised treatment. *British Medical Bulletin, 65,* 193–207.

McDonald, A. J. (1991). Organization of amygdaloid projections to the prefrontal cortex and associated striatum in the rat. *Neuroscience, 44,* 1–14.

McDonald, A. J., Mascagni, F., & Guo, L. (1996). Projections of the medial and lateral prefrontal cortices to the amygdala: A Phaseolus vulgaris leucoagglutinin study in the rat. *Neuroscience, 71,* 55–75.

McEwen, B. S. (2003). Mood disorders and allostatic load. *Biological Psychiatry, 54,* 200–207.

McLaughlin, J., Skaggs, H., Churchwell, J., & Powell, D. A. (2002). Medial prefrontal cortex and pavlovian conditioning: trace versus delay conditioning. *Behavioral Neuroscience, 116,* 37–47.

Milad, M. R., Quinn, B. T., Pitman, R. K., Orr, S. P., Fischl, B., & Rauch, S. L. (2005). Thickness of ventromedial prefrontal cortex in humans is correlated with extinction memory. *Proceedings of the National Academy of Sciences USA, 102,* 1070–1071.

Milad, M. R., & Quirk, G. J. (2002). Neurons in medial prefrontal cortex signal memory for fear extinction. *Nature, 420,* 70–74.

Milad, M. R., Rauch, S. L., & Quirk, G. J. (2006). Fear extinction in rats: Implications for human brain imaging and anxiety disorders. *Biological Psychology, 73,* 61–71.

Milad, M. R., Vidal-Gonzalez, I., & Quirk, G. J. (2004). Electrical stimulation of medial prefrontal cortex reduces conditioned fear in a temporally specific manner. *Behavioral Neuroscience, 118,* 389–394.

Milner, B. (1964). Some effects of frontal lobectomy in man. In J. M. Warren & K. Akert (Eds.), *The frontal granular cortex and behavior.* New York: McGraw-Hill.

Miracle, A. D., Brace, M. F., Huyck, K. D., Singler, S. A., & Wellman, C. L. (2006). Chronic stress impairs recall of extinction of conditioned fear. *Neurobiology of Learning and Memory, 85,* 213–218.

Miserendino, M. J., Sananes, C. B., Melia, K. R., & Davis, M. (1990). Blocking of acquisition but not expression of conditioned fear-potentiated startle by NMDA antagonists in the amygdala. *Nature, 345,* 716–718.

Mitra, R., Jadhav, S., McEwen, B. S., Vyas, A., & Chattarji, S. (2005). Stress duration modulates the spatiotemporal patterns of spine formation in the basolateral amygdala. *Proceedings of the National Academy of Sciences USA, 102,* 9371–9376.

Morgan, M. A., Romanski, L. M., & LeDoux, J. E. (1993). Extinction of emotional learning: contribution of medial prefrontal cortex. *Neuroscience Letter, 163,* 109–113.

Myers, K. M., & Davis, M. (2002). Behavioral and neural analysis of extinction. *Neuron, 36,* 567–584.

Nader, K., Majidishad, P., Amorapanth, P., & LeDoux, J. E. (2001). Damage to the lateral and central, but not other, amygdaloid nuclei prevents the acquisition of auditory fear conditioning. *Learning and Memory, 8,* 156–163.

Nitecka, L., & Ben Ari, Y. (1987). Distribution of GABA-like immunoreactivity in the rat amygdaloid complex. *Journal of Comparative Neurology, 266,* 45–55.

Ongur, D., & Price, J. L. (2000). The organization of networks within the orbital and medial prefrontal cortex of rats, monkeys and humans. *Cerebral Cortex, 10,* 206–219.

Pare, D., Quirk, G. J., & LeDoux, J. E. (2004). New vistas on amygdala networks in conditioned fear. *Journal of Neurophysiology, 92,* 1–9.

Pare, D., & Smith, Y. (1993). The intercalated cell masses project to the central and medial nuclei of the amygdala in cats. *Neuroscience, 57,* 1077–1090.

Pare, D., Smith, Y., & Pare, J. F. (1995). Intra-amygdaloid projections of the basolateral and basomedial nuclei in the cat: Phaseolus vulgaris-leucoagglutinin anterograde tracing at the light and electron microscopic level. *Neuroscience, 69,* 567–583.

Pavlov, I. (1927). *Conditioned reflexes.* London: Oxford University Press.

Paxinos, G., & Watson, C. (1998). *The rat brain in stereotaxic coordinates* (4th ed.) San Diego, CA: Academic Press.

Pezawas, L., Meyer-Lindenberg, A., Drabant, E. M., Verchinski, B. A., Munoz, K. E., Kolachana, B. S., et al. (2005). 5-HTTLPR polymorphism impacts human cingulate-amygdala interactions: a genetic susceptibility mechanism for depression. *Nature Neuroscience, 8,* 828–834.

Phelps, E. A., Delgado, M. R., Nearing, K. I., & LeDoux, J. E. (2004). Extinction learning in humans: Role of the amygdala and vmPFC. *Neuron, 43,* 897–905.

Pickens, C. L., Saddoris, M. P., Gallagher, M., & Holland, P. C. (2005). Orbitofrontal lesions impair use of cue-outcome associations in a devaluation task. *Behavioral Neuroscience, 119,* 317–322.

Pitkanen, A., Savander, V., & LeDoux, J. E. (1997). Organization of intra-amygdaloid circuitries in the rat: An emerging framework for understanding functions of the amygdala. *Trends in Neuroscience, 20,* 517–523.

Ponnusamy, R., Nissim, H. A., & Barad, M. (2005). Systemic blockade of D2–like dopamine receptors facilitates extinction of conditioned fear in mice. *Learning and Memory, 12,* 399–406.

Quirk, G. J. (2002). Memory for extinction of conditioned fear is long-lasting and persists following spontaneous recovery. *Learning and Memory, 9,* 402–407.

Quirk, G. J., Garcia, R., & Gonzalez-Lima, F. (2006). Prefrontal mechanisms in extinction of conditioned fear. *Biological Psychiatry, 60,* 337–343.

Quirk, G. J., & Gehlert, D. R. (2003). Inhibition of the amygdala: Key to pathological states? *Annals of the New York Academy of Science, 985,* 263–272.

Quirk, G. J., Likhtik, E., Pelletier, J. G., & Pare, D. (2003). Stimulation of medial prefrontal cortex decreases the responsiveness of central amygdala output neurons. *Journal of Neuroscience, 23,* 8800–8807.

Quirk, G. J., Repa, C., & LeDoux, J. E. (1995). Fear conditioning enhances short-latency auditory responses of lateral amygdala neurons: Parallel recordings in the freely behaving rat. *Neuron, 15,* 1029–1039.

Quirk, G. J., Russo, G. K., Barron, J. L., & Lebron, K. (2000). The role of ventromedial prefrontal cortex in the recovery of extinguished fear. *Journal of Neuroscience, 20,* 6225–6231.

Radley, J. J., Rocher, A. B., Janssen, W. G., Hof, P. R., McEwen, B. S., & Morrison, J. H. (2005). Reversibility of apical dendritic retraction in the rat medial prefrontal cortex following repeated stress. *Experimental Neurology, 196,* 199–203.

Radley, J. J., Rocher, A. B., Miller, M., Janssen, W. G., Liston, C., Hof, P. R., et al. (2006). Repeated stress induces dendritic spine loss in the rat medial prefrontal cortex. *Cerebral Cortex, 16,* 313–320.

Radley, J. J., Sisti, H. M., Hao, J., Rocher, A. B., McCall, T., Hof, P. R., et al. (2004). Chronic behavioral stress induces apical dendritic reorganization in pyramidal neurons of the medial prefrontal cortex. *Neuroscience, 125,* 1–6.

Rauch, S. L., Milad, M. R., Orr, S. P., Quinn, B. T., Fischl, B., & Pitman, R. K. (2005). Orbitofrontal thickness, retention of fear extinction, and extraversion. *Neuroreport, 16,* 1909–1912.

Rauch, S. L., Shin, L. M., Segal, E., Pitman, R. K., Carson, M. A., McMullin, K., et al. (2003). Selectively reduced regional cortical volumes in post-traumatic stress disorder. *Neuroreport, 14,* 913–916.

Repa, J. C., Muller, J., Apergis, J., Desrochers, T. M., Zhou, Y., & LeDoux, J. E. (2001). Two different lateral amygdala cell populations contribute to the initiation and storage of memory. *Nature Neuroscience, 4,* 724–731.

Rescorla, R. A. (2002). Comparison of the rates of associative change during acquisition and extinction. *Journal of Experimental Psychology: Animal Behavior Processes, 28,* 406–415.

Rescorla, R. A. (2004). Spontaneous recovery. *Learning and Memory, 11,* 501–509.

Rescorla, R. A., & Heth, C. D. (1975). Reinstatement of fear to an extinguished conditioned stimulus. *Journal of Experimental Psychology: Animal Behavior Processes, 1,* 88–96.

Rhodes, S. E., & Killcross, S. (2004). Lesions of rat infralimbic cortex enhance recovery and reinstatement of an appetitive Pavlovian response. *Learning and Memory, 11,* 611–616.

Rogan, M. T., Leon, K. S., Perez, D. L., & Kandel, E. R. (2005). Distinct neural signatures for safety and danger in the amygdala and striatum of the mouse. *Neuron, 46,* 309–320.

Rolls, E. T., Critchley, H. D., Mason, R., & Wakeman, E. A. (1996). Orbitofrontal cortex neurons: role in olfactory and visual association learning. *Journal of Neurophysiology, 75,* 1970–1981.

Romanski, L. M., & LeDoux, J. E. (1992). Bilateral destruction of neocortical and perirhinal projection targets of the acoustic thalamus does not disrupt auditory fear conditioning. *Neuroscience Letters, 142,* 228–232.

Rosenkranz, J. A., & Grace, A. A. (2001). Dopamine attenuates prefrontal cortical suppression of sensory inputs to the basolateral amygdala of rats. *Journal of Neuroscience, 21,* 4090–4103.

Rosenkranz, J. A., Moore, H., & Grace, A. A. (2003). The prefrontal cortex regulates lateral amygdala neuronal plasticity and responses to previously conditioned stimuli. *Journal of Neuroscience, 23,* 11054–11064.

Rothbaum, B. O., & Schwartz, A. C. (2002). Exposure therapy for posttraumatic stress disorder. *American Journal of Psychotherapy, 56,* 59–75.

Royer, S., Martina, M., & Pare, D. (1999). An inhibitory interface gates impulse traffic between the input and output stations of the amygdala. *Journal of Neuroscience, 19,* 10575–10583.

Royer, S., & Pare, D. (2002). Bidirectional synaptic plasticity in intercalated amygdala neurons and the extinction of conditioned fear responses. *Neuroscience, 115,* 455–462.

Runyan, J. D., Moore, A. N., & Dash, P. K. (2004). A role for prefrontal cortex in memory storage for trace fear conditioning. *Journal of Neuroscience, 24,* 1288–1295.

Sacchetti, B., Lorenzini, C. A., Baldi, E., Tassoni, G., & Bucherelli, C. (1999). Auditory thalamus, dorsal hippocampus, basolateral amygdala, and perirhinal cortex role in the consolidation of conditioned freezing to context and to acoustic conditioned stimulus in the rat. *Journal of Neuroscience, 19,* 9570–9578.

Santini, E., Ge, H., Ren, K., Pena, D. O., & Quirk, G. J. (2004). Consolidation of fear extinction requires protein synthesis in the medial prefrontal cortex. *Journal of Neuroscience, 24,* 5704–5710.

Santini, E., Muller, R. U., & Quirk, G. J. (2001). Consolidation of extinction learning involves transfer from NMDA-independent to NMDA-dependent memory. *Journal of Neuroscience, 21,* 9009–9017.

Schafe, G. E., & LeDoux, J. E. (2000). Memory consolidation of auditory pavlovian fear conditioning requires protein synthesis and protein kinase A in the amygdala. *Journal of Neuroscience, 20,* RC96.

Schoenbaum, G., & Roesch, M. (2005). Orbitofrontal cortex, associative learning, and expectancies. *Neuron, 47,* 633–636.

Sechenov, I. M. (1866). *Refleksy Golovnago Mozga (Reflexes of the brain).* St. Petersburg, Russia: St. Petersburg.

Sesack, S. R., Deutch, A. Y., Roth, R. H., & Bunney, B. S. (1989). Topographical organization of the efferent projections of the medial prefrontal cortex in the rat: An anterograde tract-tracing study with Phaseolus vulgaris leucoagglutinin. *Journal of Comparative Neurology, 290,* 213–242.

Shin, L. M., Orr, S. P., Carson, M. A., Rauch, S. L., Macklin, M. L., Lasko, N. B., et al. (2004). Regional cerebral blood flow in the amygdala and medial prefrontal cortex during traumatic imagery in male and female Vietnam veterans with PTSD. *Archives of General Psychiatry, 61,* 168–176.

Shin, L. M., Whalen, P. J., Pitman, R. K., Bush, G., Macklin, M. L., Lasko, N. B., et al. (2001). An fMRI study of anterior cingulate function in posttraumatic stress disorder. *Biological Psychiatry, 50,* 932–942.

Shumyatsky, G. P., Tsvetkov, E., Malleret, G., Vronskaya, S., Hatton, M., Hampton, L., et al. (2002). Identification of a signaling network in lateral nucleus of amygdala important for inhibiting memory specifically related to learned fear. *Cell, 111,* 905–918.

Sierra-Mercado, Jr., D., Corcoran, K. A., Lebron, K., & Quirk, G. J. (2006). Inactivation of ventromedial prefrontal cortex reduces expression of conditioned fear and impairs subsequent recall of extinction. *European Journal of Neuroscience, 24,* 1751–1758.

Sotres-Bayon, F., Bush, D. E., & LeDoux, J. E. (2004). Emotional perseveration: An update on prefrontal-amygdala interactions in fear extinction. *Learning and Memory, 11,* 525–535.

Starr, M. A. (1884). Cortical lesions of the brain. *American Journal of Medical Sciences, 88,* 114–141.

Szapiro, G., Vianna, M. R., McGaugh, J. L., Medina, J. H., & Izquierdo, I. (2003). The role of NMDA glutamate receptors, PKA, MAPK, and CAMKII in the hippocampus in extinction of conditioned fear. *Hippocampus, 13,* 53–58.

Takita, M., Izaki, Y., Jay, T. M., Kaneko, H., & Suzuki, S. S. (1999). Induction of stable long-term depression *in vivo* in the hippocampal–prefrontal cortex pathway. *European Journal of Neuroscience, 11,* 4145–4148.

Vertes, R. P. (2004). Differential projections of the infralimbic and prelimbic cortex in the rat. *Synapse, 51,* 32–58.

Vianna, M. R., Szapiro, G., McGaugh, J. L., Medina, J. H., & Izquierdo, I. (2001). Retrieval of memory for fear-motivated training initiates extinction requiring protein synthesis in the rat hippocampus. *Proceedings of the National Academy of Sciences, USA, 98,* 12251–12254.

Vyas, A., Mitra, R., Shankaranarayana Rao, B. S., & Chattarji, S. (2002). Chronic stress induces contrasting patterns of dendritic remodeling in hippocampal and amygdaloid neurons. *Journal of Neuroscience, 22,* 6810–6818.

Vyas, A., Pillai, A. G., & Chattarji, S. (2004). Recovery after chronic stress fails to reverse amygdaloid neuronal hypertrophy and enhanced anxiety-like behavior. *Neuroscience, 128,* 667–673.

Walker, D. L., & Davis, M. (2002). The role of amygdala glutamate receptors in fear learning, fear-potentiated startle, and extinction. *Pharmacology, Biochemistry, and Behavior, 71,* 379–392.

Walker, D. L., Ressler, K. J., Lu, K. T., & Davis, M. (2002). Facilitation of conditioned fear extinction by systemic administration or intra-amygdala infusions of D-cycloserine as assessed with fear-potentiated startle in rats. *Journal of Neuroscience, 22,* 2343–2351.

Weber, E. F. W., & Weber, E. H. W. (1846). Experiences qui prouvent que les nerfs vagues peuvent retarder le mouvement. *Archives Générales de Medecine, Suppl. 12.*

Wilensky, A. E., Schafe, G. E., & LeDoux, J. E. (1999). Functional inactivation of the amygdala before but not after auditory fear conditioning prevents memory formation. *Journal of Neuroscience, 19,* RC48.

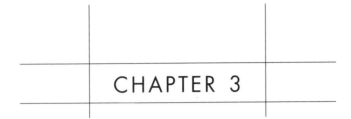

CHAPTER 3

Neural Bases of Emotion Regulation in Nonhuman Primates and Humans

RICHARD J. DAVIDSON
ANDREW FOX
NED H. KALIN

One of the most important characteristics that distinguish between humans and other species is our capacity to regulate our emotions. Emotion regulation clearly reaches its pinnacle in humans. This capacity provides important flexibility to our behavioral repertoire and it also confers significant risk (see, e.g., Davidson, Putnam, & Larson, 2000c). More than any other species, our emotional reactions are under some degree of voluntary control. However, it appears that the same substrate that confers this flexible competence also can become dysfunctional and lead to abnormalities of emotional regulation that can result in psychopathology. Many psychiatric disorders in humans involve abnormalities in our emotion regulatory skills, and it is likely that the naturally occurring incidence of such pathology is greater in humans than in other species, in part because of our increased capacity to regulate our emotions. Notwithstanding these important species differences, the study of nonhuman primates clearly provides us with an important and powerful window to study some of the basic neural substrates of emotion regulation. And as we note below, there are certain components of emotion regulation that can be more crisply examined in an animal model and that shed important new light on issues that have been difficult to empirically address in the study of emotion regulation in humans. The study of the nonhuman primate we would argue is essential in furthering our understanding of emotion regulation because it sits between rodent models and human studies. Rodent models have provided powerful new data on the molecular machinery underlying some aspects of emotion regulation (e.g., Rumpel,

LeDoux, Zador, & Malinow, 2005). However, the prefrontal cortical territories and the amygdala of the rodent are anatomically distinct from the primate and argue for the need to develop a primate model that has a prefrontal cortex that more closely resembles what we have in humans (see, e.g., Stefanacci & Amaral, 2002).

Our work on emotion regulation in both humans and nonhuman primates has emphasized the important role of individual differences. In many prior publications, we have suggested that affective style or individual differences in the subcomponents of emotional reactivity, are importantly determined by variations in emotion regulation (see, e.g., Davidson, 2000a; Davidson, Jackson, & Kalin, 2000a). We have suggested that many features of affective style are in fact determined by individual differences in emotion regulation and thus it is critical to develop a better and more complete understanding of individual differences in emotion regulation to enable us to understand affective style.

Elsewhere in this handbook (Gross & Thompson, this volume) the many varieties of emotion regulation are described. One continuum along which emotion regulation varies is from fully automatic and nonconscious to voluntary, effortful, and conscious processing. Gross and Thompson (this volume) also call attention to *intrinsic* and *extrinsic* forms of emotion regulation. The former refers to strictly internal influences on emotion regulation within the individual while the latter refers to social and contextual influences that serve to regulate emotion. We have devoted considerable attention to developing experimental paradigms to probe both automatic and voluntary emotion regulation in humans (see, e.g., Jackson, Malmstadt, Larson, & Davidson, 2000; Jackson et al., 2003; Urry et al., 2006). In our nonhuman studies we have emphasized *extrinsic* influences on emotion regulation, in part because such influences are likely more significant than *intrinsic* influences in nonhuman primates and, second, because they are readily amenable to experimental manipulation.

This chapter begins with a brief summary of some of the key components of the neural circuitry of emotion and emotion regulation, drawing on a broad literature including human and nonhuman studies. After the circuitry of emotion- regulation is described, we then focus on key issues in the study of the neural bases of emotion regulation in nonhuman primates with an emphasis on the contextual regulation of emotion.

A SELECTIVE REVIEW OF KEY NEURAL CIRCUITRY FOR EMOTION AND EMOTION REGULATION

In many recent publications Davidson and colleagues (e.g., Davidson, 2000a, 2000b, 2004a, 2004b; Davidson, Jackson, et al., 2000), have suggested, along with others that emotions serve to facilitate adaptive behavior and decision making in response to salient events. Emotions that are poorly regulated and/or occur out of context can impair functioning. Over the past decade, tremendous progress has been made in delineating the neural circuitry of emotion and more recently, emotion regulation. What is particularly gratifying about these developments is the convergence that is occurring between basic research at the animal level and translational research at the human level. We have proposed that individual differences in emotion regulation are fundamental to understanding variations in affective style (Davidson, 2000a, 2004a). Moreover, we have also suggested that abnormalities especially in the capacity to downregulate negative affect, but perhaps also in the capacity to upregulate, maintain and enhance positive affect, are crucial in determining vulnerability to psychopathology, particularly mood and anxiety disorders. In this brief section, we review some of the key pertinent findings in the literature to set the stage for our own program of research that is reviewed in more detail in the subsequent section.

Neural Circuitry of Emotion

Affective neuroscience (Davidson & Sutton, 1995) refers to the study of the neural substrates of emotion-relevant processes that underlie emotional reactivity, emotion regulation, and other emotion-relevant subcomponents. Work in this area, relying on animal models, lesion studies, and electrophysiological and neuroimaging studies has identified a number of key structures that together form the brain's emotion circuitry, structures that include dorsolateral and ventral regions of prefrontal cortex (including the anterior cingulate cortex [ACC]), amygdala, hippocampus, and insula (see, e.g., Davidson, 2000b). Here we focus primarily on prefrontal cortex and amygdala because these components are most pertinent to our research, though we make selective references to other key structures in this circuitry.

Prefrontal Cortex

Although the prefrontal cortex (PFC) is often considered to be the province of higher cognitive control, it has also consistently been linked to various features of affective processing (see, e.g., Nauta, 1971, for an early preview). Miller and Cohen (2001) have recently outlined a comprehensive theory of prefrontal function based on nonhuman primate anatomical and neurophysiological studies, human neuroimaging findings and computational modeling. The core feature of their model holds that the PFC maintains the representation of goals and the means to achieve them. Particularly in situations that are ambiguous, the PFC sends bias signals to other areas of the brain to facilitate the expression of task-appropriate responses in the face of competition with potentially stronger alternatives. If a signal of competition emerges, this output signals the need for controlled processing. The dorsolateral PFC (Brodmann's area [BA] 9 and 46) is assumed to be critical for this form of controlled processing, in that it represents and maintains task demands necessary for such control and inhibits (see, e.g., Garavan, Ross, & Stein, 1999) or increases neural activity in brain regions implicated in the competition. The most rostral zone of the PFC, the frontopolar region or rostral PFC (BA 10), has been identified specifically as subserving a system that somehow weights the priority between internally generated, stimulus-independent thought versus stimulus-oriented thought or current sensory input (see, e.g., Burgess, Simons, Bumontheil, & Gilbert, 2005). Because voluntary emotion regulation clearly represents a balance between internally generated versus externally elicited processing, it is likely that BA 10 will be involved. Interestingly, BA 10 is the zone of PFC that shows the greatest increase in size across primate species with humans showing the largest relative size (relative to the remainder of the brain) compared with apes (Semendeferi, Armstrong, Schleicher, Ziles, & Van Hoesen, 2001). The structure that has been implicated in monitoring is a region of medial PFC called the ACC, which some have proposed acts as a bridge between attention and emotion (Devinsky, Morrell, & Vogt, 1995; Vogt, Nimchinsky, Vogt, & Hof, 1995; Ebert & Ebmeier, 1996; Mayberg et al., 1997).

Amygdala

Although a link between amygdala activity and negative affect has been a prevalent view in the literature, particularly when examined in response to exteroceptive aversive stimuli (e.g., LeDoux, 2000), recent findings from invasive animal studies and human lesion and functional neuroimaging studies are converging on a broader view that regards the amygdala's role in negative affect as a special case of its more general role in directing attention to affectively salient stimuli and issuing a call for further processing of stimuli that have major significance for the individual. Extant evidence is consistent with the argument that the amygdala is critical for recruiting and coordinating cortical arousal and vigilant attention for optimizing sensory and perceptual processing of stimuli associated with underdetermined contingencies, such as novel, "surprising," or "ambiguous" stimuli (Whalen, 1998; Holland & Gallagher, 1999; see also Davis & Whalen, 2001). Most, though not all, stimuli in this class may be conceptualized as having an aversive valence as we tend to have a negativity bias in the face of uncertainty (Taylor, 1991), though at least parts of the amygdala have also been implicated in appetitive processes (Holland & Gallagher, 1999). Importantly, by way of the central nucleus, the amygdala contributes to mobilization of behavioral, autonomic, and endocrine outputs (LeDoux, 2000). Additional detail regarding the contribution of the amydala to individual differences in aspects of emotion regulation are provided below.

Neural Correlates of Regulation and Dysregulation

An important component of disorders of emotion that was highlighted in a National Institute of Mental Health report on the neural and behavioral substrates of mood and mood regulation is abnormalities in the regulation of emotion (Davidson et al., 2002a). We (e.g., Davidson et al., 2000a, 2000b) and others (e.g., Ochsner & Gross, 2005) have proposed that prefrontal activity may be particularly important for emotion regulation and in some of our work, we have found that individuals with high levels of baseline left-prefrontal activation in particular (as assessed with electrophysiological methods) are particularly skilled in the downregulation of negative affect. The correlates of individual differences in asymmetric prefrontal function may derive at least in part from a fundamental difference in the capacity to regulate negative affect, differences that appear to be consequential for positive psychological adaptation (Urry et al., 2004a). According to this formulation, subjects with relative hypoactivation of left prefrontal function may be impaired in the ability to regulate negative affect (Jackson et al., 2003). While this electrophysiological work provides important and cost-effective information about regional cortical contributions to emotion regulation, the spatial resolution of these scalp-recorded signals is relatively coarse. To date, only a handful of studies using measures with high spatial resolution, such as functional, magnetic resonance imaging (fMRI), have been reported (Beauregard, Levesque, & Bourgouin, 2001; Schaefer et al., 2002; Ochsner, Bunge, Gross, & Gabrieli, 2002; Ochsner et al., 2004; Levesque et al., 2003; see review in Ochsner & Gross, 2005).

In one of the first studies of its kind, Schaefer et al. (2002) performed an fMRI study in which participants were instructed to regulate ("maintain" or "passive") negative affect in response to pictures. As hypothesized, results showed greater amygdala activation while subjects were maintaining their negative emotion compared to when they were passively experiencing negative affect. Using an adapted version of the Jackson et al. (2000) paradigm, Ochsner et al. (2002) asked participants to reinterpret negative photos such that their negative response was diminished in one condition ("reappraise"), and to pay attention to but not to modify their feelings in any way ("attend") in another condition. Supporting the prediction that regulation of negative affect should draw on brain regions implicated in cognitive control, they found that voluntarily reducing negative affect was associated with activation in the left superior, middle, and inferior frontal gyri and dorsomedial PFC. They also found reduced signal in the left medial orbital frontal cortex and the right amygdala, suggesting that these regions are sensitive to reductions in unpleasantness or significance arising in the wake of regulatory efforts. Finally, they found that subjects with higher activation of dorsal ACC were more successful at reducing negative affect as measured via subjective ratings. More recently, Ochsner et al. (2004) reported on the effects of both increasing and decreasing negative affect. Compared to control trials in which subjects simply responded naturally, increasing and decreasing negative affect evoked greater activation in numerous frontal regions, including dorsal and ventral lateral PFC, dorsal medial PFC, and dorsal ACC. In addition, the amygdala tracked changes in affect, such that subject-initiated increases in negative affect resulted in greater left amygdalar activation relative to a control condition and decreases with less activation. In one of the few studies examining the neural correlates of regulating positive affect, Beauregard et al. (2001) found that males, instructed to inhibit sexual arousal by taking the perspective of a detached observer and distancing oneself in response to erotic film clips, produced activation in the right superior frontal (SFG; BA 10), left inferior frontal (IFG; BA 44), and right anterior cingulate (BA 32) gyri. In a second study, this group (Levesque et al., 2003) found that females suppressing sadness displayed activation in the right dorsolateral PFC (BA9), right orbitofrontal cortex (OFC; BA 47), and left IFG (BA 44).

More recently, we (Urry et al., 2006) have adapted a more faithful replica of the Jackson et al. (2000) for the scanner to interrogate the circuitry associated with the down-regulation of negative affect specifically. In this experiment, negative and neutral stimuli were presented. In response to negative pictures, subjects were randomly presented with instructions to enhance, suppress, or maintain their emotional response using cognitive reappraisal strategies that were taught to them in a preexperimental practice session. In response to the neutral pictures, subjects always received the instruction to maintain. A total of 17 participants between the ages of 63–66 years were tested.

We measured pupillometry in the scanner in order to provide a continuous real-time measure of autonomic activation that is generally thought to reflect "cognitive effort" (e.g., Tursky, Shapiro, Crider, & Kahnman, 1969). We wanted to establish that there were not differences in effort between the Enhance and Suppress conditions. If such differences did exist, then at least some of the difference between these conditions in levels of magnetic resonance (MR) signal change could be attributed to differences in effort. The pupillometry data reveals that both the Enhance and Suppress conditions produce comparable and significantly larger changes in pupil diameter compared with the Maintain condition. These findings indicate that there were not any major differences in effort between our critical emotion regulation conditions.

Our first major question was to determine whether the downregulation results in decreased BOLD signal in the amygdala relative to the Maintain condition and whether the Enhance condition leads to an increase in BOLD signal in the amygdala relative to the Maintain condition. Figure 3.1 presents the main effects for the left and right amygdalae for the condition contrast (Enhance, Suppress, Maintain) and reveals a reliable change in MR signal in the amygdala as a function of regulation instruction.

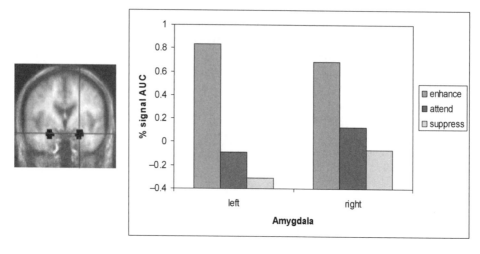

FIGURE 3.1. Amygdala regions of interest and signal change in response to the three regulation conditions during the presentation of negative pictures. Data from Urry et al. (2006).

Although we obtained a main effect for regulation condition on amygdala activation, there was considerable variation in the magnitude of amygdala signal reduction during the downregulate condition (compared with the Maintain condition). To better understand this variation, we asked what other regions of the brain are activated when subjects downregulate negative affect. This analysis was performed across subjects to enable us to address the nature and correlates of the individual differences in facility at downregulation of the amygdala.

We determined which areas of the brain were reciprocally coupled to signal change in the amygdala. The results of this analysis revealed a large and significant bilateral cluster in ventromedial prefrontal cortex (vmPFC) as displayed in Figure 3.2. These data indicate that subjects who show greater reductions in amygdala activation in response to the Suppress compared with the Maintain conditions show greater activation in the vmPFC prefrontal cortex during these respective conditions.

We next asked whether individual differences in amygdala and vmPFC signal change during instructed downregulation of negative affect predict another regulatory process that occurs in everyday life. Specifically, we asked whether the individual differences in MR signal change we observed were related to individual differences in the diurnal slope of cortisol. This question was of interest in light of other evidence indicating that subjects with flatter cortisol profiles (primarily contributed by higher cortisol values late in the day) do worse on a variety of outcomes (Abercrombie et al., 2004). In the week following the scan, subjects provided six saliva samples each day for 7 consecutive days. Our assay method employed the Salimetrics (State College, PA) cortisol enzyme immunoassay (EIA) kit. In light of prior data on the functional significance of individual differences in cortisol slope, we specifically focused on relations between MR signal change in the Suppress versus Maintain conditions. We predicted that those subjects who are relatively less able to decrease signal in the amygdala during the Suppress versus Maintain conditions should have a flatter cortisol slope. As Figure 3.3 reveals, those subjects who showed the smallest decrease in MR signal change in the

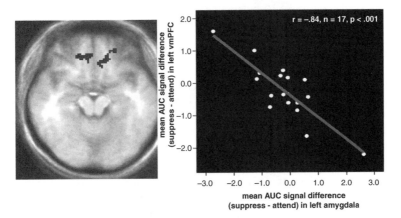

FIGURE 3.2. Increased vmPFC activation that is inversely correlated with activation in the amygdala during the Suppress versus Maintain conditions. Two regions in left and right vmPFC, maximum $t(16) = -4.79$ at Talairach coordinates $x = -23$, $y = 43$, $z = -10$, and maximum $t(16) = -5.28$ at $x = 5$, $y = 37$, $z = -12$, respectively, demonstrate an inverse functional association with the left amygdala. Data from Urry et al. (2006).

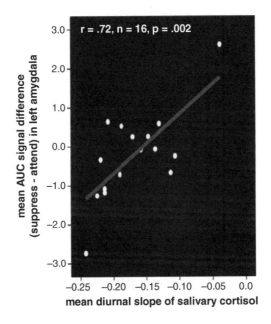

FIGURE 3.3. Relations between MR signal change in the amygdala during Suppress versus Maintain regulation conditions on the ordinate and mean of diurnal cortisol slope calculated within subjects across 7 consecutive days of sampling. Data from Urry et al. (2006).

amygdala in response to the Suppress versus Maintain conditions show the flattest cortisol slope.

The inverse of this effect was obtained for the vmPFC cluster, as the amygdala and vmPFC clusters were themselves highly inversely correlated. Further examination of these effects reveals that it is specifically cortisol levels in the evening that are associated with MR signal change. Thus, poor regulators (i.e., those with less vmPFC and higher levels of amygdala activity during the voluntary downregulation of emotion) are the ones with the highest levels of cortisol in the evening, suggesting that short-term laboratory measures of voluntary regulation are related to longer-term neuroendocrine regulation.

A variety of other data at both the animal and human levels implicates territories in PFC, particularly vmPFC, in the modulation of limbic activity, especially activity in the amygdala during tasks and contexts where regulation can be inferred. For example, Phelps, Delgado, Nearing, and LeDoux (2004) have provided compelling evidence in humans for activation of vmPFC during extinction of conditioned fear, a finding that is consistent with rodent evidence implicating this region in extinction learning and the modulation of amygdala activity (Quirk, Russo, Baron, & LeBron, 2000; Quirk, Likhtik, Pelletier, & Pare, 2003). In addition, Amat et al. (2005) have recently demonstrated the importance of vmPFC in the rodent for the modulation of the dorsal raphe nucleus in response to a stressor.

Evidence suggests that dysfunction in PFC and amygdala are common in depression (see Davidson et al., 2002b for review). Recent data suggest that depressed patients require significantly greater lateral PFC activation than controls to maintain the same level of performance on a working-memory n-back task (Harvey et al., 2005). Other evidence suggests that the polymorphism in the human serotonin transporter gene that has been found to confer susceptibility for affective disorders (Caspi et al., 2003; though see Surtees et al., 2006, for a nonreplication) also is associated with accentuated functional activity in the amygdala (Hariri et al., 2005), and related evidence indicates that this polymorphism may be specifically associated with abnormalities in coupling between vmPFC and amygdala (Heinz et al., 2005). In addition, we have speculated that PFC abnormalities may lead to difficulties in regulating negative affect and may be expressed as increased rumination in depression (see Davidson, Pizzagalli, Nitschke, & Putnam, 2002b; Davidson et al., 2003a). Finally, failure to sustain PFC activity in positive contexts may be associated with anhedonic symptoms and lack of motivation (Pizzagalli, Sherwood, Henriques, & Davidson, 2005).

There are several key outstanding issues that have not been addressed in the extant literature. Of central importance is the issue of individual differences. Little work has focused on the nature and correlates of individual differences in emotion regulation and even less work has addressed possible differences in the neural substrates of emotion regulation in patients with various forms of mood and/or anxiety disorders. A second key issue concerns the correlates of variations in emotion regulation in endocrine and autonomic output though our recent findings described earlier begin to provide a window on this question. We know that the central nucleus of the amygdala provides an important bridge to both autonomic and endocrine outputs, but there has been little study to directly address this issue. A third issue is whether individual differences in basic mechanisms of cognitive control (i.e., the ability to orchestrate thought and action in accordance with internal goals) predict individual differences in emotion regulation. There are no data in the literature that directly bear on this important question, though some theoretical accounts strongly suggest this to be the case (see Barrett, Mugade, & Engle, 2004, for review). Virtually no data are available on relations between short-term measures of regulation in the laboratory and longer-term regulatory processes. Such longer-term regulatory processes may have consequences for peripheral biology that are health-relevant (e.g., Davidson, 2004a). Finally, what few data are available on individual differences in emotion regulation do not rigorously separate the contributions of variations in emotional reactivity from those associated with emotional reactivity. This is a difficult conceptual and methodological problem.

Summary

The existing work points to the importance of prefrontal and amygdalar circuits in the regulation of negative affect and suggests that the functioning of these circuits might be consequential for adapting to adversity. We suggest that prefrontal and amygdalar circuits play an important role in regulating emotion and in modulating vulnerability to psychopathology. This framework, though indirectly supported in the studies described previously, has yet to be tested explicitly. Moreover, while the extant literature on the brain bases of emotion regulation provides important insights into the roles of prefrontal cortex and amygdala, there are limitations to the work to date. For one, there are inconsistencies with regard to the timing of regulation instruction delivery. In some studies, regulation instructions are provided prior to the appearance of the emotion-eliciting stimulus. The consequence is that one cannot verify that the emotion-eliciting stimulus actually provoked an emotion prior to the application of regulatory processes. In addition, some studies are limited to all males or all females or the sample size is too small, and only one study has so far reported on the neural substrates of regulating positive affect. These issues call into question the generalizability of some of the findings. Finally, while the studies in humans have emphasized intrinsic emotion regulatory processes, they have devoted considerably less attention to extrinsic factors that modulate emotion regulation. Here the development of a nonhuman primate model is particularly important. In addition, studies in nonhuman primates provide a powerful opportunity for the examination of individual differences in emotion regulation because animals at the extremes of distributions can be selected for more intensive study.

CONTEXT AND REGULATION
IN A NONHUMAN PRIMATE MODEL

The role of context in the regulation of affective reactivity is relatively understudied, particularly at the human level. Numerous studies at the animal level have demonstrated the importance of context in the regulation of affective behavior and have highlighted the role of the hippocampus (Anagnostaras, Maren, & Fanselow, 1999) and interconnected structures (bed nucleus of the stria terminalis: Davis & Lee, 1998) in this type of process. The contextual regulation of emotion is assumed to proceed relatively automatically. The organism apprehends context and based on the output of an analysis of current context, behavior is adjusted in a contextually appropriate manner. To study the role of context in emotion regulation, it is necessary to evaluate aspects of emotional responsivity in two or more contexts so that a comparison across context can be made.

   Some forms of psychopathology that involve disorders of affect may be best conceptualized as disorders of the context regulation of affect. For example, both mood
and anxiety disorders typically involve the expression of normal emotion in inappropriate contexts. That is, the emotion expressed in these disorders would be normative and
appropriate in certain contexts. In the diagnostic criteria for major depression following bereavement, the depression must persist for more than 2 months to be labeled
major depression according to the fourth edition of the *Diagnostic and Statistical Manual
of Mental Disorders* (DSM-IV; American Psychiatric Association, 1994). In other words,
the continued expression of depressed affect beyond the context in which it is deemed
appropriate is central to the diagnosis. In many of the anxiety disorders, the fear and
other emotions that might be experienced are perfectly normal emotions. They are simply expressed at inappropriate times in nonnormative contexts. Thus, the fear that a
social phobic might experience in the course of interacting with a group of people is
not in itself pathological. What makes the expression of the fear pathological is the fact
that it is expressed in contexts in which most other individuals do not experience such
fear.
   In an effort to investigate context-inappropriate emotion in nonhuman primates,
Kalin (Kalin & Shelton, 2000) examined 100 rhesus monkeys in a series of behavioral
tests called the Human Intruder Paradigm that have been used extensively in his laboratory (see Kalin & Shelton, 1989). These tests involve exposure of a monkey to three specific conditions. In one condition, the animal is alone; in a second condition, a human
enters the room and exposes his profile to the animal (the No Eye Contact condition);
in a third condition, the human enters the room and stares at the animal. Each of these
conditions is presented for 10 minutes. During each condition, various behaviors of the
animal are coded. In previous work, Kalin has demonstrated the differential sensitivity
of the different behaviors to specific pharmacological manipulations (Kalin & Shelton,
1989). Normatively, monkeys freeze when exposed to the human profile. Interestingly,
there are individual differences in freezing duration and these differences are stable
over time (Kalin, Shelton, Rickman, & Davidson, 1998). In response to both the Alone
and the Stare conditions, the normative response of monkeys is to display little if any
freezing, with other behaviors increasing in frequency during these conditions. When a
very large group of animals is tested ($N = 100$), the pattern of normative behavior previously observed is confirmed at the group level. There is a highly significant difference
in freezing duration among the conditions such that freezing is significantly higher during the No Eye Contact (NEC) condition compared with the other two conditions. However, there are also marked individual differences, not only in the duration of freezing
during the normative condition (No Eye Contact) but also in the duration of freezing
during the other conditions. There were three animals in this group of 100 that displayed levels of freezing during the Stare condition that were very high and indistinguishable from their freezing duration during the normative NEC condition (see Figure 3.4). Note that the freezing of this small subgroup of three was high during the No
Eye Contact condition, but there were quite a few other animals who displayed levels of
freezing that were comparable during this condition. However, all but these three animals turned off this response during the other conditions. These three animals can be
said to be displaying context-inappropriate freezing. In analyses of biological data
(prefrontal activation asymmetry and cortisol) it was found that these three animals had
markedly more extreme patterns than their counterparts who froze for an identical
duration of time during the normative context (Kalin & Shelton, 2000).

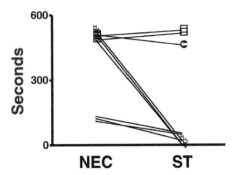

FIGURE 3.4. Freezing duration in seconds (out of a total of 600 seconds) in response to the No Eye Contact (NEC—exposure of the monkey to a profile of a human) and the Stare (ST) conditions in three groups of animals: One group shows very long durations of freezing during the normative context (NEC) but then freezes little during ST. A second group shows virtually no freezing during either NEC or ST. Finally, the third group exhibits high levels of freezing in response to both NEC and ST. This is the group that displays out-of-context freezing (i.e., during ST). The group of three animals who show the out-of-context freezing are the only animals in a group of 100 to exhibit this pattern. From Kalin and Shelton (2000). Copyright 2000 by Oxford University Press. Reprinted by permission.

While a mechanistic understanding of such context-inappropriate affective responding is not yet available, there are several issues that warrant comment. First, given the role of the hippocampus and bed nucleus of the stria terminalis that have been featured in rodent models of context conditioning (Davis & Lee, 1998), it is likely that these brain regions play a role in the context regulation of affective responding in humans. It is noteworthy that in several disorders that are known to involve context-inappropriate affective responding, morphometric study of hippocampal volume with high-resolution MRI has revealed significant atrophy (e.g., Sheline, Wang, Gado, Csernansky, & Vannier, 1996; Sheline, Sanghavi, Mintung, & Gado, 1999; Bremner et al., 1995, 1997). Such atrophy may arise as a consequence of exposure to elevated levels of cortisol, as several authors have hypothesized (Gold, Goodwin, & Chrousos, 1988; McEwen, 1998), though recent twin research has suggested that smaller hippocampal volume may be a predisposing vulnerability factor in the development of at least some of these disorders, in this case posttraumatic stress disorder (Gilbertson et al., 2002). At the human level, age-related declines in hippocampal volume have been related to elevated cortisol levels. The consequences of such age-related changes have been examined in the cognitive domain, specifically measures of declarative memory that are thought to be hippocampally mediated (Lupien et al., 1998). However, there has been no study of which we aware that has specifically related hippocampal morphometric differences to context-dependent affective responding. Based on the issues described previously, it is likely that variations in hippocampal structure and in connectivity between hippocampus and PFC will also be accompanied by profound affective changes and will impair an organism's ability to adaptively regulate emotion in a context-appropriate fashion. The affective consequences of hippocampal dysfunction may be as, if not more, important to the adaptive functioning of the organism as the cognitive changes that have been featured so prominently in the human literature. One of the important challenges in this area for the future is to develop a better understanding of context from a human perspective because most previous studies have been conducted at the nonhuman level (and mostly in the rodent) and have relied on simple manipulations of housing conditions to alter context.

The second issue that deserves emphasis here is the implications of the work on context and its role in shaping affective responding for assessing certain behavioral traits. We use behavioral inhibition as our example here in part because the studies we have conducted in nonhuman primates have been designed to model human behavioral inhibition. In the developmental literature on human infants and toddlers, this temperamental characteristic has typically been assessed by observing behavioral signs of fearfulness and wariness in contexts of novelty and unfamiliarity (e.g., Kagan, Reznick, & Snidman, 1988). Thus, for example, behavioral inhibition (one measure of which is freezing) has been coded when toddlers are approached by unfamiliar strangers or bizarre-looking robots. These are situations in which it is normative to show some wariness. In fact, the display of high levels of approach behavior in this context is the nonnormative, context-inappropriate response. As we noted earlier, there appear to be important differences between monkeys who express identically high levels of freezing during the normative context (exposure to the human profile) but differ in their duration of freezing during a nonnormative context (exposure to the human staring). Were the assessment period with these monkeys restricted to the normative context, the group of high freezing animals would have been classified identically. Only by including an assessment of their behavior in a nonnormative context were behavioral differences revealed, which helped to account for some of the variance in basal levels of prefrontal activation asymmetry and cortisol (Kalin & Shelton, 2000). These findings imply that our assessments of human behavioral inhibition may not be nearly as sensitive as they might. Rather than performing such assessments in the context-appropriate conditions of novelty and unfamiliarity, perhaps we should be measuring these temperamental characteristics in nonnormative contexts. We would hypothesize that individuals who habitually fail to regulate their affective responses in a context-sensitive fashion may have functional impairment of the hippocampus and/or stria terminalis. Such functional impairment may arise as a consequence of plastic changes in these regions as a function of cumulative exposure to elevated glucocorticoids (McEwen, 1998) or they may arise from a genetic predisposition to have compromised hippocampal structure and function (e.g., Gilbertson et al., 2002).

It has been known for some time that neurogenesis (the growth of new neurons), primarily in the dentate region of the hippocampus, can occur in the postnatal period in rodents (see Gould & McEwen, 1993, for review). However, it has only recently been demonstrated that such plastic changes can occur in the adult human hippocampus as well (Eriksson et al., 1998). The fact that such neurogenesis can occur in adult humans raises the possibility that both salubrious as well as stressful conditions might influence this process and that these experience-induced hippocampal changes, in turn, can have significant affective and cognitive consequences. Kempermann, Kuhn, and Gage (1997) have demonstrated that exposure of adult mice to an enriched environment produced a 15% increase in granule cell neurons in the dentate gyrus of the hippocampus compared with littermates housed in standard cages. This basic phenomenon has been recently replicated in rats (Nilsson, Perfilieva, Johansson, Orwar, & Eriksson, 1999) and extended by demonstrating that the rats raised in an enriched environment who showed neurogenesis in the dentate gyrus also demonstrate improved performance in a spatial learning test. Conversely, it has been shown that stress diminishes proliferation of granule cell precursors in the dentate region of adult marmoset monkeys (Gould,

Tanapat, McEwen, Flugge, & Fuchs, 1998). Collectively, these findings highlight the plasticity of certain regions of the brain that persist into adulthood and raise the possibility that interventions, even those occurring during adulthood, not only can have effects on neuronal function but can also literally influence neurogenesis. The fact that the focus of this work is in the hippocampus indicates that a major substrate of context-dependent emotional responding is a key target for these experientially induced changes. It is likely that other brain regions as well will exhibit plastic changes. Whether these will involve neurogenesis or will favor other mechanisms is a question that must be addressed in future work. For now, the extant findings provide a rationale for examining the impact of therapeutic interventions, both pharmacological as well as behavioral, as well as naturally occurring environmental stressors and stress buffers, on neuronal structure and the central circuitry of emotion regulation, that might underlie changes in affective style.

In more recent work on our nonhuman primate model of emotion regulation, we have used microPET with fluorolabeled deoxyglucose (FDG) to label regional glucose metabolism in the monkey brain. This procedure is ideally suited to study whole-brain changes in activation in response to naturalistic challenges in monkeys. In this procedure, animals are exposed to standardized behavioral challenges. In our case here, we used the Human Intruder paradigm described earlier. Animals are injected with FDG prior to exposure to these challenges. FDG is taken up in the brain over the course of an approximately 30-minute period. After this 30-minute period has elapsed, the FDG is trapped in the neurons for a couple of hours before it is metabolized. Thus, the integrated activity over the course of an approximately 30-minute period produced by the behavioral challenge will be reflected in the distribution of FDG in the brain. Following this initial 30-minute period, the animals are then anesthetized and placed in the microPET scanner. The images we obtain reflect the integrated activity from the prior 30-minute period.

Using this method, we (Kalin et al., 2005) recently showed that glucose metabolism in a region that includes the bed nucleus of the stria terminalis (BNST) and the nucleus accumbens is highly correlated with the duration of freezing both in the normative context (i.e., during the NEC condition) as well as in the nonnormative context (in this case, while the animal was alone; see Figure 3.5).

We next addressed the question of which brain regions changed their pattern of activation in different contexts and predicted behavioral changes in the two contexts. To address this question, we examined relations between the change in freezing from the Alone to the NEC condition and changes in glucose metabolism between these two conditions. There were several regions that emerged from this analysis but the most important one was the dorsal anterior cingulate cortex (dACC) region. There was a very strong relation between change in dACC activity and change in freezing such that animals who showed higher durations of freezing during the NEC compared with the Alone conditions showed higher levels of glucose metabolism during NEC compared with Alone in the dACC.

Collectively the findings from this study demonstrate that the BNST region, previously linked to anxiety by Davis and colleagues (Davis & Lee, 1998) is strongly associated with freezing across contexts. However, alterations in metabolic rate in this region was not associated with changes in freezing between contexts. The dACC was very strongly associated with changes in freezing between contexts. This region of dACC (BA 24c) has direct projections to motor cortex (Dum & Strick, 2002) and has been linked to conflict monitoring and error detection when divergent motor responses are

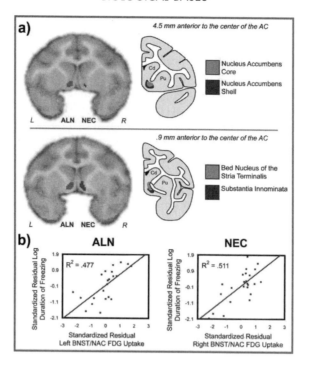

FIGURE 3.5. The BNST/nucleus accumbens (NAC) regions that are correlated with freezing duration in the NEC (red) and Alone (ALN; blue) conditions are displayed. (A) more anterior region of the BNST/NAC; (B) a more posterior region. Scatter plots represent the relation between log freezing duration and brain activity in the BNST/NAC regions of interest for the ALN and NEC conditions. Both variables are standardized and residualized for age. From Kalin et al. (2005). Copyright 2005 by the Society for Biological Psychiatry. Reprinted by permission.

required, as would appear to be the case in shifting between contexts that normatively have very different signatures of motor output.

Another important feature of contextual regulation of emotion in nonhuman primates concerns the manner in which contextual support is used or requested. Regions of the PFC likely play a role guiding behavior in a goal-directed manner to reduce distress and regulate negative affect. This process can be effectively studied in monkeys by using microPET in conjunction with another naturalistic challenge—separation of an infant from its mother. In much earlier research conducted in Davidson's laboratory, Davidson and Fox (1989) separated 10-month-old infants from their mothers for a brief 30-second period and examined the extent to which they cried in response to this challenge. Prior to the separation period, baseline levels of prefrontal activation were assessed with brain electrical measures. They found that infants who cried in response to maternal separation had higher levels of right-sided prefrontal activation during the prior baseline period compared with infants who did not cry. One interpretation of these findings is that right PFC is playing some role in guiding behavior toward the reduction of the negative affect elicited by separation. In this case, the crying can be viewed as a signal to reinstate contact with the mother. On the other hand, if infants were extremely fearful and hypervigilant for threat-related cues in response to this challenge, we might expect that they would be less likely to cry. Crying in this case provides a clear signal to possible predators about one's location.

Based on the aforementioned conjectures, we designed a study in monkeys to test some of the hypotheses to have emerged from a consideration of the human data (Fox et al., 2005). Our experiment was based on earlier observations from the Kalin lab (Kalin & Shelton, 1989) indicating that in response to separation, the normative response of monkeys is to coo, though there are large individual differences in the duration of cooing displayed. To explain the variation across individuals, we hypothesized that animals who perceived this challenge as a threat and thus would strongly activate the amygdala would show less cooing while those animals who directed their behavior toward reinstating contact with the mother and thus cooing more would show increased activation in the right dorsolaeratal PFC. In this experiment, we adopted the same strategy that we used in the other microPET studies with monkeys. In this case, we injected FDG prior to period of separation and then anesthetized the animals and scanned their brain after a 30-minute separation period. We specifically hypothesized that we would find a positive correlation between metabolic rate in the right dorsolateral PFC (dLPFC) and cooing and a negative correlation between metabolic rate in the amygdala and cooing. Figure 3.6a presents the data for the right dlPFC and amygdala.

As can be seen from this figure, animals with higher levels of glucose metabolism in the amygdala show decreased cooing in response to separation while those with higher levels of activation in the right dlPFC show higher levels of cooing. Interestingly, these two neural systems are relatively orthogonal in response to this challenge because when they are added in separate steps of a higherarchical regression, they explain 76% of the variance in cooing behavior (see Figure 3.6b).

In a very recent study we used the Human Intruder paradigm to select extreme groups of monkeys based on the duration of freezing they exhibited in response to the NEC challenge. We hypothesized that animals with the highest levels of freezing, akin to human behavioral inhibition, would show the highest levels of amygdala activity. In addition, we further predicted that in response to separation, the most behaviorally inhibited animals would show the least amount of cooing. Figure 3.7 presents the data on freezing behavior in three groups of animals that we tested further. Figure 3.8 shows the PET data and illustrates that the high-freezer group exhibits the highest levels of glucose metabolism in the amygdala compared with the other two groups. For reasons we do not yet understand, the middle group actually showed the lowest levels of amygdala activation compared with the high and the low group freezer groups. Figure 3.9 presents the data in a continuous fashion across groups and reveals that animals with the highest levels of amygdala activation (who have the highest levels of freezing in the nonnormative context of being alone) show the least amount of cooing. These findings indicate that the group of animals with the most nonnormative affective expression, in this case high levels of freezing during the Alone condition, were the least effective in calling for help during the Alone condition.

SUMMARY AND CONCLUSIONS

This chapter has selectively reviewed recent empirical studies of the neural bases of emotion regulation in humans and nonhuman primates. The human studies have

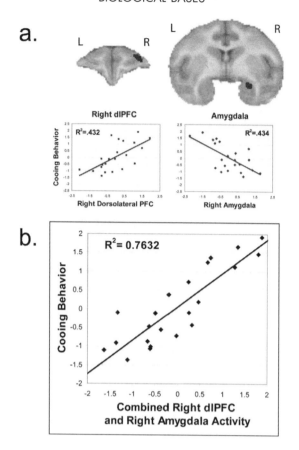

FIGURE 3.6. Relations between glucose metabolic activity in the right dorsolateral PFC and the amygdala and duration of cooing during separation. From Fox et al. (2005). Copyright 2005 by Proceedings of the National Academy of Sciences. Reprinted by permission.

emphasized voluntary emotion regulation, a competence that appears to be if not uniquely human, certainly much more well developed in humans than other species. It was shown that individual differences in the neural correlates of voluntary emotion regulation are related to endogenous regulatory processes in everyday life. We specifically presented new evidence to indicate that those individuals who were poor emotion regulators as reflected in less vmPFC activation and more amygdala activation when attempting to voluntarily downregulate negative affect using cognitive strategies show a flatter slope of the cortisol rhythm. This flatter slope was found to be primarily a function of higher evening levels of cortisol. These findings suggest that laboratory probes of the neural correlates of emotion regulation reflect longer-term regulatory processes that may have important consequences for mental and physical health and illness.

The studies in nonhuman primates highlight the utility and power of studying emotion regulation at this level. There are certain questions primarily related to extrinsic influences on emotion regulation that are very well suited for addressing at the nonhuman primate level, particularly the role of context in shaping automatic emotion regula-

□ Screening 1 ■ Screening 2

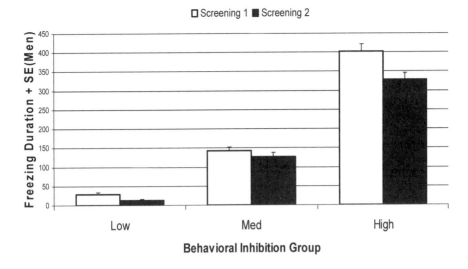

FIGURE 3.7. Durations of freezing at first assessment and follow-up in three groups of animals selected to show extremely high, low, or middle durations of freezing in response to the NEC condition in the Human Intruder paradigm.

tion as well as the recruitment of conspecifics to facilitate emotion regulation. We provided evidence to show that there are important individual differences in the extent to which context regulates emotion. The failure to regulate emotion in a context-appropriate fashion may reflect unique neurobiological processes. We believe these findings have important implications for human studies that assess emotion reactivity in normative contexts. Furthermore, there is a critical need to develop novel paradigms in humans that address the contextual regulation of emotion and that characterize individual differences in such processes. We believe that individual differences in the

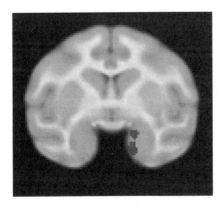

FIGURE 3.8. Region of the amygdala where the high-freezer group shows significantly greater amygdala metabolism compared with the other two groups in response to the Alone condition.

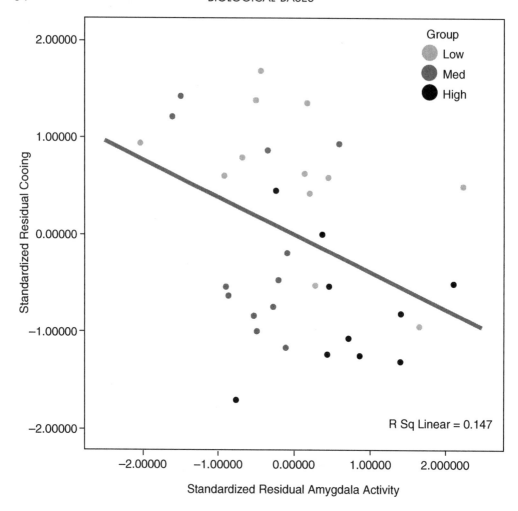

FIGURE 3.9. Relation between glucose metabolism in the amygdala and cooing. Animals who show the highest level of glucose metabolism in the amygdala coo the least.

context-dependent automatic regulation are crucially important in governing vulnerability to psychopathology; assessment procedures that capture such individual differences in humans require development. In animals whose environments are highly controlled, it is easier to manipulate context compared with the human case where the very term "context" is difficult to operationalize. Our capacity for top-down control, to voluntarily cast our attentional spotlight selectively to certain features of our environment enables context to be changed through the endogenous regulation of attention. This is clearly an area in which additional research is required and in which creative new strategies inspired by the nonhuman work are needed.

It is clear that advances in the understanding of the neural bases of emotion regulation will be greatly facilitated by combining the insights derived from both human and nonhuman studies and that both approaches are necessary to fully characterize the complexities of emotion regulation and dysregulation.

REFERENCES

Abercrombie, H. C., Giese-Davis, J., Sephton, S., Epel, E. S., Turner-Cobb, J. M., & Spiegel, D. (2004). Flattened cortisol rhythms in metastatic breast cancer patients. *Psychoneuroendocrinology, 29,* 1082–1092.

Amat, J., Baratta, M. V., Paul, E., Bland, S. T., Watkins, L. R., & Mauer, S. F. (2005). Medial prefrontal cortex determines how stressor controllability affects behavior and dorsal raphe nucleus. *Nature Neuroscience, 8,* 365–371.

American Psychiatric Association. (1994). *Diagnostic and statistical manual of mental disorders* (4th ed.). Washington, DC: Author.

Anagnostaras, S. G., Maren, S., & Fanselow, M. S. (1999). Temporally graded retrograde amnesia for contextual fear after hippocampal damage in rats: Within-subjects examination. *Journal of Neuroscience, 19,* 1106–1114.

Barrett, L. F., Mugade, M. M., & Engle, R. W. (2004). Individual differences in working memory capacity and dual-process theories of mind. *Psychological Bulletin, 130,* 553–573.

Beauregard, M., Levesque, J., & Bourgouin, P. (2001). Neural correlates of conscious self-regulation of emotion. *Journal of Neuroscience, 21,* 165.

Bremner, J. D., Randall, P., Scott, T. M., Bronen, R. A., Seibyl, J. P., Southwick, S. M., et al. (1995). MRI-based measurement of hippocampal volume in patients with combat-related posttraumatic stress disorder. *American Journal of Psychiatry, 152,* 972–981.

Bremner, J. D., Randall, P., Vermetten, E., Staib, L. H., Bronen, R. A., Mazure, C., et al. (1997). Magnetic Resonance imaging-based measurement of hippocampal volume in posttraumatic stress disorder related to childhood physical and sexual abuse: A preliminary report. *Biological Psychiatry, 41,* 23–32.

Burgess, P. W., Simons, J. S., Dumontheil, I., & Gilbert, S. J. (2005). The gateway hypothesis of rostral prefrontal cortex (area 10) function. In J. Duncan & P. McLeod (Eds.), *Measuring the mind: Speed, control, and age* (pp. 217–248). Oxford, UK: Oxford University Press.

Caspi, A., Sugden, K., Moffitt, T. E., Taylor, A., Craig, I. W., Harrington, H., et al. (2003). Influence 0of life stress on depression: Moderation by a polymorphism in the 5-HTT gene. *Science, 301,* 386–389.

Davidson, R. J. (2000a). Affective style, psychopathology, and resilience: Brain mechanisms and plasticity. *American Psychologist, 55,* 1196–1214.

Davidson, R. J. (2000b). Cognitive neuroscience needs affective neuroscience (and vice versa). *Brain and Cognition, 42,* 89–92.

Davidson, R. J. (2004a). Well-being and affective style: Neural substrates and biobehavioral correlates. *Philosophical Transactions of the Royal Society of London, B, 359,* 1395–1411.

Davidson, R. J. (2004b). What does the prefrontal cortex "do" in affect: Perspectives in frontal EEG asymmetry research. *Biological Psychology, 67,* 219–234.

Davidson, R. J., & Fox, N. A. (1989). Frontal brain asymmetry predicts infants' response to maternal separation. *Journal of Abnormal Psychology, 98,* 127–131.

Davidson, R. J., Irwin, W., Anderle, M. J., & Kalin, N. H. (2003a). The neural substrates of affective processing in depressed patients treated with venlafaxine. *American Journal of Psychiatry, 160,* 64–75.

Davidson, R. J., Jackson, D. C., & Kalin, N. H. (2000a). Emotion, plasticity, context, and regulation: Perspectives from affective neuroscience. *Psychological Bulletin, 126,* 890–909.

Davidson, R. J., Kabat-Zinn, J., Schumacher, J., Rosenkranz, M. A., Muller, D., Santorelli, S. F., et al. (2003b). Alterations in brain and immune function produced by mindfulness meditation. *Psychosomatic Medicine, 65,* 564–570.

Davidson, R. J., Lewis, D., Alloy, L., Amaral, D., Bush, G., Cohen, J., et al. (2002a). Neural and behavioral substrates of mood and mood regulation. *Biological Psychiatry, 52,* 478–502.

Davidson, R. J., Pizzagalli, D., Nitschke, J. B., & Putnam, K. M. (2002b). Depression: Perspectives from affective neuroscience. *Annual Review of Psychology, 53,* 545–574.

Davidson, R. J., Putnam, K. M., & Larson, C. L. (2000c). Dysfunction in the neural circuitry of emotion regulation: A possible prelude to violence. *Science, 289,* 591–594.

Davidson, R. J., & Sutton, S. K. (1995). Affective neuroscience: The emergence of a discipline. *Current Opinion in Neurobiology, 5,* 217–224.

Davis, M., & Lee, Y. L. (1998). Fear and anxiety: Possible roles of the amygdala and the bed nucleus of the stria terminalis. *Cognition and Emotion, 12,* 277–306.

Davis, M., & Whalen P. J. (2001). The amygdala: Vigilance and emotion. *Molecular Psychiatry, 6,* 13–34.

Devinsky, O., Morrell, M. J., & Vogt, B. A. (1995). Contributions of anterior cingulate cortex to behaviour. *Brain, 118,* 279–306.

Dum, R. P., & Strick, P. L. (2002). Motor areas in the frontal lobe of the primate. *Physiology and Behavior, 77,* 677–682.

Ebert, D., & Ebmeier, K. P. (1996). The role of the cingulate gyrus in depression: From functional anatomy to neurochemistry. *Biology, 39,* 1044–1050.

Eriksson, P. S., Perfilieva, E., Bjork-Eriksson, T., Alborn, A., Nordborg, C., Peterson, D. A., et al. (1998). Neurogenesis in the adult human hippocampus. *Nature Medicine, 4,* 1313–1317.

Fox, A. S., Oakes, T. R., Shelton, S. E., Converse, A. K., Davidson, R. J., & Kalin, N. H. (2005). Calling for help is independently modulated by brain systems underlying goal-directed behavior and threat perception. *Proceedings of the National Academy of Sciences, USA, 102,* 4176–4179.

Garavan, H., Ross, T. J., & Stein, E. A. (1999). Right hemispheric dominance of inhibitory control: An event-related functional MRI study. *Proceedings of the National Academy of Sciences, USA, 96,* 8301–8306.

Gilbertson, M. W., Shenton, M. E., Ciszewski, A., Kasai, K., Lasko, N. B., Orr, S. P., et al. (2002). Smaller hippocampal volume predicts pathologic vulnerability to psychological trauma. *Nature Neuroscience, 5,* 1242–1247.

Gold, P. W., Goodwin, F. K., & Chrousos, G. P. (1988). Clinical and biochemical manifestations of depression: Relation to the neurobiology of stress (Parts 1&2). *New England Journal of Medicine, 314,* 348–353.

Gould, E., & McEwen, B. S. (1993). Neuronal birth and death. *Current Opinion in Neurobiology, 3,* 676–682.

Gould, E., Tanapat, P., McEwen, B. S., Flugge, G., & Fuchs, E. (1998). Proliferation of granule cell precursors in the dentate gyrus of adult monkeys is diminished by stress. *Proceedings of the National Academy of Sciences, USA, 95,* 3168–3171.

Gross, J. J., & Thompson, R. A. (2007). Emotion regulation: Conceptual foundations. In J. J. Gross (Ed.), *Handbook of emotion regulation* (pp. 3–24). New York: Guilford Press.

Hariri, A. R., Drabant, E. M., Munoz, K. E., Kolachana, B. S., Mattay, V. S., Egan, M. F., et al. (2005). A susceptibility gene for affective disorders and the response of the human amygdala. *Archives of General Psychiatry, 62,* 146–152.

Harvey, P. O., Fossati, P., Pochon, J. B., Levy, R., Lebastard, G., Lehericy, S., et al. (2005). Cognitive control and brain resources in major depression: An fMRI study using the n-back task. *NeuroImage, 26,* 860–869.

Heinz, A., Braus, D. F., Smolka, M. N., Wrase, J., Puls, I., Hermann, D., et al. (2005). Amygdala-prefrontal coupling depends upon a genetic variation of the serotonin transporter. *Nature Neuroscience, 8,* 20–21.

Holland, P. C., & Gallagher, M. (1999). Amygdala circuitry in attentional and representational processes. *Trends in Cognitive Sciences, 3,* 65–73.

Jackson, D. C., Malmstadt, J. R., Larson, C. L., & Davidson, R. J. (2000). Suppression and enhancement of emotional responses to unpleasant pictures. *Psychophysiology, 37,* 515–522.

Jackson, D. C., Mueller, C. J., Dolski, I., Dalton, K. M., Nitschke, J. B., Urry, H. L., et al. (2003). Now you feel it, now you don't: Frontal EEG asymmetry and individual differences in emotion regulation. *Psychological Science, 14,* 612–617.

Kagan J., Reznick, J. S., & Snidman, N. (1988). Biological bases of childhood shyness. *Science, 240,* 167–171.

Kalin, N. H., & Shelton, S. E. (1989). Defensive behaviors in infant Rhesus monkeys: Environmental cues and neurochemical regulation. *Science, 243,* 1718–1721.

Kalin, N. H., & Shelton, S. E. (2000). The regulation of defensive behaviors in rhesus monkeys: Implications for understanding anxiety disorders. In R. J. Davidson (Ed.), *Anxiety, depression and emotion* (pp. 50–68). New York: Oxford University Press.

Kalin, N. H., Shelton, S. E., Fox, A. S., Oakes, T. R., & Davidson, R. J. (2005). Brain regions associated with the expression and contextual regulation of anxiety in primates. *Biological Psychiatry, 58,* 796–804.

Kalin, N. H., Shelton, S. E., Rickman, M., & Davidson, R. J. (1998). Individual differences in freezing and cortisol in infant and mother rhesus monkeys. *Behavioral Neuroscience, 112,* 251–254.

Kempermann, G., Kuhn, H. G., & Gage, F. H. (1997). More hippocampal neurons in adult mice living in an enriched environment. *Nature, 386,* 493–495.

LeDoux, J. E. (2000). Emotion circuits in the brain. *Annual Review of Neuroscience, 23,* 155–184.

Levesque, J., Eugene, F., Joanette, Y., Paquette, V., Mensour, B., Beaudoin, G., et al. (2003). Neural circuitry underlying voluntary suppression of sadness. *Society of Biological Psychiatry, 53,* 502–510.

Lupien, S. J., de Leon, M., de Santi, S., Convit, A., Tarshish, C., Nair, N. P., et al. (1998). Cortisol levels during human aging predict hippocampal atrophy and memory deficits. *Nature Neuroscience, 1,* 69–73.

Mayberg, H. S., Brannan, S. K., Mahurin, R. K., Jerabek, P. A., Brickman, J. S., Tekell, J. L., et al. (1997). Cingulate function in depression: A potential predictor of treatment response. *Neuroreport, 8,* 1057–1061.

McEwen, B. S. (1998). Protective and damaging effects of stress mediators. *New England Journal of Medicine, 338,* 171–179.

Miller, E. K., & Cohen, J. D. (2001). An integrative theory of prefrontal cortex function. *Annual Review of Neuroscience, 24,* 167–202.

Nauta, W. J. (1971). The problem of the frontal lobe: A reinterpretation. *Journal of Psychiatry Research, 8,* 167–87.

Nilsson, M., Perfilieva, E., Johansson, U., Orwar, O., & Eriksson, P. S. (1999). Enriched environment increases neurogenesis in the adult rat dentate gyrus and improves spatial memory. *Journal of Neurobiology, 39,* 569–578.

Ochsner, K., Bunge, S. A., Gross, J. J., & Gabrieli, J. D. E. (2002). Rethinking feelings: An fMRI study of the cognitive regulation of emotion. *Journal of Cognitive Neuroscience, 14,* 1215–1229.

Ochsner, K. N., & Gross, J. J. (2005). The cognitive control of emotion. *Trends in Cognitive Sciences, 9,* 242–249.

Ochsner, K. N., Ray, R. D., Cooper, J. C., Robertson, E. R., Chopra, S., Gabrieli, J. D., et al. (2004). For better or for worse: Neural systems supporting the cognitive down- and up-regulation of negative emotion. *NeuroImage, 23,* 483–499.

Phelps, E. A., Delgado, M. R., Nearing, K. I., & LeDoux, J. E. (2004). Extinction learning in humans: Role of the amygdala and vmPFC. *Neuron, 43,* 897–905.

Pizzagalli, D. A., Sherwood, R., Henriques, J. B., & Davidson, R. J. (2005). Frontal brain asymmetry and reward responsiveness: A source localization study. *Psychological Science, 16,* 805–813.

Quirk, G. J., Likhtik, E., Pelletier, J. G., & Pare, D. (2003). Stimulation of medial prefrontal cortex decreases the responsiveness of central amygdala output neurons. *Journal of Neuroscience, 23,* 8800–8807.

Quirk, G. J., Russo, G. K., Barron, J. L., & Lebron, K. (2000). The role of ventromedial prefrontal cortex in the recovery of extinguished fear. *Journal of Neuroscience, 20,* 6225–6231.

Rumpel, S., LeDoux, J., Zador, A., & Malinow, R. (2005). Postsynaptic receptor trafficking underlying a form of associative learning. *Science, 14,* 234–235.

Schaefer, S. M., Jackson, D. C., Davidson, R. J., Aguirre, G. K., Kimberg, D. Y., & Thompson- Schill, S. L. (2002). Modulation of amygdalar activity by the conscious regulation of negative emotion. *Journal of Cognitive Neuroscience, 14,* 913–921.

Semendeferi, K., Armstrong, E., Schleicher, A., Zilles, K., & Van Hoesen, G. W. (2001). Prefrontal cortex in humans and apes: A comparative study of area 10. *American Journal of Physical Anthropology, 114,* 224–241.

Sheline, Y. I., Sanghavi, M., Mintun, M. A., & Gado, M. H. (1999). Depression duration but not age predicts hippocampal volume loss in medically healthy women with recurrent major depression. *Journal of Neuroscience, 19,* 5034–5043.

Sheline, Y. I., Wang, P. W., Gado, M. H., Csernansky, J. G., & Vannier, M. W. (1996). Hippocampal atrophy in recurrent major depression. *Proceedings of the National Academy of Sciences, USA, 93,* 3908–3913.

Stefanacci, L., & Amaral, D. G. (2002). Some observations on cortical inputs to the macaque monkey amygdala: An anterograde tracing study. *Journal of Comparative Neurology, 30,* 301–323.

Surtees, P. G., Wainwright, N. W. J., Willis-Owen, S. A. G., Luben, R., Day, N. E., & Flint, J. (2006).

Social adversity, the serotonin transporter (5-HTTLPR) polymorphism and major depressive disorder. *Biological Psychiatry, 59,* 224–229.

Taylor, S. E. (1991). Asymmetrical effects of positive and negative events: The mobilization–minimization hypothesis. *Psychological Bulletin, 110,* 67–85.

Tursky, B., Shapiro, D., Crider, A., & Kahnman, D. (1969). Pupilary, heart rate, and skin resistance changes during a mental task. *Journal of Experimental Psychology, 79,* 164–167.

Urry, H. L., Nitschke, J. B., Dolski, I., Jackson, D. C., Dalton, K. M., Mueller, C. J., et al. (2004). Making a life worth living: Neural correlates of well-being. *Psychological Science, 15,* 367–372.

Urry, H. L., van Reekum, C. M., Johnstone, T., Kalin, N. H., Thurow, M. E., Schaefer, H. S., et al. (2006). Amygdala and ventromedial prefrontal cortex are inversely coupled during regulation of negative affect and predict the diurnal pattern of cortisol secretion among older adults. *Journal of Neuroscience, 26,* 4415–4425.

Whalen, P. J. (1998). Fear, vigilance, and ambiguity: Initial neuroimaging studies of the human amygdala. *Current Directions in Psychological Science, 7,* 177–188.

Vogt, B. A., Nimchinsky, E. A., Vogt, L. J., & Hof, P. R. (1995). Human cingulate cortex: Surface features, flat maps, and cytoarchitecture. *Journal of Comparative Neurology, 359,* 490–506.

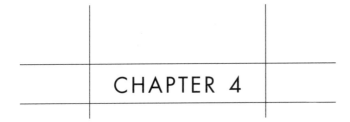

CHAPTER 4

Insights into Emotion Regulation from Neuropsychology

JENNIFER S. BEER
MICHAEL V. LOMBARDO

As the individual who laughs at a funeral or fails to show guilt after committing a crime will tell us, there are few quicker routes to social scorn than inappropriate emotion (or absence of an emotional expression) (see Beer & Keltner, 2004, for a review). While emotions may sometimes be helpful (e.g., Ekman, 1992; Levenson, 1999), it is not the case that their free expression is always adaptive. What biological systems are in place to permit flexibility in the evolved emotion system and what can they tell us about the psychological phenomena involved in emotion regulation?

Specific answers to these questions necessitate a clear definition of emotion and emotion regulation. Emotions can be considered a set of physiological, phenomenological, and facial expressions changes evoked in relation to appraisals of situations (e.g., Levenson, 1999). Emotion regulation is a diverse set of control processes aimed at manipulating when, where, how, and which emotion we experience and express (e.g., Gross, 1998; Gross & Thompson, this volume); these control processes take time to develop and subsets may be emphasized at different stages of life (e.g., Lockenhoff & Carstensen, 2004; Thompson, 1994; Zelazo, 2004). In addition, these control processes are theorized to occur at both automatic and conscious levels of processing. Emotion may be regulated to accomplish various goals. For example, from an intrapersonal perspective, we regulate our emotions in at least two ways to maximize opportunities for positive emotions and minimize opportunities for negative emotions. First, we may automatically or more deliberately attend to information, events, and people that make us feel good and avoid or ignore those who evoke negative emotions. We control which emotions we experience through the selection or creation of particular situations. Second, once an emotional experience has arisen, we may manipulate the magnitude of our response in order to quickly suppress negative emotions and amplify or perpetuate positive emotions. From an interpersonal perspective, we regulate our emotions in at least two ways. People need to regulate the magnitude of their emotional expression in reference to display rules. There are societal norms for how much one should express certain emotions (e.g., extreme pride is mostly acceptable only in politics and sports). Many clinical disorders of emotion or mood are characterized by otherwise "normal" emotions that have lasted too long or are too extreme given the external environment. In addition, one may need to produce a facial expression of emotion in the absence of a phenomenological emotional experience when the situation demands it (e.g., smiling in response to the poor humor of your boss). In summary, emotion regulation can involve a diverse set of cognitive processes that occur both automatically and with effort. Such processes permit individuals to enjoy mostly positive emotions while avoiding negative emotions (Taylor, 1991) and to increase or decrease its intensity or even manufacture emotional facial expression in reference to social norms.

Although most people might claim they know emotion regulation when they see it, the foregoing definition makes independent measurement of emotion regulation and emotion generation a tricky proposition. Emotion regulation paradigms typically measure participants' emotional responses after they are instructed to reappraise stimuli to change their emotional state, to manipulate the magnitude of their emotion, or to prevent their emotions from influencing decisions (e.g., behavioral: Beer, in press; Gross & Levenson, 1993; functional magnetic resonance imaging [fMRI]: Beer, Knight, & D'Esposito, 2006; Ochsner et al., 2004; Phan et al., 2005). Other studies have examined spontaneous emotion regulation by assessing recovery after being startled (e.g., eye blink: Jackson et al., 2003; acoustic: Roberts et al., 2004). However, the measurement of emotion as a dependent variable makes it difficult to distinguish between a primary emotional response and a regulated emotional response. Many emotion regulation strategies are antecedent-focused, meaning that they occur before appraisals generate emotional experiences (Gross & Thompson, this volume). For example, emotion regulation occurs when individuals subconsciously attend selectively to certain information to promote good feelings about the self. If we only measure an emotional response, how can we distinguish between regulated emotion resulting from selective attention and primary emotion generated from genuine but failed attempts at equivocal information processing? Do low levels of emotion mean that the response has been downregulated or did the stimulus not elicit a strong emotional response from the start? In the most extreme case, if self-perception is generally characterized by a drive to focus on the good and ignore the bad (e.g., Robins & Beer, 2001; Taylor & Brown, 1994), then it is possible that cognitive gymnastics influence most information processing and almost any emotional expression might be considered the result of some emotion regulation.

Unfortunately, the state of neuropsychological research on emotion regulation is unlikely to help resolve the distinction between emotion generation and emotion regulation. Very little research on human neuropsychological populations has been conducted in order to address questions of emotion regulation. This limitation notwithstanding, a survey of the literature suggests that neuropsychological research may indirectly address the neural and psychological basis of three processes associated with emotion regulation: (1) motivation towards reward and away from punishment, (2) manipulating the magnitude of emotional response, and (3) producing facial expressions of emotion (see Table 4.1 and Figure 4.1). Motivation toward reward and away from punishment is similar to the situation selection and situation modification strate-

TABLE 4.1. Areas of Damage Associated with Emotion Regulatory Deficits

Emotion regulation deficit	Area of damage	Citations
Motivation toward reward and away from punishment		
Lack of knowledge of social rewards	Temporal lobe, OFC, DlPFC	Anderson et al. (1999); Barrash, Tranel, & Anderson (2000); Beer et al. (2003, in press); Blair & Cipolotti (2000); Cicerone & Tanenbaum (1997); Grattan & Eslinger (1991); Mateer & Williams (1991); Price et al. (1990)
Impaired filtering of emotional information	OFC	Rule, Shimamura, & Knight (2002)
Failure to maximize positive emotion	OFC	Rahman et al. (2001); Sanfey et al. (2003); Shiv, Lowenstein, & Bechara (2005)
Impaired reversal learning	OFC	Bechara et al. (1999); Fellows & Farah (2005a); Rolls et al. (1994)
Failure to accomplish goals	DlPFC, OFC	Goel et al. (1997); Gomez-Belderrai et al. (2004); Saver & Damasio (1991); Shallice & Burgess (1991)
Impaired response to anticipated startle	OFC	Roberts et al. (2004)
Manipulating magnitude of response		
Aberrant sexual behaviors	Temporal lobe, amygdala, OFC	Ghika-Schmid et al. (1995); Hayman et al. (1999); Jha & Patel (2004); Lilly et al. (1983); Pradhan, Singh, & Pandey (1998); Yoneoka et al. (2004)
Increased rage, violence, explosive temper, aggression, hostility, anger, irritability, irreverence, lability	Temporal lobe, amygdala, caudate, ACC, OFC	Barrash, Tranel, & Anderson (2000); Berlin, Rolls, & Kischka (2004); Cicerone & Tanenbaum (1997); Ghika-Schmid et al. (1995); Grafman et al. (1986); Hayman et al. (1998); Jha & Patel (2004); MacMillan (1986); Mateer & Williams (1991); Max et al. (2001); Tateno, Jorge, & Robinson (2004)
Increased anxiety	OFC, PFC	Grafman et al. (1986); Paradiso et al. (1999); Tateno, Jorge, & Robinson (2004)
Increased pride	OFC	Beer et al. (2003)
Impulsiveness	VMPFC	Bechara, Dolan, & Hindes (2002); Berlin, Rolls, & Kischka (2004); Rolls et al. (1994); Sanfey et al. (2003)
Change in subjective emotional experience	OFC, ACC	Hornak et al. (2003)
Placidity, passivity, apathy	Temporal lobe, amygdala, caudate, ACC, OFC, lateral PFC	Barrash, Tranel, & Anderson (2000); Hayman et al. (1998); Lilly et al. (1983); Paradiso et al. (1999); Pradhan, Singh, & Pandey (1998); Yoneoka et al. (2004)

(continued)

TABLE 4.1. *(continued)*

Emotion regulation deficit	Area of damage	Citations
Manipulating magnitude of response (continued)		
Depression, less happiness	OFC, DlPFC	Berlin, Rolls, & Kischka (2004); Grafman et al. (1986); Paradiso et al. (1999); Tateno, Jorge, & Robinson (2004)
Blunted affect	Temporal lobe, OFC, DlPFC	Barrash, Tranel, & Anderson (2000); Grafman et al. (1986); Pradhan, Singh, & Pandey (1998)
Loss/reduction of anger or fear	Temporal lobe, amygdala, thalamus, ACC, OFC	Cohen et al. (2001); Sprengelmeyer et al. (1999); Yoneoka et al. (2004)
Lack of embarrassment	OFC	Beer et al. (2003, in press)
Producing facial expressions		
Impaired reflexive smiling	Corticomotor strip, corticobulbar connections	Rinn (1984)
Inappropriate crying or laughing	OFC, lateral PFC, caudate, temporal lobe	Max et al. (2001); Tateno, Jorge, & Robinson (2004)
Impaired posed facial expressions	Extrapyramidal system (basal ganglia)	Rinn (1984)

Note. ACC, anterior cingulate cortex; DlPFC, dorsolateral prefrontal cortex; OFC, orbitofrontal cortex; PFC, prefrontal cortex.

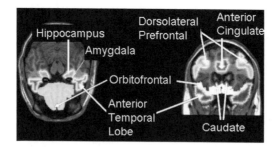

FIGURE 4.1. Neural areas implicated in emotion regulation processes.

gies discussed by Gross and Thompson (this volume). Individuals may regulate their emotions by either selecting or creating situations that are likely to generate positive emotions and decrease negative emotions. Manipulating the magnitude of emotional response and producing facial expressions are both similar to the response modulation strategy discussed by Gross and Thompson (this volume). Manipulating the magnitude of emotional response refers to the modification of an emotional response once an emotion has been generated. In contrast, producing facial expressions refers to the generation of a facial expression in the absence of a phenomenological emotional experience. These processes are not intended as an exhaustive list of emotion regulation processes; rather, the limited human neuropsychological research only permits speculations about these three.

The study of neuropsychological populations, or patients with (semi) focal brain damage, has several advantages over populations with psychiatric or progressive neurological disorders (Beer & Lombardo, in press; Beer, Shimamura, & Knight, 2004). Lesion patient methodology is deficit-focused. Patients with selective brain damage are studied to determine how a specific region of brain dysfunction impairs (or does not) specific behaviors. If a behavioral deficit is observed in relation to damage to a specific brain region, then scientists consider that brain region to be critically involved (i.e., necessary) for that behavior. In contrast, both psychiatric disorders and progressive neurological disorders such as dementia affect the brain and behavior in a diffuse manner. Diffuse damage makes it difficult to isolate behavioral deficits in relation to a specific brain region. Furthermore, psychiatric populations may be confounded by medication that affects brain function and may have different neurological developmental histories. Differential development and medication make it difficult to generalize findings from these populations to healthy populations. Moreover, studies of neuropsychological populations provide complementary information to animal lesion studies and human brain-imaging studies. While brain-imaging studies provide specific regional information about brain areas that may be recruited for a given task, studies of neuropsychological patients and nonhuman animals provide information about human brain areas that are critically involved in a given task.

MOTIVATION TOWARD REWARD AND AWAY FROM PUNISHMENT

If you wanted to ensure that you would feel good most of the time and feel bad very little of the time, what might you do? Would you enter into a business arrangement that is sure to lead to a bankruptcy? Engage in risky sexual practices? Fail to hold a job because of your preference to spend the day watching television, listening to music, and eating uncooked frozen meals? Although these suggestions may seem unreasonable, they are all examples of choices made by patients with brain damage (Anderson, Bechara, Damasio, Tranel, & Damasio, 1999; Saver & Damasio, 1991). In contrast, most people select or create situations that maximize their opportunities for positive feelings and minimize their opportunities for negative feelings. This type of emotion regulation is similar to the antecedent-focused strategies of situation selection and situation modification discussed by Gross and Thompson (this volume). Although emotion regulation may be most often associated with reappraising a stimulus or controlling a facial expression, emotion regulation may occur well before that. Specifically, people can regulate or modify what kinds of emotions they feel by choosing or changing situations. Human neuropsychological research suggests that a host of brain areas, including the temporal lobes, amygdala, frontal lobes, and anterior cingulate, help individuals increase their positive emotions and decrease their negative emotions by selecting or creating rewarding situations in favor of punishing situations.

Temporal Lobes

The history of brain damage and emotion regulation begins in the temporal lobes of monkeys (see Davidson, Fox, & Kalin, this volume; Quirk, this volume). Klüver–Bucy syndrome, a syndrome which includes emotion regulatory deficits, was initially described in monkeys with anterior and/or medial temporal lobe damage extending into the amygdala (Klüver & Bucy, 1939). A similar syndrome can arise in humans with damage to the anterior and medial temporal lobes, amygdala, and orbitofrontal cortices in both adults and children (e.g., adults: Ghika-Schmid, Assal, De Tribolet, & Regalit, 1995; Hayman et al., 1998; Jha & Patel, 2004; Lilly, Cummings, Benson, & Frankel, 1983; Yoneoka et al., 2004; children: Pradhan, Singh, & Pandey, 1998). In most studies of human Klüver–Bucy syndrome, clinician observation or family-member reports are used to assess deficits. This syndrome is associated with placidity and lowered levels of fear and anger. In addition, patients may become hypersexual, indiscriminately approaching people and objects with sexual desire, excessively manipulating the genital area, making abnormal sexual vocalizations, and inappropriately displaying body parts to strangers. This syndrome may be a dysfunction of emotion generation. Specifically, reward and punishment are incorrectly attributed to emotional stimuli, and, therefore, appropriate emotions are not generated. However, it could also be that the anterior and medial temporal lobes are part of a network that helps individuals recognize and *avoid* threat situations normally evoking anger or fear as well as recognizing and *selecting* appropriate, rewarding opportunities for mating.

Amygdala

The amygdala has long been implicated in appraising the environment for threat and stimuli of biological significance (Whalen, 1998). Unfortunately for students of emotion regulation, most research on focal amygdala damage has focused on recognition of emotional facial expressions rather than emotion regulation. While some studies suggest that these patients have difficulty in recognizing fear, studies involving larger samples suggest that amygdala damage impairs emotional face perception more generally (e.g., Adolphs et al., 1999; Broks et al., 1998; Rapcsak et al., 2000; Sprengelmeyer et al., 1999). If the amygdala plays an important role in understanding what other people are feeling, then in a distal sense this structure is involved in helping individuals recognize when their emotional expression may be offending others and requires regulation (However, the same could be said about the visual, auditory, and language system in general).

A more proximal role of the amygdala for emotion regulation is suggested by research examining amygdala damage in situations in which emotional information should influence subsequent behavior. In gambling tasks, patients with amygdala damage cannot learn which responses are rewarded and which are punished (Bechara, Damasio, Damasio, & Lee, 1999). One possibility is that these patients gamble disadvantageously because they do not generate positive emotion responses to winning and negative emotional responses to losing. However, another study found that patients with amygdala damage do not show enhanced attention and memory for negative stimuli even though they accurately report the affective valence of the stimuli (Anderson & Phelps, 2001). Moreover, other studies have found that amygdala damage does not impair the generation of emotion, in terms of either subjective emotional experiences (Anderson & Phelps, 2002) or production of facial expression of emotions (posed facial expressions: Anderson & Phelps, 2000). For example, a longitudinal study of subjective emotional experience found no differences in the magnitude and frequency of positive, negative, and fear/anxiety-related affect (i.e., the Positive and Negative Affect Scale: PANAS) among unilateral amygdala patients, a bilateral amygdala patient, and normal controls (Anderson & Phelps, 2002). Similarly, a case study found that bilateral amygdala damage does not impair the ability to express fear, disgust, sadness, and happiness in a manner consistent with control subjects (Anderson & Phelps, 2000). Therefore, the amygdala may not be involved in generating emotional experience but enables individuals to use positive and negative emotions to select situations and responses which maximize reward and minimize punishment.

Frontal Lobes

As gatekeepers of the neural world, the frontal lobes are another prime candidate to underlie the processes that maximize positive feelings and reduce negative feelings (Beer et al., 2005; see Zelazo & Cunningham, this volume). Portions of the frontal lobes have been shown to have higher rates of activity at rest; it has been suggested that this activity is related to a default mode of brain function designed to continuously and automatically monitor the environment for threat (Gusnard & Raichle, 2001). Research on neuropsychological populations suggests that damage to the orbitofrontal cortex results in impaired preferences for reward over punishment. For example, patients with orbitofrontal damage do not normally maximize their performance in gambling tasks. In comparison to healthy controls and participants with other forms of brain damage, orbitofrontal patients are characterized by failures to take contextual factors into account which increases their risk taking in some cases (e.g., Bechara, Damasio, & Damasio, 2000; Bechara, Dolan, & Hindes, 2002; Fellows & Farah, 2005a; Rolls, Hornake, Wade, & McGrath, 1994; Sanfey, Hastie, Colvin, & Grafman, 2003) and decreases risk taking in others (e.g., Rahman, Sahakian, Cardinal, Rogers, & Robbins, 2001; Shiv, Lowenstein, & Bechara, 2005; Sanfey et al., 2003). In one study, patients with orbitofrontal damage were unable to recognize that their previous gambling strategy was no longer optimal and failed to switch their strategies to maximize winnings (Fellows & Farah, 2005a). Similarly, orbitofrontal damage has been associated with an inability to prioritize solutions that are most likely to reduce interpersonal conflict quickly (Saver & Damasio, 1991) and accomplish goals (Goel, Grafman, Tajik, Gana, & Danto, 1997; Gomez-Beldarrain, Harries, Garcia-Manco, Ballus, & Grafman, 2004; Shallice & Burgess, 1991). In one study, participants were asked to perform a series of tasks to assess their ability to accomplish novel goals (Multiple Errands task; Shallice & Burgess, 1991). In comparison to healthy controls, patients with frontal lobe damage failed to complete many of the tasks, broke rules for carrying out the tasks, and were generally inefficient in completing the tasks. In another study, orbitofrontal and dorsolateral prefrontal patients failed to use advice to optimize their completion of a financial planning task and performed poorly in comparison to control subjects (Gomez-Belderrain et al., 2004). A case study found that orbitofrontal damage does not impair the ability to generate solutions to a problem (i.e., two roommates want to watch different television programs at the same time) but may impair the ability to prioritize solutions that are most feasible or most likely to result in reward (Optimal Thinking Test; Saver & Damasio, 1991). Finally, orbitofrontal damage impairs the ability to use past experience to avoid negative emotion. Orbitofrontal patients and healthy controls were presented with an acoustic startle and then told they would hear the startle again at the end of a countdown (Roberts et al., 2004). Orbitofrontal patients physiologically responded to the anticipated startle as if it were a novel stimulus in comparison to control participants who prepared themselves for the threatening stimulus.

The exact impairment underlying the failure to prioritize reward over punishment is the subject of some controversy and is further complicated by developmental issues (Beer et al., 2004; see Zelazo & Cunningham, this volume). In cases of orbitofrontal damage incurred in adulthood, the failure to prioritize reward in favor of punishment is most likely accounted for by poor online insight into discrepancies between actual behavior and intact knowledge about rewarding behaviors (Beer, John, Scabini, & Knight, 2006; Gomez-Belderrain et al., 2004). It is also likely that even if patients are made aware of their poor choices, they may not be able to prevent themselves from executing an action that is unlikely to bring reward if it was previously rewarded (e.g., Fellows & Farah, 2005a; Berlin, Rolls, & Kischka, 2004). In contrast, some research suggests that orbitofrontal damage incurred in childhood may impair the ability initially to learn which behaviors ensure reward and which ensure punishment. For example, childhood damage to this area results in impaired understanding of social rules (e.g., Anderson et al., 1999; Grattan & Eslinger, 1991; Mateer & Williams, 1991). Therefore, these children cannot select social responses that will be rewarded as they are not aware of the rules they need to follow.

Anterior Cingulate

The anterior cingulate may also be involved in directing individuals away from punishment. This area has been associated with the monitoring of errors and detecting competition of responses (Carter et al., 1998; see McClure, Botrinick, Young, Greene, & Cohen, this volume; Gehring & Knight, 2000) as well as the reappraisal of negative emotional stimuli (see Ochsner & Gross, this volume). To avoid punishment, individuals need to know when a negative emotion is about to arise or when an emotional expression is in conflict with social norms. Although focal damage to this area is rare, some studies have found a relation between anterior cingulate damage and reduced tension, anger, and pain (Cohen et al., 2001) as well as more general changes in subjective emotional state (damage extended into BA [Brodmann's area] 9; measure conflated emotional increases and decreases: Hornak et al., 2003). In one study, self-reports and clinical interviews were used to assess emotional changes in cingulotomy patients. In comparison to patients with chronic pain, patients with surgically removed cingulate tissue had reduced pain, tension, and anger. No differences were found for fatigue, anxiety, confusion, or vigor (Cohen et al., 2001). In another study, patients with damage extending from the anterior cingulate to the orbitofrontal cortex reported more changes in their aggregate emotional experiences of sadness, anger, happiness, fear, and disgust in comparison to subjects with dorsolateral and orbitofrontal damage (Hornak et al., 2003). No distinction was made in this study between increases or decreases in emotion, nor were data for discrete emotions provided. From the standpoint of cingulate lesion research, it might be tempting to conclude that anterior cingulate damage results in reduced emotion because this area is important for the generation of emotion. However, this explanation would not account for the increased emotions found in some cingulate patients (Hornak et al., 2003). From the combined viewpoint of the cingulate lesion research and the neuroimaging research, it is possible that the anterior cingulate may be involved in emotion regulation processes by motivating people away from punishment (i.e., pain, tension, and anger) by increasing the salience of errors. In this case, anterior cingulate damage may be associated with increased or decreased negative emotion because the faulty monitoring system impairs the ability to accurately identify non-punishing situations.

It is important to note that the critical involvement of the anterior cingulate in error and conflict detection has recently been called into question. If so, any involvement of the anterior cingulate in emotion regulation may not be associated with detecting errors. Although anterior cingulate activity has often been associated with classic tests of conflict and error detection, focal anterior cingulate damage may not impair these abilities. For example, one study found that anterior cingulate damage did not impair performance on the Stroop task (Fellows & Farah, 2005b). Therefore, damage to this area does not impair the ability to overcome a prepotent response if it is irrelevant for the task at hand. Nor does damage extending into the anterior cingulate impair awareness of errors on an Eriksen flanker task (Stemmer, Segalowitz, Witzke, & Schonle, 2003). In other words, anterior cingulate damage does not impair the ability to recognize when an incorrect response has been selected from a set of competing responses. Although no research has directly examined anterior cingulate damage in relation to emotion regulation, these studies suggest that anterior cingulate damage may not impair performance on emotion regulation paradigms that require participants to overcome a prepotent emotional response or to recognize when one has failed to maximize the possibilities for positive emotion and minimize the possibilities for negative emotions.

In summary, a host of brain regions may help individuals direct themselves toward positive feelings and away from negative feelings through the selection of environments. The temporal lobes and amygdala may be helpful for using learned emotional responses to choose subsequent behaviors or environments. The frontal lobes may be helpful for selecting behaviors that are associated with rewards rather than punishment. The anterior cingulate may be involved in detecting situations that are potentially punishing so that they may be avoided.

MANIPULATING MAGNITUDE OF RESPONSE

Imagine you are in a particularly good mood. How would you express it? Would you sweep a hospital staff member off her feet to hug and kiss her? Or if you were angry at a driver who hit your car, would you plan to kill the driver and ask the police to help you? Although these examples may appear extreme, they are representations of ways in which patients with orbitofrontal damage have expressed their emotion (Rolls et al., 1994). In contrast, most people regulate their emotional responses in order to (1) inhibit negative feelings and amplify or perpetuate positive feelings once they have arisen or (2) to conform to social norms regarding emotional expressions. This type of emotion regulation is similar to the response-focused strategy of response modulation discussed by Gross and Thompson (this volume). Specifically, people can regulate or modify how they experience and/or express their emotions by manipulating the magnitude of their emotional response. This includes the inhibition or suppression of undesirable emotions and amplification of desirable emotions. The psychological processes by which individuals modify the magnitude of their emotional responses once emotion has been generated are informed by research on the frontal and medial temporal lobes.

Frontal Lobes

Damage to the frontal lobes has long been associated with impaired control over the magnitude of emotional expression (Anderson et al., 1999; Blair & Cipolotti, 2000; Cicerone & Tanenbaum, 1997; Grattan & Eslinger, 1991; Hornak et al., 2003; MacMillan, 1986; Mateer & Williams, 1991; Stuss & Benson, 1984). Although the classic case of Phineas Gage (MacMillan, 1986) has often been described as evidence for the relation between frontal lobe damage and personality change, it can also be construed as an example of emotion regulatory deficits. Specifically, after Gage's frontal lobes (and parts of anterior cingulate: Damasio, Grabowski, Frank, Galaburden, & Damasio, 1994) were punctured by a tamping iron, he was described by his doctors as irritable and irreverent. Recent cases of frontal damage are consistent with this classic case. In comparison to healthy controls, patients with frontal lobe damage have been associated with increased general irritability (orbitofrontal: Barrash, Tranel, & Anderson, 2000; orbitofrontal and temporal lobe: Cicerone & Tanenbaum, 1997) and increases in specific emotions such as pride (orbitofrontal: Beer, Heerey, Kelfner, Scabini, & Knight, 2003), anger, and hostility (orbitofrontal: Berlin et al., 2004; Grafman Vance, Weingartner, Salazar, & Amin, 1986) and anxiety and depression (lateral frontal: Grafman et al., 1986; Paradiso, Chemerinski, Yazici, Tartaro, & Robinson, 1999). For example, in comparison to healthy controls, patients with orbitofrontal damage be- haved inappropriately during a teasing task but reported greater levels of pride after completing the task (Beer et al., 2003). In comparison to patients with other kinds of brain damage, patients with orbitofrontal damage are viewed by their relatives as expe- riencing increased irritability, emotional lability, and inappropriate affect (Barrash et al., 2000; Cicerone & Tannenbaum, 1997). Patients with orbitofrontal damage report that they feel more anger after their trauma (Berlin et al., 2004). One study used the Profile of Mood States Inventory (POMS: measures fatigue, anger, depression, vigor, and confusion) to assess emotion and found evidence for laterality effects (Grafman et al., 1986). Right orbitofrontal lesions were associated with increased anger and depres- sion compared to bilateral or left-sided orbitofrontal damage. In contrast, patients with left dorsal lateral damage showed significantly more anger than patients with left-sided orbitofrontal damage or left nonprefrontal damage.

In contrast, damage to the frontal lobes has also been associated with blunted emo- tional experience (lateral frontal: Barrash et al., 2000; Paradiso et al., 1999) or the absence of an expected emotion such as feeling embarrassment after violating social norms (Beer et al., 2003; Beer, John, et al., 2006). For example, clinical observations of frontal lobe patients suggest that lateral frontal lobe damage is associated with blunted affect and reduced motivation (Paradiso et al., 1999). Still other studies have not found deficits; for example, orbitofrontal damage does not dampen or enhance response to emotional stimuli in a laboratory setting (see Beer, in press), nor does frontal lobe dam- age necessarily change trait levels of emotions (Paradiso et al., 1999).

Why might damage to the frontal lobes both increase and decrease emotional experience? These findings are less paradoxical than they may appear at first. A large body of research on frontal lobe function has characterized this region as primarily response for executive functioning and this may extend to the emotion domain (Beer et al., 2004; Shimamura, 2000). The frontal lobes have been traditionally associated with a variety of executive functions or control processes, including the direction of attention, maintaining information in working memory, revising information in relation to envi- ronmental changes, and suppressing irrelevant information. From the perspective of dynamic filtering theory, the frontal lobes determine whether incoming emotional information will be operated on or inhibited through executive function processes used in nonemotional tasks (Shimamura, 2000). Specifically, the magnitude of an emotional response will depend on whether incoming emotional information (1) becomes the subject of attention (selection), (2) is kept active in short-term memory (maintenance), (3) is revised as contexts change (updating), and/or (4) inhibited (rerouting). From this perspective, frontal lobe damage does not necessarily result in unidirectional deficits of too little or too much emotion. Damage to the filtering system may result in too little emotion if emotional information does not become the focus of attention or is not kept active in memory. However, damage to this filtering system might also result in too much emotion if emotional information is not discarded as contexts change or inhibited when it is irrelevant to the task at hand. Empirical support for this view is suggested by a study that found that patients with frontal lesions exhibit larger event-related potentials (ERPs) (P3a) to loud bursts of noise and electric shocks and show lower levels of habituation in response to these irritating stimuli when compared to healthy control participants (Rule, Shimamura, & Knight, 2002). Therefore, the general control function of the frontal lobes may also be recruited for controlling the intensity of emotional responses as well as how quickly emotional responses habituate. In other words, the control processes involved in modifying emotion are similar to "cold" control processes (i.e., nonemotional control processes).

Temporal Lobes

Research on damage to a portion of the temporal lobe different than that associated with Klüver–Bucy syndrome suggests that manipulation of emotional response regulation may occur without awareness. Specifically, amnesiac patients, some who have severe hippocampal damage, engage in dissonance reduction (Lieberman, Ochsner, Gilbert, & Schacter, 2001). Amnesics and control participants show equal magnitudes of attitude change after a discrepancy between their original attitude and behavior arises. One interpretation of dissonance reduction is that individuals strive to reduce a discrepancy between their attitudes and behavior because this discrepancy creates a negative feeling state. In the case of amnesic patients, dissonance reduction occurs even though they could not have explicitly remembered any aversive state that may have arisen. This suggests that regulating aversive emotions may not require explicit awareness of the discrepancy.

In summary, research on human neuropsychological populations suggests that people may influence how intensely they experience or express an emotion by recruiting regions in the frontal lobes. The executive function or control processes associated with frontal lobe function may be recruited to control both nonemotional and emotional information. In addition, control processes through the executive function of the frontal lobes do not necessarily require the engagement of memory systems in the medial temporal lobes.

PRODUCING FACIAL EXPRESSIONS

What if you received a gift you did not like? Would you stare blankly at the gift giver? A patient with corticobulbar damage, bereft of the ability to produce an emotional facial expression in the absence of an emotional experience, might do just that. In contrast, most people would simply produce a smile in order to conform to social norms. This type of emotion regulation is similar to the response-focused strategy of response modulation discussed by Gross and Thompson (this volume). Specifically, people can regulate or modify when they express an emotion even in the absence of a phenomenological emotional experience. Human neuropsychological research suggests that motor systems and possibly the frontal lobes help individuals produce emotional facial expressions in the absence of an internal emotional experience.

Motor Systems

Research on selective damage to the pathways controlling facial muscle movement suggests that spontaneous emotional facial expressions and posed emotional facial expressions are distinct from one another (see Rinn, 1984, for a review). For example, patients with damage to the cortical motor strip or corticobulbar projections are unable to execute instructions to smile but smile spontaneously in reaction to positive stimuli. In contrast, patients with damage to the extrapyramidal motor system, especially the basal ganglia, have the reverse problem. These patients can manipulate their face in response to instruction but do not express spontaneously arising emotional experiences on their face. These studies suggest that the ability to flexibly produce an emotional facial expression in the absence of actual emotional experience is supported by a system different than facial expressions arising in concert with an emotional experience.

Frontal Lobes

The separation between expressions of emotion and internal experience of emotion is also reinforced by the syndrome of pathological crying or laughing (also known as emotional incontinence or pseudobulbar affect). Pathological laughing and crying is a period of intense laughter or crying that results from a stimulus that would not normally result in an emotional response. The outbursts are not true reflections of the individual's internal emotional state. In other words, the laughing and crying are not associated with phenomenological experiences of joy or sadness, respectively. Although pathological laughing and crying are typically associated with neurological or psychiatric disorders, it can be associated with traumatic brain injury. In these cases, the damage is usually in the left lateral frontal lobes and is often comorbid with depression or anxiety disorders (Max, Robertson, & Lansing, 2001; Tateno, Jorge, & Robinson, 2004). Therefore, the study of these populations is subject to the problems outlined in Chapter 1 (Gross & Thompson, this volume). However, the research on motor systems and the existence of pathological crying and laughing suggests that regulating expressions of emotion and the internal experience of emotion may recruit distinct neural systems.

SUMMARY AND FUTURE DIRECTIONS

Perhaps the strongest conclusion that can be drawn from this research is that more research on emotion regulation in neuropsychological populations is needed. Few extant studies have been conducted and even fewer have been driven by questions of emotion regulation. The dearth of studies makes it difficult to evaluate evidence for the critical involvement of specific neural networks in particular emotional regulatory processes. A review of Table 4.1 suggests that the frontal lobes, the anterior cingulate, the temporal lobes, and possibly the amygdala and caudate may be involved in emotion regulation in the form of motivating individuals toward reward and away from punishment and/or regulating how emotion is expressed. In some sense, these studies have only served to reinforce the role of "the usual (neural) suspects" in emotional processes seen in research on humans and nonhuman animals (see Figure 4.1 and Davidson, Fox, & Kalin, this volume; Ochsner & Gross, this volume; Quirk, this volume). Many of these areas are anatomically connected to one another and many are included in the limbic system. However, the putative role of the caudate reinforces the claim that confining the study of emotional processes to limbic structures is imprecise and unhelpful (LeDoux, 1993).

Some tentative insights into the psychological structure of emotion regulatory processes can be gleaned from these studies of brain damage. First, the manipulation of the magnitude of emotional expression may not be completely distinct from the control systems used in "cold" or nonemotional tasks. In other words, behavioral control for the purpose of maximizing reward and avoiding punishment as well as for purposes other than emotion regulation (i.e., focusing attention on a task) are both likely handled by the frontal lobes. It may also be that the nonemotional control processes are building blocks in emotion regulation. In this case, damage to the frontal lobes impairs emotion regulation in a distal, rather than a proximal, sense. Future research should explore the possibility that the orbitofrontal region of frontal cortex, with its tighter connections to areas such as the amygdala and caudate, may be most proximally involved in controlling emotional processes. Second, the manipulation of emotion magnitude may occur without explicit awareness of the aversive emotion. Amnesiac patients with temporal lobe damage may be not be able to remember a negative emotion associated with a discrepancy between their attitudes and behavior but they do engage in regulatory processes to reduce this discrepancy. Third, regulating emotional facial expressions is distinct from regulating the internal emotional experience. Posed emotional facial expressions recruit a different neural system than the system supporting spontaneous emotional facial expressions. Although some conclusions can be drawn, much more attention has been paid to executive functioning in relation to "cold" regulation processes than emotion regulation in studies of neuropsychological populations. For example, a variety of standardized neuropsychological tests measure the executive functions of the frontal lobes (see Kolb & Whishaw, 2003) but none specifically measure the ability to control emotion. Future research needs to incorporate several different factors to directly address emotion regulation.

Future studies of neuropsychological populations should focus on specific questions regarding emotion regulation. For example, how different are automatic and effortful emotion regulation processes? What can brain damage tell us about how emotion regulation systems may or may not differ depending on the valence, cognitive complexity, or intensity of the primary emotional experience? How might developmental differences in emotion regulatory ability be explained by the developmental trajectories of brain areas involved in these processes? What can be said about individual differences in emotion regulatory ability or strategy preference in relation to various kinds of brain damage? There are many questions remaining in research on emotion regulation and neuropsychological populations are an important method for addressing these issues.

Future lesion research should also include the careful emotional suppression and amplification paradigms used in behavioral studies and in imaging studies (e.g., Beer et al., 2006; Gross & Levenson, 1993, 1995; Ochsner et al., 2004; Phan et al., 2005). For example, in an emotional suppression paradigm, participants are presented with an emotion-eliciting stimulus (such as a film) and told to behave "in such a way that a person watching you would not know you were feeling anything" (Gross & Levenson, 1993).

An amplification paradigm might present participants with an emotion-eliciting stimulus and ask them to increase their emotions either by imaging themselves in the situation or the situation getting worse (Ochsner et al., 2004). The inclusion of standardized emotion regulation paradigms across lesion and imaging studies will permit direct comparisons across these approaches. At the moment, it is difficult to make sense of results from lesion studies in relation to imaging studies. For example, the involvement of the frontal lobes in controlling the magnitude of emotional response is consistent with imaging studies that have shown frontal activity in relation to emotional reappraisals and changes in emotional magnitude (e.g., Ochsner et al., 2004; see Ochsner & Gross, this volume; Phan et al., 2005). Furthermore, frontal activity has been shown to modulate amygdala activity during emotional reappraisal. This finding might be interpreted as an indication that the amygdala is responsible for emotion generation and needs to be "shut off" in order to change or decrease emotion. However, patients with amygdala damage do not report any change in their trait emotional experiences (Anderson & Phelps, 2002). Therefore, emotional experience may not be critically generated in the amygdala but activity in this area must be modulated to change an already elicited emotional state. The use of standardized paradigms across levels of analyses will move the field closer to answers rather than only raising new questions.

Finally, it is important to recognize the limitations of research with neuropsychological populations (Beer & Lombardo, in press). First, this type of experimentation capitalizes on accidents of nature which do not always (in fact, do not usually) result in damage to precise subregions or a particular subregion of interest. For example, some of the research reviewed in this chapter suggests that anterior cingulate and the caudate may be involved in emotion regulation yet focal damage to these areas is rare. In contrast, traumatic events and strokes are much more likely to result in focal damage to portions of the frontal lobes. Ideally, studies should involve patients with damage that is as circumscribed to a particular area as possible. Studies involving patients with diffuse damage or grossly defined damage (e.g., Kim & Choi-Kwon, 2000; Weddell, Miller, & Trevarthen, 1990) suffer from many of the same problems as studies of psychiatric and progressive neurological populations mentioned in the introduction of this chapter. Furthermore, lesion volume must also be quantified across patients and correlated with behavioral performance. It may be that lesion volume rather than particular location accounts for emotion regulatory deficits. Second, nonrandom assignment may be a particular concern for scientists interested in individual differences of emotion regulation. Lesion patients may have differed on personality traits that may have made them more likely to sustain trauma (i.e. risk-seeking). In this case, any differences in regulation of risk between these patients and healthy controls may be accounted for by brain damage or individual differences. Finally, it is impossible to know whether "critical involvement" means that area is important for sending or receiving a necessary neural signal. The damaged region may affect emotion regulation because signals from the region directly affect an emotion regulation process. The damaged region may also affect emotion regulation because damaged fibers of passage preclude the relay of a message between the damaged brain area and another brain area.

In conclusion, the prevalence of emotion regulation in daily life warrants investigation of its underlying processes. In contrast to traditional executive functioning, little attention has been paid to emotion regulation, particularly in the study of neuropsychological populations. Future research should draw on extant frameworks of emotion regulation, employ standardized paradigms, and use patients with focal damage to rigorously investigate unanswered questions about emotion regulation.

REFERENCES

Adolphs, R., Tranel, D., Hamann, S., Young, A. W., Calder, A. J., Phelps, E. A., et al. (1999). Recognition of facial emotion in nine individuals with bilateral amygdala damage. *Neuropsychologia, 37,* 1111–1117.

Amaral, D. G., Capitanio, J. P., Jourdain, M., Mason, W., Mendoza, S. P., & Prather, M. (2003). The amygdala: Is it an essential component of the neural network for social cognition? *Neuropsychologia, 41,* 235–340.

Anderson, A. K., & Phelps, E. A. (2000). Expression without recognition: Contributions of the human amgydala to emotional communication. *Psychological Science, 11,* 106–111.

Anderson, A. K., & Phelps, E. A. (2001). Lesions of the human amygdala impair enhanced perception of emotionally salient events. *Nature, 411,* 305–309.

Anderson, A. K., & Phelps, E. A. (2002). Is the human amygdale critical for the subjective experience of emotion? Evidence of intact dispositional affect in patients with amygdale lesions. *Journal of Cognitive Neuroscience, 14,* 709–720.

Anderson, S. W., Bechara, A., Damasio, H., Tranel, D., & Damasio, A. R. (1999). Impairment of social and moral behavior related to early damage in human prefrontal cortex. *Nature Neuroscience, 2,* 1032–1037.

Barrash, J., Tranel, D., & Anderson, S. W. (2000) Acquired personality disturbances associated with bilateral damage to the ventromedial prefrontal region. *Developmental Neuropsychology, 18,* 355–381.

Bechara, A., Damasio, H., & Damasio, A. R. (2000). Emotion, decision making, and the orbitofrontal cortex. *Cerebral Cortex, 10,* 295–307.

Bechara, A., Damasio, H., Damasio, A. R., & Lee, G. P. (1999). Different contributions of the human amygdala and ventromedial prefrontal cortex to decision-making. *The Journal of Neuroscience, 19,* 5473–5481.

Bechara, A., Dolan, S., & Hindes, A. (2002). Decision-making and addiction (part II): Myopia for the future of hypersensitivity to reward? *Neuropsychologia, 40,* 1690–1705.

Beer, J. S. (in press). The importance of emotion-cognition interactions for social adjustment: Insights from the orbitofrontal cortex. In E. Harmon-Jones & P. Winkielman (Eds.), *Social neuroscience: Integrating biological and psychological explanations of social behavior.* New York: Guilford.

Beer, J. S., Heerey, E. H., Keltner, D., Scabini, D., & Knight, R. T. (2003). The regulatory function of self-conscious emotion: Insights from patients with orbitofrontal damage. *Journal of Personality and Social Psychology, 85,* 594–604.

Beer, J. S., John, O. P., Scabini, D., & Knight, R. T. (2006). Orbitofrontal cortex and social behavior: Integrating self-monitoring and emotion–cognition interactions. *Journal of Cognitive Neuroscience, 18,* 871–880.

Beer, J. S., & Keltner, D. (2004). What is unique about self-conscious emotions?: Comment on Tracy & Robins' "Putting the self into self-conscious emotions: A theoretical model." *Psychological Inquiry, 15,* 126–129.

Beer, J. S., Knight, R.T., & D'Esposito, M. (2006). Integrating emotion and cognition: The role of the frontal lobes in distinguishing between helpful and hurtful emotion. *Psychological Science, 17,* 448–453.

Beer, J. S., & Lombardo, M. V. (in press). Patient and neuroimaging methodologies in the study of personality and social processes. In R. W. Robins, R. C. Fraley, & R. Krueger (Eds.), *Handbook of research methods in personality psychology.* New York: Guilford Press.

Beer, J. S., Shimamura, A. P., & Knight, R. T. (2004). Frontal lobe contributions to executive control of cognitive and social behavior. In M. S. Gazzaniga (Ed.), *The cognitive neurosciences* (3rd ed., pp. 1091–1104). Cambridge, MA: MIT Press.

Berlin, H. A., Rolls, E. T., & Kischka, U. (2004). Impulsivity, time perception, emotion, and reinforcement sensitivity in patients with orbitofrontal cortex lesions. *Brain, 127,* 1108–1126.

Blair, R. J., & Cipolotti, L. (2000). Imapired social response reversal: A case of "acquired sociopathy." *Brain, 123,* 1122–1141.

Broks, P., Young, A. W., Maratos, E. J., Coffey, P. J., Calder, A. J., Isaac, C. I., et al. (1998). Face processing impairments after encephalitis: Amygdala damage and recognition of fear. *Neuropsychologia, 36,* 59–70.

Carter, C. S., Braver, T. S., Barch, D. M., Botvinick, M. M., Noll, D., & Cohen, J. D. (1998). Anterior cingulate cortex, error detection, and the online monitoring of performance. *Science, 280,* 747–749.

Cicerone, K. D., & Tanenbaum, L. N. (1997). Disturbance of social cognition after traumatic orbitofrontal brain injury. *Archives of Clinical Neuropsychology, 12,* 173–188.

Cohen, R. A., Paul, R., Zawacki, T. M., Moser, D. J., Sweet, L., & Wilkinson, H. (2001). Emotional and personality changes following cingulotomy. *Emotion, 1,* 38–50.

Damasio, H., Grabowski, T., Frank, R., Galaburda, A. M., & Damasio, A. R. (1994). The return of Phineas Gage: Clues about the brain from the skull of a famous patient. *Science, 264,* 1102–1105.

Davidson, R. J., Fox, A., & Kalin, N. H. (2007). Neural bases of emotion regulation in nonhuman primates and humans. In J. J. Gross (Ed.), *Handbook of emotion regulation* (pp. 47–68). New York: Guilford Press.

Ekman, P. (1992). An argument for basic emotions. *Cognition and Emotion, 6,* 169–200.

Ekman, P. (1993). Facial expression and emotion. *American Psychologist, 48,* 384–392.

Fellows, L. K., & Farah, M. J. (2005a). Different underlying impairments in decision-making following ventromedial and dorsolateral frontal lobe damage in humans. *Cerebral Cortex, 15,* 58–63.

Fellows, L. K., & Farah, M. J. (2005b). Is anterior cingulate cortex necessary for cognitive control? *Brain, 128,* 788–796.

Gehring, W. J., & Knight, R. T. (2000). Prefrontal–cingulate interactions in action monitoring. *Nature Neuroscience, 3,* 516–520.

Ghika-Schmid, F., Assal, G., De Tribolet, N., & Regli, F. (1995). Klüver–Bucy syndrome after left anterior temporal resection. *Neuropsychologia, 33,* 101–113.

Goel, V., Grafman, J., Tajik, J., Gana, S., & Danto, D. (1997). A study of the performance of patients with frontal lobe lesions in a financial planning task. *Brain, 120,* 1805–1822.

Gomez-Beldarrain, M., Harries, C., Garcia-Monco, J. C., Ballus, E., & Grafman, J. (2004). Patients with right frontal lesions are unable to assess and use advice to make predictive judgements. *Journal of Cognitive Neuroscience, 16,* 74–89.

Grafman, J., Vance, S. C., Weingartner, H., Salazar, A. M., & Amin, D. (1986). The effects of lateralized frontal lesions on mood regulation. *Brain, 109,* 1127–1148.

Grattan, L. M., & Eslinger, P. J. (1991). Frontal damage in children and adults: A comparative review. *Developmental Neuropsychology, 7,* 283–326.

Gross, J. J. (1998). The emerging field of emotion regulation: An integrative review. *Review of General Psychology, 2,* 271–299.

Gross, J. J., & Levenson, R. W. (1993). Emotional suppression: Physiology, self-report, and expressive behavior. *Journal of Personality and Social Psychology, 64,* 970–986.

Gross, J. J., & Levenson, R. W. (1995). Emotion elicitation using films. *Cognition and Emotion, 9,* 87–108.

Gross, J. J., & Thompson, R. A. (2007). Emotion regulation: Conceptual foundations. In J. J. Gross (Ed.), *Handbook of emotion regulation* (pp. 3–24). New York: Guilford Press.

Gusnard, D. A., & Raichle, M. E. (2001). Searching for a baseline: Functional imaging and the resting human brain. *Nature Reviews Neuroscience, 2,* 685–694.

Hayman, A. L., Rexer, J. L., Pavol, M. A., Strite, D., & Meyers, C. A. (1999). Klüver–Bucy syndrome after bilateral selective damage of amygdale and its cortical connections. *Journal of Neuropsychiatry and Clinical Neurosciences, 10,* 354–358.

Hornak, J., Bramham, J., Rolls. E. T., Morris, R. G., O'Doherty, J., Bullock, P. R., et al. (2003). Changes in emotion after circumscribed surgical lesions of the orbitofrontal and cingulated cortices. *Brain, 126,* 1691–1712.

Jackson, D. C., Mueller, C. J., Dolski, I., Dalton, K. M., Nitschke, J. B., Urry, H. L., et al. (2003). Now you feel it, now you don't: Frontal brain electrical asymmetry and individual differences in emotion regulation. *Psychological Science, 14,* 612–617.

Jha, S., & Patel, R. (2004). Klüver–Bucy syndrome: An experience with six cases. *Neurology India, 52,* 369–371.

Kim, J. S., & Choi-Kwon, S. (2000). Poststroke depression and emotional incontinence: Correlation with lesion location. *Neurology, 54,* 1805–1810.

Klüver, H., & Bucy, P. C. (1939). Preliminary analysis of functions of the temporal lobes in monkeys. *Archives of Neurology and Psychiatry, 42,* 979–1000.

Kolb, B., & Whishaw, I. Q. (2003). *Fundamentals of human neuropsychology*. New York: Worth.

LeDoux, J. E. (1993). Emotional networks in the brain. In M. Lewis & J. M. Haviland (Eds.), *Handbook of emotions* (pp. 109–118). New York: Guilford Press.

Levenson, R. W. (1999). The intrapersonal functions of emotion. *Cognition and Emotion*, *13*, 481–504.

Lieberman, M. D., Ochsner, K. N., Gilbert, D. T., & Schacter, D. L. (2001). Do amnesics exhibit cognitive dissonance reduction? The role of explicit memory and attention in attitude change. *Psychological Science*, *12*, 135–140.

Lilly, R., Cummings, J. L., Benson, D. F., & Frankel, M. (1983). The human Klüver–Bucy syndrome. *Neurology*, *33*, 1141–1145

Lockenhoff, C. E., & Cartensen, L. L. (2004). Socioemotional selectivity theory, aging, and health: The increasingly delicate balance between regulating emotions and making tough choices. *Journal of Personality*, *72*, 1395–1424.

MacMillan, M. B. (1986). A wonderful journey through skull and brains: The travels of Mr. Gage's tamping iron. *Brain and Cognition*, *5*, 67–107.

Mateer, C. A., & Williams, D. (1991). Effects of frontal lobe injury in childhood. *Developmental Neuropsychology*, *7*, 359–376.

Max, J. E., Robertson, B. A. M., & Lansing, A. E. (2001). The phenomenology of personality change due to traumatic brain injury in children and adolescents. *Journal of Neuropsychiatry and Clinical Neuroscience*, *31*, 161–170.

McClure, S. M., Botvinick, M. M., Young, N., Greene, J. D., & Cohen, J. D. (Chapter 10, this volume).

Ochsner, K. N., & Gross, J. J. (2007). The neural architecture of emotion regulation. In J. J. Gross (Ed.), *Handbook of emotion regulation* (pp. 87–109). New York: Guilford Press.

Ochsner, K. N., Ray, R. D., Cooper, J. C., Robertson, E. R., Chopra, S., Gabrieli, J. D. E., & Gross, J. J. (2004). For Better or for worse: Neural systems supporting the cognitive down- and up-regulation of negative emotion. *NeuroImage*, *23*, 483–499.

Paradiso, S., Chemerinski, E., Yazici, K. M., Tartaro, A., & Robinson, R. G. (1999). Frontal lobe syndrome reassessed: Comparison of patients with lateral and medial frontal brain damage. *Journal of Neurology, Neurosurgery, and Psychiatry*, *67*, 664–667.

Phan, K. L., Fitzgerald, D. A., Nathan, P. J., Moore, G. J., Uhde, T. W., & Tancer, M. E. (2005). Neural substrates for voluntary suppression of negative affect: A functional magnetic resonance imaging study. *Biological Psychiatry*, *57*, 210–219.

Pradhan, S., Singh, M. N., & Pandey, N. (1998). Klüver–Bucy syndrome in young children. *Clinical Neurology and Neurosurgery*, *100*, 254–258.

Price, B. H., Daffner, K. R., Stowe, R. M., & Marsel-Mesulam, M. (1990). The comportmental learning disabilities of early frontal lobe damage. *Brain, 113*, 1383–1393.

Quirk, G. J. (2007). Prefrontal–amygdala interactions in the regulation of fear. In J. J. Gross (Ed.), *Handbook of emotion regulation* (pp. 27–46). New York: Guilford Press.

Rahman, S., Sahakian, B. J., Cardinal, R. N., Rogers, R. D., & Robbins, T. W. (2001). Decision making and neuropsychiatry. *Trends in Cognitive Sciences*, *5*, 271–277.

Rapcsak, S. Z., Galper, S. R., Comer, J. F., Reminger, S. L., Nielsen, L., Kaszniak, A. W., Verfaellie, M., Laguna, J. F., Labiner, D. M., & Cohen, R. A. (2000). Fear recognition deficits after focal brain damage: A cautionary note. *Neurology*, *54*, 575–581.

Rinn, W. E. (1984). The neuropsychology of facial expression: A review of the neurological and psychological mechanisms for producing facial expressions. *Psychological Bulletin*, *95*, 52–77.

Roberts, N. A., Werner, K. H., Beer, J. S., Scabini, D., Levens, S., Knight, R. T., et al. (2004). The impact of orbital prefrontal cortex damage on emotional reactivity during acoustic startle. *Cognitive, Affective, and Behavioral Neuroscience*, *4*, 307–316.

Robins, R. W., & Beer, J. S. (2001). Positive illusions about the self: Short-term benefits and long-term costs. *Journal of Personality and Social Psychology*, *80*, 340–352.

Rolls, E. T., Hornak, J., Wade, D., & McGrath, J. (1994). Emotion-related learning in patients with social and emotional changes associated with frontal lobe damage. *Journal of Neurology, Neurosurgery, and Psychiatry*, *57*, 1518–1524.

Rule, R. R., Shimamura, A. P., & Knight, R. T. (2002). Orbitofrontal cortex and dynamic filtering of emotional stimuli. *Cognitive, Affective, and Behavioral Neuroscience*, *2*, 264–270.

Sanfey, A. G., Hastie, R., Colvin, M. K., & Grafman, J. (2003). Phineas gauged: Decision-making and the human prefrontal cortex. *Neuropsychologia*, *41*, 1218–1229.

Saver, J. L., & Damasio, A. R. (1991). Preserved access and processing of social knowledge in a patient with acquired sociopathy due to ventromedial frontal damage. *Neuropsychologia, 29*, 1241–1249.

Shallice, T., & Burgess, P. W. (1991). Deficits in strategy application following frontal lobe damage in man. *Brain, 114*, 727–741.

Shimamura, A. P. (2000). The role of the prefrontal cortex in dynamic filtering. *Psychobiology, 28*, 207–218.

Shiv, B., Loewenstein, G., & Bechara, A. (2005). The dark side of emotion in decision-making: When individuals with decreased emotional reactions make more advantageous decisions. *Cognitive Brain Research, 23*, 85–92.

Sprengelmeyer, R., Young, A. W., Schroeder, U., Grossenbacher, P. G., Federlein, J., Buettner, T., et al. (1999). Knowing no fear. *Philosophical Transactions of the Royal Society of London, B, Biological Sciences, 266*, 2451–2456.

Stemmer, B., Segalowitz, S. J., Witzke, W., & Schonle, P. W. (2003). Error detection with lesions to the medial prefrontal cortex: An ERP study. *Neuropsychologia, 42*, 118–130.

Stuss, D. T., & Benson, D. F. (1984). Neuropsychological studies of the frontal lobes. *Psychological Bulletin, 95*, 3–28.

Tateno, A., Jorge, R. E., & Robinson, R. G. (2004). Pathological laughing and crying following traumatic brain injury. *Journal of Neuropsychiatry and Clinical Neurosciences, 16*, 426–434.

Taylor, S. E. (1991). Asymmetrical effects of positive and negative events: The mobilization–minimization hypothesis. *Psychological Bulletin, 110*, 67–85.

Taylor, S. E., & Brown, J. D. (1994). Positive illusions and well-being revisited: Separating fact from fiction. *Psychological Bulletin, 116*, 21–27.

Thompson, R. A. (1994). Emotion regulation: A theme in search of definition. In N. A. Fox (Ed.), The development of emotion regulation: biological and behavioral considerations. *Monographs of the Society for Research in Child Development, 59*, 25–52.

Weddell, R. A., Miller, D. J., & Trevarthen, C. (1990). Voluntary emotional facial expressions in patients with focal cerebral lesions. *Neuropsychologia, 28*, 49–60.

Whalen, P. J. (1998). Fear, vigilance, and ambiguity: Initial neuroimaging studies of the human amygdala. *Current Directions in Psychological Science, 7*, 177–188.

Yoneoka, Y., Takeda, N., Inoue, A., Ibuchi, Y., Kumagai, T., Sugai, T., et al. (2004). Human Klüver–Bucy syndrome following acute subdural haematoma. *Acta Neurochirurgica, 146*, 1267–1270.

Zelazo, P. D. (2004). The development of conscious control in childhood. *Trends in Cognitive Sciences, 8*, 12–17.

Zelazo, P. D., & Cunningham, W. A. (2007). Executive function: Mechanisms underlying emotion regulation. In J. J. Gross (Ed.), *Handbook of emotion regulation* (pp. 135–158). New York: Guilford Press.

CHAPTER 5

The Neural Architecture of Emotion Regulation

KEVIN N. OCHSNER
JAMES J. GROSS

Churchill once said of Russia that it was "a riddle wrapped in a mystery inside an enigma." He could as easily have been describing the topic of emotion regulation. Emotions are nothing if not a riddle, at once substantial and fleeting and always the subject of much debate. Our capacity to regulate emotions is something of a mystery, at once ubiquitous and deeply puzzling, particularly when our ability to regulate emotion fails us. And emotion and emotion regulation involve social, psychological, and biological factors, whose interplay can be somewhat enigmatic. In this chapter, we draw on recent human neuroimaging studies to offer a framework for analyzing the neural systems that give rise to our emotion regulatory abilities.

Toward that end, our chapter is divided into five parts. The first part provides an initial working model for understanding the brain bases of emotion and cognitive control that integrates insights from both human and animal research. The second and third parts review recent functional imaging research that examines the use of two different types of cognitive control to regulate emotional responses. The fourth part uses this review to update and elaborate the initial model, and the final section explores how it can be used as a foundation for future research.

MODELS OF THE BRAIN BASES OF EMOTION AND EMOTION REGULATION

A century of animal research has examined the neural bases of emotion and emotional learning (Davidson, Fox, & Kalin, this volume; Quirk, this volume). However, it has only been in the past decade that human research has begun to examine the neural bases of our emotion regulatory abilities. As a consequence, until recently models of the brain systems involved in emotion and emotion regulation were derived from a bottom-up approach to understanding emotion that emphasizes the affective properties of stimuli and gives relatively short shrift to higher-level cognitive processes and individual differences in emotion and regulatory abilities.

The Bottom-Up Approach

The bottom-up approach characterizes emotion as a response to stimuli with intrinsic or learned reinforcing properties (e.g., Rolls, 1999). This view has roots in both common sense and academic theories of emotion that treat emotions as the inevitable consequence of perceiving specific kinds of stimuli. This view was memorably propounded by William James (1890) who wrote, "The organism is like a lock to which is matched certain parts of the environment as if they are keys. And among these 'nervous anticipations' are the emotions which are such that they are 'called forth directly by the perception of certain facts' " (p. 250).

Early nonhuman research on the brain systems involved in emotion seemed to support this view. Numerous experiments suggested that both aggressive and prosocial behaviors could be triggered by direct electrical stimulation of either subcortical brain structures, such as the hypothalamus and amygdala, or the "limbic" cortical systems with which they were connected (Cannon, 1915; Kaada, 1967; Maclean, 1955). Modern lesion and recording studies have built on these early studies by elaborating complementary roles for subcortical and cortical systems in emotional learning. For example, research has shown that the amygdala is important for learning initially which events predict the occurrence of intrinsically unpleasant stimuli (e.g., electric shock), whereas the medial and orbital frontal cortex support extinction and alteration of these stimulus–reinforcer associations (LeDoux, 2000; Quirk & Gehlert, 2003; Rolls, 1999). Taken together, both past and present nonhuman work is motivated by the view that emotions are generated by bottom-up processes that encode two kinds of associations: those between actions and the pleasant or unpleasant outcomes that are a consequence of them (as in operant conditioning) and those between stimuli and the pleasant or unpleasant responses they evoke (as in classical conditioning).

This view was echoed by the first cognitive neuroscience studies of emotion in healthy humans, which followed the advent of functional imaging research in the early 1990s. These initial studies treated emotion as a response to stimulus properties that could be perceived directly and encoded in a bottom-up fashion. Participants were simply asked to passively view, hear, smell, taste, or touch purportedly affective stimuli while brain responses were recorded in a scanner. This approach reflected the influence of successful prior nonhuman research. But it also reflected the influence on human imaging work of vision and memory research that involved passive perception of words and objects whose processing was thought to be driven by the bottom-up encoding of stimulus properties such as shape, size, and color.

Although the emotion-as-stimulus-property view was sensible given prior work, problems with this view soon became apparent as imaging studies failed to consistently confirm predictions based on studies with nonhuman populations. For example, amygdala activation in response to emotional stimuli was found inconsistently (Phan, Wager, Taylor, & Liberzon, 2002), and prefrontal systems not important in animal work were often activated in human studies (for review, see Ochsner & Gross, 2004). As described in the next section, studying emotion in humans involves something more than mapping the neural correlates of bottom-up processing of affective stimuli.

The Top-Down Approach

That something more was explained by appraisal theories of emotion. Such theories describe emotion as the product of cognitive processes that interpret the meaning of stimuli in the context of an individual's current goals, wants and needs (Scherer, Schorr, & Johnstone, 2001). A critical feature of appraisal theories is that the same stimulus can be appraised as threatening or not, or rewarding or not, depending on the circumstances. For example, seeing someone draw his fist back and prepare to strike might elicit fear or anger if appraised as aggressive but might elicit laughter if appraised as playful and harmless.

Although appraisals may be generated automatically by bottom-up processes, they may also be controlled by top-down control processes that enable one to deliberately attend to and appraise a situation in different ways. Unlike rodents and perhaps many other primates, humans possess the capacity to make conscious choices about the way they construe and respond to emotionally evocative situations. Rather than responding on the basis of automatically activated stimulus–response linkages, humans can regulate their emotions by relying on higher cognitive processes such as, selective attention, working memory, language, and long-term memory. It should be noted that for many appraisal theorists, bottom-up appraisal processes are not rigid reflexes, but flexible interpretations may be influenced by situational factors and individual differences in personality and emotion. Top-down processes do allow an individual, however, to actively control the appraisal process using various kinds of higher cognitive processes.

These higher cognitive processes have been associated with regions of lateral and medial prefrontal cortex (PFC) thought to implement processes important for regulatory control, and regions of dorsal anterior cingulate cortex (ACC) thought to monitor the extent to which control processes are achieving their desired goals (e.g., Botvinick, Braver, Barch, Carter, & Cohen, 2001; Miller & Cohen, 2001). The use of top-down control processes may help explain some of the apparent inconsistency of the early emotion imaging literature. The spontaneous use of cognitive regulatory strategies by participants is quite common in behavioral research (Erber, 1996) and may be as common in imaging studies. If participants are controlling their attention to, and appraisal of, emotionally evocative stimuli, that could explain at least some instances of PFC activity, and potentially failures to observe amygdala activity as well. This hypothesis provided a springboard for developing our working model of the cognitive control of emotion.

Integrating Bottom-Up and Top-Down Approaches

Building on prior findings and integrating previous approaches, we have formulated an initial working model of the cognitive control of emotion. According to this model, emotion generation and regulation involve the interaction of appraisal systems, such as the amygdala, that encode the affective properties of stimuli in a bottom-up fashion, with control systems implemented in prefrontal and cingulate cortex that support controlled top-down stimulus appraisals (Ochsner, Bunge, Gross, & Gabrieli, 2002; Ochsner & Gross, 2005; Ochsner et al., 2004b). It should be emphasized that the distinction between top-down and bottom-up processing is relative and not absolute. It is likely, for example, that there is a continuum along which processes can be arrayed with bottom-up and top-down as the end-point extremes. Nonetheless, this distinction serves a heuristic function for guiding thinking about the way in which different types of processes interact and combine during emotion regulation.

Our model posits that emotions can be generated and modulated either by bottom-up or top-down processes. Top-down processes can be used to place particular stimuli in the focus of attention and, in so doing, have the capacity to generate and regulate emotions by determining which stimuli have access to bottom-up processes that generate emotions. Once bottom-up generation has begun (and sometimes even before, if one anticipates a negative event), top-down processes can regulate, redirect, and alter the way in which triggering stimuli are being (or will be) appraised. Top-down processes also can initiate emotion generation directly, as beliefs, expectations, and memories guide the appraisal and interpretation of stimuli. In many cases, no external stimulus need be present—an individual can generate an emotion using top-down-generated memories of past experiences or the construction of possible future events.

Figure 5.1 illustrates the interaction between bottom-up and top-down processes in emotion generation and regulation. As shown in Figure 5.1a, the bottom-up generation of an emotional response may be triggered by the perception of stimuli with intrinsic or learned affective value. Appraisal systems such as the amygdala, ventral portions of the striatum (also known as the nucleus accumbens), and insula encode the affective properties of stimuli (Calder, Lawrence, & Young, 2001; Ochsner, Feldman, & Barrett, 2001; Phillips, Drevets, Rauch, & Lane, 2003). These systems then send outputs to hypothalamic and brainstem nuclei that control autonomic and behavioral responses, and also to cortical systems that may represent in awareness the various features of an emotional response. The top-down generation of an emotional response begins with the perception of situational cues that lead an individual either to anticipate the occurrence of a stimulus with particular kinds of emotional properties (e.g., shock) or, as shown in Figure 5.1b, to have the goal of thinking about a neutral stimulus in emotional (in this case negative) terms. At this point, an anticipatory or a manufactured emotional response may be generated. In either case, top-down beliefs alter the way in which the stimulus is appraised and subsequently experienced (e.g., leading one to experience something neutral as emotional). The top-down regulation of an emotional response is triggered by the perception (or anticipation) of an affective stimulus but transforms the initial affective appraisal through the use of cognitive control. As shown in Figure 5.1c, the active generation and application of a cognitive frame alters the way in which a stimulus is appraised. In this way, emotional responses are altered in accordance with one's current goals.

To ground this process account of emotion regulation in the brain, we have found it useful to draw on models of cognitive control in humans (e.g., Beer, Shimamura, & Knight, 2004; Miller & Cohen, 2001) and animal models of emotion (e.g., LeDoux, 2000; Quirk & Gehlert, 2003; Schultz, 2004). As illustrated in Figure 5.2, emotion regulation is thought to follow from interactions between prefrontal and cingulate systems that implement control processes and subcortical systems such as the amygdala and basal ganglia that implement various types of affective appraisal processes (Ochsner & Gross, 2004, 2005).

Five principles form the foundation of this model. The first is that emotional responses arise from interactions between multiple types of bottom-up and top-down appraisal processes, each of which may be associated with different neural systems. For example, there are debates about the putative regulatory functions of dorsal versus ventral PFC (D'Esposito, Postle, Ballard, & Lease, 1999; Roberts & Wallis, 2000) or lateral

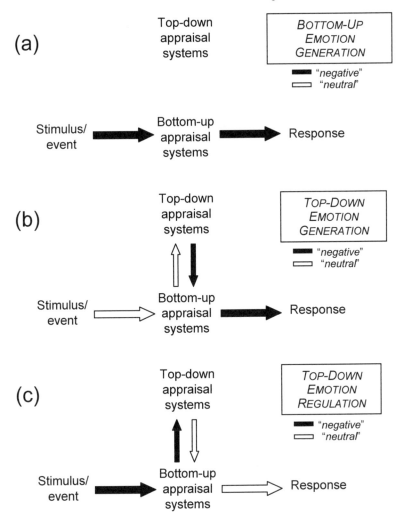

FIGURE 5.1. Schematic diagram of processes implicated in our initial model of emotion regulation. Three panels illustrate how emotional responses may evolve out of interactions between processes involved in the bottom-up and top-down generation and regulation of emotion. Although the diagram illustrates the processes involved in generating/regulating negative emotions, the processes may work in much the same way for positive emotions as well. (a) The bottom-up generation of an emotional response is triggered by the perception of stimuli with intrinsic or learned affective value. (b) In the top-down generation of an emotional response, beliefs lead one to appraise an otherwise neutral stimulus as emotionally evocative, in this case as negative. (c) In the top-down regulation of an emotional response, one actively generates and applies a cognitive frame that alters the way in which the stimulus is appraised, in this case transforming a negative appraisal into a neutral one. See text for details.

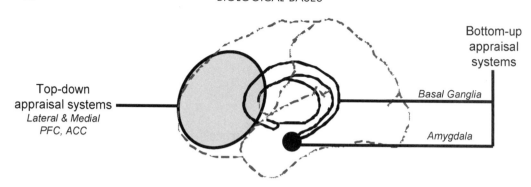

FIGURE 5.2. Schematic illustration of brain systems implicated in our initial model of emotion regulation. Each brain system shown here can be associated with a different kind of processing shown in Figure 5.1. According to this model, emotions evolve out of interactions between prefrontal and cingulate systems (not shown) that implement top-down appraisal processes, which in turn control bottom-up appraisals generated by subcortical systems like the amygdala (which may signal the affective salience of both negative and positive stimuli) and basal ganglia/ striatum (which may be particularly important for learning about rewarding stimuli). Other brain systems, such as the insula (which lies underneath the junction of the frontal and temporal lobes), also may play important roles in encoding the affective properties of stimuli but are not shown here. See text for details.

and medial orbitofrontal cortex (Elliott, Dolan, & Frith, 2000; Roberts & Wallis, 2000), and there are likely different, if overlapping, sets of neural systems implicated in primarily negative emotion (e.g., the insula), positive emotion (e.g., the basal ganglia) or both (e.g., the amygdala) (for reviews see Calder et al., 2001; Ochsner & Barrett, 2001). The second is that emotional responses are defined by their valence, degree of intensity, and potential to initiate changes across multiple response systems (Cacioppo & Berntson, 1999; Feldman Barrett, Ochsner, & Gross, in press). Third, following definitions of regulation or control in the cognitive neuroscience literature (e.g., Miller & Cohen, 2001), emotion regulation occurs when the use of goal-directed controlled processing alters one's emotional response. Importantly, this means that emotion regulation may occur in two different ways: (1) when one has the explicit goal of changing one's emotional state—as when attempting to reduce stress by actively reinterpreting an aversive situation in unemotional terms (this is known as reappraisal, as described in a following section)—and (2) when one is engaging control processes to achieve some other type of task-related goal, and emotion regulation occurs as a consequence—as when attempting to predict when a potentially painful event will occur generates anxiety in anticipation of it. Fourth, when considering how control processes may shape the appraisal process, it is important to understand what type of response (experiential, physiological, or behavioral) is being changed, in what way (whether it is to start, stop, or alter a response) and which appraisal systems are being modulated to achieve that effect. Fifth, regulatory strategies differ in the extent to which they rely on different types of control processes instantiated in different parts of PFC and ACC. An understanding of all five principles is necessary for building a model of the functional architecture supporting emotion regulation.

The remainder of this chapter uses this initial model as its starting point for organizing a review of current and potential future directions for research. Our focus is on studies that investigate *attentional deployment* or *cognitive change* (see Gross & Thompson, this volume). This focus is motivated by the facts that these two types of emotion control are quite common and to date have received the greatest amount of empirical attention. Because work on the neural bases of emotion regulation per se has only begun to appear, this review also considers studies involving the regulation of other types of valenced responses as well, including affective evaluations and motivational impulses such as pain (for discussion of relationship between different types of affective impulses, see Gross & Thompson, this volume).

ATTENTIONAL DEPLOYMENT

Attention is one of the most fundamental cognitive processes, acting as an all-purpose "gatekeeper," that allows passage of goal-relevant information for further processing. By definition, processes unaffected by attentional manipulations are deemed automatic, and those influenced by attention generate enhanced behavioral and neural responses when attention is directed toward them. Although numerous cortical and subcortical systems participate in appraising the affective properties of stimuli (see, e.g., Ochsner & Barrett, 2001), to date most cognitive neuroscience research has focused on the amygdala.

According to our model, attentional deployment in the context of emotion should work in much the same way it works in "cold" cognitive contexts. For example, directing attention to photographs of faces enhances activation in the cortical systems supporting processing of them (i.e., the fusiform face area), whereas directing attention to other stimuli decreases activation in these systems (e.g., Anderson, Christoff, Panitz, De Rosa, & Gabrieli, 2003). In the case of emotion, the question is whether directing attention to emotionally evocative stimuli influences amygdala activity. The underlying assumption of many studies is that attention should not impact the amygdala, which would suggest that its processing is automatic. Two ways in which controlled attention can be used to regulate emotion have been investigated.

Selective Attention

Selective attention can be used to select some stimuli or stimulus features for further processing while limiting the processing of other stimuli or stimulus features. For example, while in line at the airport, one's emotions can be controlled by paying attention to the smiling face and familiar voice of a traveling companion and ignoring the ranting and raving of an irate traveler standing nearby. To date, neuroimaging studies have been concerned primarily with the impact of attention on the perception of negatively valenced stimuli, which typically are faces that do not elicit strong emotional responses when presented in isolation (as has been typical in studies done to date).

Unfortunately, results have shown contradictory patterns of amygdala response when participants pay attention to the emotional features of stimuli. For example, some studies have reported amygdala activity decreases when participants pay greater attention to emotional properties of stimuli and process them with a greater degree of cognitive elaboration. Thus, amygdala activity is diminished by judging the facial expression rather than gender of fearful, angry, or happy faces (Critchley et al., 2000), matching emotional faces or scenes based on semantic labels rather than perceptual features (Hariri, Bookheimer, & Mazziotta, 2000; Lieberman, Hariri, Jarcho,

Eisenberger, & Bookheimer, 2005), viewing supra- as compared to subliminal presentations of African American faces (Cunningham, Raye, & Johnson, 2004), or rating one's
emotional response to aversive scenes rather than passively viewing them (Taylor, Phan,
Decker, & Liberzon, 2003). By contrast, other studies have found amygdala activity to
be *invariant* with respect to attention to emotional stimulus features. In these studies,
amygdala responses were unchanged when participants attended to and judged the gender of fearful faces and ignored simultaneously presented houses (Anderson et al.,
2003; Vuilleumier, Armony, Driver, & Dolan, 2001); judged the gender as compared to
expression of happy and disgust (Gorno-Tempini et al., 2001) or happy, sad, disgusted,
and fearful faces (Winston, O'Doherty, & Dolan, 2003); judged either the age or trustworthiness of normatively untrustworthy faces (Winston, Strange, O'Doherty, & Dolan,
2002); or judged whether photos showed individuals from the past or present as compared to judging whether they were good (e.g., Martin Luther King) versus bad people
(e.g., Osama bin Laden) (Cunningham, Johnson, Gatenby, Gore, & Banaji, 2003).

    Although the precise reasons for the discrepant results of these studies are not
clear, there appear to be at least three methodological possibilities. First, because most
studies seems to implicitly assume that emotion is a stimulus property that can be perceived bottom-up, like shape size or color, they failed to provide behavioral (e.g., subjective reports of experience or facial expression) or physiological measures (e.g., measures of heart rate, respiration, or skin conductance) that could be used to verify that
emotional responses were, in fact, generated. Instead, they relied only on brain activation changes to support the inference that modulation of an emotional response has
taken place, which provides little leverage for understanding why activation of an
appraisal system was or was not observed.

    Second, the studies typically used face stimuli presented in isolation, devoid of
important contextual information that may determine their emotional power. In everyday encounters, facial expressions may have the capacity to trigger emotions in large
part because of additional situational and contextual information available to a
perceiver that supports inferences about why a person is smiling (he or she is in love),
frowning (he or she failed an exam), or looks angry (I just insulted them). Behavioral
research suggests that contextual information plays a key role in determining what emotion is attributed to facial expression in the first place (Carroll & Russell, 1996), and a
recent imaging study indicates that manipulations of context can determine whether or
not a face is perceived as expressing surprise or fear, with amygdala activation evident
only if the face is perceived as expressing fear (cf. Kim, Somerville, Johnstone, Alexander, & Whalen, 2003).

    A third problem also stems from the tendency to treat emotion as a stimulus prop-
erty perceived directly like color. From this strongly bottom-up perspective, it makes
sense to examine how diminished attention impacts emotion, which essentially becomes
a form of perceptual processing. If this view of emotion is correct, then the results
reviewed previously could fail to cohere because they each used a different attentional
manipulation, each of which may impose a differing degree of (as of yet unquantified)
attentional load. However, if emotion results from an often very rapid—but partially
controllable—appraisal process, then manipulations of attention may impact not only
what perceptual features are encoded but what kinds of controlled top-down appraisal
processes are engaged (Erber, 1996). In keeping with this suggestion, Cunningham,
Raye, and Johnson (2004) found right ventral lateral activation (LPFC) when making
good/bad evaluations of attitude targets (e.g., abortion) on trials where they reported
in postscan ratings that they had exerted control. Although many of the studies

described earlier did not report PFC activations, some did report an inverse relation-ship between PFC and amygdala activity (e.g., Hariri et al., 2000; Lieberman et al., 2005; Taylor et al., 2003). This suggests that in some cases (e.g., when explicitly paying attention to emotional stimulus features), participants may be using available cognitive resources to actively reappraise stimuli. As discussed later, reappraisal is thought to involve PFC–amygdala interactions.

Attentional Distraction

Attentional distraction refers to the engagement of a secondary task that diverts attention from processing a primary target stimulus. It differs from selective attention in that it does not involve screening out unwanted distractions per se, but involves managing the competing demands of doing two things at once. Most studies using this approach have examined the impact of performing a cognitive task on responses to aversive painful stimulation. These studies avoid some of the methodological problems described ear-lier because they use a highly arousing stimulus that can elicit strong changes in multi-ple response channels, and they collect subjective reports to confirm that distraction has impacted pain experience.

Studies have shown that while experiencing painful stimulation, performing a ver-bal fluency task (Frankenstein, Richter, McIntyre, & Remy, 2001), the Stroop task (Bantick et al., 2002; Valet et al., 2004), or simply being asked to "think of something else" (Tracey et al., 2002) diminishes the aversiveness of pain and may reduce activity in cortical and subcortical pain-related regions, including mid-cingulate cortex, insula, thalamus, and periacqueductal gray. Regions of orbitofrontal cortex (OFC), medial PFC (MPFC), ACC, and dorsolateral PFC (dlPFC) may be more active during distrac-tion (Frankenstein et al., 2001; Tracey et al., 2002; Valet et al., 2004), although it is not yet clear whether these activations reflect processes supporting performance of the sec-ondary task, active attempts to regulate pain, or both. To date, no studies have attempted to address this issue directly.

Only one distraction study has used fear faces as stimuli, and it found results com-patible with the pain studies: Amygdala responses dropped when participants per-formed a line orientation judgment task (Pessoa, McKenna, Gutierrez, & Ungerleider, 2002).

Summary and Critique

Studies examining how attentional control regulates emotional responses have pro-vided mixed results. On one hand, studies of *selective attention* suggest ambiguously that paying attention to, and making judgments about, emotional stimulus features either does or does not have an impact on amygdala response. On the other hand, studies of *attentional distraction* demonstrate more consistently that responses in appraisal systems may drop when participants devote attention to performing a concurrent cognitive task. Thus, these studies do provide support for the hypothesis that prefrontal and cingulate control systems may modulate activity in appraisal systems, but this support is some-what inconsistent. In addition to the problems noted previously, because *selective atten-tion* and *attentional distraction* studies have tended to use such different kinds of stimuli—faces and photos as compared to pain—it is difficult to know how much the discrepant results are attributable to variability in the emotional responses elicited by stimuli. It will be important for future work to use comparable emotionally evocative stimuli, manipulate or measure the way in which stimuli are being appraised, and assess behavioral and physiological changes in emotional response to verify that emotion regulation has taken place.

COGNITIVE CHANGE

If attention is the "gatekeeper" for an information-processing kingdom, then our capacities for higher cognitive function are the engineers and architects that keep the kingdom functioning. Various higher cognitive abilities, such as working memory, language, and mental imagery, enable us to think about the past, plan for the future, and reason about problems more generally. As described earlier, all these abilities are thought to depend on interactions of prefrontal and cingulate control systems with posterior cortical systems that encode, represent, and store various types of perceptual information (McClure, Botvinick, Yeung, Greene, & Cohen, this volume; Zelazo & Cunningham, this volume).

In the context of emotion regulation, studies have begun to examine whether and how these control systems may modulate activity in emotional appraisal systems by enabling one to *cognitively change* the meaning of a stimulus or event. For example, one might transform anger into compassion by judging that the apparently aggressive behavior of a drunk partygoer is the unintended consequence of an attempt to drown his sorrows after receiving bad news. *Cognitive change* can be used either to generate an emotional response in the absence of an external trigger, as when one feels eagerness or anxiety in anticipation of an event, or to alter a response that was triggered by an external stimulus, as when one reinterprets the meaning of the drunken partygoer's actions. According to our model, cognitive change should depend on prefrontal and cingulate control systems that use top-down processes to modulate bottom-up activity in emotional appraisal systems such as the amygdala or striatum.

Controlled Generation

Cognitive control processes can be used to form beliefs and expectations about the emotional properties of stimuli. Four different approaches have been taken to studying how these expectations and beliefs generate emotional responses from the top down.

The first approach concerns the emotional impact of beliefs about the nature of upcoming events. If we believe that a pleasant or unpleasant event is about to occur, we may generate a pleasant or unpleasant emotion in anticipation of it. This emotion may reflect either fears or worries about the upcoming event or adaptive attempts to prepare for it. The maintenance of these pleasant or unpleasant expectations has been associated with activation of dorsal mPFC regions (Hsieh, Meyerson, & Ingvar, 1999; Knutson, Fong, Adams, Varner, & Hommer, 2001; Ploghaus et al., 1999; Porro et al., 2002) that have been implicated in making inferences about one's own or other people's emotional states (Ochsner et al., 2004a). Recruitment of MPFC during the anticipation of a pleasant or unpleasant experience may reflect beliefs about how one will feel or could feel when the expected event occurs. Also activated during anticipation are regions important for appraising the affective properties of stimuli, which might differ for positive and negative stimuli. For example, anticipating primary reinforcers that elicit pain activates regions implicated in appraising painful and aversive stimuli, including cingulate, insula, and amygdala (Hsieh et al., 1999; Jensen et al., 2003; Phelps et al.,

2001; Ploghaus et al., 1999). Similarly, anticipating either pleasant primary (e.g., a sweet taste) or secondary (e.g., money) reinforcers activates some combination of amygdala, NAcc, cingulate, insula, and/or OFC (Knutson et al., 2001; O'Doherty, Deichmann, Critchley, & Dolan, 2002). It remains to be clarified how activation of each of the systems contributes to the generation of a pleasant or unpleasant emotion. However, it is clear that anticipatory activation may reflect priming of systems to more rapidly encode expected stimulus properties, which is a function of top-down processes in vision and spatial attention (Kosslyn, Ganis, & Thompson, 2001). In some cases this priming may contribute directly to the experience of anxiety, eagerness, or other anticipatory emotions.

The second approach also concerns the emotional impact of beliefs about upcoming events but instead of examining an anticipatory interval focuses on how we respond to the stimulus when it appears. To date, this issue has been addressed only in studies of expectations about potentially painful stimuli. When participants expect a painful stimulus will be delivered but receive only a nonpainful one, they nonetheless show activation of pain-related regions of midcingulate cortex (Sawamoto et al., 2000), rostral cingulate/MPFC regions likely related to expectations about how it might feel, and medial temporal regions related to memory (Ploghaus et al., 2001).

The third approach is not concerned with expectations per se but, rather, with contrasting the use of beliefs to generate emotion in a top-down fashion with the generation of emotion via the bottom-up encoding of intrinsically affective stimuli. To date, only a single study has investigated this issue. Participants were asked either to passively perceive highly arousing aversive images—a bottom-up route to emotion generation—or to actively appraise neutral images as conveying an aversive meaning—a top-down route to emotion generation. Although both routes to emotion generation activated the amygdala, only top-down generation activated systems associated with cognitive control, such as ACC, LPFC, and MPFC (Ochsner & Gross, 2004). This suggests that appraisal systems participate in both types of emotion generation, but that higher cognitive processes come into play when generation proceeds top-down.

The fourth approach concerns appraisals of one's ability to control one's response to a stimulus. The perception that one may exert control over a situation can have an important impact on one's emotional response to it (Sapolsky, this volume). To date, only a single imaging study has investigated the neural correlates of top-down beliefs about the ability to control (Salomons, Johnstone, Backonja, & Davidson, 2004). This study found that when painful stimuli were presented, the perception one could limit the duration of pain diminished activation of systems (such as the midcingulate cortex) related to the experience of pain and controlling behavioral responses to it.

Controlled Regulation

In contrast to *controlled generation*, which concerns the initiation of an emotional response in the absence of affective cues, *controlled regulation* refers to the use of higher cognitive processes to alter or change a response triggered by a stimulus with innate or acquired emotional properties. Broadly speaking, higher cognitive processes may be used to regulate emotion in two ways—by either (1) using top-down processes to change the way one mentally describes a stimulus, which leads appraisal systems to respond to this new description, or (2) directly experiencing a change in the emotional outcomes associated with an action or stimulus event and subsequently using top-down processes to update these predictive relationships. In both cases, top-down processes change the way in which one represents the relationship between a stimulus and one's emotional response to it.

The first type of cognitive regulation is exemplified by *reappraisal*, which entails actively reinterpreting the meaning of an emotionally evocative stimulus in ways that lessen its emotional punch. Colloquially, reappraisal involves "looking on the bright side," by cognitively reframing the meaning of an aversive event in more positive terms. For instance, one can reappraise an initially sad image of a sick individual in the hospital as depicting a hearty person who is temporarily ill and soon will be well. A growing number of studies are using functional imaging to investigate the neural bases of reappraisal and in general have provided consistent results. Reappraisal activates dorsal ACC and PFC systems that presumably support the working memory, linguistic, and long-term memory processes used to select and apply reappraisal strategies. Activation of these control systems leads to decreases, increases, or sustained activity in appraisal systems such as the amygdala and/or insula in accordance with the goal of reappraisal to decrease, increase, or maintain negative affect (Beauregard, Levesque, & Bourgouin, 2001; Levesque et al., 2003; Ochsner et al., 2002, 2004b; Phan et al., 2005; Schaefer et al., 2002). Some of the variability in activation of prefrontal and appraisal systems may be attributable to differences in the types of stimuli employed, which have ranged from sexually arousing or sad film clips to disgusting and disturbing photos.

Perhaps more interestingly, some of the variability also may be attributable to differences in the kinds of reappraisal strategies used in each study. Most studies have left relatively unconstrained the way in which participants are asked to reappraise, which leaves open the possibility that different strategies depend on different types of controlled processes. To date, only a single study has investigated this possibility, by systematically instructing participants to reappraise stimuli using either a self-focused or a situation-focused reappraisal strategy to decrease negative emotion (Ochsner et al., 2004b). Self-focused reappraisal involves decreasing the sense of personal relevance of an image by becoming a detached, distant, objective observer. Situation-focused reappraisal involves reinterpreting the affects, dispositions, and outcomes of pictured persons in a more positive way. Although both strategies recruited overlapping PFC and cingulate systems, self-focused reappraisal more strongly activated MPFC whereas a situation-focused reappraisal more strongly activated LPFC. This pattern may reflect the use of systems that track the personal motivational significance of the stimulus, as compared to accessing alternative meanings for an event in memory.

The placebo effect is another form of controlled regulation that may involve mentally redescribing the meaning of a stimulus. In a typical placebo study, participants are led to believe that creams or pills will exert a regulatory effect on experience when, in fact, they contain no active drug compounds that could have an impact on bottom-up appraisal. Thus far, this has been studied only in the context of pain. Three studies have led participants to believe that placebos should blunt pain experience and have observed that stimuli elicit less pain and produce decreased activation of amygdala and pain-related cingulate, insula, and thalamic regions (Lieberman et al., 2004; Petrovic, Kalso, Petersson, & Ingvar, 2002; Wager et al., 2004). Although the precise nature of the cognitive processes mediating placebo effects is not yet clear, it is noteworthy that placebo effects are associated with activation of lateral prefrontal regions related to cognitive control and implicated in reappraisal, including ACC and right LPFC (Lieberman et al., 2004; Wager et al., 2004). This suggests that like reappraisal, placebo effects involve the active maintenance of beliefs about placebo compounds that in turn change the way in which stimuli are appraised top-down (Wager et al., 2004).

The second type of cognitive regulation concerns changes in the emotional value of a stimulus as a function of learning that associations between stimuli and emotional outcomes have changed. This work employs classical and instrumental conditioning techniques like those used in animal models of emotion. Perhaps not surprisingly, the results of the studies are very consistent with results from the animal literature. For example, as was the case for animal studies (e.g., LeDoux, 2000; Quirk & Gehlert, 2003; Rolls, 1999), instrumental avoidance of aversive stimuli (Jensen et al., 2003), extinction of classically conditioned fear responses (Gottfried & Dolan, 2004; Phelps, Delgado, Nearing, & LeDoux, 2004), and reversal of stimulus–reward associations (Cools, Clark, Owen, & Robbins, 2002; Kringelbach & Rolls, 2003; Morris & Dolan, 2004; Rogers, Andrews, Grasby, Brooks, & Robbins, 2000) depend on interactions between the amygdala, NAcc, and ventral PFC, OFC, and/or ACC. Consistent with these findings, neuropsychological studies have shown impairments of stimulus-reinforcer reversal learning in patients with lesions of ventral and orbital but not dorsolateral PFC (Fellows & Farah, 2003, 2004; Hornak et al., 2004).

Although this general pattern of interaction between control and appraisal systems has been consistent, there has been significant interstudy variability in the specific prefrontal systems activated and the particular ways in which appraisal systems are modulated. For example, amygdala activation may either drop (Phelps et al., 2004) or increase (Gottfried & Dolan, 2004) during extinction, and both striatal (Cools et al., 2002) and amygdala activation have been observed during reversal learning (Morris & Dolan, 2004). Some of these discrepancies may result from differences in the way that emotional associations initially were learned. But some discrepancies may follow from problems of methodology noted earlier for studies of attentional control. Just as many studies of attentional control failed to manipulate or measure the way in which stimuli were appraised, classical and instrumental conditioning paradigms do not control the way in which a participant appraises the meaning of a stimulus. Although this is likely not a problem when the participant is a rodent, it may very well be a problem when the participant is a human. During reversal or extinction a participant may form expectations about whether and when choosing a stimulus will lead to a reward or a conditioned stimulus (CS) will be followed by an unconditioned stimulus (US), which could involve the cognitive generation of an emotional response. In addition, in some cases participants may reappraise the meaning of undesired outcomes, such as picking the wrong stimulus during reversal or receiving an unexpected shock during extinction. These factors may influence whether or not participants use the mechanisms of classical instrumental conditioning to regulate their emotions, or whether they use the mechanisms supporting description-based reappraisal of the meaning of a stimulus. As argued in the next section, these two forms of cognitive change may depend differentially on ventral and dorsal PFC, respectively.

Summary and Critique

Studies examining the use of cognitive change consistently have demonstrated that (1) regions of lateral and medial prefrontal cortex as well as anterior cingulate are activated when participants generate or regulate emotional responses top-down, and (2) that top-down control may modulate activity in a variety of appraisal systems, including the amygdala, midcingulate cortex, and insula. These data are more consistent than the results described for studies of attentional deployment in part because cognitive change studies consistently employ strongly emotionally evocative stimuli, provide behavioral indices of emotional response, and explicitly manipulate the way in which participants appraise stimuli. That being said, there are at least two noteworthy ambiguities in this literature. First, the strategy used and the time course over which it is deployed are confounded for studies of cognitive regulation: Effects of reappraisal or placebo are studied only in the short-term, whereas the effects of reversal learning or extinction are measured over longer spans of time. In principle, both types of strategies can be employed in both the short and long term, although descriptive strategies such as reappraisal may be more easily and flexibly deployed as immediate needs arise. It remains to be seen, therefore, whether some of the differences in brain activation across the two types of studies reflect differences in training, learning, and even automaticity in the application of regulatory strategies that only emerge long term. The second ambiguity also concerns the use of strategies and the fact that even within studies examining a single type of strategy, such as reappraisal, different control systems often are activated. Part of this variability may be attributable to differences in participants and analysis, but a more important factor may be differences in the way each strategy may be implemented. Whether it is reappraisal, extinction, or reversal, there may be multiple ways in which cognitive control may achieve the goal of describing differently an emotional event or learning to place different emotional value on a given outcome. Unpacking these differences will be an important focus for future research.

SPECIFYING A FUNCTIONAL ARCHITECTURE FOR THE COGNITIVE CONTROL OF EMOTION

We began with an initial working model of the cognitive control of emotion derived from prior human and animal work. Although the preceding review supports the general model of interactions between control and appraisal systems, it also suggests some important ways in which the model can be elaborated in greater detail. Here we describe one way in which our initial model can be elaborated and acknowledge that there may be many additions and modifications to the working model that may depend on the nature of the regulatory strategy in question, emotion to be regulated, or other variables to be identified in future work.

Taken together, studies examining attentional control and cognitive change converge to suggest that two different types of systems are involved in the cognitive control of emotion (Figure 5.3). The first may be termed the top-down "description-based appraisal system" (DBAS), which consists of dorsal PFC and cingulate regions important for generating mental descriptions of one's emotional states and the emotional properties and associations of a stimulus. These descriptions re-represent nonspecific feeling states in a symbolic format that often is verbalizable. Top-down appraisals, expectations, and beliefs are composed in large part of these descriptions, which allow us to categorize the nature and kind of emotional response we are experiencing or wish to experience. The controlled generation of emotion via expectation, and the controlled regulation of emotion via reappraisal and placebo all tend to strongly recruit this system. Importantly, the DBAS has few direct reciprocal connections with (subcortical) emotional appraisal systems. As illustrated in Figure 5.3, it must influence bottom-up appraisal systems indirectly by either (1) using working memory, mental imagery, and long-term memory to generate alternative representations in perceptual appraisal systems that then send neutralizing inputs to affective appraisal systems, or (2) communicating directly with the top-down Outcome-Based Appraisal System.

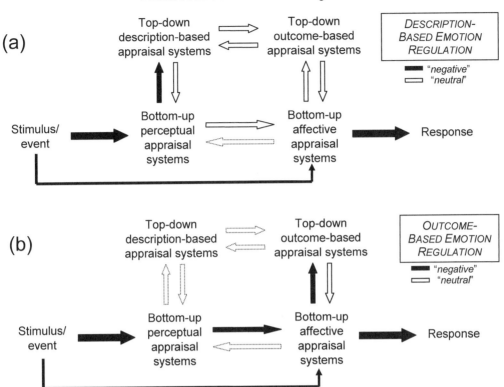

FIGURE 5.3. Schematic diagram of processes implicated in an elaborated model of emotion regulation that expands the initial model shown in Figure 5.1 based on review of the current imaging literature. This figure illustrates two different types of top-down appraisal systems that may be involved in generating and regulating emotion via interactions with multiple types of posterior cortical systems that represent different types of auditory, visual, linguistic, or spatial information. For simplicity, and because the current literature provides the strongest support for this model only in the case of emotion regulation, this figure expands only panel c of Figure 5.1 to show how each type of top-down appraisal system may be involved in emotion regulation. (a) The *top-down description-based appraisal system* consists of dorsal medial and lateral prefrontal systems important for generating mental descriptions of one's emotional states and the emotional properties and associations of a stimulus. This system is implicated in the use of controlled appraisals and reappraisals, top-down expectations, and beliefs to regulate emotion. (b) The *top-down outcome-based appraisal system* consists of orbital and ventral prefrontal regions important for learning associations between emotional outcomes and the choices or percepts that predict their occurrence. This system is implicated in the use of extinction or stimulus-reinforcer reversal learning to alter emotional associations. See text for details.

The top-down "outcome-based appraisal system" (OBAS) consists of orbitofrontal and ventral PFC and cingulate regions important for representing associations between emotional outcomes and the choices or percepts that predict their occurrence. Various types of classically conditioned and instrumental learning depend on these stimulus-reinforcer associations, which are acquired as an organism experiences the reinforcing contingencies of their environment through direct experience. The controlled regulation of emotion by extinction or stimulus-reinforcer reversal learning both tend to strongly recruit the OBAS. Figure 5.3b diagrams the direct path by which representations of alternative affective outcomes may bias appraisal systems.

Working together, the DBAS and OBAS enable us to exert various types of control over our emotional responses. Figure 5.4 illustrates the neural bases for each type of regulatory system. The DBAS supports the use of higher cognitive functions to regulate emotion, and most of our knowledge concerning its function comes from human imaging studies. By contrast, the OBAS supports the regulation of emotional responses through passive conditioning and instrumental choice, and many components of the OBAS appear to function similarly in humans and nonhuman primates and rodents. It will be important for future research to investigate how different components of each system implement different types of cognitive control processes, how these systems interact with one another, how they are involved with nonemotional forms of "cold" cognitive control, and how they come into play for the regulation of positive emotion, which has been comparatively understudied.

IMPLICATIONS FOR DEVELOPMENT, INDIVIDUAL DIFFERENCES, AND PSYCHOPATHOLOGY

According to the functional architecture we have developed in this chapter, variability in emotion regulation can be accounted for by differences in the relative strength of bottom-up emotional responses and/or in the capacity to control them using top-down processes.

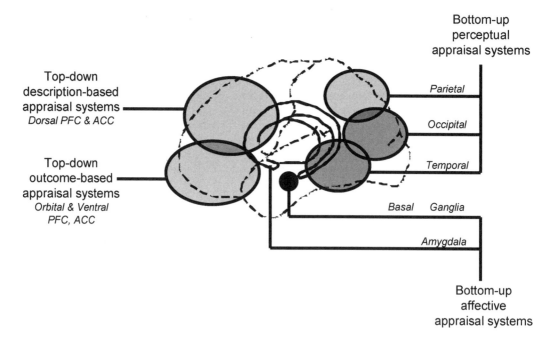

FIGURE 5.4. Schematic illustration of brain systems implicated in our elaborated model of emotion regulation. Each brain system shown here can be associated with a different kind of processing shown in Figure 5.3. This figure indicates the relative locations of the description-based appraisal system in dorsal medial and lateral prefrontal cortex, the outcome-based appraisal system in ventral and orbital prefrontal cortex, and the bottom-up perceptual and affective processing systems in posterior cortical and subcortical regions. See text for details.

Development

Developmental changes in emotion and emotion regulation across the lifespan can be analyzed in terms of differences between the strength of bottom-up emotional impulses and the top-down capacity to control them. Biological components of temperament, as well as early epigenetic influences such as quality of maternal care early in life, may exert an important influence on the ease with which negative emotional responses are generated in adulthood. For example, children at 2 years of age may be characterized as having an inhibited temperament characterized by strong and negative emotional responses to potentially threatening novel stimuli. A recent study has shown that as adults these children show greater amygdala responses to novel as compared to familiar faces (Schwartz, Wright, Shin, Kagan, & Rauch, 2003), suggesting that temperament may have an impact on responsivity in bottom-up affective appraisal systems. One's environment may shape amygdala sensitivity as well. An absence of positive social inter-actions early in life, especially those involving physical contact with caregivers, helps set a low threshold for activating the amygdala in response to potential threats that may persist throughout the lifespan (Meaney, 2001). Imaging studies have not yet investi-gated maternal shaping of the amygdala response in humans.

These and other affective predispositions may interact with the emotion regulatory norms prevalent in one's dominant culture, which may prescribe—and provide de facto training in—the use of specific kinds of emotion regulatory strategies. For example, in Asian cultures social norms dictate the regular restraint of facial expressions of emo-tion and the experience of particular social emotions, such as shame (Tsai, Levenson, & Carstensen, 2000). It is possible that these norms reflect themselves in the tendency to generate certain emotions bottom up, and the capacity to use particular top-down regu-latory strategies with greater efficacy.

The ability to implement any given regulatory strategy may initially depend on development of prefrontal regions that implement control processes. PFC is known to undergo a rapid growth spurt between the ages of 8 and 12 that continues into one's late 20s (Luna et al., 2001), and behavioral development of "cold" forms of cognitive control is known to track these structural developments (Casey, Giedd, & Thomas, 2000). This suggests that the development of emotion control may show a similar rela-tionship, although this question remains to be explored. Changes in cortical structure and function later in life may also impact the capacity to regulate emotion. It is known, for example, that older adults tend to experience a greater proportion of positive, and a smaller proportion of negative, emotions as they age (Carstensen, Isaacowitz, & Charles, 1999). It is not yet clear, however, whether these differences relate to changes in the tendency to generate positive emotions bottom-up (Mather et al., 2004) or whether they represent an enhanced ability to generate or regulate them top down.

Individual Differences

People may differ in the strength of bottom-up processing in a number of ways. Some of these are reflected in the broad personality dimensions such as extraversion and neuroticism (Barrett, 1997; Costa & McCrae, 1980). Recent imaging work suggests that these personality differences may reflect differences in the tendency to generate emotions bottom-up, as indicated by enhanced reactivity in structures such as the amygdala to positively and negatively valenced stimuli (Hamann & Canli, 2004; Kim et al., 2003).

The top-down capacity to control or shape appraisal processes also may differ across individuals in numerous ways. Some differences may derive from the knowledge an individual possesses about how and when their emotions can be regulated. These differences in emotion knowledge may be reflected in differing beliefs about whether emotions are controllable in the first place and the different strategies that may to be deployed in different circumstances. Assuming a given strategy is available, individuals may differ in their ability to implement it. One of the most important determinants of performance on "cold" cognitive control tasks is working-memory capacity (Barrett, Tugade, & Engle, 2004), and it is possible that individual differences in this capacity may determine one's ability to reappraise or distract oneself from an aversive experience. Individuals may also differ in their tendencies to use specific types of regulatory strategies, which may in turn affect their ability to regulate activation in bottom-up appraisal systems. For example, individual differences in the ability to identify and describe one's emotions may be useful for deciding how to regulate them (Barrett, Gross, Christensen, & Benvenuto, 2001), and the habitual tendency to reappraise emotional events in everyday life (as compared, for example, to suppressing one's behavioral responses to them) may affect the efficacy with which prefrontal systems implement descriptive regulatory strategies and downregulate activation in appraisal systems (Gross & John, 2003). In support of this hypothesis, we observed that individuals who tend to ruminate about negative life events, turning them over and over in their mind, showing greater ability to regulate activation of the amygdala up or down using reappraisal (Ray et al., 2005). Interestingly, this ability was not associated with differences in prefrontal activation, suggesting that ruminators may get "more affective bang for their regulatory buck" when attempting to control their emotions.

Psychopathology

One important extension of our heuristic framework for understanding the normative functional architecture for emotion control is to clinical populations suffering from various kinds of emotional disorders. More than half of the clinical disorders described in DSM-IV are characterized by emotion dysregulation. What is more, resting metabolic and structural imaging studies have suggested abnormalities in emotional appraisal and cognitive control systems in numerous disorders, ranging from depression and anxiety to posttraumatic stress disorder and sociopathy (Drevets, 2000; Rauch, Savage, Alpert, Fischman, & Jenike, 1997).

Each of these disorders may be characterized as reflecting an imbalance, or dysregulation, of interactions between bottom-up and top-down processes involved in emotion control. For example, resting brain metabolic studies of depressed individuals often show relative hyper activation of the amygdala and hypoactivation of left prefrontal cortex (Drevets, 2000). Strikingly, this pattern is the opposite of the pattern of brain activation shown when normal participants effectively downregulate negative emotion using reappraisal (Ochsner et al., 2002, 2004b). Future work may determine whether depression reflects an increased strength of bottom-up negative responses, weakened capacity to regulate these responses top down, or some combination of the two.

Bottom-up and top-down processing in depression also may differ qualitatively. Thus, depressed individuals may not differ in the strength of bottom-up, or the capacity to use top-down, processes but in the way in which they use specific kinds of top-down control to modulate negative emotion. For example, the capacity to reappraise may be normal in depression. But depressed individuals may typically use reappraisal to upregulate negative emotion using self-focused strategies rather than downregulating negative emotion using situation-focused strategies. This hypothesis is supported by a recent finding that was described earlier: Normal variability in the tendency to ruminate, which is a risk factor for depression, is associated with greater ability to upregulate and downregulate the amygdala using situation-focused reappraisal strategies (Ray et al., 2005).

CONCLUDING COMMENT

Any model of the neural architecture of emotion regulation depends on the quality of the data available to use as construction material. The preceding review highlighted a number of conceptual and methodological problems in the existing literature. With these in mind, we conclude by offering five recommendations for future research on emotion regulation.

It is important (1) to recognize that emotional responses are driven in part by the bottom-up encoding of affective stimulus properties and in part by top-down processes that can guide, shape, and alter the phase of initial stimulus-driven encoding. This means that investigators (2) should manipulate and/or measure, as much as possible, the way in which stimuli are being appraised, and not assume that emotions are driven by the passive encoding of stimulus properties. This will help track the extent to which participants spontaneously choose to regulate their emotional responses and more generally appraise stimuli in emotional versus unemotional terms. Because emotions are valenced responses that may include changes in experience, behavior, and physiology, researchers should be sure (3) to employ stimuli that elicit strong emotional responses and (4) to measure changes in one or more of these response channels to verify that emotion regulation has taken place *independent* of observed changes in brain activity. Finally, experiments (5) should be guided by a theoretical conception of the way in which specific types of cognitive control may interact with different kinds of emotional appraisal processes. For example, different types of emotionally evocative stimuli (e.g., those that elicit sadness as compared to fear) may involve different types of appraisal processes (Scherer et al., 2001), and different psychological operations may be involved when an individual uses different types of reappraisal strategies to regulate emotions generated in different stimulus contexts.

As we see it, one of the major goals for future research should be to refine our methods and our experiments in ways that will allow us to determine exactly how, when, and with the support of which brain systems we are able to effectively regulate different types of emotions.

ACKNOWLEDGMENTS

The completion of this chapter was supported by National Science Foundation Grant No. BCS-93679 and National Institute of Health Grant Nos. MH58147 and MH66957.

REFERENCES

Anderson, A. K., Christoff, K., Panitz, D., De Rosa, E., & Gabrieli, J. D. (2003). Neural correlates of the automatic processing of threat facial signals. *Journal of Neuroscience, 23*(13), 5627–5633.

Bantick, S. J., Wise, R. G., Ploghaus, A., Clare, S., Smith, S. M., & Tracey, I. (2002). Imaging how attention modulates pain in humans using functional MRI. *Brain, 125*(Pt. 2), 310–319.

Barrett, L. F. (1997). The relationships among momentary emotion experiences, personality descriptions, and retrospective ratings of emotion. *Personality and Social Psychological Bulletin, 23*(10), 1100–1110.

Barrett, L. F., Gross, J., Christensen, T. C., & Benvenuto, M. (2001). Knowing what you're feeling and knowing what to do about it: Mapping the relation between emotion differentiation and emotion regulation. *Cognition and Emotion, 15*(6), 713–724.

Barrett, L. F., Tugade, M. M., & Engle, R. W. (2004). Individual differences in working memory capacity and dual-process theories of the mind. *Psychological Bulletin, 130*(4), 553–573.

Beauregard, M., Levesque, J., & Bourgouin, P. (2001). Neural correlates of conscious self-regulation of emotion. *Journal of Neuroscience, 21*(18), RC165.

Beer, J. S., Shimamura, A. P., & Knight, R. T. (2004). Frontal lobe contributions to executive control of cognitive and social behavior. In M. S. Gazzaniga (Ed.), *The cognitive neurosciences: III* (pp. 1091–1104). Cambridge, MA: MIT Press.

Botvinick, M. M., Braver, T. S., Barch, D. M., Carter, C. S., & Cohen, J. D. (2001). Conflict monitoring and cognitive control. *Psychological Review, 108*(3), 624–652.

Cacioppo, J. T., & Berntson, G. G. (1999). The affect system: Architecture and operating characteristics. *Current Directions in Psychological Science, 8*(5), 133–137.

Calder, A. J., Lawrence, A. D., & Young, A. W. (2001). Neuropsychology of fear and loathing. *Nature Reviews Neuroscience, 2*(5), 352–363.

Cannon, W. B. (1915). *Bodily changes in pain, hunger, fear, and rage: An account of recent researches into the function of emotional excitement.* New York: Appleton.

Carroll, J. M., & Russell, J. A. (1996). Do facial expressions signal specific emotions? Judging emotion from the face in context. *Journal of Personality and Social Psychological, 70*(2), 205–218.

Carstensen, L. L., Isaacowitz, D. M., & Charles, S. T. (1999). Taking time seriously: A theory of socioemotional selectivity. *American Psychologist, 54*, 165–181.

Casey, B. J., Giedd, J. N., & Thomas, K. M. (2000). Structural and functional brain development and its relation to cognitive development. *Biological Psychiatry, 54*(1–3), 241–257.

Cools, R., Clark, L., Owen, A. M., & Robbins, T. W. (2002). Defining the neural mechanisms of probabilistic reversal learning using event-related functional magnetic resonance imaging. *Journal of Neuroscience, 22*(11), 4563–4567.

Costa, J. P. T., & McCrae, R. R. (1980). Influence of extraversion and neuroticism on subjective well-being. *Journal of Personality and Social Psychological, 38*, 668–678.

Critchley, H., Daly, E., Phillips, M., Brammer, M., Bullmore, E., Williams, S., et al. (2000). Explicit and implicit neural mechanisms for processing of social information from facial expressions: A functional magnetic resonance imaging study. *Human Brain Mapping, 9*(2), 93–105.

Cunningham, W. A., Johnson, M. K., Gatenby, J. C., Gore, J. C., & Banaji, M. R. (2003). Neural components of social evaluation. *Journal of Personality and Social Psychology, 85*, 639–649.

Cunningham, W. A., Raye, C. L., & Johnson, M. K. (2004). Implicit and explicit evaluation: fMRI correlates of valence, emotional intensity, and control in the processing of attitudes. *Journal of Cognitive Neuroscience, 16*(10), 1717–1729.

Davison, R. J., Fox, A., & Kalin, N. H. (2007). Neural bases of emotion regulation in nonhuman primates and humans. In J. J. Gross (Ed.), *Handbook of emotion regulation* (pp. 47–68). New York: Guilford Press.

D'Esposito, M., Postle, B. R., Ballard, D., & Lease, J. (1999). Maintenance versus manipulation of information held in working memory: An event-related fMRI study. *Brain and Cognition, 41*(1), 66–86.

Drevets, W. C. (2000). Neuroimaging studies of mood disorders. *Biological Psychiatry, 48*(8), 813–829.

Elliott, R., Dolan, R. J., & Frith, C. D. (2000). Dissociable functions in the medial and lateral orbitofrontal cortex: Evidence from human neuroimaging studies. *Cerebral Cortex, 10*(3), 308–317.

Erber, R. (1996). The self-regulation of moods. In L. L. Martin & A. Tesser (Eds.), *Striving and feeling: Interactions among goals, affect, and self-regulation* (pp. 251–275). Mahwah, NJ: Erlbaum.

Feldman Barrett, L., Ochsner, K. N., & Gross, J. J. (in press). Automaticity and emotion. In J. A. Bargh (Ed.), *Automatic processes in social thinking and behavior.* New York: Psychology Press.

Fellows, L. K., & Farah, M. J. (2003). Ventromedial frontal cortex mediates affective shifting in humans: evidence from a reversal learning paradigm. *Brain, 126*(Pt. 8), 1830–1837.

Fellows, L. K., & Farah, M. J. (2004). Different underlying impairments in decision-making following ventromedial and dorsolateral frontal lobe damage in humans. *Cerebral Cortex, 15*(1), 58–63.

Frankenstein, U. N., Richter, W., McIntyre, M. C., & Remy, F. (2001). Distraction modulates anterior cingulate gyrus activations during the cold pressor test. *NeuroImage, 14*(4), 827–836.

Gorno-Tempini, M. L., Pradelli, S., Serafini, M., Pagnoni, G., Baraldi, P., Porro, C., et al. (2001). Explicit and incidental facial expression processing: an fMRI study. *NeuroImage, 14*(2), 465–473.

Gottfried, J. A., & Dolan, R. J. (2004). Human orbitofrontal cortex mediates extinction learning while accessing conditioned representations of value. *Nature Neuroscience, 7*(10), 1144–1152.

Gross, J. J., & John, O. P. (2003). Individual differences in two emotion regulation processes: Implications for affect, relationships, and well-being. *Journal of Personality and Social Psychology, 85,* 348–362.

Gross, J. J., & Thompson, R. A. (2007). Emotion regulation: Conceptual foundations. In J. J. Gross (Ed.), *Handbook of emotion regulation* (pp. 3–24). New York: Guilford Press.

Hamann, S., & Canli, T. (2004). Individual differences in emotion processing. *Current Opinion in Neurobiology, 14*(2), 233–238.

Hariri, A. R., Bookheimer, S. Y., & Mazziotta, J. C. (2000). Modulating emotional responses: Effects of a neocortical network on the limbic system. *Neuroreport, 11*(1), 43–48.

Hornak, J., O'Doherty, J., Bramham, J., Rolls, E. T., Morris, R. G., Bullock, P. R., et al. (2004). Reward-related reversal learning after surgical excisions in orbito-frontal or dorsolateral prefrontal cortex in humans. *Journal of Cognitive Neuroscience, 16*(3), 463–478.

Hsieh, J. C., Meyerson, B. A., & Ingvar, M. (1999). PET study on central processing of pain in trigeminal neuropathy. *European Journal of Pain, 3*(1), 51–65.

James, W. (1890). *The principles of psychology* (Vol. 1). New York: Holt.

Jensen, J., McIntosh, A. R., Crawley, A. P., Mikulis, D. J., Remington, G., & Kapur, S. (2003). Direct activation of the ventral striatum in anticipation of aversive stimuli. *Neuron, 40*(6), 1251–1257.

Kaada, B. (1967). Brain mechanisms related to aggressive behavior. *UCLA Forum Medical Sciences, 7,* 95–133.

Kim, H., Somerville, L. H., Johnstone, T., Alexander, A. L., & Whalen, P. J. (2003). Inverse amygdala and medial prefrontal cortex responses to surprised faces. *Neuroreport, 14*(18), 2317–2322.

Knutson, B., Fong, G. W., Adams, C. M., Varner, J. L., & Hommer, D. (2001). Dissociation of reward anticipation and outcome with event-related fMRI. *Neuroreport, 12*(17), 3683–3687.

Kosslyn, S. M., Ganis, G., & Thompson, W. L. (2001). Neural foundations of imagery. *Nature Reviews Neuroscience, 2*(9), 635–642.

Kringelbach, M. L., & Rolls, E. T. (2003). Neural correlates of rapid reversal learning in a simple model of human social interaction. *NeuroImage, 20*(2), 1371–1383.

LeDoux, J. E. (2000). Emotion circuits in the brain. *Annual Review of Neuroscience, 23,* 155–184.

Levesque, J., Eugene, F., Joanette, Y., Paquette, V., Mensour, B., Beaudoin, G., et al. (2003). Neural circuitry underlying voluntary suppression of sadness. *Biological Psychiatry, 53*(6), 502–510.

Lieberman, M. D., Hariri, A., Jarcho, J. M., Eisenberger, N. I., & Bookheimer, S. Y. (2005). An fMRI investigation of race-related amygdala activity in African-American and Caucasian-American individuals. *Nature Neuroscience, 8*(6), 720–722.

Lieberman, M. D., Jarcho, J. M., Berman, S., Naliboff, B. D., Suyenobu, B. Y., Mandelkern, M., et al. (2004). The neural correlates of placebo effects: A disruption account. *NeuroImage, 22*(1), 447–455.

Luna, B., Thulborn, K. R., Munoz, D. P., Merriam, E. P., Garver, K. E., Minshew, N. J., et al. (2001). Maturation of widely distributed brain function subserves cognitive development. *NeuroImage, 13*(5), 786–793.

Maclean, P. D. (1955). The limbic system ("visceral brain") and emotional behavior. *AMA Archives of Neurological Psychiatry, 73*(2), 130–134.

Mather, M., Canli, T., English, T., Whitfield, S., Wais, P., Ochsner, K., et al. (2004). Amygdala responses to emotionally valenced stimuli in older and younger adults. *Psychological Science, 15*(4), 259–263.

McClure, S. M., Botvinick, M. M., Yeung, N., Greene, J. D., & Cohen, J. D. Conflict monitoring in cognition–emotion competition. In J. J. Gross (Ed.), *Handbook of emotion regulation* (pp. 204–226). New York: Guilford Press.

Meaney, M. J. (2001). Maternal care, gene expression, and the transmission of individual differences in stress reactivity across generations. *Annual Review of Neuroscience, 24,* 1161–1192.

Miller, E. K., & Cohen, J. D. (2001). An integrative theory of prefrontal cortex function. *Annual Review of Neuroscience, 24,* 167–202.

Morris, J. S., & Dolan, R. J. (2004). Dissociable amygdala and orbitofrontal responses during reversal fear conditioning. *NeuroImage, 22*(1), 372–380.

O'Doherty, J. P., Deichmann, R., Critchley, H. D., & Dolan, R. J. (2002). Neural responses during anticipation of a primary taste reward. *Neuron, 33*(5), 815–826.

Ochsner, K. N., & Barrett, L. F. (2001). A multiprocess perspective on the neuroscience of emotion. In T. J. Mayne & G. A. Bonanno (Eds.), *Emotions: Currrent issues and future directions* (pp. 38–81). New York: Guilford Press.

Ochsner, K. N., Bunge, S. A., Gross, J. J., & Gabrieli, J. D. (2002). Rethinking feelings: An fMRI study of the cognitive regulation of emotion. *Journal of Cognitive Neuroscience, 14*(8), 1215–1229.

Ochsner, K. N., & Gross, J. J. (2004). Thinking makes it so: A social cognitive neuroscience approach to emotion regulation. In R. F. Baumeister & K. D. Vohs (Eds.), *Handbook of self-regulation: Research, theory, and applications* (pp. 229–255). New York: Guilford Press.

Ochsner, K. N., & Gross, J. J. (2005). The cognitive control of emotion. *Trends in Cognitive Sciences, 9*(5), 242–249.

Ochsner, K. N., Knierim, K., Ludlow, D., Hanelin, J., Ramachandran, T., & Mackey, S. (2004a). Reflecting on feelings: An fMRI study of neural systems supporting the attribution of emotion to self and other. *Journal of Cognitive Neuroscience, 16*(10), 1746–1772.

Ochsner, K. N., Ray, R. D., Cooper, J. C., Robertson, E. R., Chopra, S., Gabrieli, J. D. E., et al. (2004b). For better or for worse: Neural systems supporting the cognitive down- and up-regulation of negative emotion. *NeuroImage, 23*(2), 483–499.

Pessoa, L., McKenna, M., Gutierrez, E., & Ungerleider, L. G. (2002). Neural processing of emotional faces requires attention. *Proceedings of the National Academy of Sciences, USA, 99*(17), 11458–11463.

Petrovic, P., Kalso, E., Petersson, K. M., & Ingvar, M. (2002). Placebo and opioid analgesia—Imaging a shared neuronal network. *Science, 295*(5560), 1737–1740.

Phan, K. L., Fitzgerald, D. A., Nathan, P. J., Moore, G. J., Uhde, T. W., & Tancer, M. E. (2005). Neural substrates for voluntary suppression of negative affect: A functional magnetic resonance imaging study. *Biological Psychiatry, 57*(3), 210–219.

Phan, K. L., Wager, T., Taylor, S. F., & Liberzon, I. (2002). Functional neuroanatomy of emotion: A meta-analysis of emotion activation studies in PET and fMRI. *NeuroImage, 16*(2), 331–348.

Phelps, E. A., Delgado, M. R., Nearing, K. I., & LeDoux, J. E. (2004). Extinction learning in humans: Role of the amygdala and vmPFC. *Neuron, 43*(6), 897–905.

Phelps, E. A., O'Connor, K. J., Gatenby, J. C., Gore, J. C., Grillon, C., & Davis, M. (2001). Activation of the left amygdala to a cognitive representation of fear. *Nature Neuroscience, 4*(4), 437–441.

Phillips, M. L., Drevets, W. C., Rauch, S. L., & Lane, R. (2003). Neurobiology of emotion perception I: The neural basis of normal emotion perception. *Biological Psychiatry, 54*(5), 504–514.

Ploghaus, A., Narain, C., Beckmann, C. F., Clare, S., Bantick, S., Wise, R., et al. (2001). Exacerbation of pain by anxiety is associated with activity in a hippocampal network. *Journal of Neuroscience, 21*(24), 9896–9903.

Ploghaus, A., Tracey, I., Gati, J. S., Clare, S., Menon, R. S., Matthews, P. M., et al. (1999). Dissociating pain from its anticipation in the human brain. *Science, 284*(5422), 1979–1981.

Porro, C. A., Baraldi, P., Pagnoni, G., Serafini, M., Facchin, P., Maieron, M., et al. (2002). Does anticipation of pain affect cortical nociceptive systems? *Journal of Neuroscience, 22*(8), 3206–3214.

Quirk, G. J. (2007). Prefrontal–amygdala interactions in the regulation of fear. In J. J. Gross (Ed.), *Handbook of emotion regulation* (pp. 27–46). New York: Guilford Press.

Quirk, G. J., & Gehlert, D. R. (2003). Inhibition of the amygdala: Key to pathological states? In P. Shinnick-Gallagher & A. Pitkänen (Eds.), *The amygdala in brain function: Basic and clinical approaches* (Vol. 985, pp. 263–325). New York: New York Academy of Sciences.

Rauch, S. L., Savage, C. R., Alpert, N. M., Fischman, A. J., & Jenike, M. A. (1997). The functional neuroanatomy of anxiety: A study of three disorders using positron emission tomography and symptom provocation. *Biological Psychiatry, 42*(6), 446–452.

Ray, R. D., Ochsner, K. N., Cooper, J. C., Robertson, E. R., Gabrieli, J. D. E., & Gross, J. J. (2005). Individual differences in trait rumination modulate neural systems supporting the cognitive regulation of emotion. *Cognitive, Affective, and Behavioral Neuroscience, 5*(2), 156–168.

Roberts, A. C., & Wallis, J. D. (2000). Inhibitory control and affective processing in the prefrontal cortex: Neuropsychological studies in the common marmoset. *Cerebral Cortex, 10*(3), 252–262.

Rogers, R. D., Andrews, T. C., Grasby, P. M., Brooks, D. J., & Robbins, T. W. (2000). Contrasting cortical and subcortical activations produced by attentional-set shifting and reversal learning in humans. *Journal of Cognitive Neuroscience, 12*(1), 142–162.

Rolls, E. T. (1999). *The brain and emotion.* Oxford, UK: Oxford University Press.

Salomons, T. V., Johnstone, T., Backonja, M. M., & Davidson, R. J. (2004). Perceived controllability modulates the neural response to pain. *Journal of Neuroscience, 24*(32), 7199–7203.

Sapolsky, R. M. (2007). Stress, stress-related disease, and emotional regulation. In J. J. Gross (Ed.), *Handbook of emotion regulation* (pp. 606–615). New York: Guilford Press.

Sawamoto, N., Honda, M., Okada, T., Hanakawa, T., Kanda, M., Fukuyama, H., et al. (2000). Expectation of pain enhances responses to nonpainful somatosensory stimulation in the anterior cingulate cortex and parietal operculum/posterior insula: An event-related functional magnetic resonance imaging study. *Journal of Neuroscience, 20*(19), 7438–7445.

Schaefer, S. M., Jackson, D. C., Davidson, R. J., Aguirre, G. K., Kimberg, D. Y., & Thompson-Schill, S. L. (2002). Modulation of amygdalar activity by the conscious regulation of negative emotion. *Journal of Cognitive Neuroscience, 14*(6), 913–921.

Scherer, K. R., Schorr, A., & Johnstone, T. (Eds.). (2001). *Appraisal processes in emotion: Theory, methods, research.* New York: Oxford University Press.

Schultz, W. (2004). Neural coding of basic reward terms of animal learning theory, game theory, microeconomics and behavioural ecology. *Current Opinion in Neurobiology, 14*(2), 139–147.

Schwartz, C. E., Wright, C. I., Shin, L. M., Kagan, J., & Rauch, S. L. (2003). Inhibited and uninhibited infants "grown up": Adult amygdalar response to novelty. *Science, 300*(5627), 1952–1953.

Taylor, S. F., Phan, K. L., Decker, L. R., & Liberzon, I. (2003). Subjective rating of emotionally salient stimuli modulates neural activity. *NeuroImage, 18*(3), 650–659.

Tracey, I., Ploghaus, A., Gati, J. S., Clare, S., Smith, S., Menon, R. S., et al. (2002). Imaging attentional modulation of pain in the periaqueductal gray in humans. *Journal of Neuroscience, 22*(7), 2748–2752.

Tsai, J. L., Levenson, R. W., & Carstensen, L. L. (2000). Autonomic, subjective, and expressive responses to emotional films in older and younger Chinese Americans and European Americans. *Psychology and Aging, 15*(4), 684–693.

Valet, M., Sprenger, T., Boecker, H., Willoch, F., Rummeny, E., Conrad, B., et al. (2004). Distraction modulates connectivity of the cingulo-frontal cortex and the midbrain during pain—An fMRI analysis. *Pain, 109*(3), 399–408.

Vuilleumier, P., Armony, J. L., Driver, J., & Dolan, R. J. (2001). Effects of attention and emotion on face processing in the human brain: An event-related fMRI study. *Neuron, 30*(3), 829–841.

Wager, T. D., Rilling, J. K., Smith, E. E., Sokolik, A., Casey, K. L., Davidson, R. J., et al. (2004). Placebo-induced changes in fMRI in the anticipation and experience of pain. *Science, 303*(5661), 1162–1167.

Winston, J. S., O'Doherty, J., & Dolan, R. J. (2003). Common and distinct neural responses during direct and incidental processing of multiple facial emotions. *NeuroImage, 20*(1), 84–97.

Winston, J. S., Strange, B. A., O'Doherty, J., & Dolan, R. J. (2002). Automatic and intentional brain responses during evaluation of trustworthiness of faces. *Nature Neuroscience, 5*(3), 277–283.

Zelazo, P. D., & Cunningham, W. A. (2007). Executive function: Mechanisms underlying emotion regulation. In J. J. Gross (Ed.), *Handbook of emotion regulation* (pp. 135–158). New York: Guilford Press.

CHAPTER 6

Genetics of Emotion Regulation

AHMAD R. HARIRI
ERIKA E. FORBES

Identifying the biological underpinnings that contribute to brain structure and complex cognitive and emotional behaviors is paramount to our understanding of how individual differences in these behaviours emerge and how such differences may confer vulnerability to neuropsychiatric disorders. Advances in both molecular genetics and noninvasive neuroimaging have provided us with the tools necessary to address these questions on an increasingly sophisticated level (Hariri & Weinberger, 2003b). With completion of a rough draft of the reference human genome sequence, a major effort is under way to identify common variations in this sequence that impact on gene function and subsequently to understand how such functional variations alter human biology.

Genetics approaches have now been applied to several topics germane to the biological bases of emotion regulation. For the purposes of the current chapter, our working definition deserves mention. We conceptualize emotion regulation as including both lower-level (e.g., autonomic and subcortical), automatic processes and higher-level, cognitive processes. We see emotion regulation as involving the enhancement of emotions as well as the reduction of emotions, and we have applied it to the experience and expression of positive emotions as well as negative emotions (Forbes & Dahl, 2005). We approach emotion regulation in terms of the brain regions and circuits likely to contribute to both reactivity and regulation, with multiple brain regions contributing to an emotion regulation response. The role of genes in emotion regulation, then, is inextricably linked to the implications of several gene systems for brain function.

Because approximately 70% of all genes are expressed in the brain, many of these functional gene variations will account for interindividual variability of brain structure and function. A variety of neuroimaging methods have the capacity to assay gene function in the brain. These methods are complementary with regard to their ability to characterize different aspects of brain structure and function and currently include structural magnetic resonance imaging (MRI), functional magnetic resonance imaging (fMRI), positron emission tomography (PET), single photon emission tomography (SPECT) as well as the two related techniques electroencephalography (EEG) and magnetoencephalography (MEG). In the near future, this list of tools will probably be extended by additional imaging methods such as diffusion tensor imaging (DTI) or magnetic resonance spectroscopy (MRS).

In this chapter, we (1) describe the conceptual basis for, and potential of, using neuroimaging in human genetics research; (2) propose guiding principles for the implementation and advancement of this research strategy; and (3) highlight recent studies that exemplify these principles. As a first step, we consider behavior association studies relevant to the genetics of emotion regulation in healthy and clinical populations. These studies, with their challenges and limitations, provide a foundation for the imaging genetics approach, which aims to examine mechanisms leading to individual variability in emotion regulation that is more proximal to genetic factors.

BEHAVIOR GENETICS

Why Study Genes?

Genes represent the "go square" on the monopoly board of life. They are the biological toolbox with which one negotiates the environment. While most human behaviors including emotion regulation cannot be explained by genes alone, and certainly much variance in aspects of brain information processing will not be genetically determined, variations in genetic sequence that impact gene function will contribute some variance to these more complex phenomena. This conclusion is implicit in the results of studies of twins, which have revealed heritabilities of from 40 to 70% for various aspects of cognition, temperament, and personality (McGuffin, Riley, & Plomin, 2001).

Our proposed approach to understanding the nature of individual differences in emotion regulation revolves around genes because these constructs have an unparalleled potential impact on all levels of biology. In the context of disease states, particularly behavioral disorders, genes not only transcend phenomenological diagnosis but represent mechanisms of disease. Moreover, genes offer the potential to identify at-risk individuals and biological pathways for the development of new treatments. In the case of psychiatric illness, genes appear to be the only consistent risk factors that have been identified across populations and the lion's share of susceptibility to major psychiatric disorders is accounted for by inheritance (Moldin & Gottesman, 1997). While the strategy for finding susceptibility genes for complex disorders, by traditional linkage and association methods, may seem relatively straightforward (albeit not easily achieved), developing a useful and comprehensive understanding of the mechanisms by which such genes increase biological risk is a much more daunting challenge. How many genes contribute to a particular complex behavior or complex disease state? What genetic overlap exists across behaviors and diseases? How large are the effects of candidate genes on particular brain functions? And, perhaps most important, how does a gene affect brain information processing to increase risk for a disorder of behavior?

Traditional Association Studies

The "candidate gene association approach" has been a particularly popular strategy for attempting to answer these questions. Genetic association is a test of a relationship between a particular phenotype and a specific allele of a gene. This approach usually begins with selecting a biological aspect of a particular condition or disease, then identifying variants in genes thought to have an impact on the candidate biological process, and next searching for evidence that the frequency of a particular variant ("allele") is increased in populations having the disease or condition. A significant increase in allele frequency in the selected population is evidence of association. When a particular allele is significantly associated with a particular phenotype, it is potentially a causative factor in determining that phenotype. There are caveats to the design and interpretation of genetic association studies, such as linkage disequilibrium with other loci and ancestral stratification, that are beyond the scope of this review and have been discussed at length elsewhere (Emahazion et al., 2001).

A starting point for personality or psychiatric genetics is the findings of genetic influence through traditional behavioral genetics studies such as twin studies. By comparing the similarity of monozygotic and dizygotic twins on individual-differences variables such as extraversion, such studies examine the extent to which variability is due to heritable (i.e., genetic) factors or to environmental factors. These studies indicate that genetic influences shape personality traits and do so across the lifespan (Nigg & Goldsmith, 1998; Plomin & Nesselroade, 1990; Rutter & Plomin, 1997; Viken, Rose, Kaprio, & Koskenvuo, 1994).

From these broad estimates of heritability stem more circumscribed association studies of personality attempting to identify relationships between specific allelic variants or genotypes of distinct genes and personality or temperament factors. These studies, which take a molecular genetics approach, identify candidate genes of interest and examine their relation to a phenotype. The candidate genes included in these studies are typically those related to the patterns of brain function that putatively underlie personality style.

Association Studies of Genes Involved in Emotion Regulation

Behavioral and molecular genetics approaches have not been applied to questions of particular emotion regulation responses as defined in studies of behavior or physiology. For instance, it would be a stretch to examine the behavioral, cognitive, or physiological components of the emotion regulation strategy of situation modification in relation to a specific gene variant. Instead, typical research in genetics has addressed the association between genes and proxy variables for emotion regulation. These proxy variables represent broad individual differences in emotional style or tendency and have generally been in the areas of personality or affective disorders. While these variables are related to emotion regulation constructs, they are more broad and heterogeneous.

Behavioral and molecular genetics approaches have been applied to two topics that are relevant to stable emotion regulatory style: personality and affective disorders. Personality refers to stable normal individual differences, many of which pertain to emotional experience and expression. Affective disorders, while more in the realm of abnormal emotional experience, can be considered examples of pathological emotion dysregulation. These disorders—which include intense and long-duration depressed, manic, or anxious emotional states—involve reduced emotional flexibility. Presumably, difficulty with modulating the frequency, intensity, or duration of affective states underlies these disorders. For example, depression is characterized by sustained sadness and unusually low-frequency, low-intensity positive affect. The genes that predispose people to experience the disorders therefore may constitute genetic influences on effective, healthy emotion regulation.

Molecular genetics approaches to emotion regulation often focus on polymorphisms leading to variability in neurotransmitter availability or neurotransmitter receptor function. For example, extraversion's characteristics of dominance, novelty seeking, and reward sensitivity are thought to be driven by variability in function of the dopamine (DA) system. There are many neurotransmitter systems, each of which has complex function and influence on brain and behavior. In addition, the influence of the various neurotransmitter systems on emotion regulation is presumably complex and interrelated. Research on the association between neurotransmitter genes and emotion regulation-related characteristics has focused on narrow aspects of specific neurotransmitter systems. Two particular systems appear to be especially relevant to questions of emotion regulation, however: the serotonin (5-HT) system, and the DA system. 5-HT has been implicated in the generation and regulation of emotional behavior (Lucki, 1998), and manipulation of 5-HT activity has effects on behaviors such as impulsivity and aggression (Manuck et al., 1999). The DA system plays a critical role in reward processing and has been linked to normal individual differences in reward traits (Depue & Collins, 1999) as well as to disorders involving enhanced reward-seeking such as addiction (Kalivas & Volkow, 2005).

We address both neurotransmitter systems in our review of association studies that follows, and we focus specifically on the 5-HT system in our discussion of imaging genetics in the remainder of the chapter. In addition, while we address genetic factors in both normal and abnormal individual differences in the review of association studies, we emphasize normal individual differences in our treatment of imaging genetics. As we explain later, the conceptual foundation for imaging genetics lends itself best to first examining normal variability in neural function.

Personality

We do not provide additional details on definitional issues on personality because those have been covered in another chapter of this volume (John & Gross, this volume). We refer to that chapter both for a description of personality and for the claim that each personality factor in the five-factor model potentially involves a style of emotion regulation. Extraversion, for example, is likely to involve an approach toward goals despite setbacks and assertion that serves to modify a current situation.

Consequently, studies of the genetic underpinnings of extraversion have focused on polymorphisms related to DA function (Ebstein, Zohar, Benjamin, & Belmaker, 2002; Noblett & Coccaro, 2005). Specifically, genetic variants of DA receptor subtypes, such as the D2 and D4 receptors, which mediate the myriad neuromodulatory effects of DA, as well as the dopamine transporter, which facilitates the active reuptake of DA from the extracellular space, have been examined in relation to the broad trait of extraversion and to one of its facets, novelty seeking. More recently, studies have begun to examine other genes that influence broader DA and other catecholamine availability, including catechol-O-methyltransferase (COMT) and monoamine oxidase A (MAOA). As recent reviews and meta-analyses have noted, the associations between specific DA polymorphisms and complex measures of personality have been inconsistent across studies, with null findings relatively common (Ebstein, 2006; Schinka, Letsch, & Crawford, 2002; Strobel, Spinathm Angkitner, Reimann, & Lesch, 2003).

Another significant line of related research from the field of personality genetics is the examination of 5-HT subsystem polymorphisms on negative emotional behaviors such as neuroticism, impulsivity, and aggression. A gene of particular interest has been a relatively frequent length variant in the promoter or regulatory region of the 5-HT transporter (5-HTT) gene. Numerous studies have indicated that the short variant of this gene, resulting in relatively reduced 5-HTT availability, is associated with higher levels of temperamental anxiety. Other investigators have established links between variation in 5-HT genes controlling biosynthesis, receptor function, and metabolic degradation with additional dimensional measures of negative emotionality such as impulsive aggression (Manuck et al., 1999; Manuck, Flory, Ferrell, Mann, & Muldoon, 2000) and suicidality (Bellivier, Chaste, & Malafosse, 2004). Despite some replication, these lines of investigation have also been marked by null findings (Glatt & Freimer, 2002), with several reports, including meta-analyses, emphasizing that the ability to detect associations depends on the personality instruments used, with "broad bandwidth" personality measures (e.g., extraversion) typically representing constructs that are too heterogeneous to map meaningfully onto biological systems (Munafo, Clark, & Flint, 2005).

Affective Disorders

The leap from studies of genetic influences on dimensional indices of normal variability in personality and temperament to studies of genetic influences on affective disorders such as depression and anxiety is understandable given the correlation of these indices with symptoms of these disorders and the genetic influences on such correlations (Carey & DiLalla, 1994). For example, depression and the personality trait of neuroticism appear to share genetic influence, and in addition, the correlation between depression and neuroticism appears to be influenced by genetic factors (Kendler, Neale, Kessler, Heath, & Eaves, 1993). Such attempts to link polymorphisms directly with clinical syndromes has been fueled by the suggestion that genes might have a more detectable influence at extreme, pathological ends of the emotional trait distribution. While any specific gene in isolation is unlikely to serve as a predisposition to a complex disorder such as major depressive disorder, the influence of a particular gene is more likely to be detected in a clinical population than in individuals with lower levels of the emotional dysfunction involved in the disorder. If neuroticism and depression share genetic influence (Kendler et al., 1993), and if depression can be seen as an extreme version of high neuroticism, then influences of 5-HT polymorphisms, for instance, may be more clear when depression is the target construct.

Studies of genetic influences on depression and anxiety in humans have emphasized the role of genes related to 5-HT and hypothalamic–pituitary–adrenal (HPA) axis function (see Leonardo & Hen, 2006, for a more thorough review). Both the 5-HT and HPA systems play a critical role in emotional reactivity and regulation and are thus prime candidates for studies of these mood disorders. Many candidate polymorphisms in these systems have been linked to increased risk for mood disorders. Moreover, the existence of an association has been demonstrated to be moderated by the environment. In particular, social stress, such as maltreatment during childhood or divorce in adulthood, appears to unmask genetic vulnerability for depression and anxiety.

Limitations of Behavioral Association Studies

All the findings from traditional behavioral association studies have been inconsistent, with an impressive amount of null findings for each gene studied. In many ways, this underscores the argument that in the context of behavior and psychiatric illness there are only susceptibility genes and not disease genes, which clearly and specifically determine affective disorders. Association studies have important limitations, not the least of which is the long chain of events from gene function to personality or psychiatric disorder. Additional limitations include the specificity of findings to particular personality instruments, the reliance on self-report rather than observed behavior, the failure to account for developmental effects, and the difficulties of defining and examining gene-by-environment effects.

IMAGING GENETICS

Overview

Because genes are directly involved in the development and function of brain regions subserving specific cognitive and emotional processes, functional polymorphisms in genes may be strongly related to the function of these specific neural systems, and in turn, mediate/moderate their involvement in behavioral outcomes. This is the underlying assumption of our investigations examining the relation between genes and neural systems, what we initially called imaging genomics (Hariri & Weinberger, 2003b) and more recently describe as "imaging genetics" (Hariri et al., 2006), because this approach is used to explore variation in specific genes and not the genome broadly. The potential for marked differences at the neurobiological level underscores the need for a direct assay of brain function. Accordingly, imaging genetics within the context of a "candidate gene association approach" provides an ideal opportunity to further our understanding of biological mechanisms potentially contributing to individual differences in behavior and personality. Moreover, imaging genetics provides a unique tool with which to explore and evaluate the functional impact of brain-relevant genetic polymorphisms with the potential to understand their impact on behavior. Of course, the relevance of imaging genetics findings for disease vulnerability will only be made once the variants under study are further associated with disease risk directly or if their impact on brain function is manifest (or even exaggerated) in the diseases of interest.

Why Functional Neuroimaging?

Traditionally, the impact of genetic polymorphisms on human behavior has been examined using indirect assays such as personality questionnaires and neuropsychological batteries. While a few such studies have reported significant associations between specific genetic polymorphisms and behaviors, their collective results have been weak and inconsistent (Malhotra & Goldman, 1999). This is not surprising given the considerable individual variability and subjectivity of such behavioral measures. Because such behavioral assays are vague and imprecise, it has been necessary to use very large samples, often exceeding several hundred subjects, to identify even small gene effects (Glatt & Freimer, 2002). In addition, behavioral probes and neuropsychological tests allow for the use of alternative task strategies by different individuals that may obscure potential gene effects on the underlying neural substrates meant to be engaged by the tests.

Because the response of brain regions subserving specific cognitive and emotional processes may be more objectively measurable than the subjective experience of these same processes, functional genetic polymorphisms may have a more robust impact at the level of brain than at the level of behavior. Thus, functional polymorphisms in genes weakly related to behaviors and, in an extended fashion, psychiatric syndromes may be strongly related to the function of neural systems involved in processing cognitive and emotional information in brain. This is the underlying assumption of imaging genetics. The potential for marked differences at the neurobiological level in the absence of significant differences in behavioral measures underscores the need for a direct assay of brain function. Accordingly, imaging genetics provides a unique opportunity to explore and evaluate the functional impact of brain-relevant genetic polymorphisms potentially more incisively and with greater sensitivity than existing behavioral assays.

Functional neuroimaging techniques, especially those that are noninvasive like fMRI, typically require no more than a few minutes of subject participation to acquire substantial data sets, reflecting the acquisition of many hundreds of repeated measures of brain function within a single subject. This is analogous to the signal detection power of EEG and MEG approaches, which also have been used to identify physiologic signals that are highly heritable (Vogel, Schalt, Kruger, Propping, & Lehnert, 1979). Thus, these techniques, in contrast to their behavioral counterparts, may require considerably fewer subjects (tens vs. hundreds) to identify significant gene effects on the response characteristics of the brain. Moreover, the efficiency of these techniques allows for the ability to investigate the specificity of gene effects by examining their influence on multiple functional systems (e.g., prefrontal, striatal, and limbic) in a single subject in one experimental session. This capacity to rapidly assay differences in the brain responses of different information-processing systems with enhanced power and sensitivity places functional neuroimaging at the forefront of available tools for the *in vivo* study of functional genetic variation.

Imaging Genetics: Three Basic Principles

Selection of Candidate Gene

Ideally, the application of functional neuroimaging techniques to the study of genetic effects should start where studying gene effects on behavior would also start (i.e., from well-defined functional polymorphisms, such as those reported for apolipoprotein E (APOE), COMT, brain-derived neurotrophic factor (BDNF) and 5-HTT. Because the genetic variation in such genes has been associated with specific physiological effects at the cellular level and their impact has been described in distinct brain regions and circuits, imaging paradigms can be developed to explore their effects on local information processing in both normal and impaired populations.

Short of well-defined functional polymorphisms, candidate genes with identified single nucleotide polymorphisms (SNPs) or other allele variants in coding or promoter regions with likely functional implications (e.g., nonconservative amino acid substitution or missense mutation in a promoter consensus sequence) involving circumscribed neuroanatomical systems would also be attractive substrates for imaging genetics. The investigation of genes and variations without well-established functional implications in brain, however, necessarily requires greater caution not only in the design of imaging tasks but also in the interpretation of differential brain responses. Recent imaging genetics studies, however, have taken the lead in exploring the functionality of candidate variants by first describing *in vivo* effects at the level of brain systems (Brown et al., 2005). As such, imaging genetics can provide the initial impetus for further characterization of molecular and functional effects of specific candidate genes in brain systems thought to be involved in behavior. In this manner, the contributions of abnormalities in these systems to complex behaviors and emergent phenomena, possibly including psychiatric syndromes, can then be understood from the perspective of their biological origins.

Control for Nongenetic Factors

The contribution of single genes to the response characteristics of brain systems, while putatively more substantial than that to emergent behavioral phenomena, is still presumably small. Furthermore, typically large effects of age, gender, and IQ as well as environmental factors such as illness, injury, or substance abuse on phenotypic variance can easily obscure these small potential gene effects. Because association studies in imaging genetics are susceptible to population stratification artifacts, as in any case-control association study, ethnic matching within genotype groups is also potentially critical. Thus, the identification and contribution of genetic variation to specific phenotypes should be limited to studies in which other potential contributing and confounding factors are carefully matched across genotype groups. If the imaging protocol involves performance of a task, the groups should also be matched for level of performance, or, at least, any variability in performance should be considered in the analysis and interpretation of the imaging data. This is because task performance and imaging responses are linked *pari passu*, and systematic differences in performance between genotype groups could either obscure a true gene effect or masquerade for one.

Task Selection

The last five years have been witness to a tremendous proliferation of functional neuroimaging studies and, with them, behavioral tasks designed specifically for this experimental setting. Many of these are modified versions of classic behavioral and neuropsychological tests (e.g., the Wisconsin Card Sorting Task; Axelrod, 2002) designed to tap neural systems critical to particular behaviors. More recent paradigms have emerged that focus on interactions of specific behaviors and disease states as these questions have become newly accessible with noninvasive imaging (e.g., the emotion Stroop and obsessive–compulsive disorder; Whalen et al., 1998).

Because of the relatively small effects of single genes, even after having controlled for nongenetic and other confounder variables, imaging tasks must maximize sensitivity and inferential value. As the interpretation of potential gene effects depends on the validity of the information processing paradigm, it is best to select well-characterized paradigms that are effective at engaging circumscribed brain regions and systems, produce robust signals in every individual, and show variance across individuals (see below). In short, imaging genetics studies are probably not the appropriate venue to design and test new functional tasks, and to do so might undermine their tremendous potential.

5-HT AND THE GENETICS OF EMOTION REGULATION

Overview

Converging evidence from animal and human studies has revealed that 5-HT is a critical neuromodulator in the generation and regulation of emotional behavior (Lucki, 1998). Serotonergic neurotransmission has also been an efficacious target for the pharmacological treatment of mood disorders including depression, obsessive–compulsive disorder, anxiety, and panic (Blier & de Montigny, 1999). Moreover, genetic variation in several key 5-HT subsystems, presumably resulting in altered central serotonergic tone and neurotransmission, has been associated with various aspects of personality and temperament (Munafo et al., 2005; Schinka, Busch, Robichaux-Keene, 2004; Sen, Burmeister, & Ghosh, 2004) as well as susceptibility to affective illness (Murphy et al., 1998; Reif & Lesch, 2003). However, enthusiasm for the potential of such genetic variation to affect behaviors and especially disease liability has been tempered by weak, inconsistent, and failed attempts at replication of specific associations with psychiatric syndromes (Glatt & Freimer, 2002).

The inability to substantiate such relationships through consistent replication in independent cohorts may simply reflect methodological issues such as inadequate control for population stratification, insufficient power, and/or inconsistency in the methods applied. Alternatively, and perhaps more important, such inconsistency may reflect the underlying biological nature of the relationship between allelic variants in serotonin genes, each of presumably small effect, and observable behaviors in the domain of mood and emotion that typically reflect complex functional interactions and emergent phenomena. Given that the biological impact of variation in a gene traverses an increasingly divergent path from cells to neural systems to behavior, the response of brain regions subserving emotional processes in humans (e.g., amygdala, hippocampus, prefrontal cortex, and anterior cingulate gyrus) represents a critical first step in their impact on behavior. Thus, functional polymorphisms in 5-HT genes may be strongly related to the integrity of these underlying neural systems and mediate/moderate their ultimate effect on behavior (Hariri & Weinberger, 2003a).

The 5-HT Transporter and 5-HTTLPR

The 5-HT plays an important role in serotonergic neurotransmission by facilitating reuptake of 5-HT from the synaptic cleft. In 1996, a relatively common polymorphism was identified in the human 5-HTT gene located on chromosome 17q11.1-q12 (Heils et al., 1996). The polymorphism is a variable repeat sequence in the promoter region (5-HTTLPR) resulting in two common alleles: the short (S) variant comprised of 14 copies of a 20–23 base pair repeat unit, and the long (L) variant comprised of 16 copies. In populations of European ancestry, the frequency of the S allele is approximately 0.40, and the genotype frequencies are in Hardy–Weinberg equilibrium (L/L = 0.36, L/S = 0.48, S/S = 0.16). These relative allele frequencies, however, can vary substantially across populations (Gelernter, Kranzler, & Cubells, 1997).

Following the identification of this polymorphism, Lesch et al. (1996) demonstrated *in vitro* that the 5-HTTLPR alters both gene transcription and level of 5-HTT function. Cultured human lymphoblast cell lines homozygous for the long allele have higher concentrations of 5-HTT mRNA and express nearly twofold greater 5-HT reuptake in comparison to cells possessing either one or two copies of the short allele. Subsequently, both *in vivo* imaging measures of radioligand binding to 5-HTT (Heinz et al., 2000) and postmortem calculation of 5-HTT density (Little et al., 1998) in humans reported nearly identical reductions in 5-HTT binding levels associated with the short allele as observed *in vitro* (but see Patkar et al., 2004; Shioe et al., 2003; van Dyck et al., 2004). These data are consistent with *in vivo* neuroimaging studies in humans and non-human primates reporting an inverse relationship between 5-HTT availability and cerebrospinal fluid concentrations of 5-hydroxyindoleacetic acid (5-HIAA), a 5-HT metabolite (Heinz et al., 1998; Heinz et al., 2002), and indicate that the 5-HTTLPR is functional and impacts on serotonergic neurotransmission.

In their initial study, Lesch et al. (1996) also demonstrated that individuals carrying the short allele are slightly more likely to display abnormal levels of anxiety in comparison to L/L homozygotes (Lesch et al., 1996). Since their original report, others have confirmed the association between the 5-HTTLPR short allele and heightened anxiety (Du, Bakish, & Hrdina, 2000; Katsuragi et al., 1999; Mazzanti et al., 1998; Melke et al., 2001) and have also demonstrated that individuals possessing the short allele more readily acquire conditioned fear responses (Garpenstrand, Annas, Ekblom, Oreland, & Fredrikson, 2001) and develop affective illness (Lesch & Mossner, 1998) in comparison to those homozygous for the long allele. Recent studies utilizing pharmacological challenge paradigms of the 5-HT system suggest that these differences in affect, mood, and temperament may reflect 5-HTTLPR driven variation in 5-HTT expression and subsequent changes in synaptic concentrations of 5-HT (Moreno et al., 2002; Neumeister et al., 2002; Whale, Clifford, & Cowen, 2000). Furthermore, reduced 5-HTT availability, as putatively indexed by the 5-HTTLPR short allele, has been associated with mood disturbances including major depression (Caspi et al., 2003; Malison et al., 1998) and the severity of depression and anxiety in various psychiatric disorders (Eggers et al., 2003; Heinz et al., 2002; Willeit et al., 2000). Intriguingly, it appears that exposure to stressful life events moderates the impact of the 5-HTTLPR for the development of depression (Caspi et al., 2003).

The Neuroanatomy of Emotion Regulation

The amygdala is a central brain structure in the generation of both normal and pathological emotional behavior, especially fear (LeDoux, 2000). Furthermore, the amygdala is densely innervated by serotonergic neurons and 5-HT receptors are abundant throughout amygdala subnuclei (Azmitia & Gannon, 1986; Sadikot & Parent, 1990; Smith, Daunais, Nader, & Porrino, 1999). Thus, the activity of this subcortical region may be uniquely sensitive to alterations in serotonergic neurotransmission and any resulting variability in amygdala excitability is likely to contribute to individual differences in emergent phenomena such as mood and temperament. However, it is essential to appreciate the importance of a distributed and interconnected network of cortical and subcortical brain regions for the generation, integration, and modulation of emotional behavior. Results from a series of landmark imaging studies (Beauregard, Levesque, & Bourgouin, 2001; Hariri, Bookheimer, & Mazziotta, 2000; Keightley et al., 2003; Lange et al., 2003; Nakamura et al., 1998; Narumoto et al., 2000) suggest that the dynamic interactions of the amygdala and prefrontal cortex may be critical in regulating emotional behavior (Hariri, Mattay, Tessitore, Fera, & Weinberger, 2003).

Imaging Genetics of the 5-HTTLPR and Amygdala Reactivity

Although the potential influence of genetic variation in 5-HTT function on human mood and temperament was bolstered by subsequent studies demonstrating increased - anxiety-like behavior and abnormal fear conditioning in 5-HTT knockout mice (Holmes, Lit, Murphy, Gold, & Crawley, 2003), the underlying neurobiological correlates of this functional relationship remain unknown. Because the physiological response of the amygdala during the processing of fearful or threatening stimuli temporally precedes the subjective experience of emotionality, the 5-HTTLPR may have a more obvious impact at the level of amygdala biology.

In 2002, our research group at the National Institute of Mental Health (NIMH) utilized an imaging genetics strategy with fMRI to directly explore the neural basis of the apparent relationship between the 5-HTTLPR and emotional behavior (Hariri et al., 2002b). Specifically, we hypothesized that 5-HTTLPR S allele carriers, who presumably have altered synaptic concentrations of 5-HT and have been reported to be more anxious and fearful, would exhibit greater amygdala activity in response to fearful or threatening stimuli than those homozygous for the L allele, who presumably have normal levels of synaptic 5-HT and have been reported to be less anxious and fearful.

In our initial study, subjects from two independent cohorts (n = 14 in each) were divided into equal groups based on their 5-HTTLPR genotype, with the groups matched for age, gender, IQ, and task performance. During scanning, the subjects performed a simple perceptual processing task involving the matching of fearful and angry human facial expressions. Importantly, this task has been effective at consistently engaging the amygdala across multiple subject populations and experimental paradigms (Hariri et al., 2000; Hariri et al., 2002a; Hariri, Tessitore, Mattay, Fera, & Weinberger, 2002c; Tessitore et al., 2002). Consistent with our hypothesis, we found that subjects carrying the less efficient 5-HTTLPR S allele exhibited significantly increased amygdala activity in comparison with subjects homozygous for the L allele (Hariri et al., 2002b). In fact, the difference in amygdala activity between 5-HTTLPR genotype groups in this study was nearly fivefold, accounting for 20% of the total variance in the amygdala response. This initial finding suggested that the increased anxiety and fearfulness associated with individuals possessing the 5-HTTLPR S allele may reflect the hyperresponsiveness of their amygdala to relevant environmental stimuli.

Replication of 5-HTTLPR Effects on Amygdala Reactivity

The gold standard in genetic association studies attempting to link any candidate genotype with a specific phenotype, regardless of its nature, remains replication of the association in independent populations. Given the enormity of the multiple comparisons issue in genetic association studies attempting to isolate a single variable (i.e., a single candidate polymorphism) from the hundreds of thousands, if not millions (i.e., all the variation in the genome), of alternatives, a simple yet effective approach is to demonstrate a distinct pattern of association between a specific genetic variant and a downstream biological or behavioral phenotype across many independent samples. When such replications are produced across samples of differing characteristics (age, sex, experience, etc.), and especially across samples of different genetic backgrounds (typically identified by race), our confidence in the causal link between genotype and phenotype is increased exponentially. As illustrated previously with the 5-HTTLPR, it is exactly this lack of consistent replication that has plagued behavioral association studies and undermined attempts to elucidate the genetic basis of behavior.

In striking contrast, every published study to date (and many additional unpublished reports) has replicated the association we first described in 2002 between the 5-HTTLPR S allele and relatively increased amygdala hyperreactivity. More than anything else, this consistent replication across different populations, imaging modalities, and challenge stimuli speaks volumes to the importance of assessing genetic effects on more proximate biological phenotypes. Seven independent functional imaging studies have reported identical 5-HTTLPR S-allele driven amygdala hyperreactivity in cohorts of healthy German (Heinz et al., 2005), Italian (Bertolino et al., 2005), and three American (Brown & Hariri, 2006; Canli et al., 2005; Hariri et al., 2005) adult volunteers as well as Dutch patients with social phobia (Furmark et al., 2004) and German patients with panic disorder (Domschke et al., 2005). In the largest of these replication studies, we again demonstrated 5-HTTLPR S effects on amygdala reactivity in a large, independent cohort of adult volunteers ($n = 92$) who were carefully screened to exclude individuals with a past history of psychiatric illness or treatment (Hariri et al., 2005). This large sample also allowed for the exploration of both sex-specific and S allele load effects on amygdala function and, in turn, dimensions of temperament associated with depression and anxiety (see below).

Specifically, we again observed that 5-HTTLPR S allele carriers exhibited significantly increased right amygdala activation in response to our fMRI challenge paradigm (Hariri et al., 2005). In addition, our latest data revealed that 5-HTTLPR S allele-driven amygdala hyperresponsivity is equally pronounced in both sexes and independent of S allele load. The equivalent effect of one or two S alleles on amygdala function is consistent with the original observations of Lesch et al. (1996) on the influence of the 5-HTTLPR on *in vitro* gene transcription efficiency and subsequent 5-HTT availability. The absence of sex differences suggests that the increased prevalence of mood disorders in females may be related to factors other than the direct risk effect of the 5-HTTLPR S allele.

Beyond the Amygdala: 5-HTTLPR Effects on Corticolimbic Circuitry

A third study from the NIMH cohort further captured the dynamic effects of the 5-HTTLPR on genes, brain, and behavior by examining effects on brain structure and corticolimbic functional connectivity (Pezawas et al., 2005). Here, we used a multimodal neuroimaging strategy to identify mechanisms on the level of neural systems contributing to behavioral and, potentially, clinical effects associated with 5-HTTLPR. We used voxel-based structural MRI techniques in a large sample ($n = 114$) to test for genetic association with the anatomical development of limbic circuitry, as might be expected from neurodevelopmental studies of animals with altered 5-HT function (Gaspar, 2004). We found that, in comparison to the long/long (LL) genotype subjects, S allele carriers showed significantly reduced gray matter volume of the perigenual anterior cingulate cortex (pACC) and amygdala. This suggests that pACC and amygdala represent a functional circuit the morphological development of which is modulated by genetic variation in the serotonergic system.

We next explored the impact of these observed structural effects on the functional interactions of the amygdala and pACC in our fMRI data set. Independent of 5-

HTTLPR genotype status, we found that the amygdala and pACC were significantly functionally connected. Two distinct regions of functional connectivity were identified within the pACC—a positive coupling between the amygdala and the subgenual cingulate and a negative coupling between the amygdala and the supragenual cingulate. This pattern of functional connectivity is consistent with anatomical tracing studies in nonhuman primates which have defined a feedback circuit from amygdala to subgenual cingulate and then from supragenual cingulate back to amygdala. These intrinsic cingulate regions also showed strong positive connectivity with each other, suggesting that the corticolimbic feedback loop is closed via local processing within the cingulate cortex. This intrinsic cingulate connection also is consistent with anatomical studies in nonhuman primates. Remarkably, 5-HTTLPR S allele carriers showed a significant reduction of amygdala–pACC functional connectivity in comparison to LL homozygotes. This difference was most pronounced in the coupling of the amygdala and subgenual anterior cingulate cortex (ACC). These findings suggest that a disruption of this amygdala–pACC feedback circuitry could underlie the earlier observation of increased amygdala activity in S carriers during the processing of biologically salient stimuli (Hariri et al., 2005; Hariri et al., 2002b). More specifically, the data suggest that the overactivation of the amygdala associated with the 5-HTTLPR S allele may reflect more a relative failure of regulation of the amygdala response than an abnormal primary response, per se. Taken together, these data show that 5-HTTLPR genotype affects the structure and putative wiring of a core region within the limbic system thought to be crucial for anxiety-related temperamental traits and depression (Mayberg, 2003a, 2003b; Phillips, Drevets, Rauch, & Lane, 2003a, 2003b). These findings thus suggest a causal mechanism linking developmental alterations in 5-HT-dependent neuronal pathways to impaired interactions in a regulatory network that has been related to emotional reactivity.

Corticolimbic Circuitry and Emotion Regulation

The collective results of these imaging genetics studies reveal that the 5-HTTLPR S allele has a robust effect on human amygdala structure and function as well as the functional interactions of corticolimbic circuitry implicated in both normal and pathological mood states. Importantly, the absence of group differences in age, gender, IQ, and ethnicity in each of these studies indicates that the observed effects are not likely due to a bias resulting from population stratification. Rather, the data suggest that heritable variation in 5-HT signaling associated with the 5-HTTLPR results in structural alterations of the amygdala and pACC, accompanied by biased amygdala reactivity and functional coupling with pACC in response to salient environmental cues. Furthermore, the emergence of these effects in samples of ethnically matched volunteers carefully screened to exclude any lifetime history of psychiatric illness or treatment argues that they represent genetically determined biological traits that are not altered by the presence of a psychiatric illness.

In contrast to the striking imaging genetics findings of 5-HTTLPR S allele effects on amygdala reactivity and limbic circuitry dynamics, initial attempts to link these effects on brain function with measures of emergent behavioral phenomena, namely, the personality trait of harm avoidance, have failed to detect any significant direct relationships. Specifically, in both our initial (Hariri et al., 2002b) and replication studies (Hariri et al., 2005) we did not find any significant 5-HTTLPR genotype association with subjective behavioral measures of anxiety-like or fear-related traits as indexed by the Harm Avoidance (HA) component of the Tridimensional Personality Question-naire, a putative personality measure related to trait anxiety and 5-HT function (Cloninger, 1986; Cloninger, Svrakic, & Przybeck, 1993). This failure to find a behavioral association is not surprising given the relatively small sample sizes of each study and thus limited power to detect likely small (e.g., 1–5%) genetically mediated differences in behavior as well as the theses of this paper: namely, that genes do not directly predict behavior and their effect on behavior is mediated/moderated by their effects on distinct brain circuitry.

However, to our surprise, there was also an absence of any predictive relationship between blood oxygen level dependent (BOLD) amygdala reactivity and HA in our initial studies. Given the critical role for the amygdala in detecting potential environmental threat and harnessing available resources for appropriate reactions, one might expect that its reactivity to such stimuli would predict individual differences in a temperamental trait such as HA. But, a convergence of evidence from animal and human studies clearly demonstrates that emotional behaviors, especially those as complex as HA, are likely influenced by a densely interconnected and distributed cortical and subcortical circuitry of which the amygdala is only one component. Thus, we were compelled to examine the relationship between HA and the observed 5-HTTLPR effects on the functional connectivity of the amygdala and pACC. We reasoned that if functional uncoupling of the amygdala–pACC affective circuit underlies reported associations of 5-HTTLPR with emotional phenotypes, functional connectivity indices between these regions should predict normal variation in temperamental trait measures related to anxiety and depression such is HA. These analyses revealed a striking pattern wherein nearly 30% of the variance in HA scores was predicted by our measure of amygdala–pACC functional connectivity (Pezawas et al., 2005). Consistent with our previous studies (Hariri et al., 2005; Hariri et al., 2002b), functional (or structural) measures of single brain regions (i.e., amygdala or pACC) were of no predictive value. Thus, 5-HTTLPR-mediated corticolimbic functional connectivity alterations are manifested in anxiety-related temperamental traits, possibly reflecting inadequate regulation and integration of amygdala-mediated arousal, leading to an increased vulnerability for persistent negative affect and eventually depression in the context of accumulating environmental adversity. While investigations of localized structural and functional abnormalities have provided insights about depression, our data underscore the importance of studying genetic mechanisms of complex brain disorders at the level of dynamically interacting neural systems. We suggest that such relationships capture more proximally the functional consequences of neurodevelopmental processes altering circuitry function implicated in human temperament and psychiatric disorders.

Diathesis–Stress and Genetic Approaches to Emotion Regulation

It is important to emphasize that the 5-HTTLPR S allele effect on amygdala structure, reactivity and connectivity in our studies as well as those by Heinz et al., Bertolino et al. and Canli et al. exist in samples of healthy adult volunteers with no history of affective or other psychiatric disorders. On one hand, this is consistent with a recent fMRI study reporting that while amygdala hyperexcitability reflects a stable, heritable trait associated with inhibited behavior, it does not by itself predict the development of affective disorders (Schwartz, Wright, Shin, Kagan, & Rauch, 2003). On the other hand, more and more evidence is accumulating which indicates that the majority of psychopathology is rooted early in life first emerging during childhood and adolescence (e.g., Kim-Cohen et al., 2003). Thus, it is possible that the relevance of 5-HTTLPR S allele effects on corticolimbic brain circuitry will be more manifest during the development of individuals predisposed to psychopathology. Moreover, it is likely that exposure to environmental stressors impacts this gene–brain pathway which in turn increases one's risk to develop psychopathology. The hallmark study of Caspi et al. (2003) and subsequent replication studies (Eley et al., 2004; Kaufman et al., 2004; Kendler, Kuhn, Vitum, Prescott, & Riley, 2005) suggest that the existence of significant stressors in the environment of individuals carrying the 5-HTTLPR S allele is necessary to further tip the balance toward the development of psychopathology. Similarly, abnormal social behavior (Champoux et al., 2002) and 5-HT metabolism (Bennett et al., 2002) have been reported in rhesus macaques with the 5-HTTLPR S allele homologue, but only in peer-reared, and thus environmentally stressed, individuals. Emerging data from studies of the 5-HTT knockout mouse implicate similar early developmental phenomena interacting with genetically driven variation in 5-HT in shaping the neurobiological landscape contributing to emotional behaviors (Ansorge, Zhou, Lira, Hen, & Gingrich, 2004; Esaki et al., 2005; Holmes & Hariri, 2003). It is pertinent to note that in many of these examples the genetic vulnerability has manifested as a consequence of environmental stressors that have occurred early in development.

This shift from normal to pathological behaviors and when during the lifespan this shift occurs may reflect the effects of cumulative environmental stress on brain regions, most notably the prefrontal cortex, critical in the regulation of amygdala activity (Hariri et al., 2003; Keightley et al., 2003; Rosenkranz, Moore, & Grace, 2003). For example, repeated exposure to environmental insults before the maturation of relatively late developing prefrontal regulatory circuits (Lewis, 1997) may result in further biased amygdala drive in S allele carriers. Such relative hyperamygdala and hypo-prefrontal activity has been documented in affective disorders (Phillips et al., 2003b; Siegle, Steinhauer, Thase, Stenger, & Carter, 2002) and, thus, may represent a critical pathway or predictive biological marker for the future development of psychopathology.

Recent imaging studies (Heinz et al., 2005; Pezawas et al., 2005) demonstrating altered functional coupling of the amygdala and medial prefrontal cortex during affective processing in adult healthy S allele carriers underscore that complex dynamic interactions of the amygdala and prefrontal cortex may be critical for normal behavioral responses in individuals possessing this risk allele. These results suggest that individual differences in indices of complex, emergent behaviors, such as harm avoidance, reflect the effects of genetic variation on a distributed brain system involved in not only mediating physiological and behavioral arousal (e.g., amygdala) but also regulating and integrating this arousal in the service of adaptive responses to environmental challenges (e.g., prefrontal cortex).

The 5-HTTLPR–SSRI Paradox

That a genetically driven relative loss of 5-HTT function is associated with increased risk for anxiety and depression appears counterintuitive to the anxiolytic and antidepressant effects of selective serotonin reuptake inhibitors (SSRIs) (Ballenger, 1999). These drugs act as 5-HTT blockers and, like the 5-HTTLPR S allele, are predicted to increase extracelluar 5-HT availability (Kugaya et al., 2003). However, recent studies have revealed that the clinical effects of SSRIs are complex, temporally graded, and dependent on alterations in several 5-HT subsystems. For example, Blier and de Montigny (1999) have argued that the anxiolytic effects of SSRIs are mediated through long-term downregulation of presynaptic 5-HT$_{1A}$ autoreceptors, resulting in normalization of 5-HT tone, and not simply through increased synaptic 5-HT resulting from 5-HTT blockade. Importantly, the SSRI-mediated 5-HT$_{1A}$ downregulation occurs approximately 2 to 3 weeks after initiation of treatment, a time course parallel to that of the drugs' anxiolytic effects. Thus, constitutive variation in 5-HT availability affecting amygdala reactivity is unlikely to be directly related to the SSRI-mediated anxiolytic response. Moreover, it is conceivable that congenital increases in synaptic 5-HT may also translate into downregulation of the postsynaptic signaling apparatus, rendering S allele carriers relatively desensitized to 5-HT. In fact, several studies have demonstrated that 5-HTTLPR S allele carriers respond poorly to SSRIs and/or require higher doses than L allele homozygotes (Lotrich, Pollock, & Ferrell, 2001; Murphy, Hollander, Rodrigues, Kremer, & Schatzberg, 2004), further supporting the hypothesis that 5-HTT availability may dictate the relative effectiveness of SSRIs to increase synaptic 5-HT, leading to negative feedback on 5-HT$_{1A}$ autoreceptors, postsynaptic adaptations, and long-term therapeutic effect.

One major difference between the 5-HTTLPR and SSRIs is that a constitutive alteration in 5-HTT function resulting from a gene variation is extant during development as well as adulthood. There is therefore the potential for alterations in the development of the neural systems subserving emotion as a result of a relative loss of 5-HTT function in S allele carriers. In this context, there is evidence that the loss of 5-HTT gene function in mice during early development disrupts the cytoarchitecture and function of cortical regions (Esaki et al., 2005; Gaspar, Cases, & Maroteaux, 2003). There is also growing evidence from studies in rodents that disruption to 5-HT function during critical periods of ontogeny produces lasting abnormalities in emotion. For example, null mutation of either Pet-1, a transcription factor guiding development of the 5-HT system, or the 5-HT$_{1A}$ receptor, produces increased anxiety-like behavior in adulthood (for reviews, see Gross & Hen, 2004; Holmes et al., 2005). In addition, a recent study found that postnatal treatment with the SSRI fluoxetine causes abnormalities on mouse tasks of emotional behavior (Ansorge et al., 2004).

A simple model would predict that putative increases in extracelluar 5-HT in S allele carriers would cause increased activation of presynaptic autoreceptors (5-HT$_{1A}$, 5-HT$_{1B}$) on 5-HT neurons, as well as postsynaptic 5-HT receptors (e.g., 5-HT$_{1A}$, 5-HT$_{2A}$, 5-HT$_{2C}$, 5-HT$_3$) on target neurons in regions including the amygdala (Hariri & Holmes, 2006). However, the consequences of these changes for 5-HT neurotransmission are likely to be highly complex, in part due to adaptive changes in 5-HT homeostasis resulting from the constitutive reduction in 5-HTT function. Indeed, studies in 5-HTT knockout (KO) mice have shown that the expression and function of various 5-HT receptors is markedly altered by the gene mutation.

Of particular relevance to the amygdala hyperreactivity associated with the S allele, 5-HTT KO mice exhibit a significant downregulation of 5-HT$_{1A}$ receptors and a corresponding upregulation of 5-HT$_{2C}$ receptors in the amygdala (Holmes et al., 2003; Li et al., 2003). Because 5-HT$_{1A}$ receptors exert inhibitory effects on postsynaptic neurons while 5-HT$_{2C}$ receptors are excitatory, these changes could conceivably shift the balance of 5-HT effects in the amygdala toward hyperexcitability. In addition, 5-HTT KO also exhibit a marked downregulation of 5-HT$_{1A}$ autoreceptor function on dorsal raphe neurons, which reduces the ability of the 5-HT neurons to self-regulate (Gobbi, Murphy, Lesch, & Blier, 2001; Kim et al., 2005). A loss of inhibitory control of 5-HT firing and release could possibly serve to further exacerbate the excitatory bias of 5-HT effects in the amygdala during emotional provocation.

These predictions remain to be tested empirically in 5-HTT KO mice. It also remains to be determined whether or not such functional alterations occur in S allele carriers. However, demonstrating that at least one important change is also seen in S allele carriers, recent PET study found that 5-HT$_{1A}$ receptor binding is significantly reduced in several brain regions, including the amygdala, dorsal raphe nucleus and prefrontal cortex (David et al., 2005). Whether the emotional abnormalities (Caspi et al., 2003; Collier et al., 1996) and corticolimbic dysfunction (Hariri et al., 2002b; Heinz et al., 2005; Pezawas et al., 2005) seen in S allele carriers also have their origins in development is currently unknown. Notwithstanding, the available evidence supports a working hypothesis in which a genetically driven relative loss of 5-HTT function might compromise the development of neural circuits necessary for effectively regulating negative affect and stress later in life. If substantiated, this model could have significant implications for devising early diagnostic and preventive treatment of emotional disorders in childhood.

Looking Forward

A growing literature from a variety of approaches ranging from noninvasive human neuroimaging studies to gene mutation studies in mice has identified an influence of the gene variation in the 5-HTT in the regulation of emotion (Hariri & Holmes, 2006). Collectively, these studies have demonstrated that genetically mediated changes in 5-HTT function affect both the structure and function of key corticolimbic pathways regulating the brain's capacity for effectively dealing with stress. Recent evidence suggests that these neural changes contribute to the emergence of individual differences in affect and temperament that are associated with 5-HTT gene variation as well as functional polymorphisms in other systems affecting the availability and action of neurotransmitters (Drabant et al., in press; Meyer-Lindenberg et al., 2006). With sufficient stress on the system, such heritable differences in corticolimbic reactivity could have a significant impact on vulnerability to affective illness.

Thus, these findings not only identify a major candidate gene in psychiatry but also speak to a fundamental concept regarding how we think about the role of genes in shaping behavior and how we study their ability to influence risk for disease. While imaging genetics in and of itself provides a powerful new approach to the study of genes, brain, and behavior, its true potential will only be realized by aggressively expanding the scope and scale of the experimental protocols within a developmental framework, especially one that is focused on examining the developmental origins of behavior and disease. Although gene effects on brain function can be readily documented in samples of adults, the contributions of these genes acting in response to variable environmental pressures across development (when these systems are arguably most malleable) must be assessed in order to understand the biological pathways that bias behavior and risk for psychiatric illness.

Moreover, the study of the 5-HTT illustrates how through close dialogue and convergence of experimental approaches, the neurobiological underpinnings of complex behavior and disease could be revealed at rates previously unimaginable. As behavioral neuroscience advances in the postgenomic era, it becomes increasingly incumbent upon investigators from diverse disciplines employing divergent methodologies to work together in a reciprocal and mutually informative fashion in the pursuit of knowledge.

Translational research that meets this challenge will be able to capitalize on developmental imaging genetics findings and in the future we will be able to document what constitute truly predictive markers for developmental outcome and disease progression as well as allow for the early identification of individuals at greater risk for emotional regulatory problems that can have long-term health-related implications.

REFERENCES

Ansorge, M. S., Zhou, M., Lira, A., Hen, R., & Gingrich, J. A. (2004). Early-life blockade of the 5-HT transporter alters emotional behavior in adult mice. *Science, 306*, 879–881.

Axelrod, B. N. (2002). Are normative data from the 64-card version of the WCST comparable to the full WCST? *Clinical Neuropsychology, 16*, 7–11.

Azmitia, E. C., & Gannon, P. J. (1986). The primate serotonergic system: A review of human and animal studies and a report on Macaca fascicularis. *Advances in Neurology, 43*, 407–468.

Ballenger, J. C. (1999). Current treatments of the anxiety disorders in adults. *Biological Psychiatry, 46*, 1579–1594.

Beauregard, M., Levesque, J., & Bourgouin, P. (2001). Neural correlates of conscious self-regulation of emotion. *Journal of Neuroscience, 21*, RC165.

Bellivier, F., Chaste, P., & Malafosse, A. (2004). Association between the TPH gene A218C polymorphism and suicidal behavior: A meta-analysis. *American Journal of Medical Genetics: B, Neuropsychiatry and Genetics, 124*, 87–91.

Bennett, A. J., Lesch, K. P., Heils, A., Long, J. C., Lorenz, J. G., Shoaf, S. E., et al. (2002). Early experience and serotonin transporter gene variation interact to influence primate CNS function. *Molecular Psychiatry, 7*, 118–122.

Bertolino, A., Arciero, G., Rubino, V., Latorre, V., De Candia, M., Mazzola, V., et al. (2005). Variation of human amygdala response during threatening stimuli as a function of 5-HTTLPR genotype and personality style. *Biological Psychiatry, 57*, 1517–1525.

Blier, P., & de Montigny, C. (1999). Serotonin and drug-induced therapeutic responses in major depression, obsessive–compulsive and panic disorders. *Neuropsychopharmacology, 21*, 91S–98S.

Brown, S. M., & Hariri, A. R. (2006). Neuroimaging studies of serotonin gene polymorphisms: Exploring the interplay of genes, brain, and behavior. *Cognitive, Affective, and Behavioral Neuroscience.*

Brown, S. M., Peet, E., Manuck, S. B., Williamson, D. E., Dahl, R. E., Ferrell, R. E., et al. (2005). A regulatory variant of the human tryptophan hydroxylase-2 gene biases amygdala reactivity. *Molecular Psychiatry, 10*, 884–888.

Canli, T., Omura, K., Haas, B. W., Fallgatter, A., Constable, R. T., & Lesch, K. P. (2005). Beyond affect: A role for genetic variation of the serotonin transporter in neural activation during a cognitive attention task. *Proceedings of the National Academy of Sciences, USA, 102*, 12224–12229.

Carey, G., & DiLalla, D. L. (1994). Personality and psychopathology: Genetic perspectives. *Journal of Abnormal Psychology, 103*, 32–43.

Caspi, A., Sugden, K., Moffitt, T. E., Taylor, A., Craig, I. W., Harrington, H., et al. (2003). Influence of life stress on depression: Moderation by a polymorphism in the 5-HTT gene. *Science, 301*, 386–389.

Champoux, M., Bennett, A., Shannon, C., Higley, J. D., Lesch, K. P., & Suomi, S. J. (2002). Serotonin transporter gene polymorphism, differential early rearing, and behavior in rhesus monkey neonates. *Molecular Psychiatry, 7*, 1058–1063.

Cloninger, C. R. (1986). A unified biosocial theory of personality and its role in the development of anxiety states. *Psychiatric Development, 4*, 167–226.

Cloninger, C. R., Svrakic, D. M., & Przybeck, T. R. (1993). A psychobiological model of temperament and character. *Archives of General Psychiatry, 50*, 975–990.

Collier, D. A., Stober, G., Li, T., Heils, A., Catalano, M., Di Bella, D., et al. (1996). A novel functional polymorphism within the promoter of the serotonin transporter gene: Possible role in susceptibility to affective disorders. *Molecular Psychiatry, 1*, 453–460.

David, S. P., Murthy, N. V., Rabiner, E. A., Munafo, M. R., Johnstone, E. C., Jacob, R., et al. (2005). A functional genetic variation of the serotonin (5-HT) transporter affects 5-HT1A receptor binding in humans. *Journal of Neuroscience, 25,* 2586–2590.

Depue, R. A., & Collins, P. F. (1999). Neurobiology of the structure of personality: Dopamine, facilitation of incentive motivation, and extraversion. *Behavioral and Brain Sciences, 22,* 491–517.

Domschke, K., Braun, M., Ohrmann, P., Suslow, T., Kugel, H., Bauer, J., et al. (2005). Association of the functional [minus sign]1019C/G 5-HT 1A polymorphism with prefrontal cortex and amygdala activation measured with 3 T fMRI in panic disorder. *International Journal of Neuropsychopharmacology, 9,* 349–355.

Drabant, E. M., Hariri, A. R., Meyer-Lindenberg, A., et al. (in press). Catechol-O-methyltransferase Val158Met genotype and neural mechanisms of emotional arousal and regulation. *Archives of General Psychiatry.*

Du, L., Bakish, D., & Hrdina, P. D. (2000). Gender differences in association between serotonin transporter gene polymorphism and personality traits. *Psychiatric Genetics, 10,* 159–164.

Ebstein, R. P. (2006). The molecular genetic architecture of human personality: Beyond self-report questionnaires. *Molecular Psychiatry, 11,* 427–445.

Ebstein, R. P., Zohar, A. H., Benjamin, J., & Belmaker, R. H. (2002). An update on molecular genetic studies of human personality traits. *Applied Bioinformatics, 1,* 57–68.

Eggers, B., Hermann, W., Barthel, H., Sabri, O., Wagner, A., & Hesse S. (2003). The degree of depression in Hamilton rating scale is correlated with the density of presynaptic serotonin transporters in 23 patients with Wilson's disease. *Journal of Neurology, 250,* 576–580.

Eley, T. C., Sugden, K., Corsico, A., Gregory, A. M., Sham, P., McGuffin, P., et al. (2004). Gene-environment interaction analysis of serotonin system markers with adolescent depression. *Molecular Psychiatry, 9,* 908–915.

Emahazion, T., Feuk, L., Jobs, M., Sawyer, S. L., Fredman, D., St. Clair, D., et al. (2001). SNP association studies in Alzheimer's disease highlight problems for complex disease analysis. *Trends in Genetics, 17,* 407–413.

Esaki, T., Cook, M., Shimoji, K., Murphy, D. L., Sokoloff, L., & Holmes, A. (2005). Developmental disruption of serotonin transporter function impairs cerebral responses to whisker stimulation in mice. *Proceedings of the National Academy of Sciences, USA, 102,* 5582–5587.

Forbes, E. E., & Dahl, R. E. (2005). Neural systems of positive affect: Relevance to understanding child and adolescent depression? *Developmental Psychopathology, 17,* 827–850.

Furmark, T., Tillfors, M., Garpenstrand, H., Marteinsdottir, I., Langstrom, B., Oreland, L., et al. (2004). Serotonin transporter polymorphism linked to amygdala excitability and symptom severity in patients with social phobia. *Neuroscience Letters, 362,* 1–4.

Garpenstrand, H., Annas, P., Ekblom, J., Oreland, L., & Fredrikson, M. (2001). Human fear conditioning is related to dopaminergic and serotonergic biological markers. *Behavioral Neuroscience, 115,* 358–364.

Gaspar, P. (2004). Genetic models to understand how serotonin acts during development. *Journal de la Société de Biologie, 198,* 18–21.

Gaspar, P., Cases, O., & Maroteaux, L. (2003). The developmental role of serotonin: News from mouse molecular genetics. *Nature Reviews: Neuroscience, 4,* 1002–1012.

Gelernter, J., Kranzler, H., & Cubells, J. F. (1997). Serotonin transporter protein (SLC6A4) allele and haplotype frequencies and linkage disequilibria in African- and European-American and Japanese populations and in alcohol-dependent subjects. *Human Genetics, 101,* 243–246.

Glatt, C. E., & Freimer, N. B. (2002). Association analysis of candidate genes for neuropsychiatric disease: The perpetual campaign. *Trends in Genetics, 18,* 307–312.

Gobbi, G., Murphy, D. L., Lesch, K., & Blier, P. (2001). Modifications of the serotonergic system in mice lacking serotonin transporters: An *in vivo* electrophysiological study. *Journal of Pharmacology and Experimental Therapeutics, 296,* 987–995.

Gross, C., & Hen, R. (2004). The developmental origins of anxiety. *Nature Reviews: Neuroscience, 5,* 545–552.

Hariri, A. R., Bookheimer, S. Y., & Mazziotta, J. C. (2000). Modulating emotional responses: Effects of a neocortical network on the limbic system. *Neuroreport, 11,* 43–48.

Hariri, A. R., Drabant, E. M., Munoz, K. E., Kolachana, B. S., Mattay, V. S., Egan, M. F., et al. (2005). A susceptibility gene for affective disorders and the response of the human amygdala. *Archives of General Psychiatry, 62,* 146–152.

Hariri, A. R., Drabant, E. M., & Weinberger, D. R. (2006). Imaging genetics: Perspectives from studies of genetically driven variation in serotonin function and corticolimbic affective processing. *Biological Psychiatry, 59,* 888–897.

Hariri, A. R., & Holmes, A. (2006). Genetics of emotional regulation: The role of the serotonin transporter in neural function. *Trends in Cognitive Science, 10,* 182–191.

Hariri, A. R., Mattay, V. S., Tessitore, A., Fera, F., Smith, W. G., & Weinberger, D. R. (2002a). Dextroamphetamine modulates the response of the human amygdala. *Neuropsychopharmacology, 27,* 1036–1040.

Hariri, A. R., Mattay, V. S., Tessitore, A., Fera, F., & Weinberger D. R. (2003). Neocortical modulation of the amygdala response to fearful stimuli. *Biological Psychiatry, 53,* 494–501.

Hariri, A. R., Mattay, V. S., Tessitore, A., Kolachana, B., Fera, F., Goldman, D., et al. (2002b). Serotonin transporter genetic variation and the response of the human amygdala. *Science, 297,* 400–403.

Hariri, A. R., Tessitore, A., Mattay, V. S., Fera, F., & Weinberger, D. R. (2002c). The amygdala response to emotional stimuli: A comparison of faces and scenes. *NeuroImage, 17,* 317–323.

Hariri, A. R., & Weinberger, D. R. (2003a). Functional neuroimaging of genetic variation in serotonergic neurotransmission. *Genes, Brain and Behavior, 2,* 314–349.

Hariri, A. R., & Weinberger, D. R. (2003b). Imaging genomics. *British Medical Bulletin, 65,* 259–270.

Heils, A., Teufel, A., Petri, S., Stober, G., Riederer, P., Bengel, D., et al. (1996). Allelic variation of human serotonin transporter gene expression. *Journal of Neurochemistry, 66,* 2621–2624.

Heinz, A., Braus, D. F., Smolka, M. N., Wrase, J., Puls, I., Hermann, D., et al. (2005). Amygdala-prefrontal coupling depends on a genetic variation of the serotonin transporter. *Nature Neuroscience, 8,* 20–21.

Heinz, A., Higley, J. D., Gorey, J. G., Saunders, R. C., Jones, D. W., Hommer, D., et al. (1998). *In vivo* association between alcohol intoxication, aggression, and serotonin transporter availability in nonhuman primates. *American Journal of Psychiatry, 155,* 1023–1028.

Heinz, A., Jones, D. W., Bissette, G., Hommer, D., Ragan, P., Knable, M., Wellek S., et al. (2002). Relationship between cortisol and serotonin metabolites and transporters in alcoholism [correction of alcolholism]. *Pharmacopsychiatry, 35,* 127–134.

Heinz, A., Jones, D. W., Mazzanti, C., Goldman, D., Ragan, P., Hommer, D., et al. (2000). A relationship between serotonin transporter genotype and in vivo protein expression and alcohol neurotoxicity. *Biological Psychiatry, 47,* 643–649.

Holmes, A., & Hariri, A. R. (2003). The serotonin transporter gene-linked polymorphism and negative emotionality: Placing single gene effects in the context of genetic background and environment. *Genes, Brain and Behavior, 2,* 332–335.

Holmes, A., le Guisquet, A. M., Vogel, E., Millstein, R. A., Leman, S., & Belzung, C. (2005). Early life genetic, epigenetic and environmental factors shaping emotionality in rodents. *Neuroscience and Biobehavioral Reviews, 29,* 1335–1346.

Holmes, A., Lit, Q., Murphy, D. L., Gold, E., & Crawley, J. N. (2003). Abnormal anxiety-related behavior in serotonin transporter null mutant mice: The influence of genetic background. *Genes, Brain and Behavior, 2,* 365–380.

John, O. P., & Gross, J. J. (2007). Individual differences in emotion regulation. In J. J. Gross (Ed.), *Handbook of emotion regulation* (pp. 351–372). New York: Guilford Press.

Kalivas, P. W., & Volkow, N. D. (2005). The neural basis of addiction: A pathology of motivation and choice. *American Journal of Psychiatry, 162,* 1403–1413.

Katsuragi, S., Kunugi, H., Sano, A., Tsutsumi, T., Isogawa, K., Nanko, S., et al. (1999). Association between serotonin transporter gene polymorphism and anxiety-related traits. *Biological Psychiatry, 45,* 368–370.

Kaufman, J., Yang, B. Z., Douglas-Palumberi, H., et al. (2004). Social supports and serotonin transporter gene moderate depression in maltreated children. *Proceedings of the National Academy of Sciences, USA, 101,* 17316–17321.

Keightley, M. L., Winocur, G., Graham, S. J., Mayberg, H. S., Hevenor, S. J., & Grady, C. L. (2003). An fMRI study investigating cognitive modulation of brain regions associated with emotional processing of visual stimuli. *Neuropsychologia, 41,* 585–596.

Kendler, K. S., Kuhn, J. W., Vittum, J., Prescott, C. A., & Riley, B. (2005). The interaction of stressful life events and a serotonin transporter polymorphism in the prediction of episodes of major depression: A replication. *Archives of General Psychiatry, 62,* 529–535.

Kendler, K. S., Neale, M. C., Kessler, R. C., Heath, A. C., & Eaves, L. J. (1993). A longitudinal twin study of personality and major depression in women. *Archives of General Psychiatry, 50,* 853–862.

Kim, D. K., Tolliver, T. J., Huang, S. J., Martin, B. J., Andrews, A. M., Wichems, C., et al. (2005). Altered serotonin synthesis, turnover and dynamic regulation in multiple brain regions of mice lacking the serotonin transporter. *Neuropharmacology, 49,* 798–810.

Kim-Cohen, J., Caspi, A., Moffitt, T. E., Harrington, H., Milne, B. J., & Palton, R. (2003). Prior juvenile diagnoses in adults with mental disorder. Developmental follow-back of a prospective-longitudinal cohort. *Archives of General Psychiatry, 60,* 709–717.

Kugaya, A., Seneca, N. M., Snyder, P. J., Williams, S. A., Malison, R. T., Baldwin, R. M., et al. (2003). Changes in human *in vivo* serotonin and dopamine transporter availabilities during chronic antidepressant administration. *Neuropsychopharmacology, 28,* 413–420.

Lange, K., Williams, L. M., Young, A. W., Bullmore, E. T., Brammer, M. J., Williams, S. C., et al. (2003). Task instructions modulate neural responses to fearful facial expressions. *Biological Psychiatry, 53,* 226–232.

LeDoux, J. E. (2000). Emotion circuits in the brain. *Annual Review of Neuroscience, 23,* 155–184.

Leonard, E. D.. & Hen, R. (2006). Genetics of affective disorders. *Annual Review of Psychology, 57,* 117–137.

Lesch, K. P., Bengel, D., Heils, A., Sabol, S. Z., Greenberg, B. D., Petri, S., et al. (1996). Association of anxiety-related traits with a polymorphism in the serotonin transporter gene regulatory region. *Science, 274,* 1527–1531.

Lesch, K. P., & Mossner, R. (1998). Genetically driven variation in serotonin uptake: Is there a link to affective spectrum, neurodevelopmental, and neurodegenerative disorders? *Biological Psychiatry, 44,* 179–192.

Lewis, D. A. (1997). Development of the prefrontal cortex during adolescence: Insights into vulnerable neural circuits in schizophrenia. *Neuropsychopharmacology, 16,* 385–398.

Li, Q., Wichems, C. H., Ma, L., Van de Kar, L. D., Garcia, F., & Murphy, D. L. (2003). Brain region-specific alterations of 5-HT2A and 5-HT2C receptors in serotonin transporter knockout mice. *Journal of Neurochemistry, 84,* 1256–1265.

Little, K. Y., McLaughlin, D. P., Zhang, L., Livermore, C. S., Dalack, G. W., McFinton, P. R., et al. (1998). Cocaine, ethanol, and genotype effects on human midbrain serotonin transporter binding sites and mRNA levels. *American Journal of Psychiatry, 155,* 207–213.

Lotrich, F. E., Pollock, B. G., & Ferrell, R. E. (2001). Polymorphism of the serotonin transporter: Implications for the use of selective serotonin reuptake inhibitors. *American Journal of Pharmacogenomics, 1,* 153–164.

Lucki, I. (1998). The spectrum of behaviors influenced by serotonin. *Biological Psychiatry, 44,* 151–162.

Malhotra, A. K., & Goldman, D. (1999). Benefits and pitfalls encountered in psychiatric genetic association studies. *Biological Psychiatry, 45,* 544–550.

Malison, R. T., Price, L. H., Berman, R., van Dyck, C. H., Pelton, G. H., Carpenter, L., et al. (1998). Reduced brain serotonin transporter availability in major depression as measured by [123I]-2 beta-carbomethoxy-3 beta-(4-iodophenyl)tropane and single photon emission computed tomography. *Biological Psychiatry, 44,* 1090–1098.

Manuck, S. B., Flory, J. D., Ferrell, R. E., Dent, K. M., Mann, J. J., & Muldoon, M. F. (1999). Aggression and anger-related traits associated with a polymorphism of the tryptophan hydroxylase gene. *Biological Psychiatry, 45,* 603–614.

Manuck, S. B., Flory, J. D., Ferrell, R. E., Mann, J. J., & Muldoon, M. F. (2000). A regulatory polymorphism of the monoamine oxidase-A gene may be associated with variability in aggression, impulsivity, and central nervous system serotonergic responsivity. *Psychiatry Research, 95,* 9–23.

Manuck, S. B., Flory, J. D., McCaffery, J. M., Matthews, K. A., Mann, J. J., & Muldoon, M. E. (1998). Aggression, impulsivity, and central nervous system serotonergic responsivity in a nonpatient sample, *Neuropsychopharmacology, 19,* 287–299.

Mayberg, H. S. (2003a). Modulating dysfunctional limbic-cortical circuits in depression: Towards development of brain-based algorithms for diagnosis and optimised treatment. *British Medical Bulletin, 65,* 193–207.

Mayberg, H. S. (2003b). Positron emission tomography imaging in depression: A neural systems perspective. *Neuroimaging Clinics of North America, 13,* 805–815.

Mazzanti, C. M., Lappalainen, J., Long, J. C., Bengel, D., Naukkarinen, H., Eggert, M., et al. (1998).

Role of the serotonin transporter promoter polymorphism in anxiety-related traits. *Archives of General Psychiatry, 55*, 936–940.

McGuffin, P., Riley, B., & Plomin, R. (2001). Genomics and behavior. Toward behavioral genomics. *Science, 291*, 1232–1249.

Melke, J., Landen, M., Baghei, F., Rosmond, R., Holm, G., Bjorntorp, P., et al. (2001). Serotonin transporter gene polymorphisms are associated with anxiety-related personality traits in women. *American Journal of Medical Genetics, 105*, 458–463.

Meyer-Lindenberg, A., Buckholtz, J. W., Kolachana, B., Hariri, A. R., Pezawas, L., Blasi, G., et al. (2006). Neural mechanisms of genetic risk for impulsivity and violence in humans. *Proceedings of the National Academy of Sciences, USA, 103*, 6269–6274.

Moldin, S. O., & Gottesman, I. I. (1997). At issue: Genes, experience, and chance in schizophrenia—Positioning for the 21st century. *Schizophrenia Bulletin, 23*, 547–561.

Moreno, F. A., Rowe, D. C., Kaiser, B., Chase, D., Michaels, T., Gelernter, J., et al. (2002). Association between a serotonin transporter promoter region polymorphism and mood response during tryptophan depletion. *Molecular Psychiatry, 7*, 213–216.

Munafo, M. R., Clark, T., & Flint, J. (2005). Does measurement instrument moderate the association between the serotonin transporter gene and anxiety-related personality traits?: A meta-analysis. *Molecular Psychiatry, 10*, 415–419.

Murphy, D. L., Andrews, A. M., Wichems, C. H., Li, Q., Tohda, M., & Greenberg, B. (1998). Brain serotonin neurotransmission: An overview and update with an emphasis on serotonin subsystem heterogeneity, multiple receptors, interactions with other neurotransmitter systems, and consequent implications for understanding the actions of serotonergic drugs. *Journal of Clinical Psychiatry, 59*(Suppl. 15), 4–12.

Murphy, G. M., Jr., Hollander, S. B., Rodrigues, H. E., Kremer, C., & Schatzberg, A. F. (2004). Effects of the serotonin transporter gene promoter polymorphism on mirtazapine and paroxetine efficacy and adverse events in geriatric major depression. *Archives of General Psychiatry, 61*, 1163–1169.

Nakamura, K., Kawashima, R., Nagumo, S., Ito, K., Sugiura, M., Kato, T., et al. (1998). Neuroanatomical correlates of the assessment of facial attractiveness. *Neuroreport, 9*, 753–757.

Narumoto, J., Yamada, H., Iidaka, T., Sadato, N., Fukui, K., Itoh, H., et al. (2000). Brain regions involved in verbal or non-verbal aspects of facial emotion recognition. *Neuroreport, 11*, 2571–2576.

Neumeister, A., Konstantinidis, A., Stastny, J., Schwarz, M. J., Vitouch, O., Willeit, M., et al. (2002). Association between serotonin transporter gene promoter polymorphism (5HTTLPR) and behavioral responses to tryptophan depletion in healthy women with and without family history of depression. *Archives of General Psychiatry, 59*, 613–620.

Nigg, J. T., & Goldsmith, H. H. (1998). Developmental psychopathology, personality, and temperament: Reflections on recent behavioral genetics research. *Human Biology, 70*, 387–412.

Noblett, K. L., & Coccaro, E. F. (2005). Molecular genetics of personality. *Current Psychiatry Reports, 7*, 73–80.

Patkar, A. A., Berrettini, W. H., Mannelli, P., Gopalakrishnan, R., Hoehe, M. R., Bilal, L., et al. (2004). Relationship between serotonin transporter gene polymorphisms and platelet serotonin transporter sites among African-American cocaine-dependent individuals and healthy volunteers. *Psychiatric Genetics, 14*, 25–32.

Pezawas, L., Meyer-Lindenberg, A., Drabant, E. M., Verchinski, B. A., Munoz, K. E., Kolachana, B. S., et al. (2005). 5-HTTLPR polymorphism impacts human cingulate-amygdala interactions: A genetic susceptibility mechanism for depression. *Nature Neuroscience, 8*, 828–834.

Phillips, M. L., Drevets, W. C., Rauch, S. L., & Lane, R. (2003a). Neurobiology of emotion perception. I: The neural basis of normal emotion perception. *Biological Psychiatry, 54*, 504–514.

Phillips, M. L., Drevets, W. C., Rauch, S. L., & Lane, R. (2003b). Neurobiology of emotion perception. II: Implications for major psychiatric disorders. *Biological Psychiatry, 54*, 515–528.

Plomin, R., & Nesselroade, J. R. (1990). Behavioral genetics and personality change. *Journal of Personality, 58*, 191–220.

Reif, A., & Lesch, K. P. (2003). Toward a molecular architecture of personality. *Behavioural Brain Research, 139*, 1–20.

Rosenkranz, J. A., Moore, H., & Grace, A. A. (2003). The prefrontal cortex regulates lateral amygdala neuronal plasticity and responses to previously conditioned stimuli. *Journal of Neuroscience, 23*, 11054–11064.

Rutter, M., & Plomin, R. (1997). Opportunities for psychiatry from genetic findings. *British Journal of Psychiatry, 171,* 209–219.

Sadikot, A. F., & Parent, A. (1990). The monoaminergic innervation of the amygdala in the squirrel monkey: An immunohistochemical study. *Neuroscience, 36,* 431–447.

Schinka, J. A., Busch, R. M., & Robichaux-Keene, N. (2004). A meta-analysis of the association between the serotonin transporter gene polymorphism (5-HTTLPR) and trait anxiety. *Molecular Psychiatry, 9,* 197–202.

Schinka, J. A., Letsch, E. A., & Crawford, F. C. (2002). DRD4 and novelty seeking: Results of meta-analyses. *American Journal of Medical Genetics, 114,* 643–648.

Schwartz, C. E., Wright, C. I., Shin, L. M., Kagan, J., & Rauch, S. L. (2003). Inhibited and uninhibited infants "grown up": Adult amygdalar response to novelty. *Science, 300,* 1952–1953.

Sen, S., Burmeister, M., & Ghosh, D. (2004). Meta-analysis of the association between a serotonin transporter promoter polymorphism (5-HTTLPR) and anxiety-related personality traits. *American Journal of Medical Genetics, 127B,* 85–89.

Shioe, K., Ichimiya, T., Suhara, T., Takano, A., Sudo, Y., Yasuno, F., et al. (2003). No association between genotype of the promoter region of serotonin transporter gene and serotonin transporter binding in human brain measured by PET. *Synapse, 48,* 184–188.

Siegle, G. J., Steinhauer, S. R., Thase, M. E., Stenger, V. A., & Carter, C. S. (2002). Can't shake that feeling: Event-related fMRI assessment of sustained amygdala activity in response to emotional information in depressed individuals. *Biological Psychiatry, 51,* 693–707.

Smith, H. R., Daunais, J. B., Nader, M. A., & Porrino, L. J. (1999). Distribution of [3H]citalopram binding sites in the nonhuman primate brain. *Annals of the New York Academy of Science, 877,* 700–702.

Strobel, A., Spinath, F. M., Angleitner, A., Riemann, R., & Lesch, K. P. (2003). Lack of association between polymorphisms of the dopamine D4 receptor gene and personality. *Neuropsychobiology, 47,* 52–56.

Tessitore, A., Hariri, A. R., Fera, F., Smith, W. G., Chase, T. N., Hyde, T. M., et al. (2002). Dopamine modulates the response of the human amygdala: A study in Parkinson's disease. *Journal of Neuroscience, 22,* 9099–9103.

van Dyck, C. H., Malison, R. T., Staley, J. K., Jacobsen, L. K., Seibyl, J. P., Laruelle, M., et al. (2004). Central serotonin transporter availability measured with [123I]beta-CIT SPECT in relation to serotonin transporter genotype. *American Journal of Psychiatry, 161,* 525–531.

Viken, R. J., Rose, R. J., Kaprio, J., & Koskenvuo, M. (1994). A developmental genetic analysis of adult personality: Extraversion and neuroticism from 18 to 59 years of age. *Journal of Personality and Social Psychology, 66,* 722–730.

Vogel, F., Schalt, E., Kruger, J., Propping, P., & Lehnert, K. F. (1979). The electroencephalogram (EEG) as a research tool in human behavior genetics: Psychological examinations in healthy males with various inherited EEG variants. I. Rationale of the study. Material. Methods. Heritability of test parameters. *Human Genetics, 47,* 1–45.

Whale, R., Clifford, E. M., & Cowen, P. J. (2000). Does mirtazapine enhance serotonergic neurotransmission in depressed patients? *Psychopharmacology (Berl.), 148,* 325–326.

Whalen, P. J., Bush, G., McNally, R. J., Wilhelm, S., McInerney, S. C., Jenike, M. A., et al. (1998). The emotional counting Stroop paradigm: A functional magnetic resonance imaging probe of the anterior cingulate affective division. *Biological Psychiatry, 44,* 1219–1228.

Willeit, M., Praschak-Rieder, N., Neumeister, A., Pirker, W., Asenbaum, S., Vitouch, et al. (2000). [123I]-beta-CIT SPECT imaging shows reduced brain serotonin transporter availability in drug-free depressed patients with seasonal affective disorder. *Biological Psychiatry, 47,* 482–489.

PART III

COGNITIVE FOUNDATIONS

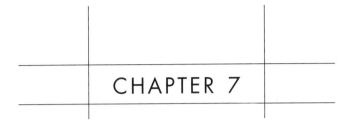
Executive Function
MECHANISMS UNDERLYING EMOTION REGULATION

PHILIP DAVID ZELAZO
WILLIAM A. CUNNINGHAM

Research on executive function (EF) is directed at understanding the conscious control of thought and action. Although EF can be understood as a domain-general construct at the most abstract functional level of analysis (i.e., as conscious goal-directed problem solving), more precise characterizations distinguish between the relatively "hot" motivationally significant aspects of EF and the more disinterested "cool" aspects (Zelazo & Müller, 2002). In this chapter, we propose a model of emotion regulation based on principles of EF (both "hot" and "cool") that spans Marr's (1982) three levels of analysis—computational (concerning what EF accomplishes), algorithmic (dealing in more detail with the way information is represented and how it is processed), and implementational (examining how the information processing is realized in the brain). This model highlights the roles of reflection (levels of consciousness) and rule use in the regulation of emotion and makes initial steps toward explaining how these processes contribute to the subjective experience of complex emotions. Presentation of this model is intended to serve as a concise summary of research on EF and as an exploration of its implications for emotion regulation.

DEFINING EMOTION AND EMOTION REGULATION

In agreement with a growing number of researchers (e.g., Barrett, Ochsner, & Gross, in press; Damasio, 1994), we suggest that a stark distinction between cognition and emotion reflects an outmoded adherence to a fundamentally moralistic world view (reason is angelic, passion beastly). Instead, we suggest that emotion corresponds to an aspect of cognition—its motivational aspect. On this view, it is possible to have cognition that is more or less emotional, more or less motivated. Thus, we use the term "emotion" to refer to an aspect of human information processing that manifests itself in multiple dimensions: subjective experience, observable behavior, and physiological activity, among them. *Emotion regulation* refers to the modulation of motivated cognition and its many manifestations. Emotion regulation can occur in a variety of ways (Gross & Thompson, this volume), but one of the most obvious varieties is the deliberate self-regulation of emotion via conscious cognitive processing, and it is this variety of emotion regulation that we address in terms of EF. It is important to note that although we focus on the aspects of emotion regulation that are directly associated with processes of EF, we are not suggesting that this is the only route to emotion regulation (cf. Fitzsimons & Bargh, 2004). As with any complex psychological phenomenon, emotion regulation may well occur in a variety of ways (some of which may be quite automatic).

EXECUTIVE FUNCTION

EF is generally recognized as an important but ill-understood umbrella term for a diverse set of "higher cognitive processes," including (but not limited to) planning, working memory, set shifting, error detection and correction, and the inhibitory control of prepotent responses (e.g., Roberts, Robbins, & Weiskrantz, 1998; Stuss & Benson, 1986; Tranel, Anderson, & Benton, 1994). These processes are recruited for the deliberate self-regulation of emotion, and in this chapter, we will attempt to explain how. First, however, we need to provide a characterization of EF. In what follows, we describe EF at each of Marr's (1982) three levels of analysis—computational (concerning what EF accomplishes), algorithmic (dealing in more detail with the way information is represented and how it is processed), and implementational (examining how the information processing is realized in the brain)—and then show in more detail how EF plays a role in emotion regulation. A new model is outlined that relies on a distinction between hot and cool EF (see below), both of which are hypothesized to be involved in emotion regulation. This model highlights what we take to be the most important aspects of EF to be considered when seeking to understand emotion regulation.

Computational Level

One way to capture the diversity of the processes associated with EF without simply listing them and without hypostasizing homuncular abilities (e.g., a Central Executive [Baddeley, 1996], or a Supervisory Attentional System [Norman & Shallice, 1986]) is to treat EF as a complex hierarchical function (Zelazo, Carter, Reznick, & Frye, 1997). In this view, which has its origins in the work of Luria (e.g., 1966) and Goldberg (e.g., Goldberg & Bilder, 1987), the function of EF is seen to be deliberate, goal-directed problem solving and functionally distinct phases of problem solving can then be flexibly and dynamically organized around this function. Figure 7.1 illustrates how different aspects of EF contribute to the eventual outcome, as well as how EF unfolds as an iterative, essentially cybernetic (Weiner, 1948), process. Although this functional characterization does not, by itself, provide an adequate explanation of EF, it provides a framework within which one can understand the hierarchical structure of EF and consider the way in which more basic cognitive processes (e.g., working memory) contribute to particular aspects of EF (e.g., the role of working memory in intending).

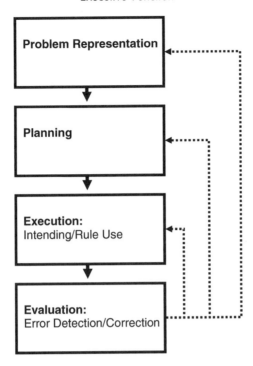

FIGURE 7.1. A problem-solving framework for understanding temporally and functionally distinct phases of executive function, considered as a functional construct. Dashed lines indicate optional recursive feedback loops. Adapted from Zelazo, Carter, Reznick, and Frye (1997). Copyright 1997 by the American Psychological Association. Adapted by permission.

To appreciate the utility of this abstract, functional characterization, consider how it applies to the Wisconsin Card Sorting Test (WCST; Grant & Berg, 1948), which is widely regarded as "the prototypical EF task in neuropsychology" (Pennington & Ozonoff, 1996, p. 55). In the WCST, participants are presented with four target cards that differ on three dimensions (number, color, and shape) and asked to sort a series of test cards that match different target cards on different dimensions. Participants must discover the sorting rule by trial and error, and after a certain number of consecutive correct responses, the sorting rule is changed. The WCST taps numerous aspects of EF, and, as a result, the origin of errors on this task is difficult to determine (but see Barceló & Knight, 2002; Delis, Squire, Bihrle, & Massman, 1992, for efforts to distinguish between different types of error). To perform correctly, one must first construct a representation of the problem space, which includes (1) one's current state, (2) one's goal state, and (3) options for reducing the discrepancy between (1) and (2). In the WCST, a key part of the problem consists in identifying the relevant dimensions. After representing the problem, one must choose a promising plan—for example, sorting according to shape. After selecting a plan, one must (1) keep the plan in mind long enough for it to guide one's thought or action, and (2) actually carry out the prescribed behavior. Keeping a plan in mind to control behavior is referred to as *intending*; translating a plan into action is *rule use*. Finally, after acting, one must evaluate the consequences of this action to determine whether one's goal state has been attained. This phase includes both error detection and, if necessary, error correction. Error correction entails revisiting earlier phases in the sequences, thereby initiating another itera-tion of the sequence—either in whole or in part. Failures of EF can occur at each problem-solving phase, so there are several possible explanations of poor performance on the WCST. For example, perseveration could occur after a rule change in the WCST either because a new plan was not formed or because the plan was formed but not car-ried out.

Notice that in this example, as in many situations, one needs to consider multiple goals simultaneously, at various levels of abstraction (Carver & Sheier, 1982). For exam-ple, one needs to pursue the relatively proximal subgoal of executing one's plan—sorting by shape—in the service of fulfilling the more distal, but still explicit, goal of performing well on the WCST. Thus, EF needs to be understood as a complex, hierar-chical function at this level of analysis.

This computational characterization of EF also applies to situations involving emo-tion regulation. Consider, for example, a child who is hit accidentally by another child on a playground. Does the first child hit back, or does he diffuse the situation as he has been told to do by his teacher? The answer may depend on whether emotion regulation is successful, and emotion regulation may fail at any of the problem-solving phases.

1. The child may fail to represent the problem adequately. For example, he may be biased to represent such situations as threatening, and he may have difficulty flexibly reinterpreting the situation.
2. Alternatively or additionally, he may fail to plan or think ahead properly. For example, he may fail to anticipate the negative consequences of responding aggressively.
3. He may understand the rules that govern the situation (e.g., "I should not hit others" or "I should do as I am asked by my teacher") but fail to use these rules, just as people fail to use rules that they know on tests of rule use (e.g., Zelazo, Frye, & Rapus, 1996; Zelazo, Müller, Frye, & Marcovitch, 2003).
4. Finally, he may have difficulty learning from past experience.

Algorithmic Level

Research on EF has generated numerous proposals regarding the cognitive processes that help fulfill the higher-order function of EF. These processes include metacogni-tion, selective attention, working memory, inhibitory control, and rule use, as well as combinations of these processes (e.g., see chapters in Roberts et al., 1998; Stuss & Knight, 2002). One approach that serves to integrate these processes has been moti-vated by research on the development of EF in childhood and across the lifespan. According to the Levels of Consciousness Model (e.g., Zelazo, 2004), EF (as defined here) is accomplished, in large part, by the ability to formulate, maintain in working memory, and then act on the basis of rule systems at different levels of complexity—from a single rule relating a stimulus to a response to a pair of rules to a hierarchical system of rules that allows one to select among incompatible pairs of rules. In this account, rules are formulated in an ad hoc fashion in potentially silent self-directed speech. These rules link antecedent conditions to consequences, as when we tell our-selves, "If I see a mailbox, then I need to mail this letter." When people reflect on the rules they represent, they are able to consider them in contradistinction to other rules and embed them under higher-order rules in the same way that we might say, "If it's before 5 P.M., then if I see a mailbox with a late pickup, then I need to mail this letter, otherwise, I'll have find a mailbox with an early morning pickup." In this example, a simple conditional statement regarding the mailbox is made dependent on the satisfaction of yet another condition (namely, the time). More complex rule systems permit the more flexible selection of certain rules for acting when multiple conflicting rules are possible. This, in turn, changes the content of one's action-oriented representations (held in working memory), resulting in the amplification and diminution of attention to potential influences on thought (inferences) and action.

Increases in rule complexity are made possible by corresponding increases in the extent that one reflects on one's representations. Rather than taking rules for granted and simply assessing whether their antecedent conditions are satisfied, reflection involves making the rules themselves an object of consideration and considering them in contradistinction to other rules at that same level of complexity. Reflection, on this account, is taken to involve the recursive reprocessing of information. Each degree of recursion results in a new "level of consciousness," and each level of consciousness allows for the integration of more information into an experience before it is replaced by new intero- or exteroceptor stimulation. Moreover, each level of consciousness allows for the formulation and use of more complex rule systems. So, we might contrast relatively automatic action at a lower level of consciousness with relatively deliberate action at a higher level of consciousness. The former type of action is performed in response to the most salient, low-resolution aspects of a situation, and it is based on the formulation of a relatively simple rule system—likely a rule describing a stereotypical response to the situation. The more deliberate action occurs in response to a more carefully considered construal of the same situation, and it is based on the formulation of a more complex and more flexible system of rules or inferences. In general, reflection is engaged as needed in the service of problem-solving goals and in the flexible, iterative way described earlier in our treatment of EF at the computational level of analysis. Details of this model (showing, for example, the cognitive implications of each level of consciousness) are presented elsewhere (e.g., Zelazo, 2004; Zelazo, Gao, & Todd, in press).

The tree diagram in Figure 7.2 illustrates the way in which hierarchies of rules can be formed through reflection—the way in which one rule can first become an object of explicit consideration at a higher level of consciousness and then be embedded under another higher-order rule and controlled by it. Rule A, which indicates that response 1 (r_1) should follow stimulus 1 (s_1), is incompatible with rule C, which connects s_1 to r_2. Rule A is embedded under, and controlled by, a higher-order rule (rule E) that can be used to select rule A or rule B, and this, in turn, is embedded under a still higher-order rule (rule F) that can be used to select the discrimination between rules A and B as opposed to the discrimination between rules C and D. This higher-order rule makes reference to setting conditions or contexts (c_1 and c_2) that condition the selection of lower-order rules, and that would be taken for granted in the absence of reflection. Higher-order rules of this type (F) are required in order to use *bivalent* rules in which the same stimulus is linked to different responses (e.g., rules A and C). Simpler rules like E suffice to select between *univalent* stimulus–response associations—rules in which each stimulus is associated with a different response.

Consider, for example, the goal of getting a letter into the mail as soon as possible. Rule A may specify that you should deposit your envelope in the first mailbox you see that has a late (e.g., 5 P.M.) pickup time. Rule B may indicate that you should refrain from depositing your envelope in mailboxes that only have early morning pickups. Reflecting on rules A and B allows you to use rule E to discriminate between mailboxes

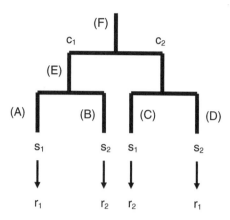

FIGURE 7.2. Hierarchical tree structure depicting formal relations among rules. c_1 and c_2 = contexts; s_1 and s_2 = stimuli; r_1 and r_2 = responses. Copyright 1995 by Elsevier. Adapted by permission.

that will help or hinder you in pursuit of your goal; A signifies approach, B avoidance. If, however, it is after 5 P.M., then you need to deposit your envelope in a mailbox with an early morning pickup and avoid mailboxes that only have late pickups. The time, therefore, is a context that needs to be considered. Reflection on this fact calls for formulation of another rule, rule F, for selecting between one context, *before 5 P.M.*, and another, *after 5 P.M.*. If it is after 5 P.M., you will want to avoid depositing your envelope in mailboxes with a 5 P.M. pickup (observing rule C instead of rule A) and proceed with another new rule, rule D: Deposit the envelope in a mailbox with an early-morning pickup.

Notice that in order to formulate a higher-order rule such as F and deliberate between rules C and D, on the one hand, and rules A and B, on the other, one has to be aware of the fact that one knows both pairs of lower order rules. Figuratively speaking, one has to view the two rule pairs from the perspective of (F). This shows how increases in reflection on lower-order rules are required for increases in embedding to occur. Each level of consciousness allows for the formulation and maintenance in working memory of a more complex rule system. A particular level of consciousness is required to use a single rule such as (A); a higher level of consciousness is required to select between two univalent rules using a rule such as (E); a still higher level is required to switch between two bivalent rules using a rule such as (F).

Implementational Level

The Levels of Consciousness Model (e.g., Zelazo, 2004) is a process model that describes the steps leading from the representation of a stimulus to the execution of a controlled response. In this model, reflection and rule use, which requires the maintenance of information in working memory, are the primary psychological processes involved in fulfilling the relatively abstract function of deliberate goal-directed problem solving (i.e., EF). The implementional level concerns how these psychological processes are realized in the brain. Considerable research remains to be conducted at this level of analysis, but there is now strong evidence that EF depends importantly on the integrity of neural systems involving the prefrontal cortex (PFC) (e.g., Luria, 1966; Miller, 1999; Stuss & Benson, 1986), although it is also clear that other brain regions are involved, and that different regions of PFC are especially important for particular aspects of EF (e.g., Bunge, 2004). A great deal of current research in cognitive neuroscience is directed at identifying specific structure–function relations in regions of the PFC (e.g., Stuss & Knight, 2002).

Bunge and Zelazo (2006) summarized a growing body of evidence that the PFC plays a key role in rule use, and that different regions of the PFC are involved in representing rules at different levels of complexity—from a single rule for responding when stimulus–reward associations need to be reversed (orbitofrontal cortex [OFC]; Brodmann's area [BA] 11[1]), to sets of conditional rules (ventrolateral prefrontal cortex [vLPFC; BA 44, 45, 47] and dorsolateral prefrontal cortex [dLPFC; BA 9, 46]), to explicit consideration of task sets (frontopolar cortex or rostrolateral prefrontal cortex [rLPFC; BA 10]; see Figure 7.4). The role of OFC in rule use can be seen in object reversal, when one learns a simple discrimination between two objects and then the discrimination is reversed (the previously unrewarded object is rewarded and vice versa). To respond flexibly and rapidly on this task, it helps to represent the new stimulus–reward association explicitly, as a simple stimulus–reward rule maintained in working memory (Schoenbaum & Setlow, 2001); damage to OFC leads to perseverative responding in both human adults (Rolls, Hornak, Wade, & McGrath, 1994) and nonhuman primates (Dias, Robbins, & Roberts, 1996). In the absence of a simple stimulus–reward association maintained in working memory, one is likely to respond to the most salient association that one has to the situation—one is likely to respond to the previously rewarded stimulus.

In contrast to the OFC, both the vLPFC and dLPFC have been consistently implicated in the retrieval, maintenance, and use of more complex sets of conditional stimulus–response rules—in lesion studies and functional magnetic resonance imaging (fMRI) studies (e.g., Wallis & Miller, 2003; see Bunge, 2004, for review). For example, using fMRI, Crone, Wendelken, Donohue, and Bunge (2006) found that both vLPFC and dLPFC are active during the maintenance of sets of conditional rules, and that they are sensitive to rule complexity, showing more activation for bivalent rules than for univalent rules. Bunge, Kahn, Wallis, Miller, and Wagner (2003) observed that these two regions are also more active for more abstract conditional rules ("match" or "non-match" rules, whereby different actions are required depending on whether two objects match or not) than for specific stimulus–response associations. However, fMRI data suggest that dLPFC may be especially important when participants must switch from one bivalent rule to another, and hence suppress the previously relevant rule (Crone et al., 2006). That is, whereas vLPFC may be necessary for representing pairs of conditional rules, dLPFC may be recruited when representing bivalent rules that place heavy demands on attentional selection (Miller, 1999) or response selection (Rowe, Toni, Josephs, Frackowiak, & Passingham, 2000). These rules may be quite general in their application, extending, for example, to the selection among competing cues in semantic memory (Thompson-Shill, D'Esposito, Aguirre, & Farah, 1997). In effect, vLPFC together with dLPFC may serve to foreground some pieces of information while backgrounding others, all in the service of a goal.

Finally, fMRI studies suggest that rLPFC plays an important role in the temporary consideration of higher-order rules (such as E and F in Figure 7.3) for selecting among task sets, as when switching between two abstract rules (Bunge et al., 2005; Crone et al., 2006), integrating information in the context of relational reasoning (Christoff et al., 2001), or coordinating hierarchically embedded goals (Koechlin, Basso, Pietrini, Panzer, & Grafman, 1999). This region may be involved in reflecting on lower-order rules and selecting among them at any level within a rule hierarchy—selecting between two univalent rules or switching between two pairs of bivalent rules. As a result, rLPFC may interact with different parts of prefrontal cortex (i.e., vLPFC or dLPFC) depending on the type of task involved (Sakai & Passingham, 2003, 2006)—and hence, we would argue, depending on the complexity of the rule systems involved.

Figure 7.3 illustrates the way in which regions of the PFC may correspond to rule use at different levels of complexity. As should be clear, the function of PFC is proposed to be hierarchical in a way that corresponds to the hierarchical complexity of the rule use underlying EF. As individuals engage in reflective processing, ascend through levels of consciousness, and formulate more complex rule systems, they recruit an increasingly complex hierarchical network of PFC regions.

One important implication of this conceptualization of EF is that it emerges from a dynamic interaction between bottom-up and top-down processes. As a result, EF takes time to occur. Information must first be processed at lower levels of consciousness and in particular parts of the PFC before it can be passed forward and processed at higher levels of consciousness and in other parts of PFC. In addition, information about a stimulus is reprocessed iteratively using the same network that was used for the original processing, with higher levels of consciousness guiding the reprocessing of information at lower levels of consciousness. Specifically, top-down PFC processes foreground specific aspects of information (hence backgrounding others), and these reweighted representations are used to "reseed" initial EF processing by influencing ongoing processing of the stimulus.

Because reflective processing takes time, the model makes predictions about the time course of EF as well as the potential consequences of requiring rapid responses (cf. White, 1965). EF can only be as effective as the amount of time allowed to complete the process. Many times, one must reach a judgment or initiate a behavioral sequence before EF processes have reached an optimal solution. In these situations, one can have partial EF—despite a person's goals.

HOT VERSUS COOL EXECUTIVE FUNCTION: TOWARD A NEW MODEL OF EMOTION REGULATION AS EXECUTIVE FUNCTION

Although EF can be understood as a domain-general construct at the most abstract, functional level (i.e., as conscious goal-directed problem solving), more precise characterizations (at the algorithmic and implementational levels) necessitate another distinction—that between the relatively "hot" motivationally significant aspects of EF more associated with ventral parts of the PFC, and the more motivationally independent "cool" aspects more associated with the lateral PFC (Zelazo & Müller, 2002; cf. Metcalfe & Mischel, 1999; Miller & Cohen, 2001). Whereas cool EF is more likely to be elicited by relatively abstract, decontextualized problems (e.g., sorting by color, number, or shape in the WCST), both hot and cool EF are required for problems that involve the regulation of motivation. Thus, hot EF is especially prominent when people really *care* about the problems they are attempting to solve, although in fact, emotion regulation involves both hot EF (control processes centered on reward representations) and cool EF (higher-order processing of more abstract information).

Interestingly, the link between EF and emotion regulation is most closely seen when the problem to be solved is that of modulating emotion, as in emotion regulation.

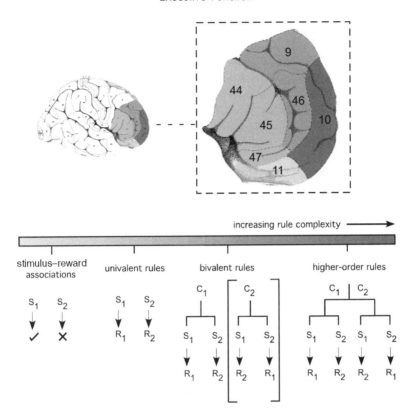

FIGURE 7.3. A hierarchical model of rule representation in the PFC. A lateral view of the human brain is depicted at the top of the figure, with regions of the PFC identified by the Brodmann's areas (BA) that comprise them: Orbitofrontal cortex (BA 11), ventrolateral PFC (BA 44, 45, 47), dorsolateral PFC (BA 9, 46), and rostrolateral PFC (BA 10). The PFC regions are shown in various shades of gray, indicating which types of rules they represent. Rule structures are depicted below, with darker shades of gray indicating increasing levels of rule complexity. The formulation and maintenance in working memory of more complex rules depends on the reprocessing of information through a series of levels of consciousness, which in turn depends on the recruitment of additional regions of PFC into an increasingly complex hierarchy of PFC activation. S, stimulus; ✓, reward; x, nonreward; R, response; C, context, or task set. Brackets indicate a bivalent rule that is currently being ignored. From Bunge and Zelazo (2006). Copyright 2006 by Blackwell Publishing. Reprinted by permission.

In such cases, EF *just is* emotion regulation—the two constructs are isomorphic. Yet, when the modulation of emotion occurs in the service of solving another problem (which we believe is the case for the majority of situations), then EF *involves* emotion regulation. It should be noted that emotion regulation in these two cases may differ. For example, when emotion regulation is a secondary goal, there may be a greater need for selecting among task sets (and hence, greater rLPFC involvement). Although it seems likely that emotion regulation occurs most often in the service other goals, research on emotion regulation has generally relied on paradigms in which emotion regulation is the participants' primary objective (e.g., Ochsner et al., 2004).

This characterization of hot EF in contradistinction to cool EF is consistent with neuroanatomical evidence that the ventral PFC differs from the lateral PFC in their patterns of connectivity with other brain regions. The OFC is part of a frontostriatal circuit that has strong connections to the amygdala and other parts of the limbic system. Consequently, the OFC is anatomically well suited for the integration of affective and nonaffective information, and for the regulation of appetitive/motivated responses (e.g., Damasio, 1994; Rolls, 1999). In contrast, these connections are less direct in the case of the lateral PFC (indeed, they are partly mediated by the OFC). In addition to its connections with the OFC, the dLPFC is connected to a variety of brain areas that would allow it to play an important role in the integration of sensory and mnemonic information and the regulation of intellectual function and action. These include the thalamus, parts of the basal ganglia (the dorsal caudate nucleus), the hippocampus, and primary and secondary association areas of neocortex, including posterior temporal, parietal, and occipital areas (e.g., Fuster, 1989).

The distinction between hot and cool EF is also consistent with a large body of research regarding the functions of the dLPFC, on the one hand, and the OFC, on the other. Traditionally, research on EF in human beings has focussed almost exclusively on dLPFC, using measures such as the WCST and the Tower of London (Shallice, 1988). Results of this research contributed our current characterization of cool EF. A good deal of early research on the OFC was conducted with nonhuman animals, using two relatively simple paradigms: object reversal learning and extinction. As noted earlier, in object reversal, animals learn a simple discrimination between two objects and then the discrimination is reversed (the previously unrewarded object is rewarded and vice versa). On this task, animals with lesions to (the inferior convexity of) the OFC fail to switch their responses and instead perseverate on the initial discrimination (e.g., Butter, 1969; Dias et al., 1996; Iversen & Mishkin, 1970; Jones & Mishkin, 1972). More recent research has demonstrated that human patients with acquired OFC damage also reveal deficits in reversal learning, including perseverative responding to the previously rewarded stimulus (Fellows & Farah, 2003; Rolls et al., 1994).

Response extinction tasks are similar to reversal learning tasks in that they also involve a change in the reinforcement contingencies after a response has been learned to criterion. In this case, a response is reinforced, and then reinforcement is withheld. In such situations, nonhuman primates with lesions to (caudal) OFC (e.g., Butter, Mishkin, & Rosvold, 1963) and human patients with OFC damage (Rolls et al., 1994) display resistance to extinction, continuing to respond to the nonreinforced stimulus.

Findings of this sort have led to suggestions that the OFC is heavily involved in the reappraisal of the affective or motivational significance of stimuli (e.g., Rolls, 1999, 2004). According to this view, while the amygdala is primarily involved in the initial learning of stimulus–reward associations (e.g., Killcross, Robbins, & Everitt, 1997; LeDoux, 1996), reprocessing of these relations is the province of the OFC. In terms of the Bunge and Zelazo (2006) model, this type of reprocessing—as assessed by relatively simple tasks such as object reversal and extinction—may rely heavily on the OFC because it requires the explicit representation of a simple stimulus–reward association to govern approach or avoidance of a concrete stimulus.

Recently, researchers have noted that human patients with OFC damage are often impaired at the self-regulation of social behavior—especially in generating appropriate emotional reactions given social norms (Beer, Heerey, Keltner, Scabini, & Knight, 2003; Damasio, 1994; Rolls et al., 1994). Researchers working with human patients have also used a variety of more complex laboratory measures of hot EF, such as the Iowa Gambling Task (e.g., Bechara, Damasio, Damasio, & Anderson, 1994), which assesses decision making about uncertain events that have emotionally significant consequences (i.e., meaningful rewards and/or losses). Although initial studies suggested that the

OFC alone (especially on the right) was important for performance on this task, more recent research has revealed an important role for the dLPFC (Fellows & Farah, 2005; Manes et al., 2002; see also Hinson, Jameson, & Whitney, 2002). This may be due to the complexity of the rules required.

In addition, however, it should be noted that the various regions of the PFC are parts of a single coordinated system and probably work together—even in a single situation. Thus, it seems likely that decision making is routinely influenced in a bottom-up fashion by affective reactions (e.g., Damasio, 1994; Gray, 2004) and the representation of reward value (e.g., Rolls, 1999). Conversely, it seems likely that a successful approach to solving hot problems is to reconceptualize the problem in relatively neutral, decontextualized terms and try to solve it using cool EF (cf. Mischel, Shoda, & Rodriguez, 1989)—reflecting on the situation, creating more complex rule systems, and recruiting more lateral regions of PFC.

Indeed, in terms of the hierarchical model of PFC function (see Figure 7.3), it is not that ventral regions such as the OFC are exclusively involved in hot EF but, rather that they remain more activated even as the hierarchy of the PFC is elaborated. Simple rules for approaching versus avoiding concrete stimuli (the provenance of the OFC) are more difficult to ignore in motivationally significant situations. Thus, in effect, hot EF involves increased bottom-up influences on PFC processing, with the result that hot EF (vs. cool EF) requires relatively more attention to (and activation of) lower levels in rule hierarchies—discriminations at that level become more salient, leading to relatively more ventral PFC (i.e., OFC and perhaps vLPFC) activation even when higher levels in the hierarchy are also involved. Rather than positing discrete systems for hot and cool EF, this model views hot–cool as a continuum that corresponds to the motivational significance of the problem to be solved, and to the degree of reflection and rule complexity made possible by the hierarchy of PFC function. These two dimensions (motivational significance and reflection or reprocessing) are understood to be correlated and to correspond to what has been called psychological distance from the situation (Carlson, Davis, & Leach, 2005; Dewey, 1931/1985; Sigel, 1993; Zelazo, 2004)—a cognitive separation from the exigencies of the situation. It should be noted, however, that it is also possible that rule complexity and motivational significance are orthogonal aspects of prefrontal organization: More anterior parts of PFC may represent more complex rules, and more ventral parts of PFC may represent reward-related information. Further research is needed to test these alternatives.

Finally, another distinction that becomes relevant when considering EF at the implementational level is that between left and right hemispheres of the brain (cf. Tucker & Williamson, 1984). A growing body of evidence suggests that the right PFC may be more likely to be involved in hot EF than cool EF. For example, damage to the right (or bilateral) OFC has a greater effect on social conduct, decision making, emotional processing, and other purported OFC functions than does damage to the left OFC (e.g., Manes et al., 2002; Rolls et al., 1994; Stuss, 1991; Stuss & Alexander, 1999; Stuss, Floden, Alexander, & Katz, 2001; Tranel, Bechara, & Denburg, 2002). As discussed by Bechara (2004; see also Tranel et al., 2002), patients with right OFC damage reveal marked impairments in everyday functioning as well as on the Iowa Gambling Task, and these effects are similar to those revealed in bilateral OFC patients. By contrast, patients with left OFC damage are relatively unimpaired, suggesting that the reliable impairments demonstrated by bilateral OFC patients may derive primarily from the right OFC.

There are several possible reasons why the right OFC may be so important for these functions. Bechara (2004) suggests that right–left hemispheric asymmetries in OFC function may derive from the differential involvement of the right and left hemispheres in avoidance (negative affect) and approach (positive affect), respectively (see also Davidson & Irwin, 1999; Davidson, Jackson, & Kalin, 2000). That is, adaptive decision making on the Iowa Gambling Task, and possibly measures of affective decision making more generally, requires avoidance of seemingly positive responses (a function for which the right OFC may be particularly well suited). The right hemisphere has also been implicated in the mapping of bodily states and the comprehension of somatic information (Davidson & Schwartz, 1976), and this too may help to explain the relative importance of right OFC to everyday decision making (Bechara, 2004; Damasio, 1994).

The hemispheric asymmetry in approach and avoidance is relevant in its own right. Building on earlier work using baseline resting electroencephalograph (EEG), research has revealed considerable evidence that processing negative information is more associated with activation in regions of the right PFC (Anderson et al. 2003; Cunningham, Johnson, Gatenby, Gore, & Banaji, 2003; Cunningham, Raye, & Johnson, 2004c; Sutton, Davidson, Donzella, Irwin, & Dottl, 1997), whereas processing positive information is more associated with activation in regions of the left PFC (Anderson et al., 2003; Cunningham et al., 2004c; Nitschke et al., 2003; Kringelbach, O'Doherty, Rolls, & Andrew, 2003; see Wager, Phan, Liberzon, & Taylor, 2003, for a meta-analysis). Given that human beings appear biased to attend to negative versus positive information (Ito, Larsen, Smith, & Cacioppo, 1998b), and that negative information is generally more arousing (Ito, Cacioppo, & Lang, 1998a), it may be the case that the right OFC is more involved in processing information with motivational significance, rather than negative information per se.

In the first part of this chapter, we suggested that EF can be understood at each of Marr's (1982) three levels of analysis—computational, algorithmic, and implementational. At the computational level, we characterized EF as an abstract, hierarchical, iterative, cybernetic function: deliberate, goal-directed problem solving. At the algorithmic level, we outlined a process model of EF that emphasizes the roles of reflection (through a series of levels of consciousness) and the formulation, maintenance in working memory, and execution of rule systems that vary in hierarchical complexity. At the implementation level, we presented a hierarchical model of PFC function. Key properties at the computational level—EF as hierarchical, iterative, and cybernetic—also apply to the algorithmic and implementational levels because these levels fulfill the function specified at the computational level.

We then distinguished between hot and cool aspects of EF and suggested that hot EF is associated with higher degrees of motivational significance. At the algorithmic level, this corresponds to attention to relatively simple discriminations between approaching and avoiding stimuli that are construed as relatively concrete. At the implementational level, this corresponds to greater activation in the ventral PFC and greater right-hemisphere involvement. This distinction is the basis of a new model of emotion regulation, which we now explore in more detail—again in terms of Marr's (1982) levels.

A NEW MODEL OF EMOTION REGULATION

Computational Level

At the computational level, one may have as a primary or secondary goal the modulation of emotion. Modulation may involve emotional upregulation (increasing the intensity of a specific emotion), emotional downregulation (decreasing the intensity of a specific emotion), maintaining an emotion, or a qualitative change in one's emotional reactions. Consider the case of downregulating anger, as a primary goal. First, one has to represent the problem, assessing (1) one's current state—a high level of anger, (2) one's goal state—a reduction in anger and, correlatively, an increase in detachment, and (3) options for reducing the discrepancy between (1) and (2). These options may include reappraisal of the anger-provoking stimulus, simple distraction, or reminding oneself about the extent to which one values detachment, among other possibilities. Second, one has to select a promising plan from among these options, considering the relative efficacy of the options as well as the effort involved. Given that one has other pressing demands, such as an article to write, distraction may be likely to work and easy to implement, so one proceeds to the third general step of executing this plan. Now, one needs to adopt a goal of focusing one's attention on the article, and one needs to keep this goal in mind and act on the basis of it despite a tendency to dwell on the anger-provoking stimulus. When absorbed in writing the article, all is well; however, when one's attention reverts to the stimulus, one has to recognize that one's efforts at downregulation have failed. That is, one has to engage in evaluation, including taking steps to correct one's errors—for example, by stepping up one's efforts to attend to a relatively engaging aspect of the distracting activity.

In most cases, one needs to consider multiple goals simultaneously, at various levels of abstraction, and one pursues them more or less automatically (Bargh, 1989; Carver & Sheier, 1982; Shallice, 1988). EF is involved in just those cases in which one is considering goals consciously and one is deliberately attempting to obtain them; normally one pursues a limited number of such goals at the same time. Nonetheless, as we saw, EF needs to be understood as a complex hierarchical function, and one inevitably needs to pursue more proximal subgoals (e.g., executing a plan) in the service of fulfilling a more distal, but still explicit, goal (e.g., solving the problem). It seems likely that emotion regulation is often a subgoal pursued in the service of another goal. That is, one strives to regulate one's emotion (e.g., upregulation or downregulation) *in order* to foster the fulfillment of some other goal about which one cares.

Algorithmic Level

At the algorithmic level, emotion regulation involves reflection and the formulation and use of rules at various levels of complexity. Reflection and rule use allow one to progress through the functional phases identified at the computational level of analysis. Whether emotion regulation is the primary goal of EF or a subgoal, it will involve the elaboration (via the reprocessing of information through levels of consciousness) of an increasingly complex rule system, or system of inferences. This more complex rule system, maintained in working memory as the activated contents of consciousness, entails a reappraisal of the emotion-relevant situation. That is, it entails contextualization of the situation; rather than accepting a relatively superficial gloss of the situation—one that extracts only its most salient, low-resolution aspects, leading to a relatively simple approach–avoidance discrimination—one's representation of the situation is reprocessed and integrated with other information about contexts in which the situation may be understood. One consequence of the ascent through levels of consciousness will be an increase in psychological distance (e.g., Dewey, 1931/1985) from the situation, which is bound to result in cooler EF. Another consequence of the more carefully considered construal of the situation, based on the formulation of a more complex system of rules, is that one can now follow higher-order rules for selecting certain aspects of the situation to which to attend. Generally speaking, attending selectively to certain aspects of the now broadly construed situation will be an effective way to modulate one's emotional reactions to the situation. For example, one may increase the intensity of one's emotional reaction by attending to more provocative aspects or decrease the intensity of one's reaction by focusing on less provocative aspects. In contrast, processing that is restricted to a relatively low level of consciousness is likely to be perseverative, and this type of processing may underlie rumination in some cases.

Implementational Level

In addition to the hierarchically arranged regions of lateral PFC depicted in Figure 7.3, emotion regulation involves a number of other neural structures, and it is instructive to show how these regions may interact with the PFC. Indeed, attempting to understand emotion regulation in terms of EF, and hence considering the interplay between top-down and bottom-up processes that occurs in emotion regulation, prompts us to develop a more comprehensive neural model of emotion regulation, albeit one that is still focused relatively exclusively on the PFC (e.g., ignoring the key roles of parietal cortex and the hippocampus) and that glosses over important distinctions within regions (within the limbic circuit: nucleus accumbens, ventral striatum, and nuclei of the amygdalae, etc.; LeBar & LeDoux, 2003).

Figure 7.4 depicts the implementational level of our model of EF as a circuit diagram. To describe the model at this level, we first follow the flow of information involved in generating an emotional reaction and triggering some efforts at emotion regulation. Perceptual information about a stimulus is processed via the thalamus and fed forward (via the direct, subcortical route) to the amygdala, which generates an initial, unreflective motivational tendency to approach or avoid the stimulus (e.g., LeDoux, 1996). This amygdala response leads to various emotional sequelae not depicted here (e.g., sympathetic activation), but it also serves as input to the OFC, which implements an initial, relatively simple level of emotion regulation by processing amygdala output relative to a learned context (and simple approach-avoidance rules). When OFC activation fails to suffice to generate an unambiguous response to the stimulus (e.g., because the stimulus is ambivalent or signals the presence of an error), this triggers activation in the anterior cingulate cortex (ACC), which responds to the motivational significance of the stimulus—as understood at this level of processing. The ACC, on this model, serves to initiate the reprocessing of information via vLPFC and then dLPFC, with rLPFC playing a key, transient role in the explicit consideration of task sets. Broca's area is depicted separately from vLPFC in Figure 7.4 in order to capture the fact that the rule use involved in these top-down regulatory processes may be intrinsically linguistic (i.e., it may be mediated by private speech; Vygotsky, 1962; Luria, 1961). At the same time, however, we note that self-directed speech may not be necessary in some cases, consistent with research on the emotional regulation of prejudice showing that the right PFC, and not the left PFC, is sometimes involved in regulation (Cunningham et al., 2004a; Richeson et al., 2004).

As in EF more generally, in emotion regulation different regions of the lateral PFC are recruited as one engages in reflection and in the retrieval, maintenance, and use of rule systems at different levels of complexity. This route to emotion regulation is tantamount to the initiation of elaborative processing of a motivationally significant stimulus; as mentioned at the algorithmic level, this entails contextualization of the situation, and it may result in ER via reciprocal suppression between levels in the hierarchy of PFC regions (e.g., Drevets & Raichle, 1998). When lateral PFC regions are engaged,

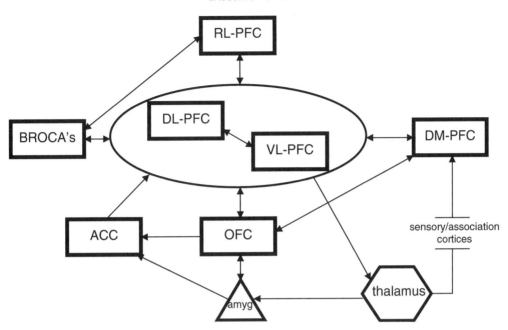

FIGURE 7.4. Neural circuitry underlying ER. Information about a sensory stimulus is processed by the thalamus and projected to the amygdala, leading to an initial motivational tendency to approach or avoid the stimulus, but also initiating further processing of the stimulus by the anterior cingulate cortex (ACC) and orbitofrontal cortex (OFC). The ACC responds to the motivational significance of the situation and may serve to recruit additional reprocessing of the stimulus via ventrolateral prefrontal cortex (vLPFC) and then dorsolateral prefrontal cortex (dLPFC), with rostrolateral prefrontal cortex (rLPFC) playing a transient role in the explicit consideration of task sets. Broca's area is involved insofar as top-down regulatory processes rely on private speech, and it is depicted separately from vLPFC, of which it is a part. Reprocessing by lateral regions of PFC corresponds to reflection (through levels of consciousness) and the elaboration of rule hierarchies, and it serves to regulate emotion by amplifying or suppressing attention to certain aspects of the situation (thalamic route) and by biasing simple approach–avoidance rules in the OFC.

rLPFC will permit reflective selection among task sets, and dLPFC and vLPFC will implement this selection, representing a reconfigured context for responding. The consequences of this new representation are propagated back down the hierarchy, biasing simple approach–avoidance rules in the OFC, which plays a more direct role in regulating amygdala activation.

The last PFC region that appears to play a critical role in ER is dorsomedial PFC (dMPFC; BA 9[medial]). Although the exact function of dMPFC is heavily debated, this region has repeatedly been shown to be involved in various aspects of reflective emotional processing. In a meta-analysis of emotion, Phan, Wager, Taylor, and Liberzon (2002) found that dMPFC was involved in many aspects of affective processing, regardless of the valence and sensory modality of the triggering stimulus. Interestingly, this region was much more likely to be activated in studies involving reflectively generated emotion, as opposed to perceptually generated emotion—for example, when people generated an emotional response in the absence of a triggering stimulus (Teasdale et al., 1999), when people monitored their emotional response (Henson, Rugo,

Shallice, Josephs, & Dolan, 1999), and when people anticipated an emotional response (Porro et al., 2002). In addition, this region appears to play an important role in the understanding of social agents (Frith & Frith, 1999; Gallagher & Frith, 2003; Mitchell, Banaji, & Macrae, 2005; Mitchell, Macrae, & Banaji, 2004), leading Cunningham and Johnson (in press) to suggest that this region may be a polymodal integration area for the complex processing and understanding of emotional information and may be involved in more complex aspects of emotion (guilt, shame, *schadenfreude*) that may drive or be a consequence of emotional regulation. This account relies on a distinction between direct, perceptual processing of stimuli (including rewards and punishers) and indirect processing that is mediated by reflective processing (e.g., *anticipated* rewards and punishers).

A series of studies from our lab that compare the more explicit to more implicit aspects of the emotional evaluation of stimuli allows for comparisons between relatively automatic emotional responses to stimuli and the emotional experience that is modified through emotion regulation. Importantly, in these studies, emotion regulation is not the person's primary goal per se but occurs in the service of other goals. For the most part in these studies, participants make either evaluative (good–bad) or non-evaluative (abstract–concrete; past–present) judgments during fMRI (Cunningham et al., 2003; Cunningham et al., 2004c, 2005b) or EEG recording (Cunningham, Espinet, DeYoung, & Zelazo, 2005a). Following scanning, participants rate each of the stimuli presented to them during scanning on several dimensions, including the extent to which they (1) had an emotional response to the stimulus, (2) experienced attitudinal ambivalence (having simultaneous positive and negative responses), and (3) attempted to regulate their initial emotional response. Using these ratings as parametric regressors, we have been able to map the relations among brain processing and specific aspects of evaluative or emotional processing.

As would be expected, emotionality ratings correlated with activation in the amygdala and the OFC for both good–bad and abstract–concrete trials—suggesting that the emotional significance of stimuli was processed relatively automatically (see Figure 7.5, left column). More critical for the discussion of emotion regulation as EF, ratings of emotion regulation correlated with activation in each of the areas in our proposed model—ACC, OFC, vLPFC, dLPFC, and rLPFC (see Figure 7.5, middle column). Providing support for the suggestion that vLPFC is involved in reweighting of the relevance of information and in selecting information for subsequent processing, we found the greatest vLPFC and ACC activity for stimuli rated as most ambivalent (Cunningham et al., 2003). In addition, self-reported emotion regulation correlated with activation in dMPFC. Interestingly, and in contrast to the correlations observed for the experience of an emotional response, the correlations between these brain regions and ratings of ambivalence and emotion regulation were found to be significantly greater for evaluative as compared to non-evaluative trials. This difference suggests that emotion regulation and the processing of complex emotions occurs primarily in the service of deliberate, goal-directed processing.

Similar results were found in an fMRI study of the regulation of prejudice—or emotion regulation in the context of attitudes about race (Cunningham et al., 2004a). In most college samples, participants are likely simultaneously to show (1) automatically activated negative behavioral responses to social outgroups and (2) motivation to suppress these feelings in order to display a more socially acceptable response (Cunningham, Nezlek, & Banaji, 2004b; Devine, 1989; Plant & Devine, 1998). Thus, on average, people are likely to adopt a goal of inhibiting or suppressing an emotional response that could potentially result in prejudice or discrimination, and they are likely

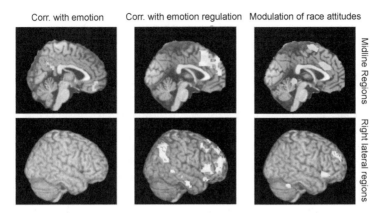

FIGURE 7.5. Data depicting the processing of emotional experience and emotion regulation. Data from the right lateral surface and the medial regions are presented for each analysis. Data for the correlation between emotion and emotion regulation are from Cunningham, Raye, and Johnson (2004c), and data for the modulation of race prejudice are from Cunningham et al. (2004a).

to use EF processes to accomplish this goal. In our study, participants were presented with black or white faces for either 30 msec or 525 msec. In the 30-msec condition, participants did not report seeing faces, whereas the 525-msec condition allowed sufficient time for the conscious recognition and processing of the face. When participants were not able to see the faces, greater amygdala activation was found to the black compared to the white faces consistent with the hypothesis that, even for individuals who claimed not to be prejudiced, there was an automatic negative emotional response to members of social outgroups. In contrast, when participants were able to see the faces and had the ability to regulate their emotional response, amygdala activation was significantly reduced and accompanied by activation in frontal regions (see Figure 7.5, right column). It is important to note that despite the vast differences between these studies, the particular PFC regions found were nearly identical to the regions found to be correlated with self-reported ER in Cunningham et al. (2004c; see Figure 7.5, middle and right columns, for comparison). Providing further evidence for the involvement of these regions in emotion regulation, we found that activity in rLPFC and ACC was significantly correlated with a reduction in amygdala activation to black compared with white faces.

It should be noted that emotion regulation does not necessarily imply the *inhibition* of a response. Similar to the fMRI studies just discussed, Cunningham et al. (2005a) presented participants with valenced stimuli and asked participants to make either good–bad or abstract–concrete judgments while high-density EEG was recorded. Consistent with hypotheses of hemispheric asymmetries in the processing of emotional stimuli (e.g., Davidson, 2004), greater anterior right sided activity was observed to stimuli rated as bad compared to stimuli rated as good. Interestingly, this effect, which began approximately 450 msec following stimulus presentation, was observed for both good–bad and abstract–concrete trials. Although the onset of the asymmetry was not influenced by task, the amplitude of the effect as measured later in processing (e.g., 1,200 msec poststimulus) was greater for the good–bad compared with the abstract–concrete trials. This suggests an automatic initiation of emotional processing followed by an amplification of a response as a result of reflective reprocessing of the stimulus (e.g., by the lateral PFC).

KEY IMPLICATIONS OF THE NEW MODEL

Reseeding

One key proposal of this model is that information about a motivationally significant stimulus is reprocessed iteratively using the same network that was used for the original processing. Specifically, PFC processes foreground specific aspects of information (hence backgrounding others), and these reweighted representations are used to "reseed" EF processing by influencing ongoing processing of the stimulus. This is accomplished, according to this model, by thalamocortical connections between the lateral PFC and the thalamus that bias attention to particular aspects of the situation as it continues to be processed in real time. As such, EF and emotion regulation should not be thought of as single processes that act in opposition to emotional processing (e.g., turning off a circuit). Rather, given the iterative nature of EF, the information is likely reprocessed multiple times before a goal state is reached. This highlights an important feature of the emotion regulation as EF model: many of the processes involved in emotion regulation are the very same processes that are used for emotion generation. Indeed, according to this model, successful emotion regulation is the deliberate, goal-directed attainment of a desired emotional state. When this state has been achieved, and the discrepancy between the goal state and the current state is reduced below some threshold, emotion regulation will cease.

Implications for Development of Emotion Regulation

The growth of the PFC follows an extremely protracted developmental course (e.g., Giedd et al., 1999; Gogtay et al., 2004; O'Donnell, Noseworthy, Levine, & Dennis, 2005; Sowell et al., 2003) that mirrors the development of EF. For example, developmental research suggests that the order of acquisition of rule types shown in Figure 7.4 corresponds to the order in which corresponding regions of the PFC mature. In particular, gray-matter volume reaches adult levels earliest in OFC, followed by the vLPFC, and then by the dLPFC (Giedd et al., 1999). Measures of cortical thickness suggest that dLPFC and rLPFC exhibit similar, slow rates of structural change (O'Donnell et al., 2005). On the basis of this evidence, Bunge and Zelazo (2006) hypothesized that the pattern of developmental changes in rule use reflects the different rates of development of specific regions within the PFC. The use of relatively complex rules is acquired late in development because it involves the hierarchical coordination of regions of the PFC—a hierarchical coordination that parallels the hierarchical structure of children's rule systems and develops in a bottom-up fashion, with higher levels in the hierarchy operating on the products of lower levels.

To the extent that the PFC is involved in emotion regulation, the development of emotion regulation should also be a protracted process and may be informed by research on the development of EF. A good deal is now known about the development of cool EF (see Zelazo & Müller, 2002, for review), but relatively little is known about the development of hot EF. One key line of work, however, comes from Overman, Bachevalier, Schuhmann, and Ryan (1996), who demonstrated age-related improvements in performance on object reversal in infants and young children. In addition, these authors found that prior to 30 months of age, boys performed better than girls—a finding consistent with work showing that performance on this task develops more slowly in female monkeys than in male monkeys, and that this sex difference is under the control of gonadal hormones (Clark & Goldman-Rakic, 1989; Goldman, Crawford, Stokes, Galkin, & Rosvold, 1974). This suggests that there may be a similar neural basis to sex differences in emotion regulation.

Kerr and Zelazo (2004) assessed hot EF in slightly older children, using a version of the Iowa Gambling Task (Bechara et al., 1994). Children chose between (1) cards that offered more rewards per trial but were disadvantageous across trials due to occasional large losses, and (2) cards that offered fewer rewards per trial but were advantageous overall. On later trials, 4-year-olds made more advantageous choices than expected by chance whereas 3-year-olds (and especially 3-year-old girls) made fewer. Three-year-olds' behavior on this task resembled that of adults with damage to the OFC, suggesting that the task may provide a behavioral index of the development of orbitofrontal function. Subsequent work explored the basis of 3-year-olds' poor performance, identifying a role for working memory (Hongwanishkul, Happaney, Lee, & Zelazo, 2005) and demonstrating that even 3-year-olds develop somatic markers as indicated by anticipatory skin conductance responses (SCRs) prior to making disadvantageous choices (DeYoung et al., 2007). Paradigms such as this one may be used to explore the role of hot EF in emotion regulation (e.g., see Lamm, Zelazo, & Lewis, 2006; Lewis, Lamm, Segalowitz, Stieben, & Zelazo, 2006).

CONCLUSION

In this chapter, we provided a new model of emotion regulation that spans Marr's (1982) three levels of analysis—computational (concerning what emotion regulation accomplishes), algorithmic (dealing in more detail with the way emotion-relevant information is represented and how it is processed during emotion regulation), and implementational (examining the neural basis of emotion regulation). Naturally, this model is overly simple; the processes involved in emotion regulation are only beginning to be understood. Nonetheless, the model makes specific claims at all three levels of analysis and may provide a useful stimulus for future research on emotion regulation. In addition to testing hypotheses derived from the model (e.g., developmental constraints on emotion regulation), future research might usefully explore whether different strategies of emotion regulation rely on different aspects of EF and how the processes underlying emotion regulation overlap with those involved in the experience of complex social emotions (i.e., emotions that likely require relatively high levels of consciousness). Overall, however, we hope that this model demonstrates how an understanding of basic processes of EF may shed light on critical aspects of emotion, including the phenomenological experience of emotion and the dynamic regulation of this experience.

ACKNOWLEDGMENTS

Preparation of this chapter was supported in part by grants from the Natural Sciences of Engineering Research Council of Canada to Philip David Zelazo and to William A. Cunningham, and the Canadian Institutes of Health Research to Philip David Zelazo. We thank Silvia Bunge, James Gross, Marc Lewis, and two anonymous reviewers for providing helpful comments on an earlier draft of this chapter, and Silvia Bunge, Doug Frye, and Ulrich Müller, with whom some of these theoretical ideas were developed. This chapter is a précis of a longer article on emotion regulation and its development in childhood.

NOTE

1. For the purposes of this chapter, we consider the OFC to be primarily the medial aspects of the orbital frontal cortex.

REFERENCES

Anderson A. K., Christoff, K., Stappen, I., Panitz, D., Ghahremani, D. G., Glover G., et al. (2003). Dissociated neural representations of intensity and valence in human olfaction. *Nature Neuroscience, 6,* 196–202.

Baddeley, A. (1996). Exploring the central executive [Special Issue: Working Memory]. *Quarterly Journal of Experimental Psychology, Human Experimental Psychology, 49A,* 5–28.

Barceló, F., & Knight, R. T. (2002). Both random and perseverative errors underlie WCST deficits in prefrontal patients. *Neuropsychologia, 40,* 349–356.

Bargh, J. A. (1989). Conditional automaticity: Varieties of automatic influence on social perception and cognition. In J. Uleman & J. Bargh (Eds.), *Unintended thought* (pp. 3–51). New York: Guilford Press.

Barrett, L. F., Ochsner, K. N., & Gross, J. J. (in press). Automaticity and Emotion. In J. Bargh (Ed.), *Automatic processes in social thinking and behavior.* New York: Psychology Press.

Bechara, A. (2004). The role of emotion in decision-making: Evidence from neurological patients with orbitofrontal damage. *Brain and Cognition (Special Issue: Development of Orbitofrontal Function), 55,* 30–40.

Bechara, A., Damasio, A. R., Damasio, H., & Anderson, S. W. (1994). Insensitivity to future consequences following damage to human prefrontal cortex. *Cognition, 50*(1-3), 7–15.

Bechara, A., Tranel, D., Damasio, H., & Anderson, S. W. (1994). Insensitivity to future consequences following damage to human prefrontal cortex. *Cognition, 50,* 7–12.

Beer, J. S., Heerey, E. H., Keltner, D., Scabini, D., & Knight, R. T. (2003). The regulatory function of self-conscious emotion: Insights from patients with orbitofrontal damage. *Journal of Personality and Social Psychology, 85,* 594–604.

Bunge, S. A. (2004). How we use rules to select actions: A review of evidence from cognitive neuroscience. *Cognitive, Affective, and Behavioral Neuroscience, 4,* 564–579.

Bunge, S. A., Kahn, I., Wallis, J. D., Miller, E. K., & Wagner, A. D. (2003). Neural circuits subserving the retrieval and maintenance of abstract rules. *Journal of Neurophysiology, 90,* 3419–3428.

Bunge, S. A., Wallis, J. D., Parker, A., Brass, M., Crone, E. A., Hoshi, E., et al. (2005). Neural circuitry underlying rule use in humans and non-human primates *Journal of Neuroscience, 9,* 10347–10350.

Bunge, S. A., & Zelazo, P. D. (2006). A brain-based account of the development of rule use in childhood. *Current Directions in Psychological Science, 15,* 118–121.

Butter, C. (1969). Perseveration in extinction and in discrimination reversal tasks following selective frontal ablations in macaca mulatta. *Physiology and Behavior, 4,* 163–171.

Butter, C. M., Mishkin, M., & Rosvold, H. E. (1963). Conditioning and extinction of a food-rewarded response after selective ablations of frontal cortex in rhesus monkeys. *Experimental Neurology, 7,* 65–75.

Carlson, S. M., Davis, A. C., & Leach, J. G. (2005). Less is more: Executive function and symbolic representation in preschool children. *Psychological Science, 16,* 609–616.

Carver, C. S., & Sheier, M. F. (1982). Control theory: A useful conceptual framework for personality—Social, clinical, and health psychology. *Psychological Bulletin, 92,* 111–135.

Christoff, K., Prabhakaran, V., Dorfman, J., Zhao, Z., Kroger, J. K., Holyoak, K. J., et al. (2001). Rostrolateral prefrontal cortex involvement in relational integration during reasoning. *NeuroImage, 14,* 1136–1149.

Clark, A. S., & Goldman-Rakic, P. S. (1989). Gonadal hormones influence the emergence of cortical function in nonhuman primates. *Behavioral Neuroscience, 103,* 1287–1295.

Crone, E. A., Wendelken, C., Donohue, S. E., & Bunge, S. A. (2006). Neural evidence for dissociable components of task switching. *Cerebral Cortex, 16,* 475–486.

Cunningham, W. A., Espinet, S. D., DeYoung, C. G., & Zelazo, P. D. (2005). Attitudes to the right—and left: Frontal ERP asymmetries associated with stimulus valence and processing goal. *NeuroImage, 28,* 827–834.

Cunningham, W. A., & Johnson, M. K. (in press). Attitudes and evaluation: Toward a component process framework. In E. Harmon-Jones & P. Winkielman (Eds.), *Fundamentals of social neuroscience*. New York: Guilford Press.

Cunningham, W. A., Johnson, M. K., Gatenby, J. C., Gore, J. C., & Banaji, M. R. (2003). Component processes of social evaluation. *Journal of Personality and Social Psychology, 85,* 639–649.

Cunningham, W. A., Johnson, M. K., Raye, C. L., Gatenby, J. C., Gore, J. C., & Banaji, M. R. (2004a). Separable neural components in the processing of Black and White faces. *Psychological Science, 15,* 806–813.

Cunningham, W. A., Nezlek, J. B., & Banaji, M. R. (2004b). Implicit and explicit ethnocentrism: Revisiting the ideologies of prejudice. *Personality and Social Psychology Bulletin, 30,* 1332–1346.

Cunningham, W. A., Raye, C. L., & Johnson, M. K. (2004c). Implicit and explicit evaluation: fMRI correlates of valence, emotional intensity, and control in the processing of attitudes. *Journal of Cognitive Neuroscience, 16,* 1717–1729.

Cunningham, W. A., Raye, C. L., & Johnson, M. K. (2005b). Neural correlates of evaluation associated with promotion and prevention regulatory focus. *Cognitive, Affective, and Behavioral Neuroscience, 5,* 202–211.

Damasio, A. R. (1994). *Descartes' error.* New York: Putnam.

Davidson, R. J. (2004). Well-being and affective style: Neural substrates and biobehavioural correlates. *Philosophical Transactions of the Royal Society of London, 359,* 1395–1411.

Davidson, R. J., & Irwin, W. (1999). The functional neuroanatomy of emotion and affective style. *Trends in Cognitive Sciences, 3,* 11–21.

Davidson, R. J., Jackson, D. C., & Kalin, N. H. (2000). Emotion, plasticity, context, and regulation: Perspectives form affective neuroscience. *Psychological Bulletin, 126,* 890–909.

Davidson, R. J., & Schwartz, G. E. (1976). The psychobiology of relaxation and related states: A multiprocess theory. In D. I. Motosky (Ed.), *Behavior control and modification of physiological activity* (pp. 399–342). Englewood Cliffs, NJ: Prentice Hall.

Delis, D. C., Squire, L. R., Bihrle, A., & Massman, P. J. (1992). Componential analysis of problem-solving ability: Performance of patients with frontal lobe damage and amnesic patients on a new sorting test. *Neuropsychologia, 30,* 683–697.

Devine, P. G. (1989). Stereotypes and prejudice: Their automatic and controlled components. *Journal of Personality and Social Psychology, 56,* 5–18.

Dewey, J. (1985). Context and thought. In J. A. Boydston (Ed.) & A. Sharpe (Textual Ed.), *John Dewey: The later works, 1925–1953* (Vol. 6, 1931–1932, pp. 3–21). Carbondale: Southern Illinois University Press. (Original work published 1931)

DeYoung, C., Prencipe, A., Happaney, K. R., Mashari, A., Macpherson, D., & Zelazo, P. D. (2005). *Development of somatic markers on the Children's Gambling Task.* Manuscript in preparation.

Dias, R., Robbins, T. W., & Roberts, A. C. (1996, March 7). Dissociation in prefrontal cortex of affective and attentional shifts. *Nature, 380,* 69–72.

Drevets, W. C., & Raichle, M. E. (1998). Reciprocal suppression of regional cerebral blood flow during emotional versus higher cognitive processes: Implications for interactions between emotion and cognition. *Cognition and Emotion, 12,* 353–385.

Fellows, L. K., & Farah, M. J. (2003). Ventromedial frontal cortex mediates affective shifting in humans: Evidence from a reversal learning paradigm. *Brain, 126,* 1830–1837.

Fellows, L. K., & Farah, M. J. (2005). Different underlying impairments in decision-making following ventromedial and dorsolateral frontal lobe damage in humans. *Cerebral Cortex, 15,* 58–63.

Fitzsimons, G. M., & Bargh, J. A. (2004). Automatic self-regulation. In R. F. Baumeister & K. D. Vohs (Eds.), *Handbook of self-regulation: Research, theory and applications* (pp. 151–170). New York: Guilford Press.

Frith, C. D., & Frith, U. (1999). Interacting minds—A biological basis. *Science, 286,* 1692–1695.

Frye, D., Zelazo, P. D., & Palfai, T. (1995). Theory of mind and rule-based reasoning. *Cognitive Development, 10,* 483–527.

Fuster, J. (1989). *The prefrontal cortex: Anatomy, physiology and neuropsychology of the frontal lobe* (2nd ed.). New York: Raven Press.

Gallagher, H. L., & Frith, C. D. (2003). Functional imaging of "theory of mind." *Trends in Cognitive Sciences, 7,* 77–83

Giedd, J. N. (2004). Structural magnetic resonance imaging of the adolescent brain. *Annals of the New York Academy of Sciences, 1021,* 77–85.

Giedd, J. N., Blumenthal, J., & Jeffries, N. O., Costellanos, F. X., Vaituzis, A. C., Fernandez, T., et al. (1999). Brain development during childhood and adolescence: A longitudinal MRI study. *Nature Neuroscience, 2*, 861–863.

Gogtay, N., Giedd, J. N., Lusk, L., Hayashi, K. M., Greenstein, D., Vaituzis, A. C., et al. (2004). Dynamic mapping of human cortical development during childhood through early adulthood. *Proceedings of the National Academy of Sciences, USA, 101*(21), 8174–8179.

Goldberg, E., & Bilder, Jr., R. M. (1987). The frontal lobes and hierarchical organization of cognitive control. In E. Perecman (Ed.), *The frontal lobes revisited* (pp. 159–187). Hillsdale, NJ: Erlbaum.

Goldman, P. S., Crawford, H. T., Stokes, L. P., Galkin, T. W., & Rosvold, H. E. (1974, November 8). Sex-dependent behavioral effects of cerebral cortical lesions in the developing rhesus monkey. *Science, 186*, 540–542.

Grant, D. A., & Berg, E. A. (1948). A behavioral analysis of degree of reinforcement and ease of shifting to new responses in a Weigl-type card-sorting problem. *Journal of Experimental Psychology, 38*, 404–411.

Gray, J. R. (2004). Integration of emotion and cognitive control. *Current Directions in Psychological Science, 13*, 46–48.

Gross, J. J., & Thompson, R. (2007). Emotion regulation: Conceptual foundations. In J. J. Gross (Ed.), *Handbook of emotion regulation* (pp. 3–24). New York: Guilford Press.

Henson, R. N., Rugo, M. D., Shallice, T., Josephs, O., & Dolan, R. J. (1999). Recollection and familiarity in recognition memory: An event-related functional magnetic resonance imaging study. *Journal of Neuroscience, 19*, 3962–3972.

Hinson, J. M., Jameson, T. L., & Whitney, P. (2002). Somatic markers, working memory, and decision making. *Cognitive, Affective, and Behavioral Neuroscience, 2*, 341–353.

Hongwanishkul, D., Happaney, K. R., Lee, W., & Zelazo, P. D. (2005). Hot and cool executive function: Age-related changes and individual differences. *Developmental Neuropsychology, 28*, 617–644.

Ito, T. A., Cacioppo, J. T., & Lang, P. J. (1998a). Eliciting affect using the International Affective Picture System: Bivariate evaluation and ambivalence. *Personality and Social Psychology Bulletin, 24*, 856–879.

Ito, T. A., Larsen, J. T., Smith, N. K., & Cacioppo, J. T. (1998b). Negative information weighs more heavily on the brain: The negativity bias in evaluative categorizations. *Journal of Personality and Social Psychology, 75*, 887–900.

Iverson, S. D., & Mishkin, M. (1970). Perseverative interference in monkeys following selective lesions of the inferior prefrontal convexity. *Experimental Brain Research, 11*, 376–386.

Jones, B., & Mishkin, M. (1972). Limbic lesions and the problem of stimulus-reinforcement associations. *Experimental Neurology, 36*, 362–377.

Kerr, A., & Zelazo, P. D. (2004). Development of "hot" executive function: The Children's Gambling Task [Special Issue: Development of Orbitofrontal Function]. *Brain and Cognition, 55*, 148–157.

Killcross, S., Robbins, T. W., & Everitt, B. J. (1997, July 24). Different types of fear-conditioned behaviour mediated by separate nuclei within amygdala. *Nature, 388*, 377–380.

Koechlin, E., Basso, G., Pietrini, P., Panzer, S., & Grafman, J. (1999). The role of the anterior prefrontal cortex in human cognition. *Nature, 399*, 148–151.

Kringelbach, M. L., O'Doherty, J., Rolls, E. T., & Andrews, C. (2003). Activation of the human orbitofrontal cortex to a liquid food stimulus is correlated with its subjective pleasantness. *Cerebral Cortex, 13*, 1064–1071.

Lamm, C., Zelazo, P. D., & Lewis, M. D. (2006). Neural correlates of cognitive control in childhood and adolescence: Disentangling the contributions of age and executive function. *Neuropsychologia, 44*, 2139–2144.

LeBar, K. S., & LeDoux, J. E. (2003). Emotional learning ciruits in animals and humans. In R. J. Davidson, K. S. Scherer, & H. H. Goldsmith (Eds.), *Handbook of affective sciences* (pp. 52–65). New York: Oxford University Press.

LeDoux, J. E. (1996). *The emotional brain.* New York: Simon & Schuster.

Lewis, M. D., Lamm, C., Segalowitz, S. J., Stieben, J., & Zelazo, P. D. (2006). Neurophysiological correlates of emotion regulation in children and adolescents. *Journal of Cognitive Neuroscience, 18*, 430–443.

Luria, A. R. (1961). *The role of speech in the regulation of normal and abnormal behaviour* (J. Tizard, Ed.). New York: Pergamon Press.

Luria, A. R. (1966). *Higher cortical functions in man* (2nd ed.). New York: Basic Books. (Original work published 1962)

Manes, F., Sahakian, B., Clark, L., Rogers, R., Antoun, N., Aitken, M., & Robbins, T. (2002). Decision-making processes following damage to the prefrontal cortex. *Brain, 125*, 624–639.

Marr, D. (1982). *Vision*. Cambridge, MA: MIT Press.

Metcalfe, J., & Mischel, W. (1999). A hot/cool-system analysis of delay of gratification: Dynamics of willpower. *Psychological Review, 106*, 3–19.

Miller, E. K. (1999). The prefrontal cortex: Complex neural properties for complex behavior. *Neuron, 22*, 15–17.

Miller, E. K., & Cohen, J. D. (2001). An integrative theory of prefrontal cortex function. *Annual Review of Neuroscience, 24*, 167–202.

Mischel, W., Shoda, Y., & Rodriguez, M. L. (1989, May 26). Delay of gratification in children. *Science, 244*, 933–938.

Mitchell, J. P., Banaji, M. R., & Macrae, C. N. (2005). General and specific contributions of the medial prefrontal cortex to knowledge about mental states. *NeuroImage, 28*, 757–762

Mitchell, J. P., Macrae, C. N., & Banaji, M. R. (2004). Encoding-specific effects of social cognition on the neural correlates of subsequent memory. *Journal of Neuroscience, 24*, 4912–4917.

Nitschke, J. B., Nelson, E. E., Rusch, B. D., Fox, A. S., Oakes, T. R., & Davidson, R. J. (2003). Orbitofrontal cortex tracks positive mood in mothers viewing pictures of their newborn infants. *NeuroImage, 21*, 583–592.

Norman, D. A., & Shallice, T. (1986). Attention to action: Willed and automatic control of behavior. In R. J. Davidson, G. E. Schwartz, & D. Shapiro (Eds.), *Consciousness and self-regulation* (Vol. 4, pp. 4–18). New York: Plenum Press.

Ochsner, K. N., Ray, R. D., Robertson, E. R., Cooper, J. C., Chopra, S., Gabrieli, J. D. E., et al. (2004). For better or for worse: Neural systems supporting the cognitive down- and up-regulation of negative emotion. *NeuroImage, 23*, 483–499.

O'Donnell, S., Noseworthy, M. D., Levine, B., & Dennis, M. (2005). Cortical thickness of the frontopolar area in typically developing children and adolescents. *NeuroImage, 24*(4), 948–954.

Overman, W. H., Bachevalier, J., Schuhmann, E., & Ryan, P. (1996). Cognitive gender differences in very young children parallel biologically-based cognitive gender differences in monkeys. *Behavioral Neuroscience, 110*, 337–344.

Pennington, B. F., & Ozonoff, S. (1996). Executive functions and developmental psychopathology. *Journal of Child Psychology and Psychiatry, 37*, 51–87.

Phan, K. L., Wager, T., Taylor, S. F., & Liberzon, I. (2002). Functional neuroanatomy of emotion: A meta-analysis of emotion activation studies in PET and fMRI. *NeuroImage, 16*, 331–348.

Plant, E. A., & Devine, P. G. (1998). Internal and external motivation to respond without prejudice. *Journal of Personality and Social Psychology, 75*, 811–832.

Porro, C. A., Baraldi, P., Pagnoni, G., Serafini, M., Facchin, P., Maieron, M., et al. (2002). Does anticipation of pain affect cortical nociceptive systems? *Journal of Neuroscience, 22*, 3206–3214.

Richeson, J. A., Baird, A. A., Gordon, H. L., Heatherton, T. F., Wyland, C. L., Trawalter, S., et al. (2003). An fMRI examination of the impact of interracial contact on executive function. *Nature Neuroscience, 6*, 1323–1328.

Roberts, A. C., Robbins, T. W., & Weiskrantz, L. (1998). *The prefrontal cortex: Executive and cognitive functions*. Oxford, UK: Oxford University Press.

Rolls, E. T. (1999). *The brain and emotion*. Oxford, UK: Oxford University Press.

Rolls, E. T. (2004). The functions of the orbitofrontal cortex [Special Issue: Development of Orbitofrontal Function]. *Brain and Cognition, 55*, 11–29.

Rolls, E. T., Hornak, J., Wade, D., & McGrath, J. (1994). Emotion-related learning in patients with social and emotional changes associated with frontal lobe damage. *Journal of Neurology, Neurosurgery and Psychiatry, 57*, 1518–1524.

Rowe, J. B., Toni, I., Josephs, O., Frackowiak, R. S., & Passingham, R. E. (2000). The prefrontal cortex: Response selection or maintenance within working memory? *Science, 288*, 1656–1660.

Sakai, K., & Passingham, R. E. (2003). Prefrontal interactions reflect future task operations. *Nature Neuroscience, 6*, 75–81.

Sakai, K., & Passingham, R. E. (2006). Prefrontal set activity predicts rule-specific neural processing during subsequent cognitive performance. *Journal of Neuroscience, 26*, 1211–1218.

Schoenbaum, G., & Setlow, B. (2001). Integrating orbitofrontal cortex into prefrontal theory: Common processing themes across species and subdivisions. *Learning and Memory, 8*, 134–147.

Shallice, T. (1988). *From neuropsychology to mental structure*. New York: Cambridge University Press.

Sigel, I. (1993). The centrality of a distancing model for the development of representational competence. In R. R. Cocking & K. A. Renninger (Eds.), *The development and meaning of psychological distance* (pp. 91–107). Hillsdale, NJ: Erlbaum.

Sowell, E. R., Peterson, B. S., Thompson, P. M., Welcome, S. E., Henkenius, A. L., et al. (2003). Mapping cortical change across the human life span. *Nature Neuroscience, 6,* 309–315.

Stuss, D. (1991). Disturbance of self-awareness after frontal system damage. In G. P. Prigatano & D. L. Schachter (Eds.), *Awareness of deficit after brain injury: Theoretical and clinical aspects.* New York: Oxford University Press.

Stuss, D. T., & Alexander, M. P. (1999). Affectively burnt in: A proposed role of the right frontal lobe. In E. Tulving (Ed.), *Memory, consciousness and the brain: The Tallinn conference* (pp. 215–227). Philadelphia: Psychology Press.

Stuss, D. T., & Benson, D. F. (1986). *The frontal lobes.* New York: Raven Press.

Stuss, D. T., & Knight, R. T. (2002). *Principles of frontal lobe function.* New York: Oxford University Press.

Stuss, D. T., Floden, D., Alexander, M. P., Levine, B., & Katz, D. (2001). Stroop performance in focal lesion patients: Dissociation of processes and frontal lobe lesion location. *Neuropsychologia, 39,* 771–786.

Sutton, S. K., Davidson, R. J., Donzella, B., Irwin, W., & Dottl, D. A. (1997). Manipulating affective state using extended picture presentations. *Psychophysiology, 34,* 217–226.

Teasdale, J. D., Howard, R. J., Cox, S. G., Ha, Y., Brammer, M. J., Williams, S. C., et al. (1999). Functional MRI study of the cognitive generation of affect. *American Journal of Psychiatry, 156,* 209–215.

Thompson-Schill, S. L., D'Esposito, M., Aguirre, G. K., & Farah, M. J. (1997). Role of left inferior prefrontal cortex in retrieval of semantic knowledge: A reevaluation. *Proceedings of the National Academy of Sciences, USA, 94,* 14792–14797.

Tranel, D., Anderson, S. W., & Benton, A. L. (1994). Development of the concept of "executive function" and its relationship to the frontal lobes. In F. Boller & J. Grafman (Eds.), *Handbook of neuropsychology* (Vol. 9, pp. 125–148). Amsterdam: Elsevier Science B.V.

Tranel, D., Bechara, A., & Denburg, N. L. (2002). Asymmetric functional roles of right and left ventromedial prefrontal cortices in social conduct, decision-making, and emotional processing. *Cortex, 38,* 589–612.

Tucker, D. M., & Williamson, P. A. (1984). Asymmetric neural control systems in human self-regulation. *Psychological Review, 91,* 185–215.

Vygotsky, L. S. (1962). *Thought and language.* Oxford, UK: Wiley.

Wager, T. D., Phan, K. L., Liberzon, I., & Taylor, S. F. (2003). Valence, gender, and lateralization of functional brain anatomy in emotion: A meta-analysis of findings from neuroimaging. *NeuroImage, 19,* 513–531.

Wallis, J. D., & Miller, E. K. (2003). Neuronal activity in primate dorsolateral and orbital prefrontal cortex during performance of a reward preference task. *European Journal of Neuroscience, 18,* 2069–2081.

Weiner, N. (1948). *Cybernetics.* Cambridge, MA: MIT Press.

White, S. H. (1965). Evidence for a hierarchical arrangement of learning processes. In L. P. Lipsitt & C. C. Spiker (Eds.), *Advances in child development and behavior* (Vol. 2, pp. 187–220). New York: Academic Press.

Zelazo, P. D. (2004). The development of conscious control in childhood. *Trends in Cognitive Sciences, 8,* 12–17.

Zelazo, P. D., Carter, A., Reznick, J. S., & Frye, D. (1997). Early development of executive function: A problem-solving framework. *Review of General Psychology, 1,* 1–29.

Zelazo, P. D., Frye, D., & Rapus, T. (1996). An age-related dissociation between knowing rules and using them. *Cognitive Development, 11,* 37–63.

Zelazo, P. D., Gao, H. H., & Todd, R. (in press). The development of consciousness. In P. D. Zelazo, M. M. Moscovitch, & E. Thompson (Eds.), *The Cambridge handbook of consciousness.* New York: Cambridge University Press.

Zelazo, P. D., & Müller, U. (2002). Executive function in typical and atypical development. In U. Goswami (Ed.), *Handbook of childhood cognitive development* (pp. 445–469). Oxford, UK: Blackwell.

Zelazo, P. D., Müller, U., Frye, D., & Marcovitch, S. (2003). The development of executive function in early childhood. *Monographs of the Society for Research in Child Development, 68*(3), vii–137.

CHAPTER 8

Explanatory Style and Emotion Regulation

CHRISTOPHER PETERSON
NANSOOK PARK

"Explanatory style" refers to how an individual habitually explains the causes of events (Peterson & Seligman, 1984). An extensive research literature links explanatory style to people's thoughts, feelings, motives, and actions in response to the events about which they make causal attributions, but virtually no studies have explored what would seem to be obvious effects of explanatory style on processes of emotional regulation. Our own PSYCInfo subject–term searches revealed only a single empirical study that simultaneously investigated explanatory style and emotion regulation, and it was an unpublished dissertation (Wheeler, 2002).

In this chapter, we discuss how explanatory style might influence emotion regulation, and we touch on reasons for the historical neglect of such inquiry. Our argument is that research into explanatory style has strayed too far from its theoretical origins in the learned helplessness model, a process account of how people respond emotionally to uncontrollable events. An explicit return to the helplessness model as a theoretical framework sheds light on the topic of emotion regulation. One of the matters potentially clarified is how people "handle" (i.e., savor) positive emotions, an issue that has received much less attention than how people "handle" (i.e., cope with) negative emotions, perhaps because people more frequently attempt to regulate negative emotions than positive ones (Gross & Thompson, this volume).

The central constructs in our chapter include emotion, emotion regulation, and of course explanatory style. By *emotion,* we mean more than mere feelings. We follow common usage in regarding an emotion as a constellation of psychological and biological characteristics that cohere around a particular affective state but also include signature thoughts, motives, response tendencies, and physiological changes.

By *emotion regulation,* we mean all the processes—intrinsic and extrinsic, conscious and nonconscious—that influence the components of emotion, their coupling, their manifestation, their grounding in particular situations, and of course their consequences. So, Frijda (1986) catalogued various types of emotion regulation, from confrontation with emotional events to appraisal of these events and the emotions they trigger to the suppression or amplification of feelings and motives to the checking, shaping, or replacement of overt responses. Other classification schemes are described throughout the present volume and elsewhere. The point is that emotion regulation can and does take place in many ways and at many points during the experience of an emotion. In describing how explanatory style affects emotion regulation, we thus need to take a broad look at the possible junctures of influence.

"Regulation" has connotations of deliberate choice, but the influences on emotion regulation—including explanatory style—often operate automatically. However, one of the important developments in explanatory style research has entailed a demonstrably effective protocol for teaching individuals to be more deliberate in how they construe the causes of events and thereby influencing the emotions they experience.

Explanatory style is sometimes described as pessimistic when bad events are explained with causes that are internal to the self and pervasive (e.g., "I am a terrible human being") versus optimistic when bad events are explained with causes that are external to the self and circumscribed (e.g., "It was a fluke"). This usage can be misleading if one starts to designate people as pessimists or optimists according to their explanatory style, not only because of the mistaken implication that there are discrete categories of people as opposed to a continuum along which people fall (usually in the middle) but also because there are everyday and scientific meanings of pessimism and optimism that are not precisely captured by the endpoints of explanatory style for bad events. Furthermore, this usage can lead researchers to overlook explanatory style for good events.

There is nonetheless a logic to the use of "pessimistic" and "optimistic" as adjectives qualifying explanatory style. Explanatory style is thought to influence the specific expectation that one's behaviors are related (or not) to important outcomes, including the occurrence of bad events (Peterson & Vaidya, 2001). A pessimistic explanatory style therefore encourages individuals to believe that they are helpless, that nothing they do matters, whereas an optimistic explanatory style encourages individuals to believe that their behaviors do affect outcomes. A pessimistic explanatory style leads people to expect bad events in the future to be frequent and inevitable, which is what pessimism has meant since it entered the lexicon (Siçinski, 1972). An optimistic explanatory style in contrast leads people to expect bad events in the future to be infrequent. This particular expectation is part of what optimism means, although neglected here is an additional and critical component of optimism: the expectation that good events will be plentiful.

In the next section, we describe the meaning and measurement of explanatory style. When we describe explanatory style as pessimistic or optimistic, the reader should keep in mind the specific meanings just explicated. We provide an overview of relevant empirical research involving explanatory style, mentioning as well topics that have not been well investigated. This overview sets the state for our concluding discussion of psychological processes possibly under the sway of explanatory style that affect how one regulates emotions, both negative and positive.

BACKGROUND

The notion of explanatory style emerged from the attributional reformulation of the learned helplessness model (Abramson, Seligman, & Teasdale, 1978), a theory that has had a much longer shelf life than most in psychology. Indeed, helplessness theory has reinvented itself frequently, sometimes in light of problematic data, more often in response to what happens when a theory is applied to problems outside the laboratory, and occasionally as an inadvertent consequence of its own popularity. The history of learned helplessness theory and research has been reviewed in detail elsewhere, but it is instructive to repeat the highlights here (Peterson, Buchanan, & Seligman, 1995; Peterson, Maier, & Seligman, 1993).

Learned Helplessness

The original helplessness model proposed that following experience with uncontrollable aversive events, animals and people become helpless—passive and unresponsive, presumably because they have "learned" that there is no contingency between actions and outcomes (Maier & Seligman, 1976). This learning is represented as a generalized expectancy that future responses will be unrelated to outcomes. It is this generalized expectation of response–outcome independence that produces helplessness.

Learned helplessness was first described several decades ago by investigators studying animal learning. Researchers immobilized a dog and exposed it to a series of brief electric shocks that could be neither avoided nor escaped. Twenty-four hours later, the dog was placed in a situation in which electric shock could be terminated by a simple response. The dog did not make this response, however, and passively endured the shock, neither moving nor whimpering nor showing other overt signs of emotionality, like defecating. If the dog did happen to make the appropriate response that terminated shock, it seemed not to learn at all from what just happened and was apt to be passive again during the next trial of shock. All this behavior was in contrast to dogs in a control group that reacted vigorously to the shock and learned readily how to turn it off.

These investigators proposed that the dog had learned to be helpless. When originally exposed to uncontrollable shock, it learned that nothing it did mattered. The shocks came and went independently of the dog's behaviors. Response–outcome independence was represented by the dogs as an expectation of future helplessness that was generalized to new situations to produce maladaptive passivity. The deficits that follow in the wake of uncontrollability are known as the *learned helplessness phenomenon,* and we want to emphasize in the present context that the learned helplessness phenomenon is typically described as a set of *deficits*—cognitive, motivational, and emotional—inferred from observed passivity. The associated cognitive explanation became known as the *learned helplessness model* (see Figure 8.1a).

Much of the early interest in learned helplessness stemmed from its clash with traditional stimulus–response theories of learning. Alternative accounts of learned helplessness were proposed that did not invoke mentalistic constructs. Many of these alternatives emphasized an incompatible motor response learned when animals were first exposed to uncontrollable shock. This response was presumably generalized to the second situation where it interfered with performance at the test task. For example, per-

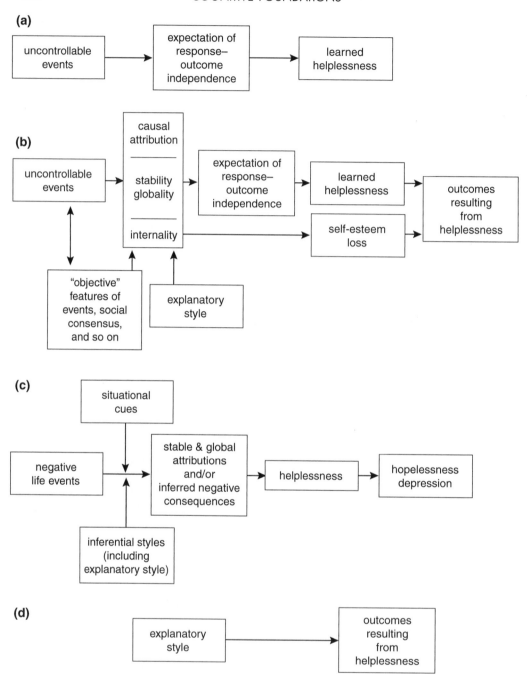

FIGURE 8.1. Process accounts: (a) original learned helplessness model; (b) attributional reformulation; (c) hopelessness theory; and (d) typical explanatory style research.

haps the dogs learned that holding still when shocked somehow decreased pain. If so, they held still in the second situation as well, because this response was previously reinforced. Studies testing the learned helplessness model versus the incompatible motor response alternatives showed that expectations were critical in producing helplessness following uncontrollable events.

Support for a cognitive interpretation of helplessness also came from studies showing that an animal could be immunized against the debilitating effects of uncontrollability by first exposing it to controllable events. The animal learns during immunization that events can be controlled, and this expectation is sustained during exposure to uncontrollable events, precluding learned helplessness.

In other studies, learned helplessness deficits were undone by forcibly exposing a helpless animal to the contingency between behavior and outcome. That is, the animal was compelled to make an appropriate response at the test task, by pushing, pulling, or otherwise prodding it into action. After several such trials, the animal notices that escape is possible and begins to respond on its own. Again, the process at work is cognitive. The animal's expectation of response–outcome independence is challenged during the therapy experience, and hence learning occurs.

Application to Human Problems

Psychologists interested in humans, and particularly human problems, were quick to see the parallels between learned helplessness as produced by uncontrollable events in the laboratory and maladaptive passivity as it exists outside the laboratory. Thus, researchers began several lines of research on learned helplessness in people (Garber & Seligman, 1980; Mikulincer, 1994).

In one line of work, helplessness in people was produced in the laboratory much as it was in animals, by exposing them to uncontrollable events and observing the effects. Unsolvable problems were usually substituted for uncontrollable electric shocks, but the critical aspects of the phenomenon remained. Following uncontrollability, people show a variety of deficits—problem-solving difficulties, motivational impairment, and negative thoughts and feelings. In other studies, researchers documented further similarities between the animal phenomenon and what was produced in the human laboratory, including immunization and therapy.

In another line of work, researchers proposed various failures of adaptation as analogous to learned helplessness and investigated the similarity between learned helplessness and such problems as academic, athletic, and vocational failure; worker burnout; unemployment; noise pollution; physical illness; chronic pain; and passivity among ethnic minorities. The best known of these applications is Seligman's (1974) proposal that reactive depression and learned helplessness share critical features: causes, symptoms, consequences, treatments, and preventions, and a large body of research has compared and contrasted the learned helplessness phenomenon and depression (Peterson & Seligman, 1985).

The fit is good but not perfect. For example, the striking gender difference in the prevalence of depression has no counterpart in laboratory-produced helplessness; males and females are equally susceptible to the damaging effects of uncontrollability (Peterson et al., 1993). For another example, helplessness as produced in the laboratory is not accompanied by thoughts of suicide, one of the hallmark symptoms of severe depression, at least in the Western world.

Some other applications have been little more than metaphorical, starting with an instance of passivity and treating it as if it must have been produced by the processes detailed in the learned helplessness model. At times this is a reasonable approach, given that uncontrollable bad life events can undercut efficacy and thereby produce difficulties in their wake. However, sometimes passivity may be produced instrumentally through processes of reward and punishment. For example, a woman beaten up or belittled by her spouse whenever she takes initiative or expresses an opinion may end up acting passively, but her helplessness is *not* of the learned variety. This point is more than an academic distinction because attempts to prevent or remediate problems may be wrong-headed if based on an incorrect assumption of the responsible mechanisms.

It is also worth returning to the point made earlier that the learned phenomenon as originally described was a set of deficits, including emotional ones. That is, helpless dogs did not act emotionally when shocked. If we can anthropomorphize, the helpless dogs—those exposed to uncontrollable shocks—appeared empty and numb. These descriptions are justified and explained by further laboratory research on learned helplessness among animals showing that uncontrollability produces an analgesia effect, meaning that helpless animals literally are anesthetized (Jackson, Maier, & Coon, 1979).

But some of the applications of helplessness theory to human problems are to phenomena in which emotions are front and center. These emotions may be unpleasant and maladaptive—consider depression and anxiety—but they are certainly not absent. None of this is to say that the learned helplessness model cannot be applied to human problems characterized by emotional excesses. The point is to be more analytic and suggest that if a complex failure of adaptation results from experience with uncontrollable events and is mediated by a belief in one's own helplessness, then learned helplessness is arguably a *mechanism* for the problem but not necessarily a *model* of it.

In other words, the processes articulated in the learned helplessness model may describe one route to some instance of passivity (i.e., a mechanism), but the learned helplessness phenomenon may not be identical to that instance (i.e., not a model). When first described, the learned helplessness phenomenon was entertained as a laboratory model of depression, just as amphetamine intoxication was once regarded as a laboratory model of the positive symptoms of schizophrenia. This strong and provocative claim is nowadays seldom encountered. The current and better question is how learned helplessness leads to depression and other failures of adaptation.

One answer may be that learned helplessness disrupts emotion regulation and leaves the helpless individual at risk for particular problems granted the presence of other predisposing factors. According to this view, the emotional deficit in learned helplessness may not reside in the emotion per se but rather in the processes that allow someone to regulate emotions, good or bad. A helpless person may be unable to "handle" his or her negative feelings, and what starts out as fleeting disappointment or annoyance may take on a life of its own and become a full-blown emotional problem.

Attributional Reformulation

These points notwithstanding, learned helplessness research ensued, and it became clear that the original learned helplessness explanation was an oversimplification in other ways. The model failed to account for the range of reactions that people display in response to uncontrollable events. Some people show the hypothesized deficits across time and situation, whereas others do not. Furthermore, failures of adaptation that the learned helplessness model was supposed to explain, and in particular depression, are often characterized by a striking loss of self-esteem, about which the model is silent.

In an attempt to resolve these discrepancies, Abramson, Seligman, and Teasdale (1978) reformulated the helplessness model as applied to people. They explained the contrary findings by proposing that people ask themselves why uncontrollable events happen. The nature of the person's answer then sets the parameters for the subsequent helplessness. If the causal attribution is *stable* ("it's going to last forever"), then induced helplessness is long-lasting; if *unstable*, then it is transient. If the causal attribution is *global* ("it's going to undermine everything"), then subsequent helplessness is manifest across a variety of situations; if *specific*, then it is correspondingly circumscribed. Finally, if the causal attribution is *internal* ("it's all my fault"), the person's self-esteem drops following uncontrollability; if *external*, self-esteem is left intact.

These hypotheses comprise the *attributional reformulation* of helplessness theory. This new theory left the original model in place, because uncontrollable events were still hypothesized to produce deficits when they gave rise to an expectation of response–outcome independence. The nature of these deficits, however, was now said to be influenced by the causal attribution offered by the individual (see Figure 8.1b).

In some cases, the situation itself provides the explanation made by the person, or the individual may draw on social consensus about operative causes. In other cases, the person relies on his or her habitual way of making sense of events that occur: *explanatory style*. All other things being equal, many people tend to offer similar explanations for disparate events. Explanatory style is therefore a distant, although important, influence on helplessness and ultimately on the failures of adaptation that involve helplessness. As already explained, an explanatory style characterized by internal, stable, and global explanations for bad events is sometimes described as pessimistic, and the opposite style—external, unstable, and specific explanations for bad events—is sometimes described as optimistic.

Hopelessness Theory

The attributional reformulation was in turn revised by Abramson, Metalsky, and Alloy (1989) in what has come to be known as *hopelessness theory*. Much of the attributional reformulation remains, although the specific focus of hopelessness theory is on depression and specifically on those instances of depression in which the cognitive processes specified by hopelessness theory are central.

In hopelessness theory, the belief in future hopelessness as opposed to the belief in past helplessness is hypothesized as the immediate cause of depression (see Figure 8.1c). Casual attributions are given less emphasis in hopelessness theory because— again—they pertain to past events. Instead, expectations about future negative consequences are emphasized in hopelessness theory. Explanatory style for bad events, especially with respect to stability and globality, is still regarded as a risk factor for depression, but hopelessness theory emphasizes that explanatory style is but a diathesis. Actual bad events must occur for depression to ensue, and there may be instances in which the features of these events—real or perceived—override habitual explanatory style to produce hopelessness and in turn depression (Johnson, 1995).

A conceptual dividend of hopelessness theory is that it offers an explanation for the comorbidity of anxiety and depression, a fact that the attributional reformulation does not address. Helplessness presumably accompanies both anxiety and depression, but hopelessness further characterizes depression. Accordingly, anxiety disorders are more common than depressive disorders, and cases of "pure" anxiety can be much more readily identified than cases of "pure" depression (Alloy, Kelly, Mineka, & Clements, 1990).

As noted, hopelessness theory builds on helplessness theory, and the differences are at times subtle. We highlight hopelessness theory because it draws our attention to the processes that lead to depression and is therefore consistent with our argument here. Hopelessness theory also makes conceptual contact with Beck's (1991) well-known cognitive account of depression, which regards negative views of the self, the world, and the future as the core of the disorder. These negative views are maintained by cognitive errors such as magnification and overgeneralization which in the present context can be described as failures of emotion regulation entailing the appraisal of events and their import. Hopelessness theory also captures the empirical fact that feelings of hopelessness robustly predict suicidal ideation and suicide attempts among depressed individuals (Beck, Steer, Beck, & Newman, 1993).

Measurement of Explanatory Style

Explanatory style took off as its own line of research when measures of explanatory style were developed. Most popular has been a self-report questionnaire called the Attributional Style Questionnaire (ASQ) (Peterson et al., 1982). In the ASQ, respondents are presented with hypothetical events involving themselves and then asked to provide "the one major cause" of each event if it were to happen. Respondents then rate these provided causes along dimensions of internality, stability, and globality. Ratings are combined. Very early on in the development of the ASQ, it became clear that the valence of the events about which causal attributions were made mattered greatly, so the questionnaire distinguishes bad events and good events and requires researchers to calculate explanatory style scores separately for them. As it turns out, explanatory style based on bad events usually has more robust correlates than explanatory style based on good events, although correlations are typically in the opposite directions (Peterson, 1991).

Why is explanatory style about bad events a more powerful predictor than explanatory style for good events? One explanation is that people become more mindful when bad things occur (and that their causal accounts have greater impact on behavior because they result from deeper processing). But another explanation is that the outcomes typically examined with respect to explanatory style have been negative ones— depression, failure, illness, and the like—and are unsurprisingly better predicted by how people think about bad events. If explanatory style researchers were to examine outcomes such as happiness, health, and success, perhaps explanatory style for good events would prove a more powerful predictor. Although only a few studies have looked at positive outcomes as a function of explanatory style for good events, the finding that internal, stable, and global attributions for good events predicts recovery from depression is consistent with this analysis (Johnson, Han, Douglas, Johannet, & Russell, 1998; Needles & Abramson, 1990).

The original ASQ requested attributions for six bad events and six good events, and the individual scales (internality, stability, and globality) were not highly reliable (Peterson et al., 1982). Revisions of the ASQ boosted reliability to satisfactory levels (αs .80) by asking about a greater number of bad events but kept the questionnaire's length manageable by no longer asking about good events (e.g., Dykema, Bergbower, Doctora,

& Peterson, 1996). In retrospect, this decision is regrettable because it further precluded the investigation of explanatory style for good events.

This modification was carried into the second common way of measuring explanatory style, a content analysis procedure—the CAVE (Content Analysis of Verbatim Explanations)—that allows written or spoken material to be scored for naturally occurring causal explanations (Peterson, Schulman, Castellon, & Seligman, 1992). Researchers identify explanations for bad events, extract them, and present them to judges who then rate them along the scales of the ASQ. The CAVE technique makes possible longitudinal studies after the fact, as long as spoken or written material can be located from early in the lives of individuals for whom long-term outcomes of interest are known.

Extensive research has followed demonstrating diverse correlates of explanatory style (for bad events) in a variety of domains—cognition, mood, behavior, physical health, and social relations (Peterson & Vaidya, 2003). Table 8.1 summarizes these findings. Some caveats should be expressed.

An optimistic explanatory style (for bad events) is associated with active coping, persistence, and delay of gratification. These are laudable characteristics as long as the

TABLE 8.1. Correlates and Consequences of Explanatory Style

Outcome variable	Correlation with pessimistic explanatory style for bad events
Cognition	
Accurate risk perception	Positive
Perception of hassle-free life	Negative
Personal control	Negative
Mood	
Absence of anxiety, depression	Negative
Absence of suicide	Negative
Behavior	
Achievement (academic, athletic, military, political, vocational)	Negative
Active (problem-focused) coping	Negative
Perseverance	Negative
Delay of gratification	Negative
Maladaptive persistence	Positive
Health	
Absence of illness	Negative
Immunocompetence	Negative
Speed of recovery from illness	Negative
Survival time with illness	Negative
Longevity	Negative
Freedom from traumatic accidents	Negative
Health promoting lifestyle	Negative
Social relations	
Absence of loneliness	Negative
Attractiveness to others	Negative
Friendships	Negative

world cooperates. But at least in principle, an optimistic explanatory style might be associated with maladaptive persistence. There is not much of a research literature here because investigators have usually studied outcomes actually attainable through perseverance. Regardless, an inflexible optimism is sometimes linked to the pursuit of the unattainable, perhaps because it leads people to overlook or ignore information that contradicts their positive expectations (Metcalfe, 1998). Constructs such as perfectionism, John Henryism, mania, and the Type A coronary-prone behavior pattern are flavored with a problematic optimism (Peterson, 1999).

Reality matters, and one's expectations about the future cannot be too much at odds with this reality. As Taylor (1989) phrased it, a beneficial optimism is illusory but not delusional. Consider findings described by Isaacowitz and Seligman (2001) that among the elderly, an *optimistic* explanatory style (for bad events) predicts depression in the wake of stressful events. Perhaps extreme optimism among the elderly is unrealistic because an indefinitely extended future orientation does not square with what will be. The occurrence of something terrible can therefore devastate optimistic older individuals when they realize that their optimism must be wrong, a realization much more infrequent for younger individuals.

Origins of Explanatory Style

What initially sets explanatory style in place? Researchers have not attempted to answer this question with a sustained line of research. What we find instead are isolated studies that document diverse influences on explanatory style. Few of these studies investigate more than one influence at a time. Hence, we cannot say what are the more important versus less important influences on explanatory style. Nor can we say how different influences interact. Finally, researchers have not studied explanatory style prior to age 8, when children are first able to respond to interview versions of the ASQ (Nolen-Hoeksema, 1986). We assume that explanatory style takes form at an earlier age, although we await appropriate assessment strategies to study the process. These shortcomings aside, here is what is known about the natural history of explanatory style.

Genetics

The explanatory styles of monozygotic twins were more highly correlated than the explanatory styles of dizygotic twins ($r = .48$ vs. $r = .00$) (Schulman, Keith, & Seligman, 1993). This finding does not necessarily mean that there is an optimism gene. Genes may be indirectly responsible for the concordance of explanatory style among monozygotic twins. For example, genes influence such attributes as intelligence and physical attractiveness, which in turn may lead to more positive (and fewer negative) outcomes in the environment, which in turn may encourage a more optimistic explanatory style.

Parents

Researchers have explored the relationship between the explanatory styles of parents and their offspring (e.g., Seligman et al., 1984). Attributions by mothers and their children are usually the focus. The relevant data prove inconclusive, with some researchers finding convergence between the causal attributions of mothers and their children and others not. Perhaps the best way to make sense of these conflicting findings is to take them at face value and conclude that explanatory style is transmitted to children by some parents but not by others. Researchers therefore must do something more than calculate simple correlations between the explanatory styles of parents and children; they need to investigate plausible moderators of this possible link. How much time do parents and children spend together? Which parent is the major caregiver? About what do they talk? Do causal explanations figure in this discourse?

We assume that the explanatory style of children can be affected by their parents through simple modeling. Children are attuned to the ways in which their parents interpret the world, and may be inclined to interpret matters in a similar manner. If, for example, children repeatedly hear their parents give internal, stable, and global explanations for bad events, they are likely to adopt these pessimistic interpretations for themselves.

Another type of parental influence involves their interpretation of their children's behaviors. Criticisms implying pessimistic causes have a cumulative effect on how children view themselves (Seligman, 1991). Related to this point, Vanden Belt and Peterson (1991) found that children whose parents had a pessimistic explanatory style vis-à-vis bad events involving them work below their potential in the classroom—perhaps because they had internalized their parents' outlook.

There is another type of parental influence that is indirect but probably quite important: whether a safe and coherent world is provided for the young child. We know that children from happy and supportive homes are more likely as adults to have an optimistic explanatory style for bad events (Franz, McClelland, Weinberger, & Peterson, 1994). Parental encouragement and support diminishes fear of failure and enables children to take the necessary risks to find and pursue their real interests and talents. Success and confidence are generated, which in turn lead to expectations of further success.

Teachers

As teachers administer feedback about children's performance, their comments may affect children's attributions about their successes and failures in the classroom. In a study by Heyman, Dweck, and Cain (1992), kindergarten students role-played scenarios in which one of their projects was criticized by a teacher. Thirty-nine percent of the students displayed a helpless response to the teacher's criticism—exhibiting negative affect, changing their original positive opinions of the project to more negative ones, and expressing disinclinations toward future involvements in that type of project. In addition, those children were more likely to make negative judgments about themselves that were internal, stable, and global. Mueller and Dweck (1998) showed that even praise can be detrimental to children when it is focused on a trait perceived to be fixed. So, children who were praised for their intelligence displayed more characteristics of helplessness in response to difficulty or failure than did children who were praised for their effort.

Trauma

Trauma also influences the explanatory style of children. For example, Bunce, Larsen, and Peterson (1995) found that college students who reported experiencing a significant trauma (e.g., death of a parent, rape, and incest) at some point in their childhood or adolescence currently had a more pessimistic explanatory style for bad events than those students who had never experienced trauma.

Media

Finally, do the media influence explanatory style? Levine (1977) reported that CBS and NBC newscasts modeled helplessness 71% of the time, thereby offering ample opportunity for the vicarious acquisition of helplessness. Gerbner and Gross (1976) also found that televised violence—whether fictional or actual—resulted in intensified feelings of risk and insecurity that promote compliance with established authority. Explanatory style was not an explicit focus, but it seems plausible that a causal message was tucked into this form of influence. Even when television viewing produces ostensibly positive feelings, helplessness may result when viewers learn to expect outcomes unrelated to behaviors (Hearn, 1991).

Although people of all ages watch television, young people may be especially susceptible to its influence. U.S. children under age 11 watch an average of 22 hours of television per week (Nielsen Media Research, 1998). Of particular concern is children's exposure to televised scenes of violence. From an explanatory style perspective, the issue is not televised violence per se but how its causes are portrayed.

Although to some extent television mirrors the world, its depictions of violence can be gratuitous. This is true not only of fictional portrayals but also of news reports. When violence erupts anywhere, television cameras arrive to record every facet of misery. Pictures of victims are displayed repeatedly; reporters review the sequence of events repeatedly; various commentators analyze the causes/effects repeatedly. Television coverage ruminates on the violence, tacitly encouraging the viewer to do the same, and such rumination may create, strengthen, and cement into place a pessimistic explanatory style.

In sum, a great deal is known about the consequences of optimistic versus pessimistic styles of explaining the causes of bad events. Far less is known about the naturally occurring origins of explanatory style. And unaddressed by any study looking at the development of explanatory style is a normative question: Does the typical person have an optimistic explanatory style, a pessimistic one, or one that is neutral or even-handed?

Deliberately Changing Explanatory Style

One practical implication of these ideas is that helplessness and its consequences can be alleviated by changing the way people think about response–outcome contingencies and how they explain the causes of bad events. Cognitive therapy for depression is effective in part because it changes these sorts of beliefs and provides clients with strategies for viewing future bad events in more optimistic ways (Seligman et al., 1988).

Another practical implication is that helplessness and its consequences can be prevented in the first place by teaching people cognitive-behavioral skills before the development of problems. One protocol based on these tenets, designed for group administration to middle-school students, is the Penn Resiliency Program (PRP), developed by Gillham, Reivich, Jaycox, and Seligman (1995). The PRP is a curriculum delivered by school teachers and guidance counselors that contains two main components, one cognitive and the other based on social problem-solving techniques. The PRP has been successfully evaluated in schools and managed care settings in both the United States and China. It succeeds in preventing later episodes of depression through at least 2 years of follow-up.

EXPLANATORY STYLE AND EMOTION REGULATION

The learned helplessness model, the attributional reformulation, and hopelessness theory are process models that articulate mechanisms thought to be involved in reactions to events, including emotions. In all these accounts, explanatory style for bad events is thought to influence these reactions. We have reviewed what is known about explanatory style, and at the risk of caricature, Figure 8.1d depicts explanatory style research as typically conducted: Administer one of the available measures of explanatory style along with some other measure and calculate the correlation. Hundreds if not thousands of such studies have been published. Readily available self-report questionnaires invite this sort of research, which means that explanatory style has taken on a life of its own as a personality construct.

We suggest that researchers return to the rich and largely untested process theories from which the explanatory style construct emerged. Doing so would broaden our understanding of the mechanisms linking explanatory style and outcomes. In particular, the potential relationship of explanatory style to emotion regulation becomes apparent and may even provide a key organizing perspective.

As noted, many of the outcomes to which explanatory style has been linked entail emotional excesses (e.g., anxiety and depression) or well-regulated emotions (e.g., those involved in achievement, perseverance, and social attractiveness). Establishing simple correlations between explanatory style and such outcomes is only a first step toward explanation. What else might be involved? We use Frijda's (1986) classification of emotion regulation processes to draw out some answers. We mainly address negative emotions because there is more relevant research in the explanatory style tradition. However, we also speculate about explanatory style and the savoring of positive emotions.

Confrontation with Emotional Events

The helplessness model, the attributional reformulation, and hopelessness theory all posit actual bad events as critical in producing emotions; explanatory style moderates these emotional reactions. This conceptualization is a diathesis–stress perspective, in which explanatory style (the diathesis) and bad life events (the stress) combine to cause outcomes. Diathesis–stress models are popular in psychopathology research but often make the simplifying assumption that the two components are not only distinguishable but independent. Indeed, researchers use multiple regression procedures that in effect force independence by examining the unique predictive power of explanatory style and bad events (e.g., Houston, 1995).

It is thoroughly implausible that people's explanatory style is independent of the events that occur to them. Buss (1987) described three kinds of interaction between personality traits and environment events which suggest potential points of mutual influence. In *evocation,* the person unintentionally elicits a particular response from the environment. In *manipulation,* people intentionally alter the world. The tactics they choose are influenced by their traits, to be sure, but the consequences of the tactics change the person. Finally, in *selection,* a person chooses to enter particular situations or avoid them, which obviously influences subsequent actions.

So how does a pessimistic explanatory style affect the world and in turn the person? Numerous influences are likely. We know that people with a pessimistic explanatory style are socially estranged—lonely and unpopular (Table 8.1). Perhaps their view of the causes of events, when expressed to others, is offputting—an instance of evocation.

A pessimistic explanatory style may create a diminished social world that in turn produces negative emotions.

From a study of gamblers at a harness race track (Atlas & Peterson, 1990), we also know that people with a pessimistic explanatory style prefer to bet on long shots, especially when they are losing—an instance of manipulation. Perhaps helplessness and hopelessness encourage them to cast their lot with chance. Alternatively or additionally, these beliefs may underlie poor impulse control and the unwillingness to delay gratification (McCormick & Taber, 1988). After all, if people believe that important life events simply happen to them, why not gamble that an immediate payoff is possible?

Finally, we know that people with a pessimistic explanatory style are at increased risk for traumatic mishaps ("accidents") in part because they are more likely to put themselves in harm's way (Peterson et al., 2001). Relative to those with an optimistic explanatory style, they prefer activities that promise to be exciting (e.g., drinking and going to wild parties) yet at the same time do not appreciate that these are potentially dangerous—an instance of selection. These findings are not fine-grained, but they invite the speculation that those with a pessimistic explanatory style try to "handle" negative feelings by overriding them with excitement.

Most generally, people with a pessimistic explanatory style are passive. In failing to engage the world, they guarantee failure at any task in which active responding would prove useful, and these failures in turn influence emotions. So, Peterson and Barrett (1987) found that college students with a pessimistic explanatory style received poor grades in part because they did not attend class or consult with their instructors. A similar finding is that college students with a pessimistic explanatory style have relatively poor health in part because they do not do the sorts of things such as exercising and eating well known to bolster wellness (e.g., Peterson, 1988).

These sorts of findings have not been the focus on much research, but they deserve more attention if we wish to understand how explanatory style influences the emotions that people experience. Emotions unfold over time in response to events, and explanatory style arguably can function as what Gross (1998) described as an antecedent-focused process of emotional regulation.

What about positive emotions? Bryant and Veroff (2006) observed that one of the chief ways to savor positive emotions is to share them with other people, either immediately or after the fact. Most of us would rather see a movie, eat dinner, or vacation with someone else because so doing makes the ensuing good feelings last. Although explanatory style has not been explicitly examined with respect to savoring, it seems likely that the documented link between an optimistic explanatory style and a rich social network would lead to increased savoring of positive emotions when they occur.

Another way to savor positive emotions is to keep souvenirs of the situations that created them, either literal things or mental snapshots that can be reexamined (Bryant & Veroff, 2006). Perhaps the keeping of souvenirs reminds the individual that positive experiences are stable and global and not just random occurrences over which there is no control.

Appraisal of Emotional Events

The causal attributions a person makes for an event are an important aspect of its appraisal, and inasmuch as explanatory style influences these attributions, it necessarily influences ensuing emotions. Indeed, appraisal is part and parcel of any emotion, which means that explanatory style can have an immediate effect on emotion. If the explanatory style entails stable and global causes for bad events, hopelessness is induced and generality of negative emotions across time and situation is encouraged (Alloy, Peterson, Abramson, & Seligman, 1984).

In a study we attempted to conduct years ago testing the diathesis–stress hypothesis of the attributional reformulation, we hypnotically suggested to research participants that they entertain either a pessimistic or optimistic explanatory style. We next imposed a bad event in the form of an unsolvable problem and looked to see if pessimistic explanatory style interacted with the bad event to produce passivity and feelings of depression. At the time, we deemed the study a failure and did not pursue it because all we could find in our pilot testing was a "main effect" of the hypnotic suggestion: Those induced to view the causes of events in a pessimistic way became (relatively) helpless and sad. With the wisdom of hindsight, we now see that these results were to be expected, showing as they did that a pessimistic appraisal of an event's causes in and of itself has an immediate and negative emotional effect. We further assume that the induction of an optimistic style would produce an immediate and positive emotional effect.

Also showing the immediacy of causal appraisals on induced emotions was a study using the symptom-context method. Available to us were psychotherapy transcripts with a patient who would at times experience sudden feelings of depression (Peterson, Luborsky, & Seligman, 1983). We looked at the topics on focus immediately prior to his shift into a depressed state and used the CAVE technique to content-analyze the causes he cited. Internal, stable, and global causes for bad events predicted increased depression mere seconds later.

Causal attributions are but one type of appraisal that influence emotions, and research suggests that explanatory style may also influence other emotion-relevant construals. For example, those with a more optimistic explanatory style see minor hassles as sources of amusement or as challenges, whereas those with a more pessimistic style see them as catastrophes (Dykema, Bergbower, & Peterson, 1995).

The reader will remember that the ASQ asks respondents to describe in their own words the causes of events and then to rate them along the dimensions of internality, stability, and globality. Our intent in asking for an actual cause to be written is to slow respondents down and encourage thoughtful attributions. What they write is rarely analyzed in its own right, but Peterson (1983) looked at these and found that some individuals turned the ostensibly good events on the ASQ into bad ones by how they explained them. For example, an event like "a friend compliments you on your appearance" might be explained by saying, "my friend felt sorry for me because I am so ugly." This tendency to find the cloud around a silver lining was infrequent but evident chiefly among those who scored high on a depression inventory.

Research in the explanatory style tradition usually focuses on external events, and these are the sorts of events included in the ASQ. However, investigations of open-ended responses to prompts such as "describe the worst thing that happened to you in the past six months" reveal that internal events are mentioned with some frequency, including in particular bouts of depression or demoralization (Peterson, Bettes, & Seligman, 1985). These negative feelings are spontaneously explained just as external events are explained, and if the explanation points to internal, stable, and global causes, then we find increased depressive symptoms even in the apparent absence of external circumstances.

Suppression or Amplification of Feelings and Motives

Stability and globality of explanatory style are thought to influence the degree to which reactions to events are generalized across time and situation. This issue has been extensively investigated with respect to the negative phenomena of helplessness and depression, and the data support the prediction. What is the mechanism? Whether we term it "catastrophizing, "magnification," "rumination," or "excessive worry," those with a pessimistic explanatory style expect further bad events to lurk around every corner. Perseverative thinking plays itself out consciously but unwillingly (Thayer & Lane, 2002), and it underlies a variety of emotional disorders (Ronan & Kendall, 1997). In the present context, perseverative thinking is a massive failure of emotion regulation—individuals cannot resist what they think and thus what they feel. They can be described as helpless with respect to their ongoing experience.

One of the features of perseverative thinking is that it is abstract (Stöber, 1998), which makes it immune to challenge by contrary experiences. This characterization helps explain the empirical fact that individuals with a pessimistic explanatory style sometimes generate more causal attributions for bad events than do their counterparts with an optimistic explanatory style (Peterson & Ulrey, 1994). By the way, this is probably not an instance of so-called attributional complexity, an often adaptive tendency (Fletcher, Danilovics, Fernandez, Peterson, & Reeder, 1986), because these attributions have a relentless similarity. They all contribute to negative feelings and presumably amplify them.

Research has explored the neurophysiological underpinnings of perseverative thinking, and it converges to implicate the breakdown of biological processes involved in inhibition (Shadmehr & Holcomb, 1999). The perseverative person is aroused but unable to regulate this arousal and do what might be needed to reduce this state. Attention becomes rigidly focused on negative feelings and not on forward-looking steps to solve the problem they represent. In general terms, these ideas are consistent with more recent investigations of the learned helplessness phenomenon, in animals and people, showing that it entails a disruption of selective attention (e.g., Barber & Winefield, 1986; Lee & Maier, 1988).

Again, contact is made with what is known about the savoring of positive emotions. Savoring occurs when the individual focuses on the details of the positive emotion and not on other matters which would necessarily detract from the pleasurable experience (Bryant & Veroff, 2006). We speculate that people with an optimistic explanatory style are more able to focus intentionally their attention on the good feelings they have.

Along these lines, one of the ways to savor positive experiences and the good feelings they produce is to believe that one deserves them (Bryant & Veroff, 2006). In attributional language, "deserving" means that successes and triumphs have internal, stable, and global causes. They are seen as likely to occur again.

Perseverative thinking has also been linked to poor health, in particular heart disease (Kubzansky et al., 1997). As noted, a pessimistic explanatory style also foreshadows poor health (Peterson & Bossio, 1991). Here is an obvious question for future research: Is the association between explanatory style and poor health mediated in part by emotion disregulation? Conversely, is wellness under the sway of an explanatory style that leads to frequent positive emotions?

Overt Responses

The striking behavioral element of learned helplessness is of course passivity, but as should now be clear, behavioral passivity needs to be described in finer detail. Learned helplessness is not to be confused with death. Helpless animals and people do behave. The deficit, as it were, lies in the ineffectuality of their behavior. Because the helpless individual expects outcomes to be independent of responses, we see a lack of goal-directed behavior.

By extrapolation, the same is true of the individual with a pessimistic explanatory style for bad events. We have described how a pessimistic explanatory style is associated with the failure of adaptive behavior in the realms of academics and health promotion. We can point to additional studies that document a link between a pessimistic explanatory style and the lack of persistence in the workplace (Seligman & Schulman, 1986), on the playing field (Martin-Crumm, Sarrazin, & Peterson, 2005), and on the stage of world politics (Zullow, Oettingen, Peterson, & Seligman, 1988). Zullow (1991) even showed that a pessimistic explanatory style manifest in popular U.S. songs foreshadowed decreased consumer spending and economic recession.

An intriguing study by Satterfield, Monahan, and Seligman (1997) seems to go against the grain of the research just cited but actually is consistent with the conclusion that a pessimistic style leads to passivity. This investigation found that a pessimistic explanatory style predicted *success* among law school students, as judged by grades and participation in law journals. The investigators speculated that the law, at least as typically practiced, requires extreme caution and sobriety—in effect, not taking chances. There may well be a downside to this phenomenon, though, in the elevated risk of depression among U.S. lawyers (Seligman, Verkuil, & Kang, 2001).

Much of the research on explanatory style has neglected the "situational" determinants of causal attributions, although these can be of overriding importance in determining actual attributions, specific expectations, ensuing helplessness, and the eventual outcomes of interest (Figures 8.1b and 8.1c). Greater attention to the situation not only would be more true to helplessness theory, in its original and revised versions, but also might shed some light on an intriguing but understudied parameter of explanatory style—the degree to which it is consistent for a given individual.

Variously referred to as the *traitedness* or *flexibility* of explanatory style, this parameter reflects the degree to which someone always offers the same sort of causal attribution for different bad events, or whether different events result in different attributions (Fresco, Williams, & Nugent, in press; Silverman & Peterson, 1993). In the present context, the flexibility of explanatory style can perhaps be described as the extent to which someone attends to the actual causal texture of events, a process which may index the degree to which antecedent-focused emotion regulation is even possible, given the person's psychological makeup. Someone with a relentlessly consistent explanatory style—pessimistic or optimistic—will simply interpret and experience all events in the same way. Someone with a more flexible style should experience a fuller and more nuanced range of emotions and as a result function better in the world.

These ideas make contact with Fredrickson's (2004) theorizing about the functions of positive emotions. According to her *broaden-and-build theory,* positive emotions signal safety, and our inherent response to them is not to narrow our options—as we do when experiencing negative emotions such as fear or anger—but to broaden and build on them. Research participants induced in the laboratory to experience positive emotion such as amusement or contentment show broader attention, greater working memory, enhanced verbal fluency, and increased openness to information. Fredrickson argued that the frequent experience of positive emotions leads to an "upward spiral" of well-being that is the feel-good counterpart of negative rumination. Whether these upward spirals are influenced by explanatory style or attributional flexibility is not known but would be an interesting topic for further investigation.

The interventions for changing explanatory style described earlier in this chapter share the strategy of making explanatory style and its emotional consequences explicit and—we assume—more under the explicit control of the individual. Current interpretations of these interventions go beyond the simple urging of "positive thinking" to champion "flexible thinking" (e.g., Reivich & Shatté, 2003). Recasting this advice in terms of deliberate emotion regulation might lead to further ways to help people flourish and thrive.

REFERENCES

Abramson, L. Y., Metalsky, G. I., & Alloy, L. B. (1989). Hopelessness depression: A theory-based subtype of depression. *Psychological Review, 96,* 358–372.

Abramson, L. Y., Seligman, M. E. P., & Teasdale, J. D. (1978). Learned helplessness in humans: Critique and reformulation. *Journal of Abnormal Psychology, 87,* 49–74.

Alloy, L. B., Kelly, K. A., Mineka, S., & Clements, C. M. (1990). Comorbidity in anxiety and depressive disorders: A helplessness/hopelessness perspective. In J. D. Maser & C. R. Cloninger (Eds.), *Comorbidity in anxiety and mood disorders* (pp. 499–543). Washington, DC: American Psychiatric Press.

Alloy, L. B., Peterson, C., Abramson, L. Y., & Seligman, M. E. P. (1984). Attributional style and generality of learned helplessness. *Journal of Personality and Social Psychology, 46,* 681–687.

Atlas, G. D., & Peterson, C. (1990). Explanatory style and gambling: How pessimists respond to lost wagers. *Behaviour Research and Therapy, 56,* 523–529.

Barber, J. G., & Winefield, A. H. (1986). Learned helplessness as conditioned inattention to the target stimulus. *Journal of Experimental Psychology: General, 115,* 236–246.

Beck, A. T. (1991). Cognitive therapy: A 30-year retrospective. *American Psychologist, 46,* 368–375.

Beck, A. T., Steer, R. A., Beck, J. S., & Newman, C. F. (1993). Hopelessness, depression, suicidal ideation and clinical diagnosis of depression. *Suicide and Life-Threatening Behavior, 23,* 139–145.

Bryant, F. B., & Veroff, J. (2006). *The process of savoring: A new model of positive experience.* Mahwah, NJ: Erlbaum.

Bunce, S. C., Larsen, R. J., & Peterson, C. (1995). Life after trauma: Personality and daily life experiences of traumatized people. *Journal of Personality, 63,* 165–188.

Buss, D. M. (1987). Selection, evocation, and manipulation. *Journal of Personality and Social Psychology, 53,* 1214–1221.

Dykema, K., Bergbower, K., Doctora, J. D., & Peterson, C. (1996). An Attributional Style Questionnaire for general use. *Journal of Psychoeducational Assessment, 14,* 100–108.

Dykema, K., Bergbower, K., & Peterson, C. (1995). Pessimistic explanatory style, stress, and illness. *Journal of Social and Clinical Psychology, 14,* 357–371.

Fletcher, G. J. O., Danilovics, P., Fernandez, G., Peterson, D., & Reeder, G. D. (1986). Attributional complexity: An individual differences measure. *Journal of Personality and Social Psychology, 51,* 875–884.

Franz, C. E., McClelland, D. C., Weinberger, J., & Peterson, C. (1994). Parenting antecedents of adult adjustment: A longitudinal study. In C. Perris, W. A. Arrindell, & M. Eisemann (Eds.), *Parenting and psychopathology* (pp. 127–144). San Diego: Academic Press.

Fredrickson, B. L. (2004). The broaden-and-build theory of positive emotions. *Philosophical Transactions of the Royal Society of London, B, Biological Sciences, 359,* 1367–1377.

Fresco, D. M., Williams, N. L., & Nugent, N. R. (in press). Flexibility and negative affect: Examining the associations of explanatory flexibility and coping flexibility to each other and to depression and anxiety. *Cognitive Therapy and Research.*

Frijda, N. H. (1986). *The emotions.* Cambridge, UK: Cambridge University Press.

Garber, J., & Seligman, M. E. P. (Eds.). (1980). *Human helplessness: Theory and applications.* New York: Academic Press.

Gerbner, G., & Gross, L. (1976). Living with television: The violence profile. *Journal of Communication, 26,* 173–199.

Gillham, J. E., Reivich, K. J., Jaycox, L. H., & Seligman, M. E. P. (1995). Prevention of depressive symptoms in schoolchildren: Two-year follow-up. *Psychological Science, 6,* 343–351.

Gross, J. J. (1998). The emerging field of emotion regulation: An integrative review. *Review of General Psychology, 2,* 271–299.

Gross, J. J., & Thompson, R. (2007). Emotion regulation: Conceptual foundations. In J. J. Gross (Ed.), *Handbook of emotion regulation* (pp. 3–24). New York: Guilford Press.

Hearn, G. (1991). Entertainment manna: Does television viewing lead to appetitive helplessness? *Psychological Reports, 68,* 1179–1184.

Heyman, G. D., Dweck, C. S., & Cain, K. M. (1992). Young children's vulnerability to self-blame and helplessness: Relationship to beliefs about goodness. *Child Development, 63,* 401–415.

Houston, D. M. (1995). Vulnerability to depressive mood reactions: Retesting the hopelessness model of depression. *British Journal of Social Psychology, 34,* 293–302.

Isaacowitz, D. M., & Seligman, M. E. P. (2001). Is pessimism a risk factor for depressive mood among community-dwelling older adults? *Behaviour Research and Therapy, 39,* 13–30.

Jackson, R. L., Maier, S. F., & Coon, D. J. (1979). Long-term analgesic effects of inescapable shock and learned helplessness. *Science, 206,* 91–94.

Johnson, J. G. (1995). Event-specific attributions and daily life events as predictors of depression symptom change. *Journal of Psychopathology and Behavioral Assessment, 17,* 39–49.

Johnson, J. G., Han, Y. S., Douglas, C. J., Johannet, C. M., & Russell, T. (1998) Attributions for positive life events predict recovery from depression among psychiatric in-patients: An investigation of the Needles and Abramson model of recovery from depression. *Journal of Consulting and Clinical Psychology, 66,* 369–376.

Kubzansky, L. D., Kawachi, I., Sparrow, D., Spiro, A., Vokonas, P., & Weiss, S. (1997). Is worrying bad for your heart?: A prospective study of worry and coronary heart disease in the normative aging study. *Circulation, 95,* 818–824.

Lee, R. K. K., & Maier, S. F. (1988). Inescapable shock and attention to internal versus external cues in a water escape discrimination task. *Journal of Experimental Psychology: Animal Behavior Processes, 14,* 302–311.

Levine, G. F. (1977). "Learned helplessness" and the evening news. *Journal of Communication, 27,* 100–105.

Maier, S. F., & Seligman, M. E. P. (1976). Learned helplessness: Theory and evidence. *Journal of Experimental Psychology: General, 105,* 3–46.

Martin-Krumm, C. P., Sarrazin, P. G., & Peterson, C. (2005). The moderating effects of explanatory style in physical education performance: A prospective study. *Personality and Individual Differences, 38,* 1645–1656.

McCormick, R. A., & Taber, J. I. (1988). Attributional style in pathological gamblers in treatment. *Journal of Abnormal Psychology, 97,* 368–370.

Metcalfe, J. (1998). Cognitive optimism: Self-deception or memory-based processed heuristics? *Personality and Social Psychology Review, 2,* 100–110.

Mikulincer, M. (1994). *Human learned helplessness: A coping perspective.* New York; Plenum Press.

Mueller, C. M., & Dweck, C. S. (1998). Praise for intelligence can undermine children's motivation and performance. *Journal of Personality and Social Psychology, 75,* 32–52.

Needles, D. J., & Abramson, L. Y. (1990). Positive life events, attributional style, and hopefulness: Testing a model of recovery from depression. *Journal of Abnormal Psychology, 99,* 156–165.

Nielsen Media Research. (1998). *1998 report on television.* New York: Author.

Nolen-Hoeksema, S. (1986). *Developmental studies of explanatory style, and learned helplessness in children.* Unpublished doctoral dissertation, University of Pennsylvania.

Peterson, C. (1983). Clouds and silver linings: Depressive symptoms and attributions about ostensibly good and bad events. *Cognitive Therapy and Research, 7,* 575–578.

Peterson, C. (1988). Explanatory style as a risk factor for illness. *Cognitive Therapy and Research, 12,* 117–130.

Peterson, C. (1991). Meaning and measurement of explanatory style. *Psychological Inquiry, 2,* 1–10.

Peterson, C. (1999). Personal control and well-being. In D. Kahneman, E. Diener, & N. Schwarz (Eds.), *Well-being: The foundations of hedonic psychology* (pp. 288–301). New York: Russell Sage.

Peterson, C., & Barrett, L. C. (1987). Explanatory style and academic performance among university freshmen. *Journal of Personality and Social Psychology, 53,* 603–607.

Peterson, C., Bettes, B. A., & Seligman, M. E. P. (1985). Depressive symptoms and unprompted causal attributions: Content analysis. *Behaviour Research and Therapy, 23,* 379–382.

Peterson, C., Bishop, M. P., Fletcher, C. W., Kaplan, M. R., Yesko, E. S., Moon, C. H., et al. (2001). Explanatory style as a risk factor for traumatic mishaps. *Cognitive Therapy and Research, 25,* 633–649.

Peterson, C., & Bossio, L. M. (1991). *Health and optimism.* New York: Free Press.

Peterson, C., Buchanan, G. M., & Seligman, M. E. P. (1995). History and evolution of explanatory style research. In G. M. Buchanan & M. E. P. Seligman (Eds.), *Explanatory style* (pp. 1–20). Hillsdale, NJ: Erlbaum.

Peterson, C., Luborsky, L., & Seligman, M. E. P. (1983). Attributions and depressive mood shifts. *Journal of Abnormal Psychology, 92,* 96–103.

Peterson, C., Maier, S. F., & Seligman, M. E. P. (1993). *Learned helplessness: A theory for the age of personal control.* New York: Oxford University Press.

Peterson, C., Schulman, P., Castellon, C., & Seligman, M. E. P. (1992). CAVE: Content analysis of verbatim explanations. In C. P. Smith (Ed.), *Motivation and personality: Handbook of thematic content analysis* (pp. 383–392). New York: Cambridge University Press.

Peterson, C., & Seligman, M. E. P. (1984). Causal explanations as a risk factor for depression: Theory and evidence. *Psychological Review, 91,* 347–374.

Peterson, C., & Seligman, M. E. P. (1985). The learned helplessness model of depression: Current status of theory and research. In E. E. Beckham & W. R. Leber (Eds.), *Handbook of depression: Treatment, assessment, and research* (pp. 914–939). Homewood, IL: Dow Jones-Irwin.

Peterson, C., Semmel, A., von Baeyer, C., Abramson, L. Y., Metalsky, G. I., & Seligman, M. E. P. (1982). The Attributional Style Questionnaire. *Cognitive Therapy and Research, 6,* 287–299.

Peterson, C., & Ulrey, L. M. (1994). Can explanatory style be scored from TAT protocols? *Personality and Social Psychology Bulletin, 20,* 102–106.

Peterson, C., & Vaidya, R. S. (2001). Explanatory style, expectations, and depressive symptoms. *Personality and Individual Differences, 31,* 1217–1223.

Peterson, C., & Vaidya, R. S. (2003). Optimism as virtue and vice. In E. C. Chang & L. J. Sanna (Eds.), *Virtue, vice, and personality: The complexity of behavior* (pp. 23–37). Washington, DC: American Psychological Association.

Reivich, K. A., & Shatté, A. (2003), *The resilience factor: Seven essential skills for overcoming life's inevitable obstacles.* New York: Random House.

Ronan, K. R., & Kendall, P. C. (1997). Self-talk in distressed youth: states-of-mind and content specificity. *Journal of Clinical Child Psychology, 26,* 330–337.

Satterfield, J. M., Monahan, J., & Seligman, M. E. P. (1997). Law school performance predicted by explanatory style. *Behavioral Science and Law, 15,* 95–105.

Schulman, P., Keith, D., & Seligman, M. E. P. (1993). Is optimism heritable? A study of twins. *Behaviour Research and Therapy, 31,* 569–574.

Seligman, M. E. P. (1974). Depression and learned helplessness. In R. J. Friedman & M. M. Katz (Eds.), *The psychology of depression: Contemporary theory and research* (pp. 83–113). Washington, DC: Winston.

Seligman, M. E. P. (1991). *Learned optimism.* New York: Knopf.

Seligman, M. E. P., Castellon, C., Cacciola, J., Schulman, P., Luborsky, L., Ollove, M., et al. (1988). Explanatory style change during cognitive therapy for unipolar depression. *Journal of Abnormal Psychology, 97,* 13–18.

Seligman, M. E. P., Peterson, C., Kaslow, N. J., Tanenbaum, R. L., Alloy, L. B., & Abramson, L. Y. (1984). Attributional style and depressive symptoms among children. *Journal of Abnormal Psychology, 93,* 235–238.

Seligman, M. E. P., & Schulman, P. (1986). Explanatory style as a predictor of productivity and quitting among life insurance agents. *Journal of Personality and Social Psychology, 50,* 832–838.

Seligman, M. E. P., Verkuil, P. R., & Kang, T. H. (2001). Why lawyers are unhappy. *Cardozo Law Review, 23,* 33–53.

Shadmehr, R., & Holcomb, H. H. (1999). Inhibitory control of competing motor memories. *Experimental Brain Research, 126,* 235–251

Siçinski, A. (1972). Optimism versus pessimism (Tentative concepts and their consequences for future research). *The Polish Sociological Bulletin, 25–26,* 47–62.

Silverman, R. J., & Peterson, C. (1993). Explanatory style of schizophrenic and depressed outpatients. *Cognitive Therapy and Research, 17,* 457–470.

Stöber, J. (1998). Worry, problem elaboration, and suppression of imagery: The role of concreteness. *Behaviour Research and Therapy, 36,* 751–756.

Taylor, S. E. (1989). *Positive illusions.* New York: Basic Books.

Thayer, J. F., & Lane, R. (2002). Perseverative thinking and health: Neurovisceral concomitants. *Psychology and Health, 17,* 685–695.

Vanden Belt, A., & Peterson, C. (1991). Parental explanatory style and its relationship to the classroom performance of disabled and nondisabled children. *Cognitive Therapy and Research, 15,* 331–341.

Wheeler, M. L. (2002). Effect of attachment and threat of abandonment on intimacy anger, aggressive behavior, and attributional style. *Dissertation Abstracts International: Section B: The Sciences and Engineering, 63*(3-B), 1579.

Zullow, H. M. (1991). Pessimistic rumination in popular songs and newsmagazines predict economic recession via decreased consumer optimism and spending. *Journal of Economic Psychology, 12,* 501–526.

Zullow, H. M., Oettingen, G., Peterson, C., & Seligman, M. E. P. (1988). Pessimistic explanatory style in the historical record: CAVing LBJ, presidential candidates, and East versus West Berlin. *American Psychologist, 43,* 673–682.

CHAPTER 9

Affect Regulation and Affective Forecasting

GEORGE LOEWENSTEIN

In the standard decision-making paradigm, people choose between alternative courses of action to maximize the desirability of experienced outcomes. Outcomes are assumed to be tightly linked to feelings—happiness and sadness, satisfaction and dissatisfaction. The study of affective forecasting, which emerged as a focus of research in the 1990s, was motivated by the recognition that, even when people can accurately predict the outcomes of their decisions, they may not be able to accurately predict the feelings associated with those outcomes (Kahneman & Snell, 1992; for a review, see Wilson & Gilbert, 2003). Indeed, research on affective forecasting has identified a number of systematic errors that people make in predicting their own feelings. For example, people tend to believe that both positive feelings associated with desirable outcomes and negative feelings associated with undesirable outcomes will last longer than they actually do—a *durability bias* in affective forecasting (see Gilbert, Pinel, Wilson, Blumberg, & Wheatley, 1998). Errors in affective forecasting complicate decision making because accurately predicting one's feelings is a virtual requirement for effective decision making. If people mispredict how different outcomes will make them feel, they are likely to take actions to secure outcomes that fail to maximize their well-being (Loewenstein, O'Donoghue, & Rabin, 2003).

If the research on affective forecasting complicates an otherwise tidy picture of decision making, the research on emotion regulation complicates it even more, by suggesting that there is an alternative route to happiness. In addition to taking *actions* that produce outcomes that will make them happy, research on affect regulation suggests, people have some ability to manipulate their emotions more directly (e.g., to view the proverbial glass as half full rather than half empty).

180

On evolutionary grounds, we should expect the potential for such mental (i.e., "internal") regulation of affect to be limited in scope.[1] We have evolved to survive and reproduce, not to feel good, and one function of feeling states is to motivate us to do what we need to do to secure these goals (Rayo & Becker, 2005). This function would be undermined if we had the ability to regulate our own affect at will.[2] Affect also serves important social functions, such as ensuring that we respond in kind to aggression even when it is no longer in our self-interest to do so (Frank, 1988). These functions, too, would be undermined if emotions (or their outward expression) could be regulated at will. Despite these evolved constraints, however, just as most people have some capacity to intentionally direct their own thoughts, most also have some capacity to manipulate their own feelings, even without taking actions that change their objective situation.

Whether people actually use affect regulation strategies that work, however, will depend not only on the effectiveness of different strategies but also on what people believe about the effectiveness of those strategies. As discussed later, the types of mental strategies that people use to regulate their own affect can be classified into two categories: those that involve altering one's appraisal of a situation, and those that involve distraction or suppression of thoughts or feelings. Moreover, the literature suggests that one of these—reappraisal—tends to be more effective than the other and to cause fewer adverse side effects. Naturally, people will tend to rely on the types of strategies that they believe are effective, and to avoid those that they believe are ineffective or counterproductive.[3] Their success in regulating their own affect will then depend on the accuracy of their "metacognitions" about the effectiveness of different mental strategies.[4,5]

Despite the breadth and depth of the literature on affective forecasting and affect regulation (the latter attested to by the existence of this volume), almost no research has addressed the intersection of these two topics (i.e., examined the content or accuracy of people's intuitions about the effectiveness of different affect regulation strategies). The goal of this chapter, therefore, is to provide a review of the very limited literature spanning the intersection between these two lines of research and, perhaps more important, to report results from what may be the first study to examine people's intuitions about the effectiveness of different affect regulation strategies.

CLASSIFICATION OF AFFECT REGULATION STRATEGIES

In classifying different affect regulation strategies, this chapter draws on Gross's process model of affect regulation (Gross, 1998b, 1999, 2002; Gross & Thompson, this volume), which details how specific strategies can be differentiated along the timeline of the unfolding emotional response.[6] A fundamental assertion of this model is that affect regulation strategies differ based on when they will have their primary impact on the emotion-generative process. At the broadest level, a distinction is made between *antecedent-* and *response*-focused affect regulation strategies.

Antecedent-focused strategies refer to tactics that are implemented before emotion response tendencies have become fully activated and have thus affected one's behavior and physiological responses. These include (1) situation selection, (2) situation modification, (3) attentional deployment, and (4) cognitive change (commonly known as reappraisal). *Response-focused strategies* refer to things that people do once an emotion is already under way and the response tendencies (behavioral and physiological) have been generated (commonly known as suppression).[7]

While the distinction between antecedent- and response-focused affect regulation strategies is both natural and useful, it could be argued that neither of the first two strategies included under the heading of antecedent strategies—situation selection and situation modification—should be subsumed under the broader category of affect regulation. Choosing situations that make us happy and modifying our situation to make us happy are the paradigmatic activities of *decision making*. Classifying these tactics under the heading of "affect regulation" blurs the distinction, discussed at the beginning of this chapter, between attempting to enhance one's subjective well-being by changing one's situation and attempting to enhance one's subjective well-being using mental strategies (i.e., in the absence of situational change). Indeed, much of the literature on affective forecasting, which makes little or no reference to the literature on affect regulation, is about the consequences of biased affective forecasts for situation selection and situation modification. "Affect regulation," as the term is used herein, therefore, is reserved for *mental* (internal) rather than behavioral strategies for regulating affect.

Limiting the scope of affect regulation to mental strategies has an important consequence for a review of affect regulation and affective forecasting—it renders the existing body of research to be reviewed almost nonexistent.[8] Not all affective forecasts are relevant to affect regulation—only forecasts about the success of affect regulation. However, as already noted, research and writing about these types of forecasts is limited. Moreover, examining the intersection of affective forecasting and affect regulation also limits the scope of relevant forms of affect regulation to a subset, and probably a small subset, of affect regulation: that which occurs consciously and deliberately. Many if not most of the processes that lead to emotional change in the absence of situational change are *not* conscious and deliberate but transpire in an unconscious, automatic, fashion (see Bargh & Williams, this volume). For example, "defense mechanisms" such as "rationalization," "denial," and "projection" (Freud, 1936/1971) operate automatically and unconsciously almost by necessity, given that they involve an element of self-deception, which is much less effective when it is conscious and deliberate. Only deliberate forms of affect regulation are, however, likely to be influenced by people's intuitions about what strategies work and do not work, so these are the sole focus of this review.[9]

Another issue that arises in the application of Gross's framework concerns the distinction between attention deployment, which Gross classifies as an antecedent-focused strategy, and suppression, which he classifies as a response-focused strategy. In principal, these two strategies can be distinguished: One involves altering the thoughts that give rise to emotions, the other the emotions themselves. In practice, however, the distinction between these two types of strategies seems blurred. For example, if, after committing a gross *faux pas*, one attempts not to think about it, would it be more accurate to say that one is distracting oneself from one's thoughts or one's feelings? Skirting such complications, I classify both of these strategies under the heading of suppression. Ultimately, therefore, I distinguish between two major categories of affect regulation: reappraisal (an antecedent-focused strategy) and suppression.

WHAT IS KNOWN ABOUT THE EFFECTIVENESS OF AFFECT REGULATION STRATEGIES?

Reappraisal

Research on reappraisal—the act of construing a potentially emotional situation in a way that enhances positive or diminishes negative affect—has generally found this to be an effective means of affect regulation (for a review, see Gross, 2002; and for a discussion of neural underpinnings, see Ochsner & Gross, this volume). For example, diverse research suggests that people who experience adverse outcomes, such as health problems or accidents, commonly discover a "silver lining" to the calamity—often some kind of new meaning from life. One study of women with breast cancer found that over half reported that the experience had caused them to reappraise their lives in a favorable fashion (Taylor, 1983), and somewhat less than half of a sample of accident victims from another study related the belief that God had intentionally (and benevolently!) selected them for victimization (Janoff-Bulman & Wortman, 1977). However, contrary to this optimistic picture, a different study of people paralyzed in auto accidents (Lehman, Wortman, & Williams, 1987) found that three-fourths of accident victims reported being unable to find any meaning in their loss. Moreover, none of this research reports whether people who discovered silver linings in calamities did so deliberately—that is, with the express intent of regulating their affect.

To the extent that people are able to direct their thoughts in such a fashion, it seems to be beneficial. Thus, Taylor (1983, p. 1163) found that women who found positive meaning in their breast cancer exhibited significantly better psychological adjustment, and Affleck, Tennen, Croog, and Levine (1987) found that men who perceived benefits from a heart attack were less likely to have a subsequent attack and exhibited lower morbidity 8 years later. However, most of the research in this vein suffers from the usual problems of assessing causality from correlational data.

Another possible reappraisal strategy involves generating advantageous counterfactuals such as "things could have turned out so much worse" or "there but for the grace of God go I." There is ample research that counterfactuals can have significant effects on emotion and well-being (see, e.g., Roese & Olson, 1995). However, again very little, if any, of the research on counterfactuals has examined whether people are able to deliberately alter their own emotions by invoking advantageous counterfactuals.

Many other forms of reappraisal are possible. For example, people might attempt to mentally "frame" outcomes in a fashion that minimizes misery and maximizes pleasure—taking gains one at a time to fully savor them but lumping losses together to digest them as quickly and efficiently as possible. Thaler and Johnson (1990) refer to such motivated mental accounting as "hedonic editing" but found that people show relatively little tendency to, in fact, mentally segregate or aggregate outcomes in a hedonically advantageous fashion. Or, as the study reported herein suggests, people may attempt to take a long-term perspective on situations that, in the short-run seem dire (e.g., "I might have failed the exam, but I'm sure I can still ace the course"). Clearly, the range of reappraisal strategies that could be used in any situation is limited only by the imagination of the individual.

Research has generally found reappraisal to be an effective strategy for affect regulation. For example, reappraisal has been found to decrease both behavioral and subjective signs of emotion following exposure to aversive stimuli without elevation in physiological responding (Gross, 1998a, 2002). In one study (Gross, 1998a), participants were shown a disgusting film (i.e., the amputation of an arm and the treatment of burn victims) while their experiential, behavioral, and physiological responses were recorded. Those who were told to reappraise (i.e., to adopt a detached and unemotional attitude while watching the film; to think about what they were seeing objectively, in terms of the technical aspects of the events they observed) reported experiencing less disgust and showed fewer behavioral signs of disgust compared to participants who were simply told to watch the film clip. There was no difference between reappraisal and uninstructed conditions in sympathetic activation of the cardiovascular or electrodermal systems.

In addition to the experiential, behavioral, and physiological consequences of reappraisal, several studies have examined the cognitive and social consequences of reappraisal. For example, Richards and Gross (2000, Study 2) examined the impact of reappraisal on cognitive performance during an emotion-eliciting situation. As participants watched a series of negative emotion-inducing slides, they were presented with information about each slide. After seeing all the slides, participants completed two memory tests—a nonverbal and a verbal memory test. Given that reappraisal occurs relatively early in the emotion-generative process and therefore should require few cognitive resources, they predicted that reappraisal would not diminish memory, which it did not; in fact, reappraisal actually enhanced nonverbal memory.

Although not addressing the effect of affect regulation per se, older research by Walter Mischel and colleagues (for a review, see Mischel & Ayduk, 2004) has also found that people are able to engage in reappraisal, and that it is an effective method of regulating behavior. In a paradigmatic study (Mischel & Baker, 1975), 4-year-old children were given a choice between a smaller earlier reward (e.g., a single marshmallow or pretzel) or a larger reward (e.g., two marshmallows or two pretzels) if they could successfully wait, without ringing a bell, for the experimenter to return. Children were either instructed to (1) simply wait until the experimenter returned; (2) cognitively restructure the situation by thinking that the marshmallows were "white, puffy clouds" or the pretzels were "little, brown logs"; or (3) cognitively restructure the situation by thinking that the marshmallows were "yummy and chewy" or the pretzels were "salty and crunchy." As expected, children who reappraised using non-affective "cool" reconstructions (e.g., "white, puffy clouds") waited significantly longer (13 minutes) than children who used affective "hot" reconstructions (e.g., "yummy and chewy"; 5 minutes). Other studies in which children reappraised the treat as if it were a picture (i.e., by "putting a frame around them in your head") (Moore, Mischel, & Zeiss, 1976) found similar results; children were able to wait almost 18 minutes in this condition compared with only 6 minutes in a control condition. Metcalfe and Mischel (1999) have proposed that thinking of the marshmallows or pretzels in a nonaffective manner "cooled" down what otherwise would have been a "hot" affective response, suggesting that reappraisal was effective at regulating affectively driven behavior.

Distraction and Suppression of Thoughts and Feelings

To an individual who is engulfed in immediate, acute fear or panic from situations such as public speaking, snakes, or heights, the use of distraction or suppression of thoughts or feelings may seem to be the fastest antidote. Indeed, several theories of affect control suggest that people can control negative affect by willfully changing the focus of their attention away from negative thoughts (Clark & Isen, 1982; Nolen-Hoeksema, 1993; Zillmann, 1988). However, even though efforts to suppress negative affect may sometimes be successful, considerable research suggests that it can also have perverse effects—prolonging and even intensifying an individual's emotional reactions (Wenzlaff, 1993; Wenzlaff et al., 1988; Wegner, Erber, & Zanakos, 1993). For example, Wenzlaff, Wegner, and Roper (1988) had dysphoric college students, who had ranked their negative thoughts as the primary contributor to their unhappy state, either suppress or not suppress their negative or positive thoughts. They found that compared to those who were not trying to control their thoughts, the dysphoric students who attempted to suppress their negative thoughts in fact failed to do so and instead ended up entertaining more negative thoughts. They observed no parallel deficit in the ability to suppress their positive thoughts.

To account for the failure of thought suppression as a strategy for controlling one's affect (and thoughts), Wegner (1992, 1994, 1997; Wegner & Wenzlaff, 1996, 2000) proposed a theory of "ironic processes" according to which thought suppression involves two mechanisms: (1) an *intentional operating process* that searches for thoughts that will promote the preferred state (i.e., anything that is not the unwanted affect/thought) and (2) an *ironic monitoring process* that searches for mental thoughts that signal the failure to achieve the preferred state (i.e., the unwanted affect/thought). The operating process is an effortful and conscious system, whereas the ironic monitoring system is unconscious and less demanding of mental effort. When the two processes function in concert (achieving successful thought suppression), the ironic monitoring process only exerts a minor influence, subtly alerting the intentional operating system of deviations from the intended goal; this is generally the case when an individual has sufficient attentional resources. However, when the intentional operating process is voluntarily terminated by the individual, or is disrupted by cognitive demands, stress, time pressure, and so on, the ironic monitoring process continues its vigilance for unwanted thoughts, thereby enhancing the mind's sensitivity to the unwanted thought and creating the "ironic effects" of thought suppression.

According to ironic process theory, therefore, the central variable dividing successful control from ironic effects is the availability of attentional resources. Supporting this idea, Wegner et al. (1993) asked participants to reminisce about a happy or sad event. They were then instructed to maintain their happy or sad state, instructed not to maintain their happy or sad state, or given no instructions. In addition, cognitive load was induced for half of the participants by having them hold in mind a nine-digit number. Participants who attempted to control their mood without an imposed cognitive load were successful (e.g., sad participants were able to reduce their sadness), but those who attempted to control their mood while under cognitive load not only failed to control their moods but reported mood changes that were opposite to what they had intended to produce. For example, sad participants who were instructed to not feel sad (i.e., to change their mood to a positive state) under cognitive load self-reported more negative moods than sad participants not under cognitive load. In a second study, Wegner et al. (1993) found that participants attempting to control their mood-related thoughts under cognitive load showed increased accessibility of those thoughts contrary to the direction of the intended control.

The ironic effects of thought suppression are not limited to emotions (e.g., sadness and happiness) but also apply to other visceral states (e.g., substance cravings and pain). Whether their habit involves drinking, eating, drugs, or smoking, individuals with substance abuse problems are highly motivated to mentally control their cravings. However, despite its potential importance, only a few studies have examined the impact of thought suppression as a strategy for dealing with addiction. Salkovskis and Reynolds (1994) found that the efforts of abstaining smokers to suppress cigarette-related thoughts yielded especially high levels of intrusions of exactly those cigarette-related thoughts. Toll, Sobell, Wagner, and Sobell (2001) similarly found a significant relationship between lack of success in quitting smoking and scores on the White Bear Suppression Inventory (WBSI; Wegner & Zanakos, 1994—a measure of people's general ability to suppress unwanted negative thoughts). The correlational nature of the study, however, precluded identification of the specific causal relationship.

With respect to pain, the common wisdom would seem to be that distraction or thought suppression is superior to attending directly to the pain. However, as already alluded to, research has shown that under some conditions attention is more effective than distraction in reducing pain experience (e.g., Ahles, Blanchard, & Leventhal, 1983; McCaul & Haugtvedt, 1982). For example, Cioffi and Holloway (1993) found that individuals who attempted to suppress pain induced by immersing their hand in cold water experienced more lingering discomfort than did individuals who deliberately monitored their pain (cf. Sullivan, Rouse, Bishop, & Johnston, 1997). Overall, the research on pain suggests that distraction is best when pain is acute, whereas attention (or "sensory monitoring") is best when pain is persistent (for a review, see Cioffi, 1993).[10]

Eliminating the Negative versus Accentuating the Positive

The vast majority of prior research on affect regulation has focused on the mitigation of negative emotions. However, affect regulation can also be applied, at least in principle, to maintaining and/or amplifying positive affective states. For example, the process of being grateful can be a fruitful strategy in eliciting and maintaining positive emotions. Emmons and McCullough (2003) randomly assigned participants to one of three conditions: listing their hassles in life, listing things for which they were thankful, or listing mundane daily activities. Participants did this either weekly for 10 weeks or daily for 21 days. In addition, they kept records of their moods, coping behaviors, health behaviors, and physical symptoms. They found that participants in the gratitude condition exhibited heightened subjective well-being and positive moods relative to those in the control conditions. Other research, however, presents a less optimistic picture. Schooler, Ariely, and Loewenstein (2003) reported two studies both of which suggest that attempts to be happy can backfire. In one laboratory study, subjects listened to a piece of classical music while they either did or did not monitor their own happiness and either did or did not attempt to be happy. Both monitoring happiness and, more important, trying to be happy produced a decline in happiness. In a second field study, Schooler et al. (2003) interviewed people in December 1999 to assess the importance they placed on having a good time during the millennium festivities, then interviewed them again a few days into the new millennium. Those who, by various measures, placed great importance on having a good time in fact reported having enjoyed themselves less than those who took a more relaxed attitude toward the celebration.

WHAT IS KNOWN ABOUT AFFECTIVE FORECASTING?

Every decision, whether large or small, is made based on the belief that it will ultimately make us happier than would an alternative choice. An integral step in the decision process of deciding between choice X versus choice Y is one's ability to predict how one would feel should a particular choice be made—which is known as affective forecasting. Unfortunately, research has documented that people routinely mispredict how much pleasure or displeasure future events will bring, and as a result, they sometimes work to bring about events that do not maximize their happiness (for reviews, see Loewenstein & Schkade, 1999; Wilson & Gilbert, 2003). Specifically, it appears that people are not adept at predicting the intensity and duration of their future emotional reactions. A variety of cognitive biases have been found to explain how and why people are not accurate forecasters of one's future emotional state.

We adopt Wilson and Gilbert's (2003) conception of affective forecasting, which is broken into four components: (1) predictions about the *valence* of one's future feelings,

(2) the *specific emotions* that will be experienced, (3) the *intensity* of the emotions, (4) and their *duration*.

In general, people make accurate predictions about the valence (i.e., positive vs. negative) a future affective experience will elicit, especially if they have had experience in that domain. For example, Wilson, Wheatley, Kurtz, Dunn, and Gilbert (2004) conducted a simulated dating game experiment where participants competed for a hypothetical date and were randomly assigned to win or lose the date. Prior to the experiment, participants were asked to forecast how they would feel if they won and lost the date. After the experiment, participants were asked to rate how they actually felt based on the outcome of the game. Without exception, all the participants forecasted that they would be in a better mood if they won than if they lost, and, perhaps not surprisingly, participants who won were, on average, in a better mood than participants who lost.

People also seem to be relatively accurate in predicting the specific emotions that they will experience (anger, fear, happy, disgust, etc.) in different situations. For example, Robinson and Clore (2001) gave participants a written description of a series of emotion-provoking pictures and asked them to forecast what specific emotions they would experience if they saw the actual pictures. Participants were generally correct about which emotion they would experience when they were presented with the actual pictures. However, people seem to be less accurate when predicting the emotional impact of situations that are likely to evoke mixed emotions, such as graduating from college, than when predicting situations that are more likely to produce more unitary feeling states (Larsen, McGraw, & Cacioppo, 2001).

Research findings are more mixed when it comes to people's accuracy in predicting the immediate intensity of their emotional reactions to events. Some research finds that people tend to overestimate the intensity of their affective reactions to events (Buehler & McFarland, 2001), but other research reaches the opposite conclusion (e.g., Rachman, 1994). This line of research is not well developed, perhaps because researchers, out of concern for subjects' feelings, are reluctant to ask people about their emotional reactions immediately after powerfully emotional events.

Finally, the most consistent finding in the literature on affective forecasting is that people have difficulty anticipating the duration of affective states, and specifically that they tend to overestimate how long both positive and negative feelings will last. The tendency to overestimate one's emotional reactions to ongoing states of affairs (Loewenstein & Frederick, 1997), dubbed the *durability bias* by Gilbert, Pinel, Wilson, Blumberg, and Wheatley (1998) has been found in a variety of populations (college students, professors, vacationers, sports fans, etc.) with a wide range of emotional events (romantic breakups, personal insults, electoral defeats, failures to lose weight, etc.). The bias seems to be "overdetermined" in the sense of being produced by multiple mechanisms.

First, people often incorrectly imagine the specifics of the future event. As several researchers have noted, if there are systematic errors in people's predictions of the objective features of events, these can lead to systematic errors in predictions of the hedonic impact of those events. One such systematic bias that can help explain the durability bias is the failure to take into account the actions one will take to mitigate negative affective states. For example, people predict that becoming paraplegic will make them more miserable than paraplegics report themselves to be, perhaps because they think about all the activities they currently do that they would no longer be able to, but do not think about new activities in which they would engage (Ubel et al., 2001).

Second, people often have incorrect intuitive theories about how future events will make them feel. Although people have frequent affective reactions to persons, places, and things, memory for moment-to-moment affective experience tends to be poor (Robinson & Clore, 2002). Instead of recalling how they actually felt, therefore, people use their intuitive theories about how events make one feel to make a guess as to how they *must have* felt (Ross, 1989). When it comes to *predicting* future feelings, moreover, the information that people have to work with is even more limited; unlike the case of past feelings, which could at least in theory be recalled, for future events, all people have to go on is their intuitive theories (which may be based only in part on past experiences). When predicting future feelings, therefore, incorrect theories are likely to result in prediction errors.

The inadequacy of people's intuitive theories can also help to explain the durability bias. If people lack intuitive theories of adaptation, they are likely to underestimate their own adaptation to positive and negative events. Given that social scientists are only starting to understand the diverse psychological processes that produce psychological adaptation (for reviews, see Frederick & Loewenstein, 1999; Wilson & Gilbert, 2005), it should come as no surprise that ordinary people tend to have an incomplete understanding of adaptive processes, to underpredict their own adaptation to events, and hence to overestimate the duration of their emotional reactions to those events.

Yet a third generic cause of affective forecasting errors has to do with the mismatch between the forecasts, which tend to be conscious, and the processes that shape affect, which tend to be unconscious and automatic. Many of the biases in affective forecasting seem to stem from the conscious brain's underappreciation of the power of unconscious processes (see, e.g., Gilbert et al., 1998, on "immune neglect"). It could be argued, in fact, that much of this research could be cast as a demonstration of the fact that people tend to underestimate the effectiveness of unconscious emotion regulation strategies. However, the fact that these processes are as likely to diminish *positive* as negative affect would seem to argue against including such automatic adaptation processes under the heading of affect regulation. In any case, the focus of the current inquiry is on people's intuitions about conscious strategies rather than unconscious processes of affect regulation.

LAY INTUITIONS ABOUT AFFECT REGULATION

While there is considerable research and writing on affective forecasting and on affect regulation, there is almost no writing about the intersection of these topics, and specifically very little research examining the types of forecasts that are most relevant to affect regulation—those dealing with the effectiveness of different affect regulation strategies.

As an initial attempt to address this gap in the research, 78 students from different public locations on the Carnegie Mellon University campus were recruited to complete a survey that assessed their intuitions and beliefs—affective forecasts—regarding their ability to regulate a variety of different emotions (e.g., shame/indignation, sadness, and disgust) in a variety of contexts (e.g., being unjustly accused, losing a friendship, and encountering a disgusting scene). Forty-seven percent of respondents were female. Ages ranged from 17 to 29, with a mean age of 20, and a standard deviation of 1.8.

The survey asked participants to imagine experiencing the situations portrayed in a series of four scenarios (for text of all the scenarios, see appendix). All scenarios were written in the first person, in what was intended to be vivid, evocative prose. The first scenario, which was intended to engender a mixture of shame and indignation, portrayed a situation in which the respondent had been falsely accused of cheating on a test. The second, which was intended to evoke sadness, described a situation in which the respondent's best friend has suddenly become unfriendly and uncommunicative. The third, which was intended to evoke anger, described a situation in which the respondent's roommate had borrowed his or her loudspeakers without permission and blown them out. The fourth, which was intended to evoke disgust, involved cleaning up the vomit of a party guest.

After each scenario respondents were asked to imagine that "there was nothing you could do about this situation in the short-run, and that you wanted to be in a positive state of mind" (three of the four scenarios continued "for someone you were about to meet"). Respondents were then asked two open-ended questions: (1a) "What types of thoughts or mental strategies would you use in this situation to try to put yourself into a positive state of mind? Please be as specific as possible" and (1b) "Do you think these methods would actually work in this situation?" and then were asked to explain why or why not.

Respondents were then presented with four prespecified affect regulation strategies that had been selected by categorizing open-ended responses to a prior pilot survey involving scenarios similar to those included in the final study. Two of the four strategies involved reappraisal: (1) "Think about the situation from a different perspective," and (2) "Reason about why the objective situation is not so bad." The other two involved distraction and suppression: (3) "Distract myself with other things; try not to the think about the situation," and (4) "Will myself to be calm, cool, and collected."[11] For each of these four strategies, respondents were asked two closed-ended questions: (1) "In this situation, would you use this strategy?" with response options: "might use" and "would probably not use," and (2) "In this situation, would it work?" with response options "probably work, "no effect," and "probably backfire."

After reading the four different scenarios involving negative affect, and answering the questions just described for each, respondents read a single positive scenario which asked them to imagine a situation in which they discovered, unexpectedly, that they had won an academic contest (see Appendix 9.1 for text). They then answered an open-ended question: "Suppose you wanted to enjoy the positive feeling as intensely and long as you possibly could. What types of thoughts or mental strategies would you use to achieve this goal?"

Open-ended responses were initially coded into a large number of categories (about 20), then these were collapsed in a process that ultimately yielded four categories. Each open-ended response was then assigned to one of these four categories or to a residual "other" category. The final categories for the open- and closed-ended responses ended up being the same, partly by design (having the same four strategies represented for both the open-ended and closed-ended responses permits an easy comparison of respondents' spontaneous ideas about how to regulate their own affect and their embracing of ideas that were presented to them), and in part because the four closed ended responses were themselves the product of a prior similar attempt to classify open-ended responses to a pilot survey into a small number of categories.

Examples of "think about the situation from a different perspective" (all taken from responses to Scenario 2, which involved being cold-shouldered by a former friend) included:

- "I would think about the time we spent together before we both became busy and the trust we put in each other. Then I would will myself to imagine that nothing has changed since then and make the phone call."
- "I would think about all the good times we had before to cheer me up."
- "I'd think about all our great memories and how close we once were."
- "Put myself in his shoes. Think of why he may not be talking."

Examples of "reason why the objective situation isn't so bad" (all taken from responses to Scenario 1, which involved being falsely accused of cheating) included:

- "I would try to convince myself that, because I actually was not cheating, I will be able to get out of the situation. If that does not put me into a positive state of mind. I may try to think about other unrelated topics." (This was coded as reasoning rather than distraction because the former was mentioned first.)
- "Knowing I did nothing wrong, I would convince myself that everything would work out in the long run and forget about things."
- "I would look to the future and realize that either I would be found innocent of the charges or that either way life would go on."

Examples of distraction, also taken from responses to Scenario 1, included:

- "I would start singing/whistling my favorite song. I would also start tapping a beat on a book or something."
- "I would think of something else."
- "Think of happy thoughts and not about the test. The situation is irreversible at the moment."

Finally, an example of "will myself to be cool calm and collected" taken from a response to Scenario 4 (which involved a disgust response to vomit) was:

- "I think the only mental strategy that I could try is to will myself to calm down, try to relax and put the situation as much out of mind as possible."

Some open-ended responses were judged not to be *mental* strategies (e.g., when a respondent proposed taking some kind of concrete action to deal with a situation). These are reported as a separate category in the tables.

Tables 9.1a and 9.1b provide summaries of the open- and closed-ended results aggregated across the four negative emotion scenarios. Collapsing respondents' classified open-ended responses to the four scenarios, Table 9.1a reveals that the two reappraisal strategies were spontaneous proposed most frequently (in 65% of cases), whereas distraction and willpower were invoked less frequently (34% of cases). Responses to closed-ended questions, however, provide a different picture. Averaging across all four negative scenarios, willing oneself to be cool, calm, and collected was actually the most commonly embraced strategy (with 68.5% stating that they might use it), whereas all the other strategies were about equally popular (51.2–54.1%) (note that respondents could embrace as many strategies as they liked in the close-ended questions). Moreover, again averaging across all four negative strategies, respondents did not generally have the intuition that exerting willpower would backfire: That strategy

TABLE 9.1a. Spontaneously Proposed Emotion Regulation Strategies (All Scenarios)

Strategy	What strategy would you use?
Think about the situation from a *different perspective*.	34%
Reason about why the objective situation isn't so bad.	31%
Distract myself with other things; try not to think about the situation.	21%
Will myself to be "cool, calm and collected."	13%
Other	2%

was judged to be the *most* likely to work (54.5% said it probably would work), and, by a small margin, *least* likely to backfire (13.2%).

Analysis of the aggregate results points to three major conclusions. First, when it comes to spontaneous ideas about what affect regulation strategies they would use, subjects embraced and reported the highest degree of confidence in the success of those strategies identified in the literature as effective. Second, however, their evaluations of strategies that were presented to them paint a very different picture. In this case, a majority of subjects reported they would use, and believed in the effectiveness of, exactly the strategies that the existing literature suggests are not effective and may even backfire. Third, and related to the second, there was little evidence that subjects were aware of the potential for such "ironic" effects.

Turning to individual scenarios in Tables 9.2–9.5b, perhaps the most important finding is that both spontaneous open-ended responses and closed-ended responses, but especially the latter, reveal that respondents thought that different types of strategies would work in different situations. When it came to Scenario 1 (being falsely

TABLE 9.1b. Individuals' Intuitions and Beliefs Regarding Specific Emotion Regulation Strategies (All Scenarios)

Strategy	In this situation, would you use this strategy?		In this situation, would it work?		
	Might use	Probably not use	Probably work	No effect	Probably backfire
Think about the situation from a *different perspective*.	53.9%	46.1%	39.3%	47.3%	13.3%
Reason about why the objective situation isn't so bad.	54.1%	45.9%	37.5%	39.2%	23.3%
Distract myself with other things; try not to think about the situation.	51.8%	48.2%	39.3%	41.6%	19.0%
Will myself to be "cool, calm, and collected."	68.5%	31.5%	54.5%	32.3%	13.2%

TABLE 9.2a. Spontaneously Proposed Emotion Regulation Strategies (Scenario 1: Falsely Accused of Cheating)

Strategy	What strategy would you use?	Effective?
Think about the situation from a *different perspective*.	21%	39%
Reason about why the objective situation isn't so bad.	30%	72%
Distract myself with other things; try not to think about the situation.	25%	60%
Will myself to be "cool, calm and collected."	21%	62%
Other	3%	
% proposing nonmental strategies (not included in above percentages)	(14%)	

TABLE 9.2b. Individuals' Intuitions and Beliefs Regarding Emotion Regulation Strategies (Scenario: Falsely Accused of Cheating)

Strategy	In this situation, would you use this strategy?		In this situation, would it work?		
	Might use	Probably not use	Probably work	No effect	Probably backfire
Think about the situation from a *different perspective*.	63%	37%	30%	51%	19%
Reason about why the objective situation isn't so bad.	63%	37%	32%	38%	30%
Distract myself with other things; try not to think about the situation.	66%	34%	46%	33%	21%
Will myself to be "cool, calm, and collected."	77%	23%	51%	30%	19%

TABLE 9.3.a. Spontaneously Proposed Emotion Regulation Strategies (Scenario 2: Spurned by an Old Friend)

Strategy	What strategy would you use?	Effective?
Think about the situation from a *different perspective*.	63%	74%
Reason about why the objective situation isn't so bad.	25%	86%
Distract myself with other things; try not to think about the situation.	9%	80%
Will myself to be "cool, calm, and collected."	2%	
Other	2%	
% proposing nonmental strategies (not included in above percentages)	(8%)	

TABLE 9.3b. Individuals' Intuitions and Beliefs Regarding Emotion Regulation Strategies (Scenario 2: Spurned by an Old Friend)

| Strategy | In this situation, would you use this strategy? | | In this situation, would it work? | | |
	Might use	Probably not use	Probably work	No effect	Probably backfire
Think about the situation from a *different perspective*.	78%	22%	70%	26%	4%
Reason about why the objective situation isn't so bad.	71%	29%	51%	36%	13%
Distract myself with other things; try not to think about the situation.	35%	65%	32%	50%	18%
Will myself to be "cool, calm, and collected."	66%	34%	51%	37%	12%

accused of cheating), respondents spontaneously thought that they would be most likely to reason about why the situation was not so bad. When it came to closed-ended responses, however, willing oneself to be cool, calm, and collected was embraced most frequently (by 77% of respondents) and was also most commonly seen as effective (by 51% of subjects).

For Scenario 2 (being spurned by an old friend), thinking about the situation from a different perspective was the most common spontaneously mentioned emotion regulation strategy (63%), the most widely embraced among the closed-ended responses (by 78% of respondents), and was most commonly seen as effective (by 70% of subjects).

For Scenario 3 (learning that their roommate had blown out their speakers), reasoning about why the situation was not so bad was again cited most commonly in open-ended responses (by 45% of respondents), but distraction and willing oneself to be cool, calm, and collected were far more popular when it came to closed-ended responses (and were also more likely to be seen as effective).

TABLE 9.4a. Spontaneously Proposed Emotion Regulation Strategies (Scenario 3: Roommate Blows Out One's Loudspeakers)

Strategy	What strategy would you use?	Effective?
Think about the situation from a *different perspective*.	14%	71%
Reason about why the objective situation isn't so bad.	45%	70%
Distract myself with other things; try not to think about the situation.	29%	87%
Will myself to be "cool, calm, and collected."	10%	60%
Other	2%	
% proposing nonmental strategies (not included in above percentages)	(19%)	

TABLE 9.4.b. Individuals' Intuitions and Beliefs Regarding Emotion Regulation Strategies (Scenario 3: Roommate Blows Out One's Loudspeakers)

Strategy	In this situation, would you use this strategy?		In this situation, would it work?		
	Might use	Probably not use	Probably work	No effect	Probably backfire
Think about the situation from a *different perspective*.	37%	63%	26%	61%	13%
Reason about why the objective situation isn't so bad.	39%	61%	31%	45%	24%
Distract myself with other things; try not to think about the situation.	57%	43%	49%	39%	12%
Will myself to be "cool, calm, and collected."	62%	38%	59%	29%	12%

For Scenario 4 (dealing with vomit at a party), respondents spontaneously thought that they would think about the situation from a different perspective, but, when confronted by the closed-ended responses, they were by far most likely to embrace willpower as the strategy that they would use and that they thought would probably work.

In sum, although responses to open-ended (spontaneous) questions revealed that reappraisal strategies were fairly consistently seen as the most likely to be used and most effective methods of affect regulation, responses to the closed-ended questions showed much greater variation across scenarios. With only four scenarios, it is difficult to discern a pattern in terms of what strategies are applied in what situations, but it is worth noting that scenarios differed on a number of dimensions, including what emotions they evoked, the likely intensity of those emotions, and the need for immediate action. Any of these differences, or others that are not immediately obvious, could be responsible for the differences in emotion strategies endorsed in the different scenarios. It is possible, for example, that suppression strategies were more likely to be evoked for Sce-

TABLE 9.5.a. Spontaneously Proposed Emotion Regulation Strategies (Scenario 4: Vomit at a Party)

Strategy	What strategy would you use?	Effective?
Think about the situation from a *different perspective*.	37%	67%
Reason about why the objective situation isn't so bad.	25%	67%
Distract myself with other things; try not to think about the situation.	20%	80%
Will myself to be "cool, calm, and collected."	18%	78%
Other	—	
% proposing nonmental strategies (not included in above percentages)	(20%)	

TABLE 9.5b. Individuals' Intuitions and Beliefs Regarding Emotion Regulation Strategies (Scenario 4: Vomit at a Party)

Strategy	In this situation, would you use this strategy?		In this situation, would it work?		
	Might use	Probably not use	Probably work	No effect	Probably backfire
Think about the situation from a *different perspective*.	38%	62%	31%	52%	17
Reason about why the objective situation isn't so bad.	43%	57%	36%	38%	26
Distract myself with other things; try not to think about the situation.	49%	51%	31%	44%	25%
Will myself to be "cool, calm, and collected."	69%	31%	58%	33%	9%

narios 1, 3, and 4 because these situations, more than the situation described in Scenario 2, called for immediate emotional calm, or it is possible that subjects believe that suppression is not effective when it comes to sadness. This is clearly a ripe area for future research.

Turning to the positive scenario, in which respondents were asked to imagine that they had won an academic competition and to propose how they might increase the intensity and duration of positive feelings, it turned out that respondents' ideas could be neatly coded into three categories (see Table 9.6).

The most popular type of strategy (endorsed by 37% of subjects) was, interestingly, the same as the most commonly spontaneously mentioned strategy for dealing with negative emotion—namely, thinking about the situation from a positive perspective. Of course, the specifics of how people planned to change their perspective were quite different for this positive scenario than they were for the negative scenarios. Examples include: "I would just remind myself of how we put in one-sixth of the effort the other teams put into their presentations, and yet we still won even after messing up so badly," and "I would have to remember, what made that feeling so good—it wasn't the actual

TABLE 9.6. Spontaneously Proposed Emotion Regulation Strategies (Scenario 5: Winning a Contest)

Strategy	What strategy would you use?	Effective?
Concentrate and savor the moment.	28%	94%
Think about the situation from a *positive perspective*.	38%	100%
Just enjoy; don't try anything	30%	95%
Other	4%	
% proposing nonmental strategies (not included in above percentages)	4%	

moment, but the hard work and months of dedication to the cause, that in this case produced a desirable result."

The second most popular strategy, *concentrate and savor the moment*, was endorsed by 27% of subjects. It can be viewed as the mirror image of the "distraction" tactic. A representative example of a response classified under this heading is: "I would recall the win, the doubts, and even the competition moments over and over in my mind and with my teammates."

Finally, despite being asked to propose mental strategies to increase the intensity and duration of their positive feelings, a surprising number of subjects (29%) rejected the premise of the question and asserted that not trying to enjoy the event was the best way to enjoy it (e.g., "Just enjoy; don't try anything"; "Enjoy the moment. Don't think about how to keep the feeling"; and "I would just be excited and not really need any mental strategy"). We did not observe any responses to the negative scenarios that rejected the premise of the question—that affect regulation strategies could potentially help to mitigate negative emotion—suggesting that accentuating the positive is seen as more problematic than minimizing the negative.

CONCLUSIONS

In recent years, researchers have rediscovered the importance of interactions between "heart" and "mind" that occupied so much of the attention of earlier philosophers and students of human psychology. The power of emotions and motivation to sway information processing is well documented, as is the complex interplay of affect and cognition in the determination of behavior. In both of these areas, people's metacognitions play an important role. Thus, for example, to the extent that one realizes that one's cognitions or behavior are being distorted by emotions, one might attempt to debias oneself or to avoid taking action in the "heat of the moment." Counting to 10 before one speaks words of anger, or waiting until the following day to respond to a hurtful email message, are commonly advocated strategies that are only likely to be implemented by individuals who are aware of the impact of emotions on their judgments and behavior.

The situation is analogous when it comes to emotion regulation. Paralleling the large literature addressing emotional influences on cognition and behavior, there is also a large literature on cognitive influences on emotion, including the extensive literature on cognitive theories of emotion, affective consequences of causal attributions, and many other lines of research. Beyond the fact that cognitions can influence emotions, as discussed in these literatures, research on affect regulation suggests that we also have some ability to regulate our emotions by intentionally directing our own cognitions. As already emphasized, however, whether we do so effectively will depend on the extent and accuracy of metacognitions about what types of affect regulation strategies do and do not work.

Given the vast amount of experience that most people inevitably amass when it comes to affect regulation, one might anticipate that people would naturally learn over time what works and what does not. Indeed, given extensive opportunities for learning from experience, where intuitions and research findings diverge one might be tempted to surmise that it is the research findings that are offbase. However, there are many reasons why experience may lead to less than acute insight (see Einhorn, 1980; Wilson, Meyers, & Gilbert, 2001).

First, a look at the specific strategies that people think would work may hint at the explanation. People generally tend to embrace fairly simplistic causal theories (Nisbett & Ross, 1980). If they recognize that being aware of, or thinking about, certain facts causes them to feel bad, it seems natural that they would believe that distracting themselves from those facts would alleviate those bad feelings.

Second, there is a strong tendency for recall to be guided by prior beliefs (Ross, 1989), which tends to impede learning from experience. When people believe something, they tend to reconstruct their memories to fit with their beliefs. For example, people who believe that small eyes on the Draw a Person test are correlated with paranoia, tend to see such a relationship even when a negative relationship is built into the data (Chapman & Chapman, 1982). Likewise, people who go on weight-reduction programs often report that the programs are helpful, even when they have no measured effect. People also seem to be, in effect, "super-Bayesians"—treating data that support their prior beliefs as supportive but finding fault with data that contradict those beliefs (Lord, Lepper, & Ross, 1979). All these factors will tend to impeded learning from experience.

Third, the feedback that people get into the success of their affect-regulation strategies is probably noisier than one might expect. Emotions change for a variety of reasons, most of them probably unrelated to attempts at regulation. Discerning the signal from the noise in such a situation is an extremely difficult inferential problem.

Finally, people might not be aware of what actually works because it never occurs to them to try the methods identified as successful in the psychology research. Thus, for example, the author had been, prior to doing research on memory for pain, unaware of the literature showing that focusing on pain can actually mitigate it; he assumed that distraction was the only possible, if seemingly ineffective, strategy for dealing with pain. Since reading an article that detailed the beneficial effects of focusing on pain, however, he has been using such a strategy with some success.

The study just presented is at best an initial step toward addressing people's intuitive understanding of affect regulation and the effect of such understanding on what strategies are actually employed. Limitations include the lack of validation data that participants actually had (or agreed they would have for) the particular emotion each scenario targeted. Perhaps even more problematical, there is no validation that subjects would actually employ the strategies that they report embracing. In any survey of this type, in which participants are asked what they "would" do, there is a substantial risk that what is really being probed are people's intuitive theories of what "should" work rather than what they would actually do in a situation. The focus of the survey is also extremely narrow, on mental, and generally very short-term, strategies of affect regulation.

Clearly, a huge void remains to be filled when it comes to systematic research on the interrelated topics of affect regulation and affective forecasting. If thoughts of this void fill you with dismay, but you have no intention of doing research on the topic, it may be more advantageous to reappraise the situation, rather than attempt to suppress your gloomy thoughts.

APPENDIX 9.1

Survey Instructions: As you read the following four scenarios in this survey, please imagine that you are experiencing this situation. Afterward, please answer the questions. Thank you in advance for participating.

Scenario 1: Shame/Indignation

You scan your test one last time just as the teacher calls time. There are more empty spaces than you would like—especially problem #2. You can remember watching the teacher explain this in class, but you can't quite remember the specifics. You walk down to the crowd of students in the front piling up their tests—your eyes never leave your test.

Then, just as you reach the pile of tests, you suddenly remember the formula. You run back to the front row of seats and hastily jot down the answer. With some relief, you stand back and attempt to return your paper to the pile, when your teacher snatches the test from your hands.

He accuses you of cheating! He claims you had seen someone's answer in the pile of tests and copied that down. Now, you are getting zero. You try to explain, but the teacher isn't listening. The teacher marks a zero on your test right in front of your face, and announces loudly for the stragglers to hear that he does not tolerate cheating in his class. You again deny the accusation when he claims he has been watching you all test period and saw your wandering eyes. You cannot remember looking at anything except the rows and rows of numbers and the clock throughout this whole stressful test, yet he demands to know who you were sitting next to. With each time he cuts you off, you find your fists clenching tighter, but still you try to talk, ask a question, say anything to be heard out. But, this time he turns his back on you and walks out with your test in his hand saying that he is going to find your academic advisor and the dean.

The other students stare at you; you hear a couple start to snicker. No one will listen even though you didn't do anything wrong!

Scenario 2: Sadness

He had been your best friend for years. When you first met him, you were surprised how easily you could talk to him. You could talk about anything, even very personal subjects, and all you ever got from him was understanding. He was willing to do whatever you wanted, even what others thought was crazy—like walk to your favorite pizza place at 2 A.M. when it was raining outside.

But now you never see him. When you call him, he's just running out or in the middle of something. He says he'll call you back, and you'll do something together, definitely. Only he does not call back. You know he is busy. You are busy too. When he does call, it seems to always be just before a huge test or project. The only way you manage to get updates about his life are through common friends. You find it upsetting that you found out that he broke up with his girlfriend from a friend of a friend of the girlfriend or that his grandfather had just passed away from the other outside channels. You thought you were his best friend and you should be there to talk to him about this stuff—just like you would have liked to talk to him about your mother having had a heart attack recently. But, you're too busy and he's too busy. So, when you call him on the phone, you wonder if this will be the last time.

Scenario 3: Anger

Where are your loudspeakers? You look over to your roommate's desk. There they are, like usual. She broke her speakers about 3 months ago, and ever since you're the one who is speakerless. Annoyed, you amble over, unknot all the wires around your speakers, reach behind her desk at an awkward angle to unplug your speakers, and then pick up your heavy speakers and carry them across the room back to your desk. You usually have to do this about three times a week. And, that is only because the other times you want your speakers, you find it is less of a hassle to just use your headphones instead. But, right now, you want to watch a movie with a friend, so you retrieve your speakers knowing full well it will be back on her desk by tomorrow.

Three months ago, it wasn't an issue. She just broke her speakers and asked to borrow your speakers to watch a movie. But soon after, she was borrowing them for longer and no longer asking. When you talked to her about it, she said she had talked to her dad about it, and she was getting new ones. Only 2 months went by and the only new speakers she has were yours. When you asked again, she said she had ordered new ones, but instead of shipping them to school she sent them home. But, it's OK because her dad was mailing them. Two weeks later, she asked to borrow them again. You're sure that the only reason she asked was because you were using them at that exact moment. When you asked what happened to hers, she said her dad wasn't going to mail them because it would be cheaper for her to bring it back when she went home for spring break. Spring break was still another 2 weeks away.

Sighing, you plug in your speakers to watch the movie. Instead, you hear static and a clicking sound. Now, your speakers are broken as well.

Scenario 4: Disgust

The party was in full swing 2 hours ago. Now, all that is left of it are empty beer cans, puddles of puke, and the smell of sweat. You search around the trashed home. The smell is disgusting. But tomorrow it will be worse if you don't clean it out of your carpets tonight. You grab some paper towels to start cleaning a puddle of vomit, but the smell is so awful you keep gagging.

Then, you hear someone in the bathroom. Apparently, not all the party crashers are gone yet. You locate the person in the bathroom. He is hunched over the toilet. As soon as you enter, you want to run out again. The smell is 50 times worse in here, and your stomach churns violently. You feel the upchuck reaction in your throat. As you approach the person, he pukes and most of it misses the toilet. You grab a paper towel so that he can clean off the vomit from his clothes.

But, when he turns to face you, you feel yourself about to vomit. The vomit is all over him. In the brown mess, you can see chucks of undigested food. Now, vomit is in the back of your throat. You can taste the acrid, sour taste in the back of your mouth. Now, it is you who needs some paper towels to clean off your clothes and feet.

Scenario 5: Joy

It was competition day. Six months ago, teams all over the state had begun preparing for this day. Now, you were sitting on the floor of a massive gymnasium with the other teams, parents, judges and spectators awaiting the result for your division's competition.

You and your team had awoken this morning early with anxious excitement. Though your team had 6 months to put together the best solution, your team had dawdled and run into problems until 1 month earlier, when suddenly things clicked and your team began to function like a team. You all brainstormed for hours around a table and rethought your entire solution. Then, things that took everyone 6 months to finish, you all managed in less than 1 month. Last week, you had found time to develop a little machine that makes bubbles, just to add effect to your presentation. And by yesterday, your runthroughs had become almost flawless.

But, this morning, the actual competition did not run as smoothly. One team member was too nervous; she rushed through her part almost incomprehensibly. Your bubble machine had stopped working. And, the faces of the judges looked set in stone.

Then, one team member made a small joke, and the judges cracked a small smile. That had an almost magical effect. The team calmed down, and you found some time to make some adjustments to the bubble machine. The judges were laughing at your well-timed jokes. The presentation was running smoothly again.

So, now on the gym floor, you and your team had some hope of placing third of second. You had 13 competitors and several that you had seen were good. No one dared to think they could get first and get to go to the World Finals Competition.

The announcement for your division began. In third place—you felt your chest tighten—the school to the left of you was announced. In second place—again your chest tightened, and you saw your teammates look up hopefully—but now a team in the back was called to collect their medals. As first place was announced, you were barely listening. You thought your entire team looked crushed. But suddenly, you heard your school's name and felt a tug from your grinning teammates. You heard the crowd cheer for you and with a thrill went up to accept your medal.

ACKNOWLEDGMENTS

I thank Liz Mullen for superb work in collecting and coding the data.

NOTES

1. It is possible that some forms of affect regulation may serve important adaptive functions. For example, in many situations, the anticipation of negative emotions such as guilt, remorse, or sadness serves the function of deterring undesirable behaviors. However, once the behavior has been done, the emotional punishment may no longer serve much of a useful function and may, in fact, be debilitating. In such cases, affect regulation may actually promote the effective functioning of the individual.
2. There is, however, some question of whether people would actually desire disembodied pleasures that are not accompanied by action and "real" experience. See, for example, Nozick's (1974) discussion of an "experience machine."
3. Other factors, such as the ease of use, may also influence the decision to use different strategies; these could potentially be subsumed as dimensions of effectiveness.
4. People's intuitive theories about psychological processes often have as big an influence on their behavior as the processes themselves, as illustrated by the vastly different effects of alcohol and marijuana on driving. Although both drugs impair driving and judgment, alcohol makes one feel more competent and aggressive, which encourages one to drive fast, while marijuana makes one feel less competent and causes one to drive more slowly (Kalant, Corrigall, Hall, & Smart, 1999). As a result, alcohol is a much larger contributor to accidents and fatalities, even after controlling for differences in use of the two drugs.
5. It should be acknowledged, however, that people could be *implicitly* aware of what works though unable to articulate their knowledge. To the extent that this is the case, studying people's conscious intuitions is unlikely to be fruitful.
6. For a review of other process models of emotion regulation see Carver and Scheier's (1982, 1990) control theory model, where affect is used as feedback regarding an individual's progress toward controlling one's goals. In addition, see Larsen's (2000) model in which he proposes that people have a setpoint for how they typically desire to feel and affect is regulated only when there is a discrepancy between their current state and their setpoint.
7. It is important to note that the type of suppression typically addressed in the emotion regulation literature is *expressive* suppression (e.g., Butler et al., 2003; Gross, 1998a; Gross & Levenson, 1993, 1997; Richards & Gross, 1999), rather than suppression of subjective feelings.
8. Limiting the definition of affect regulation in this fashion also tends to limit the focus of inquiry to *short-term* strategies that can be implemented in the midst of an affect-inducing experience.
9. It is possible that before rationalizing an act of unethical behavior one's brain might engage in some form of implicit, unconscious, affective forecast to the effect that the rationalization will make one feel better. However, it seems more likely that rationalization tends to be a more reflexive reaction to the immediate feeling of guilt or shame.
10. In addition to the experiential, behavioral, and physiological consequences of suppressing emotions, several studies have examined the cognitive and social consequences of *expressive* suppression (e.g., Richards & Gross, 1999, 2000; Butler et al., 2003). Most of these have obtained results parallel to those focusing on thought and emotion suppression; although expressive suppression is often possible, it appears to be an ineffective, and indeed possibly counterproductive, means of inhibiting the emotions themselves.
11. Not that strategies 3 and 4 could be interpreted as antecedent- and emotion-focused forms of suppression.

REFERENCES

Affleck, G., Tennen, H., Croog, S., & Levine, S. (1987). Causal attribution, perceived benefits, and morbidity after a heart attack: An 8-year study. *Journal of Consulting and Clinical Psychology, 55,* 29–35.

Ahles, T., Blanchard, E., & Leventhal, H. (1983). Cognitive control of pain: Attention to the sensory aspects of the cold pressor stimulus. *Cognitive Therapy and Research, 7,* 159–177.

Bargh, J. A., & Williams, L. E. (2007). The nonconscious regulation of emotion. In J. J. Gross (Ed.), *Handbook of emotion regulation* (pp. 429–445). New York: Guilford Press.

Buehler, R., & McFarland, C. (2001). Intensity bias in affective forecasting: The role of temporal focus. *Personality and Social Psychology Bulletin, 27,* 1480–1493.

Butler, E. A., Egloff, B. Wilhelm F. H., Smith, N. C., Erickson, E. A., & Gross, J. J. (2003). The social consequences of expressive suppression. *Emotion 3,* 48–67.

Carver, C. S., & Scheier, M. F. (1982). Control theory: A useful conceptual framework for personality-social, clinical, and health psychology. *Psychological Bulletin, 92,* 111–135.

Carver, C. S., & Scheier, M. F. (1990). Origins and functions of positive and negative affect: A control-process view. *Psychological Review, 97,* 19–35.

Cioffi, D. (1993). Sensate body, directive mind: Physical sensations and mental control. In D. M. Wegner & J. W. Pennebaker (Eds.), *Handbook of mental control* (pp. 410–442). Englewood Cliffs, NJ: Prentice Hall.

Cioffi, D., & Holloway, J. (1993). Delayed costs of suppressed pain. *Journal of Personality and Social Psychology, 64,* 247–282.

Chapman, L. J., & Chapman, J. (1982). Test results are what you think they are. In D. Kahneman, P. Slovic, & A. Tversky (Eds.), *Judgment under uncertainty: Heuristics and biases* (pp. 239–248). Cambridge, UK: Cambridge University Press.

Clark, M. S., & Isen, A. M. (1982). Toward understanding the relationship between feeling states and social behavior. In A. Hastorf & A. M. Isen (Eds.), *Cognitive social psychology* (pp. 73–108). New York: Elsevier/North-Holland.

Einhorn, H. (1980). Learning from experience and suboptimal rules in decision making. In T. Wallsten (Ed.), *Cognitive processes in choice and decision behavior* (pp. 1–20). Hillsdale, NJ: Erlbaum.

Emmons, R. A., & McCullough, M. E. (2003). Counting blessings versus burdens: An experimental investigation of gratitude and subjective well-being in daily life. *Journal of Personality and Social Psychology, 84,* 377–389.

Frank, R. H. (1988). *Passions within reason: The strategic role of emotion.* New York: W. W. Norton.

Frederick, S., & Loewenstein, G. (1999). Hedonic adaptation. In D. Kahneman, E. Diener, & N. Schwarz (Eds.), *Well-being: The foundations of hedonic psychology* (pp. 302–329). New York: Russell Sage.

Freud, A. (1971). *Ego and the mechanisms of defense.* Madison, CT: International Universities Press. (Original work published 1936)

Gilbert, D. T., Pinel, E. C., Wilson, T. D., Blumberg, S. J., & Wheatley, T. P. (1998). Immune neglect: A source of durability bias in affective forecasting. *Journal of Personality and Social Psychology, 75,* 617–638.

Gross, J. J. (1998a). Antecedent- and response-focused emotion regulation: Divergent consequences for experience, expression, and physiology. *Journal of Personality and Social Psychology, 74,* 224–237.

Gross, J. J. (1998b). The emerging field of emotion regulation: An integrative review. *Journal of General Psychology, 2,* 271–299.

Gross, J. J. (1999). Emotion and emotion regulation. In L. A. Pervin & O. P. John (Eds.), *Handbook of personality: Theory and research* (2nd ed., pp. 525–552). New York: Guilford Press.

Gross, J. J. (2002). Emotion regulation: Affective, cognitive, and social consequences. *Psychophysiology, 39,* 281–291.

Gross, J. J., & Levenson, R. W. (1993). Emotional suppression: Physiology, self-report, and expressive behavior. *Journal of Personality and Social Psychology, 64,* 970–986.

Gross, J. J., & Levenson, R. W. (1997). Hiding feelings: The acute effects of inhibiting negative and positive emotion. *Journal of Abnormal Psychology, 106,* 95–103.

Gross, J. J., & Thompson, R. A. (2007). Emotion regulation: Conceptual foundations. In J. J. Gross (Ed.), *Handbook of emotion regulation* (pp. 3–24). New York: Guilford Press.

Janoff-Bulman, R., & Wortman, C. (1977). Attributions of blame and coping in the "real world": Severe accident victims react to their lot. *Journal of Personality and Social Psychology, 35*(5), 351–363.

Kahneman, D., & Snell, J. (1992). Predicting a changing taste. *Journal of Behavioral Decision Making, 5*, 187–200.

Kalant, H., Corrigall, W., Hall, W., & Smart, R. (Eds.). (1999). *The health effects of cannabis.* Toronto, ON, Canada: Addiction Research Foundation.

Larsen, R. J. (2000). Toward a science of mood regulation. *Psychological Inquiry, 11*, 129–141.

Larsen, J. T., McGraw, P., & Cacioppo, J. T. (2001). Can people feel happy and sad at the same time? *Journal of Personality and Social Psychology, 81*, 684–698.

Lehman, D. R., Wortman, C. B., & Williams, A. F. (1987). Long-term effects of losing a spouse or child in a motor vehicle crash. *Journal of Personality and Social Psychology, 52*(1), 218–231.

Loewenstein, G., & Frederick, S. (1997). Predicting reactions to environmental change. In M. H. Bazerman, D. M. Messick, A. E. Tenbrunsel, & K. A. Wade-Benzoni (Eds.), *Environment, ethics, and behavior* (pp. 52–72). San Francisco: New Lexington Press.

Loewenstein, G., O'Donoghue, T., & Rabin, M. (2003). Projection bias in predicting future utility. *Quarterly Journal of Economics, 118*, 1209–1248.

Loewenstein, G., & Schkade, D. (1999). Wouldn't it be nice?: Predicting future feelings. In D. Kahneman, E. Diener, & N. Schwarz (Eds.), *Well-being: The foundations of hedonic psychology* (pp. 85–105). New York: Russell Sage.

Lord, C., Lepper, M. R., & Ross, L. (1979). Biased assimilation and attitude polarization: The effects of prior theories on subsequently considered evidence. *Journal of Personality and Social Psychology, 37*, 2098–2110.

Metcalfe, J., & Mischel, W. (1999). A "hot/cool-system" analysis of delay of gratification: Dynamics of willpower. *Psychological Review, 106*, 3–19.

McCaul, K. D., & Haugtvedt, C. (1982). Attention, distraction, and cold-pressor pain. *Journal of Personality and Social Psychology, 43*, 154–162.

Mischel, W., & Ayduk, O. (2004). Willpower in a cognitive–affective processing system: The dynamics of delay of gratification. In R. F. Baumeister & K. D. Vohs (Eds.), *Handbook of self-regulation: Research, theory, and applications* (pp. 99–129). New York: Guilford Press.

Mischel, W., & Baker, N. (1975). Cognitive appraisals and transformations in delay behavior. *Journal of Personality and Social Psychology, 31*(2), 254–261.

Moore, B., Mischel, W., & Zeiss, A. (1976). Comparative effects of the reward stimulus and its cognitive representation in voluntary delay. *Journal of Personality and Social Psychology, 34*, 419–424.

Nisbett, R., & Ross, L. (1980). *Human inference: Strategies and shortcomings of human judgment.* Englewood Cliffs, NJ: Prentice Hall.

Nolen-Hoeksema, S. (1993). Sex differences in control of depression. In D. M. Wegner & J. M. Pennebaker (Eds.), *Handbook of mental control* (pp. 306–324). Englewood Cliffs, NJ: Prentice Hall.

Nozick, R. (1974). *Anarchy, state and utopia.* New York: Basic Books.

Ochsner, K. N., & Gross, J. J. (2007). The neural architecture of emotion regulation. In J. J. Gross (Ed.), *Handbook of emotion regulation* (pp. 87–109). New York: Guilford Press.

Rachman, S. J. (1994). The overprediction of fear: A review. *Behaviour Research and Therapy, 32*, 683–690.

Rayo, L., & Becker, G. (2005). *Evolutionary efficiency and happiness* [Mimeo]. University of Chicago, Graduate School of Business [Online]. Available: http://gsbwww.uchicago.edu/fac/luis.rayo/research/HappinessJanuary05.pdf.

Richards, J. M., & Gross, J. J. (1999). Composure at any cost? The cognitive consequences of emotion suppression. *Personality and Social Psychology Bulletin, 25*, 1033–1044.

Richards, J. M., & Gross, J. J. (2000). Emotion regulation and memory: The cognitive costs of keeping one's cool. *Journal of Personality and Social Psychology, 79*, 410–424.

Robinson, M. D., & Clore, G. L. (2001). Simulation, scenarios, and emotional appraisal: Testing the convergence of real and imagined reactions to emotional stimuli. *Personality and Social Psychology Bulletin, 27*, 1520–1532

Robinson, M. D., & Clore, G. L. (2002). Belief and feeling: Evidence for an accessibility model of emotional self-report. *Psychological Bulletin, 128*, 934–960.

Roese, N. J., & Olson, J. M. (1995). *What might have been: The social psychology of counterfactual thinking.* Mahwah, NJ: Erlbaum.

Ross, M. (1989). Relation of implicit theories to the construction of personal histories. *Psychological Review, 96,* 341–357.

Salkovskis, P. M., & Reynolds, M. (1994). Thought suppression and smoking cessation. *Behaviour Research and Therapy, 32,* 193–201.

Schooler, J., Ariely, D., & Loewenstein, G. (2003). The pursuit of happiness can be self-defeating. In J. Carrillo & I. Brocas (Eds.), *The psychology of economic decisions* (pp. 41–70). Oxford, UK: Oxford University Press.

Sullivan, M. J. L., Rouse, D., Bishop, S., & Johnston, S. (1997). Thought suppression, catastrophizing, and pain. *Behaviour Research and Therapy, 36,* 751–756.

Taylor, S. (1983). Adjustment to threatening life events: A theory of cognitive adaptation. *American Psychologist, 38,* 1161–1173.

Thaler, R. H., & Johnson, E. J. (1990). Gambling with the house money and trying to break even: The effects of prior outcomes on risky choice. *Management Science, 36*(6), 643–660.

Toll, B. A., Sobell, M. B., Wagner, E. F., & Sobell, L. C. (2001). The relationship between thought suppression and smoking cessation. *Addictive Behavior, 26,* 509–515.

Ubel, P. A., Loewenstein, G., Hershey, J., Baron, J., Mohr, T., Asch, D. A., et al. (2001). Do nonpatients underestimate the quality of life associated with chronic health conditions because of a focusing illusion? *Medical Decision Making, 21,* 190–199.

Wegner, D. M. (1992). You can't always think what you want: Problems in the suppression of unwanted thoughts. *Advances in Experimental Social Psychology, 25,* 195–225.

Wegner, D. M. (1994). Ironic process of mental control. *Psychological Review, 101,* 34–52.

Wegner, D. M., Erber, R., & Zanakos, S. (1993). Ironic processes in the mental control of mood and mood-related thought. *Journal of Personality and Social Psychology, 65,* 1093–1104.

Wegner, D. M., & Wenzlaff, R. M. (1996). Mental control. In E. T. Higgins & A. W. Kruglanski (Eds.), *Social psychology: Handbook of basic principles* (pp. 466–492). New York: Guilford Press.

Wegner, D. M., & Wenzlaff, R. M. (2000). Thought suppression. *Annual Review of Psychology, 51,* 59–91.

Wegner, D. M., & Zanakos, S. (1994). Chronic thought suppression. *Journal of Personality, 62,* 615–640.

Wenzlaff, R. (1993). The mental control of depression: Psychological obstacles to emotional well-being. In D. M. Wegner & J. W. Pennebaker (Eds.), *Handbook of mental control* (pp. 239–257). Englewood Cliffs, NJ: Prentice Hall.

Wenzlaff, R., Wegner, D. M., & Roper, D. (1988). Depression and mental control: The resurgence of unwanted negative thoughts. *Journal of Personality and Social Psychology, 55,* 882–892.

Wilson, T. D., & Gilbert, D. T. (2003). Affective forecasting. *Advances in Experimental Social Psychology, 35,* 345–411.

Wilson, T. D., & Gilbert, D. T. (2005). *A model of affective adaptation* (Working paper). Department of Psychology, University of Virginia.

Wilson, T. D., Meyers, J., & Gilbert, D. T. (2001). Lessons from the past: Do people learn from experience that emotional reactions are short lived? *Personality and Social Psychology Bulletin, 27,* 1648–1661.

Wilson, T. D., Wheatley, T. P., Kurtz, J., Dunn, E., & Gilbert, D. T. (2004). Ready to fire: preemptive rationalization versus rapid reconstrual after positive and negative outcomes. *Personality and Social Psychology Bulletin, 30,* 340–351.

Zillman, D. (1988). Mood management: Using entertainment to full advantage. In L. Donohew, H. E. Sypher, & E. T. Higgins (Eds.), *Communication, social cognition, and affect* (pp. 147–171). Hillsdale, NJ: Erlbaum.

CHAPTER 10

Conflict Monitoring
in Cognition–Emotion Competition

SAMUEL M. McCLURE
MATTHEW M. BOTVINICK
NICK YEUNG
JOSHUA D. GREENE
JONATHAN D. COHEN

Sometime between 2:00 A.M. and 3:00 A.M., a man is being rushed through a hallway on a gurney to be treated for a gunshot wound. He has massive internal bleeding and will die soon if not treated. He is also the only person who knows the location of a stolen nuclear warhead that terrorists are threatening to detonate in a major U.S. city before dawn. As the government agent hurries the man into the operating room, he sees the one available doctor in the middle of a heart surgery necessary to save the life of the person who, only hours before, saved this agent's life. Jack Bauer is confronted with a moral dilemma, the likes of which are common fare in TV dramas (in this case, Fox's television show *24*), if not everyday life. Does Bauer sacrifice the life of the man to whom he is emotionally tied and to whom he owes his life in order to potentially save the millions of people threatened by the terrorists? Or, does he allow his friend's heart surgery to continue, running the risk that the sole connection to the stolen warhead will be lost?

While this example is clearly dramatized, it highlights a set of problems that have proven beguiling to moral philosophers (Greene, Sommerville, Nystrom, Darley, & Cohen, 2001). The utilitarian solution to Jack's dilemma is obvious: He should sacrifice the one life—no matter how cherished it is to him—for the sake of the millions of lives threatened by the terrorists. However, when dilemmas involve sacrificing the life of a person to whom you have a close personal link, then emotional reactions, and common moral intuitions, may run counter to the utilitarian solution; that is, the one that would do good for the greatest number of people. Jack is faced with a moral judgment that involves a true conflict (Greene et al., 2004). We propose that the occurrence and detection of such conflicts are used explicitly by the brain to determine when emotion regulation is necessary, and to engage regulatory control processes. In Jack's case, emotion regulation is needed to constrain and/or override his emotional response, so that the optimal course of action can be determined and executed.

In this chapter, we review recent work addressing decisions similar to the one in the preceding example, in which cognition and emotion are simultaneously involved and have opposing effects on behavior. Competition between cognitive and emotional processes arises in many domains beyond moral judgment. We review two additional examples from behavioral economics, one involving social exchange (the ultimatum game; Sanfey, Riling, Aronson, Nystrom, & Cohen, 2003), and the other time discounting and intertemporal choice (McClure et al., 2004a). Both correspond to situations that arise commonly in the world. The ultimatum game models situations such as the following: You are selling an item but have only one offer that is well below what you consider to be the fair price. One the one hand, your desire to sell motivates you to consider the offer and at least recoup some of your investment (cognitive). On the other hand, your sense of fairness pushes you to decline the offer out of sheer indignation (emotional). Studies of intertemporal choice—having to choose between two options, one of which is worth less but available sooner, and the other of which is worth more but not available until later—address an experience that we encounter almost daily: the need to resist an immediate temptation in the service of a longer-term good. Dieting is a clear example. One may wish to lose weight to improve long-term health (cognitive) but struggle at the sight of an appetizing dessert (emotional).

Recent experimental work on these three classes of problem—moral decisions, fairness in social exchange (the ultimatum game), and impulsiveness (intertemporal choice)—has produced a strikingly consistent, if still coarse-grained, picture about the neural mechanisms involved in decision making when cognitive and emotional processes come into competition. In each of the experimental examples we review, functional magnetic resonance imaging (fMRI) data have revealed regions of brain activity that respond separately to the engagement of cognitive and emotional processes. Furthermore, the relative degree of activity in these areas correlates closely with behavioral outcome. When neural activity is elevated in emotion-related brain areas, principally limbic and closely linked cortical areas, choices tend to be resolved in favor of the emotional demand. When neural activity is relatively greater in cognition-related areas, including dorsolateral prefrontal cortex (dLPFC) and posterior parietal cortex, the outcome favors what is often considered to be the more rational (or, in the case of moral decisions, utilitarian) choice.

An important question concerning the interaction between cognitive and emotional systems is how competition is detected when it occurs, and how this is resolved. This question is closely related to questions about "emotional regulation," the topic of this volume (e.g., Ochsner & Gross, 2005). The findings we review suggest that at least one set of mechanisms is involved that is similar, if not identical, to those that have been linked to other forms of competition and conflicts in processing that do not directly involve emotional regulation. Such circumstances have been consistently associated with activity in a dorsal region of the anterior cingulated cortex (ACC) and subsequent engagement of structures associated with cognitive control and the resolution of conflict, including dLPFC (Carter et al., 1998; Botvinick, Braver, Barch, Carter, & Cohen, 2001; Kerns et al., 2004). Similarly, as we shall see, conflict between cognitive and emotional processes engages similar regions. This suggests that mechanisms thought to detect and resolve conflicts in domains traditionally considered to be primarily cognitive (e.g., between color naming and word reading in the Stroop task; Stroop, 1935) may also be important for carrying out similar functions when conflict involves cognitive and emotional processes.

We begin with a brief section describing our working use of the terms "emotion" and "cognition," as well as an operational definition of "conflict." We then turn to a review of the experimental work examining moral decision making as well as economic decision making in the ultimatum game and in intertemporal choice. To interpret the consistent finding of ACC activity in these cases, we review the conflict-monitoring theory of ACC function. Finally, we highlight several predictions derived from conflict monitoring that we speculate may hold for cognitive–emotional interactions as well.

DEFINITIONS

In each of the problems to be discussed, we draw a distinction between emotional and cognitive task demands, as well as emotion- and cognition-related brain systems. These distinctions have an almost irresistible intuitive appeal and have been used to divide entire fields of inquiry, both within science and beyond. They also raise legitimate concern at both the psychological and the neurobiological levels. At the psychological level, it has long been recognized that there is there is little meaning to reason without motivation (e.g., Hume, 1739/2000), while, at the same time, emotions reflect information processing in the service of a goal, just like any other computation carried out by the brain. Furthermore, it seems likely that well-adapted behavior usually involves close interactions and tight integration between emotional and cognitive processes. So, what purpose does a distinction between cognition and emotion serve? We believe, like many others, that this distinction recognizes the fact that different forms of mental and computational processes have developed to serve different types of functions and challenge us to identify and better understand their distinguishing characteristics. Below, we outline these, as working definitions for how we use the terms "emotion" and "cognition" in the remainder of this chapter.

We use "emotion" to signify a set of valenced behavioral and concomitant physiological responses that correlate with specific subjective experiences. This is very similar to the definition employed by others (e.g., Frijda, 1986). From a psychological perspective, it is useful to think about emotional processes as a subset of automatic processes, in that they are quick to respond and produce stereotyped effects on behavior. They can be differentiated from other automatic processes in that they are valenced; that is, that they have valuative significance, carrying a level of attraction or aversion to the events that evoke them. The functions of emotion-related brain areas in limbic and paralimbic brain regions exhibit these properties (LeDoux, 1996). This includes regions of the striatum and amygdala, as well as regions of the frontal cortex that encompass the insula, orbital, and medial frontal cortex. Activity in these areas can occur within a very short delay following a stimulus, is typically associated with valenced stimuli (i.e., rewarding or aversive), and often is accompanied by stereotyped responses. Fast, strong, automatic processes of this sort provide obvious benefit for identifying and responding advantageously to a fleeting opportunity or an imminent threat. It seems reasonable, therefore, to assume that emotions represent processing mechanisms that have proven to be adaptive over the course of development, whether of the species, specific cultures, or the individual.

We contrast emotions with cognitive processes that are more deliberative and support a wider range of behaviors. Such processes appear to rely on a different set of brain structures, typically including dorsolateral and anterior regions of the prefrontal cortex (PFC), as well as the posterior parietal cortex. These systems are consistently observed to be involved in a variety of cognitive processes such as working memory (e.g., Cohen et al., 1997), abstract reasoning (e.g., Kroger et al., 2002), and general problem solving (e.g., Duncan et al., 2000). There is growing consensus that these systems are central to the brain's ability to flexibly respond to rapidly changing task demands, as well as the pursuit of longer-term, goal-directed behavior, especially when this faces competition from more immediate or compelling stimuli or behaviors (e.g., Miller & Cohen, 2001).

This distinction between emotional and cognitive processes aligns closely with the long-standing distinction that psychologists have made between automatic and controlled processing (Posner & Snyder, 1975; Shiffrin & Schneider, 1977), and the distinction made more recently by behavioral economics between hot and cold or System 1 and System 2 processes (Chaiken & Trope, 1999; Lieberman, Gaunt, Gilbert, & Trope, 2002; Mischel, Ayduk, & Mendoza-Denton, 2003; Kahneman, 2003; Loewenstein & O'Donoghue, 2004). All these models share the distinction between a fast, automatic, efficient, but rigid type of processing and slower, more effortful, and capacity-limited but more flexible type of processing.

EMOTION AND COGNITION IN DECISION MAKING: THREE EXAMPLES

Separate emotional and cognitive processes are likely to be engaged in many behaviors. When we meet someone we form a quick, emotion-based impression of them that is subsequently refined cognitively (Fiske & Neuberg, 1988). Responding to fearful events involves a fast, stereotyped, emotional response followed by a slower reaction subject to cognitive assessment (LeDoux, 1996; Fox et al., 2005). Buying behaviors are rife with automatic, emotional influences as well as deliberative ones (Hoch & Loewenstein, 1991). Even deciding between two drinks depends on both emotional and cognitive processes (McClure et al., 2004b; Adolphs, Tranel, Koenigs, & Damasio, 2005). These observations have received support from neuroimaging studies. Activation of reward and evaluative mechanisms (such as the ventral striatum, orbitofrontal cortex, and amygdala) is commonly observed in tasks that also engage cognitive processing (e.g., LeDoux, 1996; Fox et al., 2005).

Under most circumstances, behavior appears to reflect a seamless integration of cognitive and emotional processes. For example, the mechanisms underlying reinforcement learning (Montague, Dayan, & Sejnowski, 1996; Schultz, Dayan, & Montague, 1997) are also believed to play a critical role in regulating working-memory function (Luciana, 1992; Williams & Goldman-Rakic, 1995; Braver & Cohen, 2000); and brain systems long thought to be involved in arousal are now thought to play an important role in regulating the balance between task-focused versus exploratory behaviors (Aston-Jones & Cohen, 2005). However, in some circumstances, emotional and cognitive processes may come into conflict, favoring different and incompatible behavioral responses. Situations of cognitive–emotional conflict are useful, as they provide an opportunity to dissociate and thereby distinguish the influence that the neural mechanisms underlying each type of process have on behavior. These circumstances also provide a window into the mechanisms that are involved in detecting and resolving such conflict. In the following three sections, we briefly review the results of three studies that have used functional neuroimaging to examine the neural mechanisms involved in decision making under conditions in which emotional and cognitive processes are placed in conflict.

Moral Judgment: Revulsion versus the Greater Good

The proper bases for deciding the moral appropriateness of actions has long been a matter of debate. One common framework derives from Jeremy Bentham's (1982) and John Stuart Mill's ultitarianism. On this view, actions should be taken that maximize overall utility, where "overall" is determined by the number of affected individuals. Thus, if a situation requires doing harm to one individual in order to achieve a greater good for others, then the action should be deemed morally acceptable. This contrasts with alternative philosophies in which the rights of affected individuals are also considered, independent of the greater good that may come from their harm. For example, according to Immanuel Kant, it is morally unacceptable to use a person as a means to an end, even if that end brings a greater good. The difference between the utilitarian and Kantian formulations of morality, and how they relate to the moral judgments of ordinary individuals, is illustrated by the trolley problem (Foot, 1978; Thomson, 1986; Greene et al., 2001).

The trolley problem is exemplified by contrasting two scenarios. In the switch scenario, a trolley car is progressing on a track that will run over and kill five unsuspecting workers unless something is done. The only way to save the workers is to flip a switch that will divert the trolley onto a side track. However, on that track there is another, single unsuspecting workman who will be killed if the switch is flipped. The question is whether it is morally acceptable to flip the switch to save the five workers at the cost of the one. In this case, utilitarianism, Kantian morality, and common intuition all agree. Diverting the train will preserve the most life (utilitarianism); the single worker on the side track is not being used as a means—the death is simply an incidental side effect of saving the lives of others—and thus is acceptable according to Kantian morality; and an overwhelming majority of respondents in empirical investigations indicate that flipping the switch to divert the trolley is morally acceptable (Petrinovich, O'Neill, & Jorgensen, 1993; Greene et al., 2001).

A second scenario, however, elicits greater conflict. In the footbridge scenario, a trolley is once again on a course that results in the death of five unsuspecting workers. In this case there is no switch; instead, you are standing on a footbridge over the tracks and there is another, large individual (assume it is another worker) who is standing near the edge of the bridge. You can save the five workers by shoving the bystander off the footbridge. He will land in front of the trolley and stop it but will be killed in the process. Let us assume that this is the only way to save the five workers (e.g., you are too slight to jump in front of the trolley yourself), and that it is guaranteed to work. From the utilitarian perspective, the critical features of the situation are the same: Sacrificing one life will save five, and thus it is morally acceptable. From the Kantian perspective, however, the situation is fundamentally different: The bystander is being used as a means, which is morally unacceptable. Most respondents agree with the judgment that it is morally unacceptable to push the bystander off the bridge to save the five workers (Petrinovich et al., 1993; Greene et al., 2001).

One interpretation of these findings might be that Kantian moral philosophy provides a good account of common moral intuitions. However, this does not appear to be correct. This is revealed by a third variant of the trolley problem. As in the switch scenario, the trolley can be diverted onto a side track. However, in this case, the side track loops back and rejoins the main track at a location before the five workers. Therefore, without the presence of a worker on the side track, the trolley will continue on and kill the five workers. Thus, in this case a workman is required, as a means, to stop the train and save the five workers. While this does not change the utilitarian analysis, it does change the Kantian one. How do people respond? A majority indicate that, as in the original switch scenario, it is acceptable to flip the switch (Thompson, 1986; Greene et al., in press, unpublished data). This poses a fundamental dilemma: Commonly held intuitions appear to follow utilitarian principles in some cases (e.g., the original and modified switch scenarios) but not in others (the footbridge scenario), and an appeal to other sorts of rational principles (e.g., Kantian morality) does not explain this behavior.

To address this conundrum, some philosophers and social theorists have suggested that moral judgments may reflect the operation of at least two different evaluative systems, one governed by deliberation and reasoning and another governed by emotional responses (e.g., Greene & Haidt, 2002; Greene, Nystrom, Engell, Darley, & Cohen, 2004). This may explain the differing intuitions that people report for the aforementioned dilemmas. Ordinarily, people may abide by utilitarian principles of morality. However, a strong emotional response may impact the decision-making process. This is particularly clear in cases such as the Jack Bauer dilemma described at the beginning of this chapter. Interestingly, such effects are observed even when it is made explicitly clear that the question is about the morality of a particular act, not whether it would feel good or bad or whether they would or would not want to do it (Greene et al., 2001, 2004). Furthermore, people typically do not report, and may not even be aware of the presumed emotional response (Wheatley & Haidt, 2005). Given these observations, the hypothesis that moral judgments engage and can be influenced by emotional responses demands independent empirical evidence.

In one test of this hypothesis, Greene et al. (2001) devised two sets of moral dilemmas and used fMRI to compare neural activity elicited in response to each. One set ("impersonal") was designed to be similar to the switch scenario of the trolley dilemma, in which the harm to an individual (required to achieve a greater good) was produced remotely or indirectly. The other set of dilemmas ("personal") involved situations similar to the footbridge scenario, in which the harm required to achieve a greater good involved more personal or direct contact with the victim. In addition, subjects were asked to consider a set of nonmoral problems (e.g., requiring simple arithmetic calculations) that were matched to the moral dilemmas for reaction time.

Two sets of brain areas were identified that were differentially activated in response to personal and impersonal dilemmas (Figure 10.1). Regions that were preferentially activated while subjects contemplated impersonal dilemmas included dLPFC and posterior parietal cortex, areas that have been consistently associated with cognitive processes, such as working memory and problem solving (Cohen et al., 1997; Duncan et al., 2000; Wager & Smith, 2003). These same areas were activated in response to the nonmoral problems. In contrast, when subjects considered personal moral dilemmas, activity was observed in a different set of areas, including the medial prefrontal cortex and the posterior cingulate cortex. These areas receive direct afferent input from limbic brain areas and have been associated with emotions in numerous other studies (Maddock, 1999; Knutson, Adams, Fong, & Hommer, 2001; Phan, Wager, Taylor, & Liberzon, 2002; Britton et al., 2006).

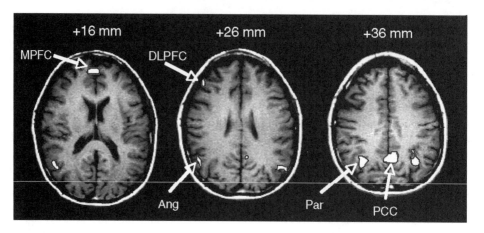

FIGURE 10.1. Neural basis of moral decision making. In Greene et al. (2001), subjects were asked to make moral judgments on a series of personal (involving direct physical contact) and impersonal (requiring causally distant interaction) moral dilemmas. Two sets of brain areas are activated when subjects make these moral judgments. One set is composed of brain areas implicated in cognitive processing and is activated preferentially by impersonal problems. This set includes the dLPFC and the angular gyrus. The other set includes brain areas commonly implicated in social and emotional processes and includes the superior temporal sulcus, the posterior cingulate cortex, and the medial prefrontal cortex. Adapted from Greene et al. (2001). Copyright 2001 by AAAS. Adapted by permission.

These results are consistent with the hypothesis that different types of moral judgments engage functionally distinct brain systems, one of which mediates the effects of deliberative processes and the other emotion responses. One question that arises with regard to these findings is the source of the negative emotional response: Why should people feel worse about pushing a person off a bridge than flipping a switch that will lead to the person's death? This question is beyond the scope of our current discussion. Another question, more directly related to the considerations in this chapter, is whether these emotional responses directly influence moral judgment or are simply correlated with the outcome of the judgment. For example, having decided that it is not acceptable to push the person off the footbridge, perhaps one feels guilty or regretful about the consequences that this would have for the five workmen who would die. Whereas it is difficult to establish causal relationships definitively without directly manipulating the systems involved, Green and colleagues addressed this question in two ways.

First, they reasoned that if emotional processing had an influence on moral decision making, it should slow responses for cases in which the emotional process favored a decision that was incongruent with the one made by the subject. For example, reaction time should be slower when a subject decides that it is acceptable to push the person off the bridge than when they make the emotionally congruent decision that it is not, or when emotions are not presumed to be involved. This is exactly what was observed (Greene et al., 2001). These findings parallel those from a large number of cognitive tasks, such as the Stroop task (Stroop 1935; MacLeod, 1991), the Simon task (Simon, 1969), and the Eriksen flanker task (Eriksen & Eriksen, 1974), in which reaction times are slower when subjects must make a response (e.g., name the color in which a word is displayed) against interference from a competing, prepotent, and automatic process (e.g., reading the word itself). In this case, the emotional response is that prepotent, automatic process.

Greene at al. (2004) also sought more direct evidence for the competition between emotional and cognitive processes. Toward this end, they focused on cases in which there was less consensus regarding the morality of an action, and therefore where there was likely to be more competition and conflict. For example, in one dilemma subjects had to decide whether it was morally acceptable to smother a crying infant in order to spare an entire village from genocide (Greene et al., 2004). In this case, and other similar ones, about half of subjects say it is acceptable and half reject this. Such dilemmas elicited activity in both the emotional and cognitive brain areas identified in the previous study. Interestingly, the relative degree of activity in these areas prior to the response was strongly and significantly correlated with the outcome of the decision, with greater activity in cognitive areas when subjects proceeded to make a utilitarian decision, and less when they made a decision consistent with the emotional response. Moreover, such decisions were associated with activity in the ACC, a finding that is consistent with the hypothesis that the ACC is responsive to conflict between competing processes—in this case, the cognitive processes favoring a utilitarian decision and the emotional response to the prospect of doing harm. We return to this finding later in the chapter.

The Ultimatum Game: Anger versus Monetary Gain

Competition between emotional and cognitive processes has also been proposed to explain behaviors that seem to deviate from the dictum of economic rationality. The ultimatum game provides a classic example of this (Thaler, 1988). In this game, two people are provided with an endowment, which is usually a sum of money. The first person, called the proposer, must make an offer which the second person, the responder, may either accept or reject. If the offer is accepted, they split the money as proposed. However, if the offer is rejected, the money is withdrawn and neither player earns anything.

According to standard economic doctrine, earning any amount of money should be preferred to earning nothing, and thus rational behavior for the proposer and responder is clear. The proposer should offer the smallest amount possible, anticipating that the responder will accept this rather than earn nothing. The responder, in turn, should accept any offer greater than zero. However, this is not how most people behave (Güth, Schmittberger, & Schwarze, 1982; Thaler, 1988). Rather, the most common offer is between 30% and 40% of the total. Furthermore, offers of less than 20% are routinely rejected, even when this means rejecting a considerable sum of money (e.g., as much as a month's pay; Hoffman, McCabe, & Smith, 1995).

One explanation for this behavior may be that subjects are sensitive to establishing a bargaining position, or maintaining their reputation (Nowak, Page, & Sigmund, 2000). If a responder is known to have accepted a small offer, this knowledge may prove disadvantageous in future interactions. However, similar behaviors are observed even when the participants know that the game will be played anonymously and only a single time (Güth et al., 1982; Kahneman, Knetch, & Thaler, 1986; Sanfey et al., 2003). An alternative explanation is that in the ultimatum game, as in the moral dilemmas discussed earlier, behavior is guided by emotional as well as cognitive processes that come into conflict in this setting. Specifically, it may be that responders have a negative emotional reaction to offers they perceive to be unfair, causing them to reject the offer. The reason for this emotion is, once again, beyond the scope of our discussion (for a consideration of this question, see Rabin, 1993; Wright, 1994; Fehr & Schmidt, 1999). What is relevant is whether rejection of remunerative, but unfair, offers is in the result of an emotional response.

Sanfey et al. (2003) investigated this question, using fMRI to examine the brain activity of responders as they considered offers in the ultimatum game. Half of the offers were presented as coming from a person that the subject had met prior to the experiment. Each of these was with a different partner, and subjects knew that their responses would be kept confidential. The other 10 offers were presented as having been produced by a computer program. In both cases, offers were fixed so that half were fair (50:50 and 70:30 splits) and the other half were unfair (80:20 and 90:10). As in earlier studies, subjects accepted nearly all of the fair offers but rejected a significant number of unfair offers. The rejection rate was significantly higher when subjects believed that the offer came from another person than a computer program. This is consistent with the observation that subjects often report being angered by unfair offers (Camerer & Thaler, 1995), something that might be expected with greater frequency or intensity when an interaction involves another person rather than a computer.

Supporting the hypothesis that anger may have contributed to the rejection of unfair offers, Sanfey et al. (2003) found (Figure 10.2) that unfair offers elicited activity in the insula, a limbic brain region tied to negative emotions (Calder, Lawrence, & Young, 2001), particularly anger and disgust (Phillips et al., 1997; Shapira et al., 2003; Britton et al., 2006). Interestingly, unfair offers were also associated with activity in the dLPFC. Furthermore, as in the case of moral judgment, behavioral outcome was closely related to the relative balance in activity in the dLPFC and emotion-related areas (in this case, the anterior insula). When activity in the insula was greater than in the dLPFC, responders rejected the unfair offer significantly more frequently than when activity in the dLPFC was greater. Finally, unfair offers were also associated with increased activity in the ACC thought to reflect, once again, the conflict between competing cognitive and emotional processes.

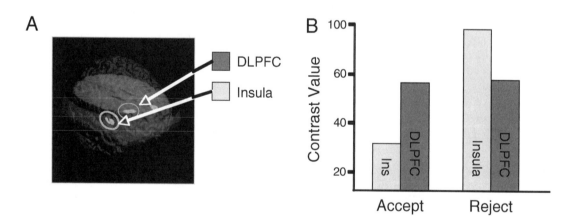

FIGURE 10.2. The ultimatum game. Responses to unfair offers in the ultimatum game are predicted by the relative activity in cognitive (dLPFC) and emotional (insula) brain areas. If activity in the insula predominates, then subjects tend to reject the offer; offers tend to be accepted when activity is greater in the dLPFC.

Intertemporal Choice: Impulsivity versus Patience

Our third example relates to intertemporal decisions, in which a choice must be made between one outcome that is available sooner, but is worth less, than a later outcome. In such cases, it must be determined whether the additional amount to be gained is worth the wait. Such choices pervade our lives, from daily decisions to ones that can have life-long consequences. Dieting is a choice between the desire to eat now and the desire to maintain long-term health. In retirement planning, we must decide how much of our current income to spend for immediate enjoyment and how much to save (Laibson, 1997). Even procrastination can be framed in these terms. Changes in intertemporal choice behavior (e.g., the ability to defer gratification) are a fundamental dimension of development (e.g., Mischel, Shoda, & Rodriguez, 1989), and disturbances in this capacity are thought to be a central feature of a number of clinical conditions, including attention-deficit disorder (e.g., Luman, Osterlan, & Sergeant, 2005) and drug addiction (Bickel & Johnson, 2003).

From a rational point of view, the optimal way to make intertemporal choices requires discounting the value of the two outcomes based on their delay and choosing the greater of the two discounted values. Preferences should also be consistent across time. If I prefer outcome *A* over an outcome *B* to occur some fixed amount of time after *A* (say a week), then I should *always* prefer *A* to *B*, whether *A* occurs today (and *B* in a week) or *A* will occur in a year (and *B* in a year and a week). Mathematically, the only discount function that ensures such consistency of preference is one that declines exponentially with delay (Samuelson, 1937; Koopmans, 1960; Frederick, Loewenstein, & O'Donoghue, 2003). However, people do not demonstrate such consistency. In a classic example, when deciding between one apple available in a year and two apples available in a year and a day, people generally prefer the latter. However, when the choice is between one apple available today and two apples available tomorrow, people generally prefer the former (Thaler, 1981). Such preference reversals indicate that humans (and other animals) discount more steeply over the near term than over the longer term. That is, people respond impulsively to goods that are immediately available.

This impulsivity has been described in terms of a hyperbolic discount function, which mathematically expresses the observation that discount rate declines with time. However, this framework does little to explain the broad range of discount rates that people exhibit for different goods and under different circumstances. People are far less impulsive for writing paper than for money or food, they discount large rewards less steeply than smaller ones, and they discount more steeply when they are in need or are aroused (Thaler, 1981; Giordano et al., 2002). While people appear to exhibit hyperbolic discounting under all these conditions, the specifics of the discount function vary substantially by circumstance.

An alternative approach has viewed discounting behavior as the engagement of separate evaluative systems, each of which uses a different discount function. The combined effect of multiple different discount functions can produce hyperbolic-like behavior. The simplest version of this account suggests that there are two types of discounting systems: one that values only goods that are immediately available, and another system that discounts more modestly over time (Laibson, 1997). This corresponds closely to a broader distinction that has been made between visceral (emotional) and deliberative (cognitive) evaluative systems involved in a wide range of economic behaviors, with the emotional system exhibiting steep discounting and the deliberative one placing greater value on future rewards (Loewenstein, 1996). This suggests why people are impulsive for certain goods and not others (such as writing paper), for which there is no associated visceral drive. Further, it may explain why large-magnitude rewards are discounted less, because these may surpass immediate visceral needs and thus come to be evaluated proportionately more by cognitive processes that discount more judiciously for time.

This two-process theory of discounting behavior has a natural interpretation in terms of neurobiological mechanisms, paralleling those identified in the moral reasoning and ultimatum game studies. That is, the steeply discounting visceral system may reflect the operation of primitive, evolutionarily conserved limbic mechanisms, while the appraisals of the more providential cognitive system may reflect the operation of higher-level cortical mechanisms involving the prefrontal cortex and associated structures. This has recently been tested in a series of fMRI experiments in which subjects chose between payoffs of different values that were available at different points in time.

In one study by McClure et al. (2004a), subjects made choices between two gift certificates with different monetary values, available either the day of the experiment or after a 2-, 4-, or 6-week delay. According to the two-process theory of intertemporal choice, the emotional system should be preferentially engaged by rewards that are available immediately. As predicted, limbic and paralimbic brains areas showed greater activity during choices that involved the opportunity for monetary rewards on the day of the experiment as contrasted with choices that involved only delayed rewards (Figure 10.3A). These areas included limbic structures such as the ventral striatum and medial orbitofrontal cortex. These areas are rich in projections from the midbrain dopamine system, have been directly tied to reward processing (e.g., Delgado, Nystrom, Fissell, Noll, & Fiez, 2001; McClure, Berns, & Montague, 2003; O'Doherty, Dayan, Friston, Critchley, & Dolan, 2003), and have been shown to scale with reward value and subjective feelings of happiness (Knutson et al., 2001). In addition, activity was observed in regions of the ventromedial prefrontal cortex and the posterior cingulate cortex, which

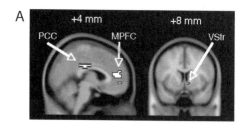
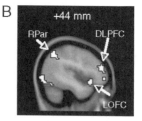

FIGURE 10.3. Cognitive and emotional systems in intertemporal choice. When people choose between different monetary payments available at different time delays, they tend to accept a larger reduction in value in order to obtain payment immediately. (A) In the brain, deciding in any intertemporal choice leads to increased activity in the lateral prefrontal cortex lateral orbitofrontal (LOFC and dLPFC) as well as in the posterior parietal cortex. (B) In addition, choices that involve immediate reward are associated with enhanced activity in several brain areas tied to reward and emotion including the ventral striatum (VStr), the orbitofrontal cortex (OFC), the posterior cingulate cortex (PCC), and the medial prefrontal cortex (mPFC). For choices involving an immediate and a delayed reward, the relative activity in the emotional (A) and cognitive (B) systems correlates with subjects' choices. Adapted from McClure et al. (2004a). Copyright 2004 by AAAS. Adapted by permission.

were tied with emotional processing in the experiments involving moral judgment and the ultimatum game.

In contrast to the emotional system, the two-system model predicts that the cognitive system should be equally engaged by all decisions, evaluating and comparing the worth of the two options presented by each choice. As predicted, typically "cognitive" brain areas were found to be activated for all choices (Figure 10.3B), including regions of the dLPFC and the posterior parietal cortex. These regions also showed greater activity for difficult than easy choices (i.e., activity greatest for choices involving options that were closest in value). We return to this observation further on.

Finally, paralleling findings from the moral judgment and ultimatum game experiments, the balance of activity observed in the cognitive and emotional systems was closely associated with behavioral outcome. For choices that engaged both systems—that is, ones involving an *opportunity* for immediate reward—increased activity in the dLPFC and the parietal cortex correlated significantly with more frequent *selection* of the later reward. These findings are consistent with the view that behavioral choice was determined by a competition between these systems. And, once again, this competition was associated with increased ACC activity (Figure 10.4).

CONFLICT MONITORING AND COGNITIVE CONTROL

The studies reviewed earlier have provided behavioral and neuroimaging evidence, suggesting that a variety of decisions are governed by a competition between cognitive and emotional processes. These findings raise important questions about how such competition is regulated and how the outcome of such decisions is determined. One simple possibility is that the strongest process wins. If this were the case, we might expect that whenever emotional processes were engaged, they would prevail. After all, we have characterized emotions as representing fast, prepotent automatic processes that are associated with strong behavioral responses. However, in the examples we have reviewed, decisions often reflected outcomes favored by more abstract, deliberative

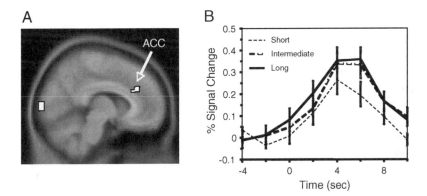

FIGURE 10.4. Response conflict in intertemporal choice. (A) Response time in intertemporal choice correlates with activity in the ACC. (B) When choices are separated into three equally sized sub-samples on the basis of response time, activity in the ACC (centered on the time of response) is seen to scale with increased deliberation time.

processes, even when these faced stiff competition from strong emotional responses. How might this come about?

There have been relatively few theories that have attempted to specify, in computationally explicit form, the neural mechanisms involved in regulating the competition between cognitive and emotional processes. However, there has been considerable work addressing the mechanisms involved in detecting and regulating competition among processes within the cognitive domain. At the very least, this work may be useful as a reference for considering the regulation of competition between cognitive and emotional processes. It is even possible that, given many close parallels to the interactions observed in the earlier examples, very similar mechanisms may be involved when competition involves emotional as well as cognitive processes. With this in mind, we review recent work addressing the mechanisms by which competition is detected and resolved within the cognitive domain. We then return to the question of whether these mechanisms may generalize to situations involving competition from emotional processes.

An Example of Cognitive Control: The Stroop Task

Perhaps the best studied example of competition between cognitive processes is the Stroop task (Stroop, 1935; see MacLeod, 1991, for a modern review of experimental findings). In this task, subjects are presented with a visual display of a word and asked either to read the word or to name the color in which it is displayed. Stroop (1935) demonstrated that when subjects are required to read the word (e.g., say "red" to the word red displayed in green), neither speed nor accuracy is affected by the color in which it is displayed. However, when the task is to name the color, response times are substantially slower (e.g., say "green" in the previous example) if the word itself and the color in which it is displayed disagree (i.e., are incongruent, as in the example) than if they agree (e.g., the word "red" is displayed in red). This has been explained in terms of the greater strength and corresponding automaticity of the word-reading process relative to the color-naming one (Posner & Snyder, 1975; Kahneman & Treisman, 1984; MacLeod & Dunbar, 1988; Cohen, Dunbar, & McClelland, 1990).

Neural network (also known as connectionist or parallel distributed processing) models have been helpful in characterizing and understanding the dynamics of the competition between cognitive processes and how these relate to behavior (e.g., Cohen, Servan-Schreiber, & McClelland, 1992). This approach has been used to study the competition between word reading and color naming in the Stroop task (Cohen et al., 1990; Cohen & Huston, 1994; O'Reilly, Munakata, & McClelland, 2000). These models assume the existence of two pathways (Figure 10.5), one for "mapping" the orthographic form of a visual stimulus onto its corresponding verbal representation (the word-reading pathway), and another for mapping the color of stimuli onto the same set of verbal representations (the color-naming pathway). Connections between mutually incompatible units are assumed to be inhibitory, capturing the fact that it is not advisable (and usually not possible) to respond in two opposing ways at the same time. This provides a mechanism for decision making and, as we shall see, for competition when conflicting inputs are provided to the two pathways.

In models of the Stroop task, connection weights are stronger in the word-reading pathway. This reflects the assumption that adult subjects have had considerable more experience reading words than naming colors out loud. In addition, printed words are more consistently associated with their verbal representations than are colors (e.g., the

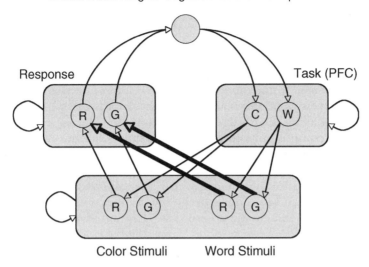

FIGURE 10.5. Response conflict and the Stroop task. In the Stroop task, words are presented to subjects written in different colored inks. Subjects are required to state the color that the word is written in as quickly and accurately as possible. When the word is different from its color (i.e., the word "green" written in red ink), interference between the two implied responses increases response time and error rate. This figure shows a model developed to capture this notion of response conflict and to adaptively adjust cognitive control to improve performance. The input layer reflects sensory input in the form of the ink color (color stimuli, either red, R, or green, G) and word meaning (word stimuli). These two inputs then bias responding, with greater strength given to word meaning to reflect the greater automaticity of this process. Cognitive control, derived from PFC activity, aids to improve performance by selectively biasing sensory inputs based on whether the task is to do color naming (C) or word reading (W). Control is gated by the detection of response conflict in the ACC.

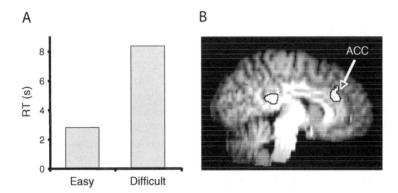

FIGURE 10.6. Conflict between emotional and cognitive brain systems. (A) Difficult and easy moral decisions were determined based on response time (RT). (B) As in the Stroop task, as moral choices become more difficult, indicating greater conflict in competing responses, increased ACC activity is evident. Greater observed ACC activity and linked increase in dLPFC response predict a greater probability of utilitarian responses. Adapted from Greene et al. (2004). Copyright 2004 by Elsevier. Adapted by permission.

color red is associated not only with the word "red" but also "fire," "embarrassment," "stopping at a light," and "communism"). The stronger connections in the word-reading pathway explain the greater automaticity of this process relative to color naming and the corresponding behavioral effects that are observed. For example, when a conflicting stimulus is presented to the model (e.g., the red input unit is activated in the word pathway, and the green input unit is activated in the color pathway), activity flows more quickly and strongly along the word-reading pathway, dominating the competition that arises among the response units to the differing inputs and producing the response corresponding to the word input (in this case, "red"). This captures the fact that when presented with a word and asked simply to respond, subjects will almost invariably read the word and not announce the color in which it is displayed.

This raises a question very similar to the one we raised earlier about the competition between emotional and emotional processes: Given that word reading is the stronger process, how can subjects ever respond by naming the color of an incongruent stimulus? In the Stroop model, this is made possible by an additional set of units that represent the two different tasks demands (color naming and word reading). More precisely, we can think of these of these as representing knowledge that subjects have about the two dimensions of the stimulus and the mapping of features in each of these dimensions onto verbal responses. By activating the appropriate task demand unit, top-down flow of activity sensitizes associative ("hidden") units in the corresponding pathway, favoring the flow of activity along that pathway. This top-down support allows information in the color-naming pathway to compete more effectively with information arriving from the otherwise stronger word-reading pathway and thereby produce a response that is consistent with the color rather than the word. In the case of word reading, this top-down support is not as essential (because it is already the stronger pathway), capturing the observation that automatic processes depend less on attention.

This model has been used to provide a conceptually unified view of the effects of attention, behavioral inhibition, and cognitive ("top-down") control, in terms of a single set of underlying mechanisms. Note that in this model, there are no mechanisms explicitly dedicated to "inhibiting" or "regulating" the competing process that is interfering with task performance. Rather, behavioral regulation is achieved through augmentation of processing in the task-relevant pathway, allowing it to compete more effectively with the offending source of interference. This is consonant with an emerging literature on the neural mechanisms underlying attention, which suggests that these operate by biasing the competition between conflicting representations (e.g., Desimone & Duncan, 1995; Maunsell & Cook, 2002; Kastner & Pinsk, 2004). This perspective also provides the foundation for the guided activation theory of cognitive control (Miller & Cohen, 2001). This posits that prefrontal representations exert control over behavior by biasing processing mechanisms in posterior pathways responsible for task execution, to guide the flow of activity along those pathways that support task-relevant behavior.

Conflict Monitoring and the Regulation of Control

The Stroop model described earlier, and related ones, has been used successfully to describe a wide range of behavioral effects in tasks probing attention, inhibition, working memory, and cognitive control (e.g., Mozer, 1988; Deheane & Changeux, 1989; Cohen et al. 1992; Cohen, Romero, Servan-Schreiber, & Farah, 1994). Recent work, building on these models, has begun to address more sophisticated questions, such as the nature of the representations in the prefrontal cortex that allow it to support such a broad and flexible range of behaviors, how these are learned, and how they are adaptively updated to ensure that goals are appropriately matched to the current environment (Braver & Cohen, 2000; Frank, Loughry, & O'Reilly, 2001; Rougier, Noelle, Braver, Cohen, & O'Reilly, 2005). Most of this work is beyond the scope of the present chapter. However, one question that is relevant here is how people dynamically change the level of control they exert in response to different task demands. It is known, for example, that when a high proportion of stimuli are incongruent, people demonstrate smaller interference effects than when incongruent stimuli are rare (Logan & Zbrodoff, 1979; Tzelgov, Henik, & Berger, 1992; Lindsay & Jacoby, 1994). Corresponding effects are also observed on a trial-to-trial basis: Responses to incongruent stimuli are faster and more accurate if the preceding stimulus was incongruent than if it was congruent, as though the level of control is dynamically adjusted to meet estimates of the ongoing demand (Gratton, Coles, & Donchin, 1992).

These adjustment effects can be explained by introducing an additional mechanism that responds to conflict in processing, and uses this information to adaptively modulate the engagement of control mechanisms (e.g., the activity of the task demand units in the Stroop model; Botvinick et al., 2001). Conflict is defined as the product of the activity of competing processing units. For example, in the Stroop model a congruent stimulus (e.g., the word "red" displayed in red) will produce strong activation of one response unit (the red one) and no activity in the other. The product of activity of the two response units will therefore be zero, indicating the absence of conflict. In contrast, competing information from the two pathways will activate both response units and the product of their activity will be positive, indicating the presence of conflict. Conflict can be reduced by augmenting activity of the unit(s), providing top-down control (e.g., the color-naming unit). This will increase activity of the task-relevant response unit, allowing it to suppress activity in the other unit, thus reducing conflict. Simulations using the Stroop model, as well as models of a number of other tasks, have shown that using a conflict-monitoring mechanism to modulate the engagement of control mechanisms accurately captures the dynamic adjustments in control that have been observed in these tasks (Botvinick et al., 2001).

A large number of studies have suggested that a dorsal region of the ACC is responsive to processing conflict (e.g., Carter et al., 1998; Botvinick, Nystrom, Fissell, Carter, & Cohen, 1999; Barch, Braver, Sabb, & Noll, 2000; Barch et al., 2001; Ullsperger & von Cramon, in press). Models of conflict monitoring have also been used to account for scalp-recorded event-related potentials (ERPs) associated with stimulus degradation (N2) and performance errors (the error-related negativity, ERN), both of which are thought to emanate from the ACC (Botvinick et al., 2001; Yeung, Botvinick, & Cohen, 2004). Furthermore, recent evidence has begun to suggest that conflict-related ACC activity on one trial correlates with increased activity in the dLPFC and improved task performance on the subsequent trial (Kerns et al., 2004). This is consistent with the hypothesis that conflict monitoring mechanisms signal the need to recruit PFC-mediated control mechanisms.

RESOLUTION OF CONFLICT BETWEEN EMOTIONAL AND COGNITIVE PROCESSES

The mechanisms described earlier, and the empirical support for them, all pertain to circumstances in which different cognitive processes compete with each other. In the first part of this chapter, we described three examples of decision making in which a strong emotional response was placed in competition with the outcome of a cognitive process. In many instances, the cognitive process prevailed. In these situations, we observed greater activity within dorsal regions of the ACC routinely associated with conflict monitoring, as well as structures consistently associated with the execution of cognitive control, such as the dLPFC. This suggests the possibility that the same mechanisms involved in monitoring and resolving conflict among cognitive processes are also involved in detecting and regulating competition between cognitive and emotional processes. This conjecture raises several interesting, and potentially important questions.

The first question concerns the specific functions of the dLPFC. Within the context of moral and economic decision making, we interpreted dLPFC activity as reflecting an evaluative function; that is, one determined by the value of the utilitarian course of action or the monetary reward. In the context of cognitive control, however, the dLPFC is believed to represent information about the demands of the current task to guide processing in the service of executing that task. One possibility is that these seemingly different functions may in fact reflect the operation of the same underlying mechanisms. For example, actively representing the value of saving five lives may serve to bias decision making in favor of that outcome, exerting control over processing in much the same way that activity of the task demand units serves to control processing in the Stroop task. This account has the appeal of parsimony. However, it is not clear that it can fully explain cognitive processing in tasks such as intertemporal choice that involve additional operations, such as calculating the discounted value of each option. In such cases, there may be a meaningful distinction between the neural mechanisms required to cognitively evaluate an outcome, and those responsible for ensuring that it exerts control over behavior. Even in the case of moral reasoning, neuroimaging evidence suggests that overlapping but distinguishable regions of prefrontal cortex may be involved in evaluation and control (Greene et al., 2004). Thus, the question of whether the same or different mechanisms are involved in evaluation and control remains an open one.

A related question is whether the same areas of prefrontal cortex are engaged in control over cognitive and emotional processes. Several of the findings reviewed in this chapter suggest that at least some common mechanisms are involved. In particular, activity in similar regions of the dLPFC has been observed in variety of tasks that demand cognitive control, including the moral and decision-making tasks reviewed here that engage emotional processes. At the same time, the study of intertemporal choice revealed a more inferior region of activity, in the lateral orbitofrontal cortex, that was associated with the more future-oriented, cognitive mechanism. One possibility is that this reflected an evaluative rather than a control function, as discussed earlier. However, an alternative is that different parts of the prefrontal cortex may represent information needed to control different types of processing and behavior, with dorsal regions responsible for the support of more cognitive processes and ventral regions associated with the support and control of social processes that often compete with emotional and appetitive processes (Miller & Cohen, 2001; Beer, Shimamura, & Knight, 2004).

This would also explain a common interpretation of ventral regions of the PFC in terms of inhibitory function, an interpretation that finds its roots in observations of the behavioral changes associated with damage to this area of the brain (e.g., Kringelbach & Rolls, 2004). Such patients often exhibit apparent "disinhibition" of emotional and appetitive responses, demonstrating behaviors that are socially inappropriate and suggesting that these behaviors are usually under the tonic inhibitory control of the ventral PFC. However, an alternative view, consistent with theories regarding the function of dLPFC in the cognitive domain, is that ventral prefrontal areas support socially appropriate behaviors against competition from more prepotent emotional and appetitive responses. This interaction would function the same way that regions of dLPFC appear to support task appropriate cognitive processes (such as color naming) against competition from otherwise stronger, prepotent processes (such as word reading). Without such top-down support, a patient will exhibit a socially inappropriate emotional response in just the same way that a patient with damage to more dorsal areas may read the word even intending to name the color of a Stroop stimulus.

Finally, similar questions can be asked about the ACC: Are the same areas of ACC involved in monitoring conflict associated with emotional processes as cognitive ones? There is scant evidence on this question. The studies reviewed in this chapter, all involving conflict between emotional and cognitive processes, elicited activity in a region of dorsal ACC very similar to the one observed when there is conflict between strictly cognitive processes. For example, Greene et al. (2004) showed that when personal moral judgments are separated into easy and difficult categories on the basis of decision time, greater ACC activity is found for difficult choices (Figure 10.6). In the ultimatum game, greater ACC activity is found for unfair offers when the cognitive motivation to make money interferes with the emotional motivation to enforce fairness (Sanfey et al., 2003). Activity in the same region of the ACC was found in intertemporal choice as well, and was observed to scale with choice difficulty (Figure 10.4). This result was found when difficulty was assessed on the basis of response time (as in moral judgment; Figure 10.6), or whether difficulty was assessed on the basis of the difference in value between the two money amounts being decided on (as in McClure et al., 2004a; not shown).

These findings suggest that similar regions of the ACC are engaged by processing conflict, whether it arises among cognitive processes or between cognitive and emotional processes. It remains to be determined whether ACC activity in response to conflict involving emotional processes serves to recruit mechanisms of cognitive control. If so, are these the same mechanisms, and are they recruited in the same manner as those recruited by conflict between cognitive processes? This would lead to the intriguing prediction that, in a manner paralleling performance in cognitive studies, increasing the frequency of difficult choices should augment cognitive control and increase the number of cognitively driven responses over emotional ones. Similarly, there should be a greater tendency to produce cognitively driven responses following a difficult versus an easy decision. These questions remain to be addressed in further empirical work.

Finally, it is important to emphasize that our focus on the conflict-monitoring function of ACC is not meant to suggest that this is the only, or even the primary, function of the ACC. We have been interested in this function in part because it is provides a neural substrate for a postulated cognitive mechanism that is otherwise difficult to measure. At the same time, we believe that this may be just one function of the ACC which may be more generally involved in signaling adverse outcomes of performance that demand corrective action. This would account for the variety of other stimuli that elicit ACC responses, including overt negative feedback (such as monetary losses) as well as physical and even social pain (Gerhing & Willoughby, 2002; Miltner, Braun, & Coles, 1997; Holroyd et al., 2004; Devinsky, Morrell, & Vogt, 1995; Wager et al., 2004; Eisenberger & Lieberman, 2004). Finally, it is tempting to speculate that just as the subjective emotional experience of pain may reflect the ACC response to physical injury (Rainville, 2002), so the experience of anxiety may reflect the phenomenological correlate of the ACC response to conflict. This possibility may have significance not only for social neuroscience studies of the mechanisms underlying emotional regulation but perhaps eventually the diagnosis and even treatment of clinical disorders involving anxiety, such as phobias, depression, and panic.

CONCLUSIONS

We have reviewed three types of decision making in which cognitive and emotional influences have discernible influences on behavior. In moral decisions, judgments about fairness in social exchange, and intertemporal choices, findings suggest that emotional and cognitive processes are correlated with activity in distinguishable brain regions. Furthermore, the relative activity in cognitive and emotional brain systems seems to anticipate behavioral outcome, with greater activity in dLPFC and associated structures closely linked to cognitive outcomes, and limbic structures associated with emotional or appetitive outcomes. Finally, when these systems favor conflicting responses, activity is observed in the dorsal ACC, a region that is also consistently associated with conflict among cognitive processes. This suggests that similar neural mechanisms, involving the dLPFC and the ACC, are involved in detecting and regulating competition between cognitive and emotional processes as when such competition arises strictly between cognitive ones. Despite the simplicity and attendant appeal of this hypothesis, it raises many questions that remain to be addressed in future research.

REFERENCES

Adolphs, R., Tranel, D., Koenigs, M., & Damasio, A. R. (2005). Preferring one taste over another without recognizing either. *Nature Neuroscience, 8*, 860–861.

Aston-Jones, G., & Cohen, J. D. (2005). An integrative theory of locus coeruleus-norepinephrine function: Adaptive gain and optimal performance. *Annual Review of Neuroscience, 28*, 403–450.

Barch, D. M., Braver, T. S., Akbudak, E., Conturo, T., Ollinger, J., & Avraham, S. (2001). Anterior cingulate cortex and response conflict: Effect of response modality and processing domain. *Cerebral Cortex, 11*, 837–848.

Barch, D. M., Braver, T. S., Sabb, F. W., & Noll, D. C. (2000). Anterior cingulate and the monitoring of response conflict: Evidence from an fMRI study of overt verb generation. *Journal of Cognitive Neuroscience, 12*, 298–309.

Beer, J. S., Shimamura, A. P., & Knight, R T. (2004). Frontal lobe contributions to executive control of cognitive and social behavior. In M. S. Gazzaniga (Ed.), *The cognitive neurosciences, III.* Cambridge, MA: MIT Press.

Bentham, J. (1982). *An introduction to the principles of morals and legislation.* London: Methuen.

Bickel, W. K., & Johnson, M. W. (2003). Delay discounting: A fundamental behavioral process of drug dependence. In G. Loewenstein, D. Read, & R. F. Baumeister (Eds.), *Time and decision* (pp. 419–440). New York: Russell Sage.

Botvinick, M. M., Braver, T. S., Barch, D. M., Carter, C. S., & Cohen, J. D. (2001). Conflict, monitoring and cognitive control. *Psychological Review, 108*, 624–652.

Botvinick, M. M., Carter, C. S., & Cohen, J. D. (2004). Conflict monitoring and anterior cingulate cortex: An update. *Trends in Cognitive Sciences, 12*, 539–546.

Botvinick, M. M., Nystrom, L., Fissell, K, Carter, C. S., & Cohen, J. D. (1999). Conflict monitoring vs. selection-for-action in anterior cingulate cortex. *Nature, 402*, 179–181.

Braver, T. S., & Cohen, J. D. (2000). On the control of control: The role of dopamine in regulating prefrontal function and working memory. In S. Monsell & J. Driver (Eds.), *Attention and performance, XVIII: Control of cognitive processes* (pp. 713–737). Cambridge, MA: MIT Press.

Britton, J. C., Phan, K. L., Taylor, S. F., Welsh, R. C., Berridge, K. C., & Liberzon, I. (2006). Neural correlates of social and nonsocial emotions: An fMRI study. *NeuroImage, 31*, 397–409.

Bunge, S. A., Hazeltine, E., Scanlon, M. D., Rosen, A. C., & Gabrieli, J. D. (2002). Dissociable contributions of prefrontal and parietal cortices to response selection. *NeuroImage, 17,* 1562–1571.

Calder, A. J., Lawrence, A. D., & Young, A. W. (2001). Neuropsychology of fear and loathing. *Nature Reviews Neuroscience, 2,* 352–363.

Camerer, C., & Thaler, R. H. (1995). Anomalies: Ultimatums, dictators, and manners. *Journal of Economic Perspectives, 9,* 209–219.

Carter, C. S., Braver, T. S., Barch, D. M., Botvinick, M. M., Noll, D., & Cohen, J. D. (1998). Anterior cingulate cortex, error detection and the on-line monitoring of performance. *Science, 280,* 747–749.

Chaiken, S. & Trope, Y. (Eds.). (1999). *Dual-process theories in social psychology.* New York: Guilford Press.

Cohen, J. D., Dunbar, K., & McClelland, J. L. (1990). On the control of automatic processes: A parallel distributed processing account of the Stroop effect. *Psychological Review, 97,* 332–361.

Cohen, J. D., & Huston, T. A. (1994). Progress in the use of interactive models for understanding attention and performance. In C. Umilta & M. Moscovitch (Eds.), *Attention and performance: XV. Conscious and nonconscious information processing* (pp. 453–476). Cambridge, MA: MIT Press.

Cohen, J. D., Perlstein, W. M., Braver, T. S., Nystrom, L. E., Noll, D. C., Jonides, J., et al. (1997). Temporal dynamics of brain activation during a working memory task. *Nature, 386,* 604–608.

Cohen, J. D., Romero, R. D., Servan-Schreiber, D., & Farah, M. J. (1994). Mechanisms of spatial attention: The relation of macrostructure to microstructure in parietal neglect. *Journal of Cognitive Neuroscience, 6,* 377–387.

Cohen, J. D., Servan-Schreiber, D., & McClelland, J. L. (1992). A parallel distributed processing approach to automaticity. *American Journal of Psychology, 105,* 239–269.

Dehaene, S., & Changeux, J. P. (1989). A simple model of prefrontal cortex function in delayed-response tasks. *Journal of Cognitive Neuroscience, 1,* 244–261.

Dehaene, S., Posner, M. I., & Tucker, D. M. (1994). Localization of a neural system for error detection and compensation. *Psychological Science, 5,* 303–305.

Delgado, M. R., Nystrom, L. E., Fissell, C., Noll, D. C., & Fiez, J. A. (2001). Tracking the hemodynamic response to reward and punishment in the striatum. *Journal of Neurophysiology, 84,* 3072–3077.

Desimone, R., & Duncan, J. (1995). Neural mechanisms of selective attention. *Annual Review of Neuroscience, 18,* 193–222.

Devinsky, O., Morrell, M. J., & Vogt, B. A. (1995). Contributions of anterior cingulate cortex to behavior. *Brain, 118,* 279–306.

Duncan, J., Seitz, R. J., Kolodny, J., Bor, D., Herzog, H., Ahmed, A., et al. (2000). A neural basis for general intelligence. *Science, 289,* 457–460.

Egner, T., & Hirsch, J. (2005). Cognitive control mechanisms resolve conflict through cortical amplification of task-relevant information. *Nature Neuroscience, 8,* 1784–1790.

Eisenberger, N. J., & Lieberman, M. D. (2004). Why rejection hurts: A common neural alarm system for physical and social pain. *Trends in Cognitive Sciences, 8,* 294–300.

Eriksen, B. A., & Eriksen, C. W. (1974). Effects of noise letters upon the identification of a target letter in a nonsearch task. *Perception and Psychophysics, 16,* 143–149.

Fehr, E., & Schmidt, K. M. (1999). A theory of fairness, competition, and cooperation. *Quarterly Journal of Economics, 114,* 817–868.

Fiske, S. T., & Neuberg, S. L. (1988). A continuum model of impression formation: From category-based to individuating processes as a function of information, motivation, and attention. *Advances in Experimental Social Psychology, 23,* 1–108.

Foot, P. (1978). *The problem of abortion and the doctrine of double effect: Virtues and vices.* Oxford, UK: Blackwell.

Fox, A. S., Oakes, T. R., Shelton, S. E., Converse, A. K., Davidson, R. J., & Kalin, N. H. (2005). Calling for help is independently modulated by brain systems underlying goaldirected behavior and threat detection. *Proceedings of the National Academy of Sciences, USA, 102,* 4176–4179.

Frank, M. J., Loughry, B., & O'Reilly, R. C. (2001). Interactions between frontal cortex and basal ganglia in working memory: A computational model. *Cognitive, Affective, and Behavioral Neuroscience, 1,* 137–160.

Frederick, S., Loewenstein, G., & O'Donoghue, T. (2003). Time discounting and time preference: A critical review. In G. Loewenstein, D. Read, & R. Baumeister (Eds.), *Decision and time* (pp. 13–86). New York: Russell Sage.

Frijda, N. (1986). *The emotions.* Cambridge, UK: Cambridge University Press.

Gehring, W. I., & Willoughby, A. R. (2002). The medial frontal cortex and the rapid processing of monetary gains and losses. *Science, 295,* 2279–2282.

Giordano, L. A., Bickel, W. K., Loewenstein, G., Jacobs, E. A., Marsch, L., & Badger, G. J. (2002). Opioid deprivation affects how opioid-dependent outpatients discount the value of delayed heroin and money. *Psychopharmacology, 163,* 174–182.

Gratton, G., Coles, M. G. H., & Donchin, E. (1992). Optimizing the use of information: Strategic control of activation and responses. *Journal of Experimental Psychology: General, 4,* 480–506.

Greene, J. D., & Haidt, J. (2002). How (and where) does moral judgment work? *Trends in Cognitive Sciences, 6,* 517–523.

Greene, J. D., Lindsell, D. A., Clarke, A. C., Lowenberg, K., Nystrom, L. E., Darley, J. M., & Cohen, J. D. (in press). *What pushes your moral buttons?: Towards a cognitive solution to the trolley problem.*

Greene, J. D., Nystrom, L. E., Engell, A. D., Darley, J. M., & Cohen, J. D. (2004). The neural bases of cognitive conflict and control in moral judgment. *Neuron, 44,* 389–400.

Greene, J. D., Sommerville, R. B., Nystrom, L. E., Darley, J. M., & Cohen, J. D. (2001). An fMRI investigation of emotional engagement in moral judgment. *Science, 293,* 2105–2108.

Guth, W., Schmittberger, R., & Schwarze, B. (1982). An experimental analysis of ultimatum bargaining. *Journal of Economic Behavior and Organization, 3,* 367–388.

Hoch, S. J., & Loewenstein, G. F. (1991). Time inconsistent preferences and consumer self-control. *Journal of Consumer Research, 17,* 492–507.

Hoffman, E., McCabe, K., & Smith, V. (1995). On expectations and the monetary stakes in ultimatum games. *International Journal of Game Theory, 86,* 653–660.

Holroyd, C. B., Yeung, N., Nieuwenhuis, S., Nystrom, L. E., Coles, M. G. H., & Cohen, J. D. (2004). Dorsal anterior cingulate cortex shows fMRI response to internal and external error signals. *Nature Neuroscience, 7,* 497–498.

Hume, D. (2000). *A treatise of human nature.* New York: Oxford University Press. (Original work published 1739)

Kahneman, D. (2003). Maps of bounded rationality: Psychology for behavioral economics. *American Economic Review, 93,* 1449–1475.

Kahneman, D., Knetsch, J. I., & Thaler, R. H. (1986). Fairness and the assumptions of economics. *Journal of Business, 59,* S285–S300.

Kahneman, D., & Triesman, A. (1984). Changing views of attention and automaticity. In R. Parasuraman & D. R. Davies (Eds.), *Varieties of attention.* Orlando, FL: Academic Press.

Kastner, S., & Pinsk, M. A. (2004). Visual attention as a multilevel selection process. *Cognitive, Affective, and Behavioral Neuroscience, 4,* 483–500.

Kerns, J. G., Cohen, J. D., MacDonald, A. W., III, Cho, R. Y., Stenger, V. A., & Carter, C. S. (2004). Anterior cingulate conflict monitoring and adjustments in control. *Science, 303,* 1023–1026.

Knutson, B., Adams, C. M., Fong, G. W., & Hommer, D. (2001). Anticipation of increasing monetary reward selectively recruits nucleus accumbens. *Journal of Neuroscience, 21,* RC159.

Koopmans, T. C. (1960). Stationary ordinal utility and impatience. *Econometrica, 28,* 287–309.

Kroger, J. K., Sabb, F. W., Fales, C. L., Bookheimer, S. Y., Cohen, M. S., & Holyoak, K. J. (2002). Recruitment of anterior dorsolateral prefrontal cortex in human reasoning: A parametric study of relational complexity. *Cerebral Cortex, 12,* 477–485.

Laibson, D. I. (1997). Golden eggs and hyperbolic discounting. *Quarterly Journal of Economics, 42,* 861–871.

LeDoux, J .E. (1996). *The emotional brain: The mysterious underpinnings of emotional life.* New York: Simon & Schuster.

Lieberman, M. D., Gaunt, R., Gilbert, D. T., & Trope, Y. (2002). Reflection and reflexion: A social cognitive neuroscience approach to attributional inference. *Advances in Experimental Social Psychology, 34,* 199–249.

Lindsay, D. S., & Jacoby, L. L. (1994). Stroop process dissociations: The relationship between facilitation and interference. *Journal of Experimental Psychology: Human Perception and Performance, 20,* 219–234.

Loewenstein, G. (1996). Out of control: Visceral influences on behavior. *Organizational Behavior and Human Decision Processes, 65,* 272–293.

Loewenstein, G., & O'Donoghue, T. (2004). Animal spirits: Affective and deliberative processes in economic behavior. *CAE Working Paper,* 4–14.

Logan, G. D., & Zbrodoff, N. J. (1979). When it helps to be misled: Facilitative effects of increasing the frequency of conflicting stimuli in a Stroop-like task. *Memory and Cognition, 7*, 166–174.

Luciana, M., Depue, R. A., Arbisi, P., & Leon, A. (1992). Facilitation of working memory in humans by a D2 dopamine receptor agonist. *Journal of Cognitive Neuroscience, 4*, 58–68.

Luman, M., Oosterlaan, J., & Sergeant, J. A. (2005). The impact of reinforcement contingencies on AD/ HD: A review and theoretical appraisal. *Clinical Psychology Review, 25*, 183–213.

Maddock, R. J. (1999). The retrosplenial cortex and emotion: New insights from functional neuroimaging of the human brain. *Trends in Neurosciences, 22*, 310–316.

MacLeod, C. M. (1991). Half a century of research on the Stroop effect: An integrative review. *Psychological Bulletin, 109*, 163–203.

MacLeod, C. M., & Dunbar, K. (1988). Training and Stroop-like interference: Evidence for a continuum of automaticity. *Journal of Experimental Psychology: Learning, Memory and Cognition, 14*, 126–135.

Maunsell, J. H., & Cook, E. P. (2002). The role of attention in visual processing. *Philosophical Transactions of the Royal Society of London B: Biological Sciences, 357*, 1063–1072.

McClure, S. M., Berns, G. S., & Montague, P. R. (2003). Temporal prediction errors in a passive learning task activate human striatum. *Neuron, 38*, 339–346.

McClure, S. M., Laibson, D. I., Loewenstein, G., & Cohen, J. D. (2004a). Separate neural systems value immediate and delayed monetary rewards. *Science, 306*, 503–507.

McClure, S. M., Li, J., Tomlin, D., Cypert, K. S., Montague, L. M., & Montague, P. R. (2004b). Neural correlates of behavioral preference for culturally familiar drinks. *Neuron, 44*, 379–387.

Miller, E. K., & Cohen, J. D. (2001). An integrative theory of prefrontal cortex function. *Annual Review of Neuroscience, 24*, 167–202.

Miltner, W. H. R., Braun, C. H., Coles, M. G. H. (1997). Event-related potentials following incorrect feedback in a time-estimation task: Evidence for a "generic" neural system for error detection. *Journal of Cognitive Neuroscience, 9*, 788–798.

Mischel, W., Ayduk, O., & Mendoza-Denton, R. (2003). Sustaining delay of gratification over time: a hot-cool systems perspective. In G. Loewenstein, D. Read, & R. Baumeister (Eds.), *Decision and time* (pp. 175–200). New York: Russell Sage.

Mischel, W., Shoda, Y., & Rodriguez, M. I. (1989). Delay of gratification in children. *Science, 244*, 933–938.

Montague, P. R., Dayan, P., & Sejnowski, T. J. (1996). A framework for mesencephalic dopamine systems based on predictive Hebbian learning. *Journal of Neuroscience, 16*, 1936–1947.

Mozer, M. (1988). A connectionist model of selective attention in visual perception. *Proceedings of the Tenth Annual Conference of the Cognitive Science Society* (pp. 195–201). Hillsdale, NJ: Erlbaum.

Nowak, M. A., Page, K. M., & Sigmund, K. (2000). Fairness versus reason in the ultimatum game. *Science, 289*, 1773–1775.

Ochsner, K. N., & Gross, J. J. (2005). The cognitive control of emotion. *Trends in Cognitive Sciences, 9*, 242–249.

O'Doherty, J. P., Dayan, P., Friston, K., Critchley, H., & Dolan, R. J. (2003). Temporal difference models and reward-related learning in the human brain. *Neuron, 38*, 329–337.

O'Reilly, R. C., & Munakata, Y. (2000). *Computational explorations in cognitive neuroscience: Understanding the mind by simulating the brain.* Cambridge, MA: MIT Press.

Petrinovich, L., O'Neill, P., & Jorgensen, M. (1993). An empirical study of moral intuitions: Towards an evolutionary ethics. *Journal of Personality and Social Psychology, 64*, 467–478.

Phan, K. L., Wager, T., Taylor, S. F., & Liberzon, I. (2002). Functional neuroanatomy of emotion: A meta-analysis of emotion activation studies in PET and fMRI. *NeuroImage, 16*, 331–348.

Phillips, M. L., Young, A. W., Senior, C., Brammer, M., Andrew, C., Calder, A. J., et al. (1997). A specific neural substrate for perceiving facial expressions of disgust. *Nature, 389*, 495–498.

Posner, M. I., & Snyder, C. R. R. (1975). Attention and cognitive control. In R. L. Solso (Ed.), *Information processing and cognition* (pp. 55–85). Hillsdale, NJ: Erlbaum.

Rabin, M. (1993). Incorporating fairness into game theory. *American Economic Review, 83*, 1281–1302.

Rainville, P. (2002). Brain mechanisms of pain effect and pain modulation. *Current Opinion in Neurobiology, 12*, 195–204.

Rougier, N. P., Noelle, D. C., Braver, T. S., Cohen, J. D., & O'Reilly, R. C. (2005). Prefrontal cortex and flexible cognitive control: Rules without symbols. *Proceedings of the National Academy of Sciences, USA, 102*, 7338–7343.

Samuelson, P. (1937). A note on the measurement of utility. *Review of Economic Studies, 4*, 155–161.

Sanfey, A. G., Rilling, J. K., Aronson, J. A., Nystrom, L. E., & Cohen, J. D. (2003). The neural basis of economic decision-making in the illtimatum Game. *Science, 300*, 1755–1758.

Schultz, W., Dayan, P., & Montague, P. R. (1997). A neural substrate of prediction and reward. *Science, 275*, 1593–1599.

Shapira, N. A., Liu, Y., He, A. G., Bradley, M. M., Lessig, M. C., James, G. A., et al. (2003). Brain activation by disgust-inducing pictures in obsessive–compulsive disorder. *Biological Psychiatry, 54*, 751–756.

Shiffrin, R. M., & Snyder, W. (1977). Controlled and automatic processing: II. Perceptual learning, automatic attending, and a general theory. *Psychological Review, 84*, 127–190.

Simon, J. R. (1969). Reactions toward the source of stimulation. *Journal of Experimental Psychology, 81*, 174–176.

Stroop, J. R. (1935). Studies of interference in serial verbal reactions. *Journal of Experimental Psychology, 18*, 643–662.

Thaler, R. H. (1981). Some empirical evidence on time inconsistency. *Review of Economic Studies, 23*, 165–180.

Thaler, R. H. (1988). Anomalies: The ultimatum game. *Journal of Economic Perspectives, 2*, 195–206.

Thomson, J. J. (1986). *Rights, restitution, and risk: Essays in moral theory*. Cambridge, MA: Harvard University Press.

Tzelgov, J., Henik, A., & Berger, J. (1992). Controlling Stroop effects by manipulating expectations for color words. *Memory and Cognition, 20*(6), 727–735.

Ullsperger, M., & von Cramon, D. Y. (in press). How does error correction differ from error signaling?: An event-related potential study. *Brain Research*.

Wager, T. D., Rilling, J. K., Smith, E. E., Sokolik, A., Casey, K. L., Davidson, R. J., et al. (2004). Placebo-induced changes in fMRI in the anticipation and experience of pain. *Science, 303*, 1162–1167.

Wager, T. D., & Smith, E. E. (2003). Neuroimaging studies of working memory: A meta-analysis. *Cognitive Affective Behavior Neuroscience, 3*, 255–274.

Wheatley, T., & Haidt, J. (2005). Hypnotically induced disgust makes moral judgments more severe. *Psychological Science, 16*, 780–784.

Williams, G. V., & Goldman-Rakic, P. S. (1995). Modulation of memory fields by dopamine D1 receptors in prefrontal cortex. *Nature, 376*, 572–575.

Wright, R. (1994). *The moral animal: Why we are the way we are*. New York: Pantheon Books.

Yeung, N., Botvinick, M. M., & Cohen, J. D. (2004). The neural basis of error detection: Conflict monitoring and the error-related negativity. *Psychological Review, 111*, 931–959.

PART IV

DEVELOPMENTAL APPROACHES

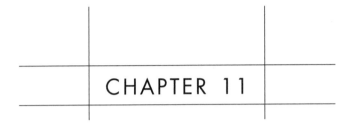

CHAPTER 11

Caregiver Influences on Emerging Emotion Regulation
BIOLOGICAL AND ENVIRONMENTAL TRANSACTIONS IN EARLY DEVELOPMENT

SUSAN D. CALKINS
ASHLEY HILL

CONCEPTUAL AND DEVELOPMENTAL CONSIDERATIONS

Defining the Construct of Emotion Regulation

Our definition of emotion regulation reflects recent theoretical and empirical work in both developmental (Cole, Martin, & Dennis, 2004; Fox & Calkins, 2003) and clinical psychology (Keenan, 2000; Sroufe, 2000) that highlights the fundamental role played by emotion processes in both child development and child functioning (Eisenberg et al., 2000). Consistent with many of our colleagues contributing to this volume (Gross & Thompson; Eisenberg, Hofer, & Vaughn; Rothbart & Sheese), we view emotion regulation processes as those behaviors, skills, and strategies, whether conscious or unconscious, automatic or effortful, that serve to modulate, inhibit, and enhance emotional experiences and expressions. We also view the dimension of emotional reactivity as part of the emotion regulation process, although we, like some of our colleagues (Gross & Thompson, this volume), see a value in examining this element of the process as distinct from the efforts to manage it, what we refer to as the control dimension (Calkins & Johnson, 1998; Fox & Calkins, 2003). The emotion regulation process is clearly a dynamic one in which reactive and control dimensions alter one another across time. Moreover, in our view, the reactive dimension, as opposed to the control dimension, is present and functional early in neonatal life, as it is strongly influenced by genetic and biological factors (Fox & Calkins, 2003; Rothbart & Sheese, this volume). Finally, we, like our colleagues, note that the display of emotional reactivity and emotion control are powerful mediators of both interpersonal relationships and socioemotional adjustment across the lifespan (Thompson & Meyer; Eisenberg et al., this volume).

The broad construct of emotion regulation has been studied in many ways across early development (Cole et al., 2004), including through the examination of the child's use of specific strategies in emotionally demanding contexts and the effects of these strategies on emotion experience and expression. For example, specific emotion regulation strategies such as self-comforting, help seeking, and self-distraction may assist the young child in managing early temperament-driven frustration and fear responses in situations in which the control of negative emotions may be necessary (Stifter & Braungart, 1995). Moreover, emotion regulation skills may be useful in situations that elicit positive affective arousal in that they allow the child to keep such arousal within a manageable and pleasurable range (Grolnick, Cosgrove, & Bridges, 1996).

Although children appear to be quite proficient in the use of such basic skills at a relatively early age, it is clear that dramatic developments occur during the infancy and toddler periods of development in terms of the acquisition and display of emotion regulation skills and abilities. The process may be described broadly as one in which the relatively passive and reactive neonate becomes a child capable of self-initiated behaviors that serve a regulatory function (Calkins, 1994; Kopp, 1982; Sroufe, 1996). The infant progresses from near complete reliance on caregivers for regulation (e.g., via, for example, physical soothing provided when the infant is held) to independent emotion regulation (e.g., choosing to find another toy to play with, rather than tantrumming, when the desired toy is taken by a companion), although the variability in such regulation across children, in terms of both style and the efficacy, is considerable (Calkins, in press). As the infant makes this transition to greater independence, the caregiver's use of specific strategies and behaviors within dyadic interactions become integrated into the infant's repertoire of emotion regulation skills, across, we presume, both biological and behavioral levels of functioning (Calkins & Johnson, 1998; Calkins & Dedmon, 2000). The child may then draw on this repertoire in a variety of contexts, in both conscious, effortful ways (e.g., walking away from a confrontation with a peer), and in nonconscious, automatic ways (e.g., averting gaze when confronted by a frightening movie scene). Because this important developmental transition occurs within the context of early relationships, we examine in some detail the ways in which caregivers, in the context of the attachment relationship, facilitate this transition, at both a biological and behavioral level.

Because the lack of adaptive emotion regulation skills may contribute to adjustment difficulties characterized by uncontrolled (i.e., acting-out) or even overcontrolled (i.e., inhibited) emotion expression (Calkins, 1994; Calkins & Dedmon, 2000; Keenan, 2000), failure to acquire these skills may lead to difficulties in areas such as social competence and school adjustment. For example, children who have difficulty managing emotion in a flexible, constructive way may be less successful in negotiating peer relationships or in managing academic challenges (Keane & Calkins, 2004; Howse, Calkins, Anastopoulos, Keane, & Shelton, 2003). Thus, the acquisition of adaptive emotion regulation skills and strategies is considered a critical achievement of early childhood (Bronson, 2000; Cole et al., 2004; Posner & Rothbart, 2000; Sroufe, 1996). Moreover, these skills may be linked, in important ways, to other dimensions of self-control or self-regulation that are also developing during early childhood. In this way, the influence of early emotion regulation on subsequent development may be considered quite pervasive (Calkins, in press). We examine this self-regulatory framework in some detail as it provides a roadmap for our discussion of the many ways in which caregiver behavior influences the child's emerging repertoire of emotion regulation skills.

A Self-Regulatory Framework for Understanding the Development of Emotion Regulation

Because we believe that emotion regulation processes are linked in fundamental ways to more basic physiological and attentional processes, and have consequences for later-developing and more sophisticated cognitive skills, we, like some of our colleagues (Eisenberg et al., this volume; Rothbart & Sheese, this volume) embed these emotion-related processes within the larger construct of self-regulation. So, for example, in our work, we routinely examine changes in children's responses to specific emotion-eliciting events; however, the level of analysis for such change includes physiological and attentional processes, as well as observable behavioral processes. Regulatory efforts occur across each of these levels, although each of these emotion regulation processes is also linked to children's responses to a variety of external events occurring everyday as they negotiate the worlds of home, school, and peers, and as they develop the skills to function independently in these worlds. So, for example, a child may be faced with the task of having to decide which of two friends to side with during a disagreement. Successful resolution of this challenge requires regulatory processes that occur across several levels of functioning, including the physiological (e.g., regulating increased heart rate that occurs as a function of the personal distress the disagreement causes), attentional (e.g., observing and processing relevant sides of the disagreement), behavioral (e.g., reaching out to restrain one friend intent on physically harming the other), and cognitive (e.g., imagining the future of each relationship depending on the resolution of the current argument).

As this example demonstrates, an emotional task may be parsed into many smaller challenges for the child, involving processes that are observable in different ways and across different levels of functioning. However, many of these same component processes might also be involved in the successful negotiation of other childhood challenges, which may not have an obvious emotion regulation demand, such as a math test, a soccer game, or a plea to a parent to attend a social event. Because of the challenge in distinguishing similar processes, which are often activated in different contexts and are components of the same or different biological and behavioral systems, in our view, it may be more useful to adopt an approach that considers multiple levels of analysis of self-regulation rather than isolating emotion regulation from related, or even integrated, processes (Calkins & Fox, 2002; Eisenberg et al., 2000; Posner & Rothbart, 2000). From this perspective, emotion regulation skills emerge during infancy and toddlerhood as a function of more basic or rudimentary regulatory processes, and they assume a central role in the development of the more complex self-regulation of behavior and cognition characteristic of early and middle childhood (Calkins & Fox, 2002; Calkins & Howse, 2004)

One rationale for examining the development and integration of these domain-specific regulatory processes emanates from recent work in the area of developmental neuroscience that has identified specific brain regions that may play a functional role in the deployment of attention and in the processing and regulation of emotion, cognition, and behavior (Posner & Rothbart, 2000; Rothbart & Sheese, this volume). This work has identified areas of the prefrontal cortex as central to the effortful regulation of behavior via the anterior attention system. This system is guided by the anterior cingulate cortex, which includes two major subdivisions. One subdivision governs cognitive and attentional processes and has connections to the prefrontal cortex. A second subdivision governs emotional processes and has connections with the limbic system and peripheral autonomic, visceromotor, and endocrine systems (Lane & McRae, 2004; Luu & Tucker, 2004). Recent research suggests that these subdivisions have a reciprocal relation (Davis, Bruce, & Gunnar, 2001; Davidson, Putnam & Larson, 2000). Moreover, the functional relation between these two areas of the cortex provides a biological mechanism for the developmental integration of specific types of self-regulatory processes in childhood.

We acknowledge that these discrete self-regulatory processes are likely to be so intertwined that once integration across levels occurs in support of more complex skills and behaviors, it is difficult to parse these complex behavioral responses into separate or independent types of control. Nevertheless, from a developmental point of view, it is useful to describe explicit types of control and how they emerge, as this specification may provide insight into nonnormative developments and problems that emerge as a result of deficits in specific components of self-regulation at particular points in development (Calkins, in press; Calkins, Graziano, & Keane, in press). So, one way to conceptualize the self-regulatory system is to describe it as adaptive control that may be observed at the level of physiological, attentional, emotional, behavioral, cognitive, and interpersonal or social processes (Calkins & Fox, 2002). Control at these various levels emerges, at least in primitive form, across the prenatal, infancy, toddler, and early childhood periods of development. Importantly, though, the mastery of earlier regulatory tasks becomes an important component of later competencies, and by extension, the level of mastery of these early skills may constrain the development of later skills. Recent developmental neuroscience work suggests that because of its dependence on the maturation of prefrontal–limbic connections, the development of self-regulatory processes is relatively protracted (Beauregard, Levesque, & Paquette, 2004), from the development of basic and automatic regulation of physiology in infancy and toddlerhood to the more self-conscious and intentional regulation of cognition emerging in middle childhood (Ochsner & Gross, 2004). Thus, understanding the development of *specific* regulatory processes, such as emotional regulation, becomes integral to understanding how regulatory deficits across multiple levels affect the emergence of childhood behavior and behavior problems (Calkins & Fox, 2002).

Embedding emotion regulation in a larger self-regulatory framework has the advantage of allowing researchers to understand the multiple levels of infant and child functioning that may be influenced by *both* intrinsic, child-driven factors, such as temperament, and extrinsic, externally imposed factors, such as caregiver behavior and the emerging attachment relationship. Because this view of emotion regulation is more expansive than narrow, in the next section, we offer in some detail a description of the normative regulatory processes involved in early emerging emotion regulation.

Normative Developments in Early Self-Regulation and Emotion Regulation

Kopp (1982; Kopp & Neufield, 2003) provides an excellent overview of the early developments in emotion regulation, with reference to other related regulatory processes that support emotion-related regulation. This description has been verified by studies of both normative development (Rothbart, Ziaie, & O'Boyle, 1992; Buss & Goldsmith, 1998) and studies of individual differences (Stifter & Braungart, 1995). These descriptions provide an explanation of how infants develop and use a rich behavioral repertoire of strategies in the service of reducing, inhibiting, amplifying, and balancing different affective responses. Moreover, it is also clear from these descriptions that functioning in a variety of nonemotional domains, including motor, language and cognition, and social development, is implicated in these changes (Kopp, 1989, 1992).

Early efforts at emotion regulation, those occurring prior to about 3 months of age, are thought to be controlled largely by innate physiological mechanisms (Kopp, 1982; Derryberry & Rothbart, 2001; Rothbart, Derryberry, & Hershey, 2000). Such efforts are characterized primarily by general reactivity to stimuli and by approach (i.e., turning toward) versus withdrawal (i.e., turning away) from pleasant versus aversive stimuli. By 3 months of age, primitive mechanisms of self-soothing such as sucking, simple motor movements such as moving away, and reflexive signaling in response to discomfort, often in the form of crying, are the primary processes operating, independent of caregiver intervention (Kopp, 1982; Rothbart et al., 1992).

The period between 3 and 6 months of age marks a major transition in infant development. First, sleep–wake cycles and eating and elimination processes have become more predictable, signaling an important biological transition. Second, the ability of the infant to use simple actions voluntarily to modify arousal levels begins to emerge. This increase in control depends largely on the development of attention mechanisms and simple motor skills (Rothbart et al., 1992; Harman, Rothbart, & Posner, 1997; Kochanska, Coy, & Murray, 2001) and leads to coordinated use of attention engagement and disengagement, particularly in contexts that evoke negative affect. When confronted by aversive stimuli, infants are now capable of engaging in self-initiated distraction, which involves moving attention from the source of negative arousal to more neutral stimuli. For example, the ability to shift attention from a negative event (e.g., something frightening) to a positive distracter (e.g., a toy, pet, or parent) may allow infants to modulate their experience of negative affect.

By the end of first year of life, infants become much more active and purposeful in their attempts to control affective arousal (Kopp, 1982). First, they begin to employ organized sequences of motor behavior that enable them to reach, retreat, redirect, and self-soothe in a flexible manner that suggests they are responsive to environmental cues. Second, their signaling and redirection become explicitly social as they recognize that caregivers and others may behave in a way that will assist them in the regulation of affective states (Rothbart et al., 1992; Diener, Mangelsdorf, McHale, & Frosch, 2002). Successful use of such behaviors is critical in making the transition from passive, caregiver-directed regulation to active self-regulation (Calkins, 2002).

During the second year of life, the transition from passive to active methods of emotion regulation is complete (Rothbart et al., 1992). Although toddlers are not entirely capable of controlling their own affective states by this age, they are capable of using specific strategies to attempt to manage different affective states, albeit sometimes unsuccessfully (Calkins & Dedmon, 2000; Calkins, Smith, Gill, & Johnson, 1998). Moreover, during this period, toddlers begin to respond to caregiver directives and, as a consequence of this responsivity, compliance and behavioral self-control begin to emerge (Kopp, 1989). This shift is supported by developments in the motor domain as well as changes in representational ability and the development of language skills. Brain maturation contributes as well, and by the end of toddlerhood, children have executive control abilities that allow for the control of arousal and the regulation of emotional reactivity in a variety of contexts (Rueda, Posner, & Rothbart, 2004). The use of more coordinated motor skills and language translates into greater skill at dealing with peers and teachers in the preschool environment and for negotiating for autonomous behavior (e.g., "I do it myself") in the home environment.

It is clear from this normative description of the emotion regulation process that multiple factors contribute to both successful acquisition of adaptive skills and to variations in the acquisition of and, perhaps, tendency to employ such skills. Next we explore the intrinsic and extrinsic sources of normative influence on early emotion regulation as well as those that produce individual variations with implications for later functioning.

THE EMERGENCE OF EMOTION REGULATION: INTRINSIC AND EXTRINSIC INFLUENCES

Like investigations of other areas of self-control (Sethi, Mischel, Aber, Shoda, & Rodriguez, 2000), understanding the development of the control of emotions necessitates examination of both intrinsic and extrinsic factors (Calkins, 1994; Fox & Calkins, 2003). Intrinsic factors include the disposition, or temperament, of the infant, and the underlying neural and physiological systems that support and are engaged in the processes of emotional control (Calkins, 1994; Fox, 1994; Fox, Henderson, & Marshall, 2001). Extrinsic factors include the manner in which caregivers shape and socialize their infant's emotional responses and the relationship that develops between infant and caregiver as a consequence of these important interactions (Calkins & Fox, 2002; Fox & Calkins, 2003; Thompson, 1994; Thompson & Meyer, this volume).

Intrinsic Factors Implicated in the Development of Emotion Regulation

One well-tested assumption of the research on intrinsic factors and early emotional regulation is that individual differences in emotionality, or temperamental reactivity, play a role in at least the display, if not the development of, emotion regulation skills (Stifter & Braungart, 1995; Calkins, 1994). From this perspective, it is assumed that the tendency of infants to become emotionally aroused influence, either directly or indirectly, the kinds of emotion regulatory skills and strategies that children develop.

With respect to this reactive dimension of temperament, Rothbart notes that the initial responses of a newborn infant may be characterized by their physiological and behavioral reactions to sensory stimuli of different qualities and intensities. This reactivity is believed to be present at birth and reflects a relatively stable characteristic of the infant (Rothbart et al., 2000). Moreover, infants will differ initially in their threshold to respond to visual or auditory stimuli as well as in their level of reactivity to stimuli expected to elicit negative affect (e.g., Calkins, Fox, & Marshall, 1996). These initial affective responses that are characterized by vocal and facial indices of negativity are presumed to reflect generalized distress. Thus, this initial reactivity has neither the complexity nor the range of later emotional responses. Rather, it is a rudimentary form of the more sophisticated and differentiated emotions that will in later infancy be labeled "fear," "anger," or "sadness." However, an infant's tendency to become distressed, or not, because external events (e.g., loud voices) may influence the initial behavioral response to such stimuli (e.g., turning toward vs. away). Early patterns of responding may become part of the infant's behavioral repertoire and influence both the level and type of regulatory response needed in a given situation.

A second area of research on the intrinsic factors involved in the emergence of emotion regulation has addressed the underlying physiological processes and functioning that may play an important role in the etiology of early regulatory behaviors (Fox,

1994; Fox & Card, 1999; Porges, 1991, 1996). Theories of emotion regulation that focus on underlying biological components of regulation assume that maturation of different biological support systems lays the foundation for the increasingly sophisticated emotional and behavioral regulation that is observed across childhood.

Fox (1989, 1994), for example, has noted that the frontal lobes of the brain are differentially specialized for approach versus avoidance and that these tendencies influence the behaviors that children engage in when emotionally and behaviorally aroused. He further notes that maturation of the frontal cortex provides a mechanism for the more sophisticated and planful regulatory behaviors of older children versus infants. Porges (1996) argues that maturation of the parasympathetic nervous system also plays a key role in regulation of state, motor activity, and emotion. One index of parasympathetic functioning is heart rate variability, which has been linked specifically to deficits in emotional and behavioral self-regulation (Calkins, 1997; Calkins & Dedmon, 2000). Moreover, behavioral and physiological research with infants and young children clearly demonstrates that control of physiological arousal eventually becomes integrated into the processes of attention engagement and disengagement (Porges, 1996; Richards, 1987), which is central to both emotional regulation and, later, to behavioral regulation (Rothbart, Posner, & Boylan, 1990; Sethi et al., 2000).

Although dimensions of children's early functioning that may be considered intrinsic play an important role in laying the foundation for subsequent development, and perhaps constraining such development, these developments are clearly occurring in a social context, and from the very earliest point in development. One important assumption of much of the research on the acquisition of emotion regulation is that parental caregiving practices may support or undermine such development and thus contribute to observed individual differences among young children's emotional skills (Calkins et al., 1998; Thompson, 1994; Thompson & Meyer, this volume). Here, we explore two related dimensions that are important in early development: caregiving behavior and attachment relationships.

Extrinsic Influences on Emerging Emotion Regulation

During infancy, successful regulation largely depends on caregiver support and flexible responding (Kopp, 1982; Calkins & Fox, 2002; Sroufe, 2000). To the extent that a caregiver can appropriately read infant signals and respond in ways that minimize distress or, alternatively, motivate positive interaction, the infant will integrate such experiences into the emerging behavioral repertoire. That is, over time, interactions with parents in emotion-laden contexts teach children that the use of particular strategies may be more useful for the reduction of emotional arousal than other strategies (Sroufe, 1996). So, for example, a parent who has successfully and repeatedly redirected a child's attention from desired but unavailable objects (e.g., the telephone) is implicitly teaching the child to engage in self-initiated redirection when faced with such situations in the future. Moreover, deviations from supportive caregiving may contribute to patterns of emotional regulation that undermine the development of appropriate skills and abilities needed for later developmental challenges (Cassidy, 1994). For example, a child who is left to cry in frustration by a parent who simply removes the desired object and walks away may be unable to generate a constructive way to deal with a similar situation in the context of a preschool classroom where greater independence is required.

One hypothesis about the way in which caregiving practices affect developing emotion regulation is through the emerging attachment relationship. Attachment processes are often activated in emotionally evocative contexts and serve specific emotion-regulatory functions. Thus, it is likely that they contribute to the acquisition of the repertoire of self-regulated emotional skills that develop in the child over the course of infancy and toddlerhood. Current theorizing about childhood attachment and its role in emotional functioning and behavioral adjustment has its roots in the work of John Bowlby (1969/1982), whose evolutionary theory of attachment emphasized the biological adaptedness of specific attachment behaviors displayed during the infancy period. Such behaviors permitted the infant to initiate and maintain contact with the primary caregiver, which served a survival purpose (Bowlby, 1988). In typical development, infants exhibit a repertoire of behaviors, including looking, crying, and clinging, that allow them to signal and elicit support from the primary caregiver in times of external threat. Bowlby argued that by the end of the first year of life, the interactive history between the infant and caregiver, including during times of stress or external threat, would produce an attachment relationship that would provide a sense of security for the infant and significantly influence the child's subsequent adaptation to a variety of developmental challenges (Bowlby, 1988).

Bowlby hypothesized that the mechanism through which early parent–child attachment affected later functioning involved a psychological construct having to do with expectations of self and other. Bowlby's notion of "internal working model" referred to cognitive representations of the self and the caregiver that were constructed out of repeated early interactions. Such representations provided the infant and young child with a guide to expectations about his or her own emotional responding and the likelihood and success of caregiver intervention in managing this affective responding. Thus, the experience of sensitive caregiving was hypothesized to lead to a secure attachment and expectations that emotional needs would either be met by the caregiver or managed with skills developed through interactions with the caregiver.

Numerous developmental scientists have conducted tests of Bowlby's theory, though Mary Ainsworth is likely the most noted. Ainsworth conducted pioneering naturalistic and observational studies of attachment processes in a longitudinal study of infants and mothers in Baltimore that focused on individual differences in mother–infant attachment relationships (Ainsworth, Blehar, Waters, & Wall, 1978). Ainsworth theorized that while all infants become attached to primary caregivers, the quality of this attachment varied as a function of the relationship history. She developed an empirical paradigm that examined infant responses as a function of this relationship history. In her "Strange Situation" laboratory procedure, she constructed a series of brief, but increasingly stressful, episodes designed to activate the infant's attachment system. On the basis of infants' behavior displayed in the Strange Situation, particularly those behaviors that reflected the dyads' ability to manage stress, she characterized infants as securely attached or insecurely attached with either resistant or avoidant profiles. She characterized secure infants as those comfortable with exploration and positive affect sharing during the low-stress context and proximity seeking and the ability to be comforted in the high-stress context of separation. In contrast, insecurity was indexed by either heightened distress or difficulty calming (referred to as resistance or ambivalence), or active avoidance, of the caregiver during the high-stress context of separation. Importantly, Ainsworth reported that the quality of different types of attachment relationships could be predicted by the quality of maternal caregiving observed in the home across the first year of life. Ainsworth argued that the experience of consistent sensitive and responsive caregiving teaches the infant about appropriate expectations regarding others as well as allows the infant to experience a reduction in arousal level as a consequence of caregiver's behaviors (Ainsworth et al., 1978). In this way, her findings provided empirical support for Bowlby's internal working model construct and supported the hypothesized link between attachment and emotion processes

This early theoretical and empirical work makes clear, then, why the recent inter-pretations of Bowlby's attachment theory attribute significance to the role of attach-ment processes in the development of emotion regulation. Sroufe (1996, 2000), for example, argues that emotional development is inextricably linked with social develop-ment, with the course of emotional development described as the transition from dyadic regulation of affect to self-regulation of affect. He argues that the ability to self-regulate arousal levels is embedded in affective interactions between the infant and caregiver. These interactions provide infants with the experience of arousal escalation and reduction as a function of caregiver interventions, distress reactions that are relieved through caregiver actions, and positive interactions with the caregiver (Sroufe, 1996, 2000). Such experiences contribute to the working model of affect-related expec-tations that will transfer from the immediate caregiving environment to the larger social world of peers and others.

Cassidy (1994) has also addressed the role of attachment processes in the develop-ment of emotion regulation. She focuses on the adaptive function of different patterns of emotional responding in the context of the attachment relationship and argues that these patterns of affective responding are actually strategies that infants use to allow their attachment needs to be met. The open and flexible emotional communication that is characteristic of a secure attachment allows the infant to comfortably and safely express both positive and negative affect within a proximal and comfortable relation-ship with a responsive caregiver. Moreover, the different strategies of insecure infants also provide these infants with a means of meeting their own needs within the context of a less-than-optimal caregiving environment. The heightened distress characterizing some insecure infants also serves as a clear signal to gain the attention of the inconsis-tent or unresponsive caregiver. In a similar manner, avoidant behavior serves the adap-tive purpose of minimizing the attachment relationship and has the effect of allowing the infant to maintain the needed proximity without threatening the relationship with the caregiver through displays of overt sadness or anger. Importantly, though, these short-term adaptations of the different patterns displayed by insecure infants may lead to long-term difficulties in other contexts. For example, heightened emotion expres-sion, in the context of peer relationships, may lead to problematic peer interactions and have implications for the development of social competence (Cassidy, 1994).

In another extension of Bowlby's theory that has implications of the development of emotion regulation, Hofer (1994) describes how the biological experience of infant–caregiver interactions becomes a representational structure that guides affective func-tioning. He argues that these early interactions are, in fact, regulatory experiences that contribute to an inner affective experience composed of sensory, physiological, and behavioral responses. Over time, these affective experiences lead to organized repre-sentations, the integration of which is the internal working model. These organized mental representations are ultimately what guide the child's behavior, rather than the individual sensory and physiological components to which the infant responded earlier in infancy (Hofer, 1994).

Schore (2000) extends these psychobiological ideas even further in arguing that the interactive experiences between caregiver and child that are the essential elements of the emerging attachment relationship also affect the development of the prefrontal cortex. The right hemisphere, in particular, he notes, is especially influenced by experiences in the social world, and, in turn, determines the regulation and coping skills that young children develop. Support for the role of the right frontal cortex in human behavioral and emotional regulation has emerged over the last several years (Fox, 1994; Fox & Card, 2000). For example, chronic exposures to stress and/or high cortisol levels may result in impaired functioning in the regions of the brain associated with inhibition and regulation, such as the prefrontal cortex (Goldsmith & Davidson, 2004).

The psychobiological explication of attachment processes offers insight into the mechanism through which interactive experiences across the first year of life become integrated into the internal working model that Bowlby articulated and, importantly, become elements of the child's emerging emotion regulation abilities. In the next section, we examine how specific dimensions of caregiver behavior and the emerging attachment relationship with the caregiver affect the development of infant emotion regulation across both biological and behavioral domains of functioning.

CAREGIVER–CHILD INTERACTIONS AND THE DEVELOPMENT OF EMOTION REGULATION

Caregiver Effects on the Biological Substrates of Emotion Regulation

In the aggregate, the number of studies examining the effects of specific caregiving behaviors on infant biological processes that may underlie emotion regulation is small; however, it is clear that these effects may place important constraints on subsequent behavioral development (Calkins, 1994; Calkins et al., 2002). Infants who have characteristically low thresholds for arousal, or who have difficulty managing that physiological arousal, are at a disadvantage because emergent emotion regulation strategies are dependent on the basic control of physiological processes that support behavioral strategies. To the extent that caregivers can provide the support for such physiological control early in early development, children should be more successful at using attentional and behavioral strategies to control emotional reactions. Moreover, it is likely that several complex caregiving practices, most of which are integral to early emerging attachment, can affect the biological aspects of emotion regulation. Here, we draw on both human and animal work to examine these interactive processes.

Because the biological underpinnings of emotion regulation are clearly evident as early as the neonatal period of development, the effects caregivers may have on the developing infant begin during the prenatal period. Moreover, these effects appear to be significant for the child's subsequent behavioral functioning. For example, in studies with both animals and humans, pregnancy stress in particular has been shown to be related to problematic outcomes such as hyperactivity, deficits in attention, and maladaptive social behavior, all of which are believed to be characterized by deficits in self-regulation and emotion regulation in particular (for reviews, see Weinstock, 1997; Koehl et al., 2001; Schneider, Coe, & Lubach, 1992). The mechanism for this effect is the increased amount of stress hormones expressed during pregnancy that may alter the fetuses' developing hypothalamic–pituitary–adrenal (HPA) axis and result in dysregulation of the stress response system (Koehl et al., 2001), a system that is clearly activated during emotion-eliciting situations (Stansbury & Gunnar, 1994).

Work with humans indicates that fetuses do indeed react to mild stressors induced during pregnancy (DiPietro, Costigan, & Gurewitsch, 2003). In this study, stress was induced using a Stroop color–word task administered to mothers at 24 and 36 gestational weeks. The fetus's responses to maternal stress, indexed by increased heart rate and motor activity, increased over gestation, even as the magnitude of mother's sympathetic response to the stressor decreased. Clearly, even mild environmental intrusions experienced by the mother may have an effect on the developing fetus's physiological systems. Moreover, at least one study has shown that prenatal stress may have long-term consequences (O'Connor, Heron, Golding, Beveridge, & Glover, 2002). Specifically, mothers' prenatal anxiety predicted behavior problems, which are characterized by difficulties in self-regulation, in boys and girls at age 4, even after controlling for postnatal maternal anxiety.

Beyond the prenatal period of development, there are multiple opportunities for caregiver behavior to influence emerging emotional regulatory processes through effects on biological functioning. Indeed, Schore (2000) suggests that across the first year of life the mother–infant dyad continues to be a mutually regulating biological unit. Moreover, evidence from animal models suggests that caregiving affects infants' biological and behavioral systems of regulation through the environment the caregiver provides rather than through shared inherited traits. For example, Meeney and colleagues have shown that high levels of maternal licking/grooming and arched-back nursing in rats affects the neurological systems associated with the stress response, a process that has a long-term influence on stress-related illness, certain cognitive functions, and physiological functions (Champagne & Meeney, 2001; Francis, Caldji, Champagne, Plotsky, & Meaney, 1999; Caldji et al., 1998). Furthermore, cross-fostering studies demonstrate convincingly that these maternal behaviors are transmitted behaviorally through the nursing mother and not through the biological mother, indicating that early caregiving is a crucial factor in early development and may affect the organism's level of emotional reactivity even when it reaches adulthood (Champagne & Meeney, 2001; Calatayud, Coubard, & Belzung, 2004).

One process that seems to have a direct impact on an infant's developing regulatory systems early in life is caregiver tactile stimulation. For example, skin-to-skin contact or "kangaroo" therapy has been shown to increase the premature infant's ability to regulate physiological processes (e.g., modulate sleep patterns, temperature, and oxygenation consumption) and has been associated with better attachment relationships with parents later in life (Anderson, Dombroski, & Swinth, 2001; Conde-Agudelo, Diaz-Rossello, & Belizan, 2003; Feldman, Weller, Sirota, & Eidelman, 2002). One hypothesis that explains these effects is that skin-to-skin contact is a mechanism for improving the functioning of the premature infant's neurobiological systems (Feldman et al., 2002).

In addition, research with normally developing human infants has shown that touch is clearly a salient feature of early care and normative development. For example, empirical work reveals that while maternal touch and affection decreased from 2- to 6-months postnatally, and the use of distraction and vocalizing increased, both holding/rocking and vocalization together served to reduced distress in infants at both ages (Jahromi, Putnam, & Stifter, 2004). Other work has shown that 3-month-olds do not respond to a still face interaction, a normally stressful experimental paradigm, unless maternal touch was allowed during the prior interaction periods, but 6-month-olds responded whether or not touch was included in the paradigm (Gusella, Muir, & Tronick, 1988). These results are consistent with Kopp's (1982, 1989) notion that the caregiver gradually reduces her external regulation of the child, and that such regulation may be more important early in life, when the infant's biological systems are maturing.

Although touch is a mode of interaction that clearly influences infant's physiological stress response as evidenced by HPA axis activity, and subsequently may play a role in the regulation of emotion, other physiological systems may be involved in emotion regulation as well. For example, caregiver behaviors seem to affect the infant's parasympathetic nervous system (PNS) regulatory processes, via the regulation of cardiac vagal tone. During homeostasis, the PNS enhances restorative and growth processes. In the context of environmental challenge, the PNS influences regulation of cardiac output through the vagal nerve pathways (Porges, 1996). Porges (1991, 1996) has proposed a hierarchical model of self-regulation in which behavioral, emotional, and motor regulation are dependent on appropriate physiological regulation, which is indexed by changes in parasympathetic responses or respiratory sinus arrythmia (RSA). Empirical research suggests that caregiver behavior may affect this physiological system, which is closely tied to emotion regulation abilities (Calkins, 1997). For example, several studies indicate that mother–infant coregulated communication patterns and more responsive parenting are positively related to good vagal regulation, and maternal intrusiveness and restrictive parenting are negatively related to such regulation (Porter, 2003; Haley & Stansbury, 2003; Calkins et al., 1998; Kennedy, Rubin, Hastings, & Maisel, 2004). And, infants who share more mutual affect regulation with their mothers (dyads that demonstrated more matched affect and synchrony of affective states) were more effective in their physiological regulation across a stress-inducing still-face paradigm (Moore & Calkins, 2004).

Although most studies of caregiver effects on infant biological development focus on individual systems, it is likely that such effects are occurring across multiple biological and behavioral systems. Hofer (1994; Polan & Hofer, 1999) addresses the multiple psychobiological roles that the caregiver plays in regulating infant's behavior and physiology early in life. Based on his research with infant rat pups, he describes these "hidden regulators" as operating at multiple sensory levels (olfactory, tactile, and oral, for example) and influencing multiple levels of behavioral and physiological functioning in the infant. So, for example, maternal tactile stimulation may have the effect of lowering the infant's heart rate during a stressful situation, which may in turn, support a more adaptive behavioral response. Moreover, removal of these regulators, during separation, for example, disrupts the infant's functioning at multiple levels as well. Clearly, then, opportunities for individual differences in the development of emotion regulation may emerge from differential rearing conditions providing more or less psychobiological regulation.

Researchers have examined whether specific attachment processes, elicited in attachment-related contexts such as the Strange Situation, also affect physiological indices of emotion regulation when the attachment system is activated. Much of this work is reviewed by Fox (Fox & Card, 1999), who notes that multiple physiological indices have been examined in relation to Strange Situation behavior, including measures of heart rate, cortisol, and brain electrical activity. One difficulty with this work, in general, is that the extent to which the measures reflect emotional tone or reactivity versus emotion regulation or control is not often clear. For example, most studies report elevated heart rate in response to both the Strange Situation and maternal separation (Donovan & Leavitt, 1985; Sroufe & Waters, 1977), but because separation distress alone is not indicative of attachment, it is difficult to know whether these measures can reveal much about individual differences in the nature of the attachment relationship and developing emotion regulation. Studies of endocrine system responding reveal similar relations to the heart rate work. Findings indicate that infants who are stressed during the Strange Situation also experience elevated cortisol. In one study, elevated cortisol was found among infants who were both highly fearful, as measured using a different empirical paradigm, and insecurely attached, suggesting, perhaps, that their experience regarding lacking of external arousal regulation has produced heightened arousal during the Strange Situation (Nachmias, Gunnar, Mangelsdorf, Parritz, & Buss, 1996).

Evidence for the role of the activation of the frontal cortex in contexts in which the attachment system is activated comes from the work on brain electrical activity (EEG) and maternal separation. This work suggests that the frontal brain regions involved in affective expression and regulation (Fox, 1994) are differentially activated during maternal separation, with the right frontal region more activated in infants who were more distressed during separation (Fox, Bell, & Jones, 1992). Again, though, the specificity of these findings to emotion regulation versus emotional reactivity is unclear, as are implications for individual differences in security of attachment.

In sum, research with human and animal subjects demonstrates that caregiver effects are observable from the prenatal period onward and influence biological functioning across several systems. However, the degree to which such functioning translates into behavioral indices of emotion regulation is often unclear. Next, we explore relations between caregiver behavior and attachment processes and indices of emotion regulation.

Caregiving Effects on the Behavioral Indices of Emotion Regulation

Much of the research on caregiving practices and the emerging observable emotion regulation skills of infants has focused on attachment-related processes. The research examining attachment and emotion regulation processes in contexts that activate the attachment system is consistent in its findings. In multiple studies, conducted in different laboratories, researchers have demonstrated that infants with secure attachment relationships use strategies that include social referencing and express a need for social intervention (Braungart & Stifter, 1991; Nachmias et al., 1996). These same researchers report that insecure/avoidant children are more likely to use self-soothing and solitary exploration with toys (Braungart & Stifter, 1991; Nachmias et al., 1996). The strategies of both secure and insecure infants seem to reflect a history of experiences and expectations regarding the availability of the caregiver as an external source of emotion regulation, expectations that are clearly important when the attachment system becomes activated during the stressful context of the Strange Situation. Such work provides direct support for the notion that patterns of emotion regulation are evident quite early in development and are an integral component of the dyadic interactions that produce secure attachment.

Interestingly, studies assessing direct relations between attachment and emotion regulation skills and strategies in contexts other than the Strange Situations paradigm are relatively rare. Three recent studies, though, support the notion that there are relations between the two domains that are observable outside the immediate dyadic context. First, Diener and colleagues (Diener et al., 2002), observed that attachment classification as observed in the Strange Situation did predict the infant's regulatory strategies in a situation in which the infant is required to regulate negative affect independently but did not explicitly activate the attachment system. Their findings were quite consistent with work examining emotion regulation within the context of the Strange Situation. Infants in secure attachment relationships with both parents used strategies emphasizing social orientation. Thus, security of attachment leads to expectations of caregivers that extend beyond the immediate parent–child interactional context. In turn, these expectations lead to the use of specific kinds of emotional regulation strategies in situations that place regulatory demands on the child.

Gilliom, Shaw, Beck, Schonberg, and Lukon (2002) conducted a study that examined specific emotion regulation strategy use beyond the infancy period. The focus of this investigation was on preschoolers' use of specific anger control strategies during a waiting paradigm. Specific strategies involving the control of attention were found to predict the anger reaction of the children in this situation. In addition, though, secure attachment in infancy was predictive of the use of specific strategies, including the use of attentional distraction, that led to successful waiting. By preschool, young children are capable of controlling their attention in a manner that leads to successful emotional and behavioral control. This study demonstrates that the effects of attachment beyond the infancy period are observable in the development and use of such strategies.

In another recent study examining the relation between attachment and emotional functioning beyond the dyadic context, Kochanska (2001) conducted an extensive longitudinal study of the development of fear, anger, and joy across the first 3 years of life. Her rationale for this investigation was that attachment processes should be implicated in the development of different emotion systems and that children with different attachment histories should display different patterns of functioning in these systems. Moreover, she argued that evidence for such a developmental process would provide an explanation of how early attachment processes might be linked to the range of outcomes and indices of adjustment that have been studied.

Differences in the emotional functioning of the secure and insecure infants in Kochanska's study were apparent at the end of the first year of life. Consistent with other research (Calkins & Fox, 1992), Kochanska found that insecure/resistant infants were more fearful than other infants. In addition, across the second and third year of life, insecure infants displayed a different pattern with respect to the display of both positive and negative affect. Secure infants showed a predictable decline in the display of negative affect, while insecure infants displayed an increase as well as a decrease in positive affect. A notable finding of this study that pertains to the development of emotion regulation concerns the pattern of the insecure/avoidant children. Recall that these children are likely to minimize their emotional reactions in the context of the Strange Situation. However, Kochanska observed that, over time, these infants display an increase in fear reactions, a finding that supports Cassidy's notion that a minimizing strategy, while effective in the short term, may lead to difficulties later in development. Clearly, the strategy of minimization is either ineffective over time or leads to repeated experiences of internal arousal that eventually become difficult to control.

Although data on the relation between attachment and emotion regulation strategies are limited, there have been a few studies examining the relations between aspects of parenting thought to be linked to attachment and emotion regulation. These studies are worth noting because they are conducted with toddlers, children for whom there are clear expectations of emerging autonomous emotional control. In one study of mothers and toddlers, for example, we examined the relations between maternal behavior across a variety of different situations and child emotional self-control in frustrating situations (Calkins et al., 1998). Our analyses indicated that maternal negative and controlling behavior (thought to be reflective of intrusive behavior characteristic of insecure attachment relationships) was related to the use of orienting to or manipulating the object of frustration (a barrier box containing an attractive toy) and negatively related to the use of distraction techniques. These data are important in light of findings that the ability to control attention and engage in distraction (such that ruminating over the object of denial is minimized) has been related to the experience of less emotional arousal and reactivity (Calkins, 1997; Grolnick et al., 1996) and to lower levels of externalizing behavior problems (Calkins & Dedmon, 2000).

From this brief review of current work in the area of caregiving practices, attachment processes, and emotion regulation, it is clear that there are multiple possible pathways to the development of emotion regulation in infancy and early childhood. Moreover, this theoretical and empirical work suggests that evidence for the role of attachment processes in the development of emotion regulation may come from a number of different directions. First, attachment processes may affect the development and functioning of physiological processes that support emotion regulation. Second, attachment processes may be predictive of specific emotional responses in the context of the relationship dyad itself and may be observed empirically in behavioral and emotional responses to the Strange Situation or in other interactions between the caregiver and the infant. Third, attachment processes may be implicated in the development and use of specific strategies outside the context of the attachment relationship such as during tasks requiring more independent self-regulation of emotion. These tentative conclusions, however, clearly suggest multiple directions for future research.

SUMMARY AND FUTURE DIRECTIONS

In this chapter, we have examined the early development of emotion regulation processes as a function of both intrinsic (temperamental, biological) factors and extrinsic (caregiving, attachment) factors. We emphasized the role of extrinsic processes because, although we acknowledge the significance of both sets of factors for adaptive development in the domain of emotion regulation, we also note that the significant developments that occur in emotion regulation, and that depend on competent physiological and attentional regulation mechanisms emerging early in development, occur in the context of significant first relationships.

Our review of research examining the effects of early attachment relationships on the development of emotion regulation demonstrates that the proximal effects of this relationship are quite evident. Evidence from the psychophysiological literature reveals that predictable biological responses can be expected from infants in contexts that activate the attachment system. Beyond this immediate dyadic context, though, there are also effects of the attachment relationship on developing emotion regulation. Secure infants and children use effective strategies when engaged in tasks that require more autonomous emotional control, rather than the anticipated external control provided in dyadic regulation. More distal effects of attachment on behavioral and emotion regulation that underlies adaptive functioning in preschool and early childhood have also been observed (Shaw, Keenan, Vondra, Delliquadri, & Giovanelli, 1997). However, clear interpretation of these data may require a more systematic evaluation of the role of mediational and moderational processes, the influence of other environmental factors on this development, and the transactional relationship between parent and child and child and parent.

First, empirical work that is more focused on process, rather than simple associations, might be more informative for elucidating the complex ways that caregiving and emotion regulation influence development. It would be important, for example, to be able to clearly specify that the physiological processes affected by early caregiving experiences are, in fact, predictive of specific skills or deficits in early self- and emotional regulation processes, rather than level general functioning, as most work now indicates. Or, it might be useful to examine the role of emotion regulation as a mediator of the relations between early attachment and other, more complex, kinds of self-regulation. In one of the few studies conducted to examine such a hypothesis, Contreras, Kerns, Weimer, Gentzler, and Tomich (2000) observed that specific dimensions of emotion regulation, including arousal and attention deployment, mediated the relation between attachment and peer social behavior.

A second step that would help illuminate these interactional processes would be to address the issues of moderators of the relation between caregiving or attachment and self-regulation. It is clear from some of the behavior problem literature, in which problem behavior is often viewed as a proxy for regulatory deficits (Shaw et al., 1997), that the direct relations are likely to be observed under some conditions but perhaps not others. For example, environmental factors that place even greater stress on the attachment relationship are also likely to have the effect of undermining the child's own efforts to develop a self-regulatory repertoire. Or, resiliency factors such as social support or positive peer relationships may offset the negative effects of a compromised caregiving experience. A focus on moderated effects will provide greater specificity in prediction while preserving the important role of attachment processes in emotional functioning.

Third, it is clear that the direction of effects in development is not always from parent to child. Transactional influences from the environment to the child and back again are clearly responsible for some pathways in development (Calkins, 2002). Moreover, it must be acknowledged that the child plays an important role in the dyadic interactions with caregivers that lead to the development of attachment relationships (Calkins, 1994). Consequently, these transactional influences may obscure the identification of longer-term effects of attachment on emotional processes but clearly are important to understanding developmental pathways (Cicchetti, 1993).

Finally, implicit in our suggestions for future research is the idea that conceptual and empirical specificity of emotion regulation processes is necessary but that such specificity depends on an appreciation that emotion regulation is integrally connected to other forms of self-regulation. Although the processes and outcomes of interest in studies of emotion regulation may center on behavioral phenomena, we are clearly advocating an approach that integrates biological and cognitive phenomena into both theoretical and empirical explications of these critical developmental processes. By adopting an expansive approach, we believe that an account of the developmental significance of emotion regulation for child and adult functioning will be greatly enhanced.

ACKNOWLEDGMENTS

The writing of this chapter was supported by National Institute of Health Grant Nos. MH 55584 and MH 74077 to Susan D. Calkins.

REFERENCES

Ainsworth, M., Blehar, M., Waters, E., & Wall, S. (1978). *Patterns of attachment*. Hillsdale, NJ: Erlbaum.
Anderson, G. C., Dombrowski, M. A., & Swinth, J. Y. (2001). Kangaroo care: Not just for stable preemies anymore. *Reflections on Nursing Leadership, 27*, 32–34.
Beauregard, M., Levesque, J., & Paquette, V. (2004). Neural basis of conscious and voluntary self-regulation of emotion. *Advances in consciousness research: Consciousness, emotional self-regulation, and the brain: Vol. 54.* (pp. 163–194). Netherlands: John Benjamins.
Bowlby, J. (1982). *Attachment and loss: Vol. 1. Attachment*. New York: Basic Books. (Original work published 1969)
Bowlby, J. (1988). *A secure base*. New York: Basic Books.
Braungart, J. M., & Stifter, C. A. (1991). Regulation of negative reactivity during the Strange Situation:

Temperament and attachment in 12–month-old infants. *Infant Behavior and Development, 14,* 349–367.

Bronson, M. B. (2000). *Self-regulation in early childhood: Nature and nurture.* New York: Guilford Press.

Buss, K. A., & Goldsmith, H. H. (1998). Fear and anger regulation in infancy: Effects on the temporal dynamics of affective expression. *Child Development, 69,* 359–374.

Calatayud, F., Coubard, S., & Belzung, C. (2004). Emotional reactivity may not be inherited but influenced by parents. *Physiological Behavior, 80,* 465–474.

Caldji, C., Tannenbaum, B., Sharma, S., Francis, D., Plotsky, P. M., & Meaney, M. J. (1998). Maternal care during infancy regulates the development of neural systems mediating the expression of fearfulness in the rat. *Neurobiology, 9,* 5335–5340.

Calkins, S. D. (1994). Origins and outcomes of individual differences in emotional regulation. In N. A. Fox (Ed.), Emotion regulation: Behavioral and biological considerations. *Monographs of the Society for Research in Child Development, 59,* 53–72.

Calkins, S. D. (1997). Cardiac vagal tone indices of temperamental reactivity and behavioral regulation in young children. *Developmental Psychobiology, 31,* 125–135.

Calkins, S. D. (2002). Does aversive behavior during toddlerhood matter? The effects of difficult temperament on maternal perceptions and behavior. *Infant Mental Health Journal, 23,* 381–402.

Calkins, S. D. (in press). Regulatory competence and early disruptive behavior problems. In S. Olson & A. Sameroff (Eds.), *Regulatory processes in the development of behavior problems: Biological, behavioral, and social-ecological interactions.* New York: Cambridge University Press.

Calkins, S. D., & Dedmon, S. A. (2000). Physiological and behavioral regulation in two-year-old children with aggressive/destructive behavior problems. *Journal of Abnormal Child Psychology, 2,* 103–118.

Calkins, S. D., Dedmon, S., Gill, K., Lomax, L., & Johnson, L. (2002). Frustration in infancy: Implications for emotion regulation, physiological processes, and temperament. *Infancy, 3,* 175–198.

Calkins, S. D., & Fox, N. A. (1992). The relations among infant temperament, security of attachment, and behavioral inhibition at twenty-four months. *Child Development, 63,* 1456–1472.

Calkins, S. D., & Fox, N. A. (2002). Self-regulatory processes in early personality development: A multilevel approach to the study of childhood social withdrawal and aggression. *Development and Psychopathology, 14,* 477–498.

Calkins, S. D., Fox, N. A., & Marshall, T. R. (1996). Behavioral and physiological antecedents of inhibited and uninhibited behavior. *Child Development, 67,* 523–540.

Calkins, S. D., Gill, K. A., Johnson, M. C., & Smith, C. (1999). Emotional reactivity and emotion regulation strategies and predictors of social behavior with peers during toddlerhood. *Social Development, 8,* 310–341.

Calkins, S. D., Graziano, P., & Keane, S. P. (in press). Cardiac vagal regulation to emotional challenge differentiates among child behavior problem subtypes. *Biological Psychology.*

Calkins, S. D., & Howse, R. (2004). Individual differences in self-regulation: Implications for childhood adjustment. In P. Philipot & R. Feldman (Eds.), *The regulation of emotion* (pp. 307–332). Mahwah, NJ: Erlbaum.

Calkins, S. D., & Johnson, M. C. (1998). Toddler regulation of distress to frustrating events: Temperamental and maternal correlates. *Infant Behavior and Development, 21,* 379–395.

Calkins, S. D., Smith, C. L., Gill, K. L., & Johnson, M. C. (1998). Maternal interactive style across contexts: Relations to emotional, behavioral and physiological regulation during toddlerhood. *Social Development, 7*(3), 350–369.

Cassidy, J. (1994). Emotion regulation: Influences of attachment relationships. In N. A. Fox (Ed.), Emotion regulation: Behavioral and biological considerations. *Monographs of the Society for Research in Child Development, 59,* 228–249.

Champagne, F., & Meeney, M. J. (2001). Like mother, like daughter: Evidence for non-genetic transmission of parental behavior and stress responsivity. *Progressive Brain Research, 133,* 287–302.

Cicchetti, D. (1993). Developmental psychopathology: Reactions, reflections, projections. *Developmental Review, 13,* 471–502.

Cole, P. M., Martin, S. E., & Dennis, T. A. (2004). Emotion regulation as a scientific construct: Methodological challenges and directions for child development research. *Child Development, 75,* 317–333.

Conde-Agudelo, A., Diaz-Rosello, J. L., & Belizan, J. M. (2003). Kangaroo mother care to reduce the morbidity and mortality in low birthweight infants. *Cochrane Database of Systematic Review, 2,* CD002771.

Contreras, J., Kerns, K. A., Weimer, B., Gentzler, A., & Tomich, P. (2000). Emotion regulation as a mediator of associations between mother–child attachment and peer relationships in middle childhood. *Journal of Family Psychology, 14,* 111–124.

Davidson, R. J., Putnam, K. M., & Larson, C. L. (2000). Dysfunction in the neural circuitry of emotion regulation: A possible prelude to violence. *Science, 289,* 591–594.

Davis, E. P., Bruce, J., & Gunnar M. R. (2001). The anterior attention network: Associations with temperament and neuroendocrine activity on 6-year-old children. *Developmental Psychobiology, 40,* 43–56.

Derryberry, D., & Rothbart, M. K. (2001). Early temperament and emotional development. In A. F. Kalverboer & A. Gramsbergen (Eds.), *Handbook of brain and behavior in human development* (pp. 967–988). Dordrecht, The Netherlands: Kluwer Academic.

Diener, M., Mangelsdorf, S., McHale, J., & Frosch, C. (2002). Infants' behavioral strategies for emotion regulation with fathers and mothers: Associations with emotional expressions and attachment quality. *Infancy, 3,* 153–174.

DiPietro, J. A., Costigan, K. A., & Gurewitsch, E. D. (2003). Fetal response to maternal stress. *Early Human Development, 7,* 125–138.

Donovan, W. L., & Leavitt, L. A. (1985). Physiologic assessment of mother–infant attachment. *Journal of the American Academy of Child Psychiatry, 24,* 65–70.

Eisenberg, N., Guthrie, I. K., Fabes, R. A., Shepard, S., Losoya, S., Murphy, B. C., et al. (2000). Prediction of elementary school children's externalizing problem behaviors from attention and behavioral regulation and negative emotionality. *Child Development, 71*(5), 1367–1382.

Eisenberg, N., Hofer, C., & Vaughan, J. (2007). Effortful control and its socioemotional consequences. In J. J. Gross (Ed.), *Handbook of emotion regulation* (pp. 287–306). New York: Guilford Press.

Feldman, R., Weller, A., Sirota, L., & Eidelman, A. I. (2002). Skin-to-skin contact (kangaroo care) promotes self-regulation in premature infants: Sleep–wake cyclicity, arousal modulation, and sustained exploration. *Developmental Psychology, 38,* 194–207.

Fox, N. A. (1989). Psychophysiological correlates of emotional reactivity during the first year of life. *Developmental Psychology, 25,* 364–372.

Fox, N. A. (1994). Dynamic cerebral process underlying emotion regulation. In N. A. Fox (Ed.), Emotion regulation: Behavioral and biological considerations. *Monographs of the Society for Research in Child Development, 59,* 152–166.

Fox, N. A., Bell, M. A., & Jones, N. A. (1992) Individual differences in response to stress and cerebral asymmetry. *Developmental Neuropsychology, 8,* 165–184.

Fox, N. A., & Calkins, S. D. (2003). The development of self-control of emotion: Intrinsic and extrinsic influences. *Motivation and Emotion, 27,* 7–26.

Fox, N. A., & Card, J. (1999). Psychophysiological measures in the study of attachment. In J. Cassidy & P. R. Shaver (Eds.), *Handbook of attachment* (pp. 226–248). New York: Guilford Press.

Fox, N. A., Henderson, H. A., & Marshall, P. J. (2001). The biology of temperament: An integrative approach. In C. A. Nelson & M. Luciana (Eds.), *The handbook of developmental cognitive neuroscience* (pp. 631–645). Cambridge, MA: MIT Press.

Francis, D. D., Caldji, C., Champagne, F., Plotsky, P. M., & Meaney, M. J. (1999). The role of cortcotropin-releasing factor-norepinephrine systems in mediating the effects of early experience on the development of behavioral and endocrine responses to stress. *Biological Psychiatry, 46,* 1153–1166.

Gilliom, M., Shaw, D., Beck, J., Schonberg, M., & Lukon, J. (2002). Anger regulation in disadvantaged preschool boys: Strategies, antecedents, and the development of self-control. *Developmental Psychology, 38,* 222–235.

Goldsmith, H., & Davidson, R. (2004). Disambiguating the components of emotion regulation. *Child Development, 75,* 361–365.

Grolnick, W., Cosgrove, T., & Bridges, L. (1996). Age-graded change in the initiation of positive affect. *Infant Behavior and Development, 19,* 153–157.

Grolnick, W., Bridges, L., & Connell, J. (1996). Emotion regulation in two-year-olds: Strategies and emotional expression in four contexts. *Child Development, 67,* 928–941.

Gross, J. J., & Thompson, R. A. (2007). Emotion regulation: Conceptual foundations. In J. J. Gross (Ed.), *Handbook of emotion regulation* (pp. 3–24). New York: Guilford Press.

Gusella, J. L., Muir, D., & Tronick, E. Z. (1988). The effect of manipulating maternal behavior during an interaction on three- and six-month olds' affect and attention. *Child Development, 59,* 1111–1124.

Haley, D. W., & Stansbury, K. (2003). Infant stress and parent responsiveness: Regulation of physiology and behavior during still-face and reunion. *Child Development, 74,* 1534–1546.

Harman, C., Rothbart, M. K., & Posner, M. I. (1997). Distress and attention interactions in early infancy. *Motivation and Emotion, 21,* 27–43.

Hofer, M. A. (1994). Hidden regulators in attachment, separation, and loss. In N. A. Fox (Ed.), Emotion regulation: Behavioral and biological considerations. *Monographs of the Society for Research in Child Development, 59,* 192–207.

Howse, R. B., Calkins, S. D., Anastopoulos, A. D., Keane, S. P., & Shelton, T. L. (2003). Regulatory contributors to children's kindergarten achievement. *Early Education and Development, 14,* 101–119.

Jahromi, L. B., Putnam, S., & Stifter, C. A. (2004). Maternal regulation of infant reactivity from 2 to 6 months. *Developmental Psychology, 40,* 477–487.

Keane, S. P., & Calkins, S. D. (2004). Predicting kindergarten peer social status from toddler and preschool problem behavior. *Journal of Abnormal Child Psychology, 32*(4), 409–423.

Keenan, K. (2000). Emotion dysregulation as a risk factor for child psychopathology. *Clinical Psychology: Science and Practice, 7,* 418–434.

Kennedy, A. E., Rubin, K. H., Hastings, P. D., & Maisel, B. (2004). Longitudinal relations between child vagal-tone and parenting behavior: 2 to 4 years. *Developmental Psychobiology, 45,* 10–21.

Kochanska, G. (2001). Emotional development in children with different attachment histories: The first three years. *Child Development, 72,* 474–490

Kochanska, G., Coy, K. C., & Murray, K. Y. (2001). The development of self-regulation in the first four years of life. *Child Development, 72*(4), 1091–1111.

Koehl, M., Lemaire, V., Vallee, M., Abrous, N., Piazza, P. V. Mayo, W., et al. (2001). Long term neurodevelopmental and behavioral effects of perinatal life events in rats. *Neurotoxicity Research, 3,* 65–83.

Kopp, C. (1982). Antecedents of self-regulation: A developmental perspective. *Developmental Psychology, 18,* 199–214.

Kopp, C. (1989). Regulation of distress and negative emotions: A developmental view. *Developmental Psychology, 25,* 243–254.

Kopp, C. (1992). Emotional distress and control in young children. In N. Eisenberg & R. Fabes, (Eds.), *Emotion and its regulation in early development* (pp. 41–56). San Francisco: Jossey-Bass/Pfeiffer.

Kopp, C. B., & Neufeld, S. J. (2003). Emotional development during infancy. In R. Davidson, K. R. Scherer, & H. H. Goldsmith (Eds.), *Handbook of affective sciences* (pp. 347–374). Oxford, UK: Oxford University Press.

Lane, R. D., & McRae, K. (2004). Neural substrates of conscious emotional experience: A cognitive-neuroscientific perspective. In B. M. Amsterdam & J. Benjamins (Eds.), *Consciousness, emotional self-regulation and the brain* (pp. 87–122). Amsterdam: John Benjamin.

Luu, P., & Tucker, D. M. (2004). Self-regulation by the medial frontal cortex: Limbic representation of motive set-points. In M. Beauregard (Ed.), *Consciousness, emotional self-regulation and the brain* (pp. 123–161). Amsterdam: John Benjamin.

Moore, G. A., & Calkins, S. D. (2004). Infants' vagal regulation in the still-face paradigm is related to dyadic coordination of mother–infant interaction. *Developmental Psychology, 40,* 1068–1080.

Nachmias, M., Gunnar, M., Mangelsdorf, S., Parritz, R., & Buss, K. (1996). Behavioral inhibition and stress reactivity: The moderating role of attachment security. *Child Development, 67,* 508–522.

Ochsner, K. N., & Gross, J. J. (2004). Thinking makes it so: A social cognitive neuroscience approach to emotion regulation. In R. F. Baumeister & K. D. Vohs (Eds.), *Handbook of self-regulation: Research, theory and applications* (pp. 229–258). New York: Guilford Press.

O'Connor, T., Heron, J., Golding, J., Beveridge, M., & Glover, V. (2002). Maternal antenatal and children's behavioral/emotional problems at 4 years. *British Journal of Psychiatry, 180,* 502–508.

Polan, H. J., & Hofer, M. A. (1999). Psychobiological origins of infants attachment and separation responses. In J. Cassidy & P. Shaver, (Eds.), *Handbook of attachment: Theory, research, and clinical applications* (pp. 162–180). New York: Guilford Press.

Porges, S. W. (1991). Vagal tone: An autonomic mediatory of affect. In J. A. Garber & K. A. Dodge (Eds.), *The development of affect regulation and dsyregulation* (pp. 11–128). New York: Cambridge University Press.

Porges, S. W. (1996). Physiological regulation in high-risk infants: A model for assessment and potential intervention. *Development and Psychopathology, 8,* 43–58.

Porter, C. L. (2003). Coregulation in mother–infant dyads: Links to infants' cardiac vagal tone. *Psychological Reports, 92,* 307–319.

Posner, M. I., & Rothbart, M. K. (2000). Developing mechanisms of self-regulation. *Development and Psychopathology, 12,* 427–441.

Richards, J. E. (1987). Infant visual sustained attention and respiratory sinus arrhythmia. *Child Development, 58,* 488–496.

Rothbart, M. K., Derryberry, D., & Hershey, K. (2000). Stability of temperament in childhood: Laboratory infant assessment to parent report at seven years. In V. J. Molfese & D. L. Malfese (Eds.), *Temperament and personality development across the lifespan* (pp. 85–119). Mahwah, NJ: Erlbaum.

Rothbart, M. K., Posner, M. I., & Boylan, A. (1990). Regulatory mechanisms in infant development. In J. T. Enns (Ed.), *The development of attention: Research and theory* (pp. 47–66). Amsterdam: Elsevier.

Rothbart, M. K., & Sheese, B. E. (2007). Temperament and emotion regulation. In J. J. Gross (Ed.), *Handbook of emotion regulation* (pp. 331–350). New York: Guilford Press.

Rothbart, M., Ziaie, H., & O'Boyle, C. (1992). Self-regulation and emotion in infancy. In N. Eisenberg, & R. Fabes, (Eds.), *Emotion and its regulation in early development* (pp. 7–23). San Francisco: Jossey-Bass/Pfeiffer.

Rueda, M. R., Posner, M. I., & Rothbart, M. K. (2004). Attentional control and self-regulation. In R. F. Baumeister & K. D. Vohs (Eds.), *Handbook of self-regulation: Research, theory, and applications* (pp. 283–300). New York: Guilford Press.

Schneider, M. L., Coe, C. L., & Lubach, G. R. (1992). Endocrine activation mimics the adverse Effects of prenatal stress on the neuromotor development of the primate. *Developmental Psychobiology, 25,* 427–439.

Schore, A. (2000). Attachment and the regulation of the right brain.. *Attachment and Human Development, 2,* 23–47

Sethi, A., Mischel, W., Aber, J. L., Shoda, Y., & Rodriguez, M. L. (2000). The role of strategic attention deployment in development of self-regulation: Predicting preschoolers' delay of gratification from mother–toddler interactions. *Developmental Psychology, 36*(6), 767–777.

Shaw, D. S., Keenan, K., & Vondra, J., Delliquadri, E., & Giovanelli, J. (1997). Antecedents of preschool children's internalizing problems: A longitudinal study of low-income families. *Journal of the American Academy of Child and Adolescent Psychiatry, 36,* 1760–1767.

Sroufe, L. A. (1996). *Emotional development: The organization of emotional life in the early years.* New York: Cambridge University Press.

Sroufe, L. A. (2000). Early relationships and the development of children. *Infant Mental Health Journal, 21,* 67–74.

Sroufe, L. A., & Waters, E. (1977). Heart rate as a convergent measures in clinical and developmental research. *Merrill–Palmer Quarterly, 23,* 3–27.

Stansbury, K., & Gunnar, M. R. (1994). The development of emotion regulation: Biological and behavioral considerations. *Monographs of the Society for Research in Child Development, 59,* 108–134.

Stifter, C. A., & Braungart, J. M. (1995). The regulation of negative reactivity in infancy: Function and development. *Developmental Psychology, 31*(3), 448–455.

Stifter, C. A., Spinrad, T., & Braungart-Rieker, J. (1999). Toward a developmental model of child compliance: The role of emotion regulation. *Child Development, 70,* 21–32.

Thompson, R. A. (1994). Emotion regulation: A theme in search of definition. In N. A. Fox (Ed.), The development of emotion regulation: Biological and behavioral considerations. *Monographs of the Society for Research in Child Development, 59*(2–3, Serial No. 240), 25–52.

Thompson, R. A., & Meyer, S. (2007). Socialization of emotion regulation in the family. In J. J. Gross (Ed.), *Handbook of emotion regulation* (pp. 249–268). New York: Guilford Press.

Weinstock, M. (1997). Does prenatal stress impair coping and regulation of the hypothalamic-pituitary–adrenal axis? *Neuroscience and Biobehavioral Review, 21,* 1–10.

CHAPTER 12

Socialization of Emotion Regulation in the Family

ROSS A. THOMPSON
SARA MEYER

Emotion regulation develops dramatically during childhood and adolescence. Although infants may cry inconsolably until parents intervene, toddlers seek the assistance of their caregivers, preschoolers talk about their feelings, older children know of the value of mental distraction for managing their emotions, and adolescents may have personal strategies (such as playing meaningful music) for doing so. These developmental changes arise from the child's growing conceptual skills, neurobiological changes in emotion control, temperamental individuality, and many social influences (Thompson, 1994).

An important contribution of a developmental approach is its emphasis on the social processes that shape the growth of emotion regulation. As any parent knows, infants are born with only the most rudimentary capacities to manage their arousal, and they depend on caregivers for soothing distress, controlling excitement, allaying fear, and even managing joyful pleasure. Although children rapidly acquire more autonomous self-regulatory capacities, emotions are managed by others throughout life as family and friends provide comfort when distressed, support when anxious, and companionship that enhances positive feelings and emotional well-being. Social influences are important to how children interpret and appraise their feelings, learn about strategies for emotion management, achieve competence and self-confidence in controlling their feelings, and acquire cultural and gender expectations for emotion regulation.

Although these social influences occur in many social contexts, we focus on family influences because these begin earliest and are thus foundational and constitute the most ubiquitous and multifaceted influences on emotional development. Our goal is to describe socialization processes in the family relevant to the development of emotion regulation, discuss their significance to developmental emotions theory, and identify future research goals. In the next section, we define emotion regulation and consider how a developmental perspective offers helpful insights into the nature of emotion regulation and individual differences in self-regulation. In the section that follows, we discuss emotion socialization processes in the family, including (1) the quality of direct parental interventions to manage the emotions of offspring (such as soothing a baby); (2) parents' sympathetic, critical, dismissive, or punitive evaluations of children's feelings that influence how children evaluate their own feelings; (3) the support or challenges presented by the broader emotional climate of family life; (4) how parents and children talk about emotions and its effects on children's developing understanding of emotion and emotion regulation; and (5) the general quality of the parent–child relationship as a source of support or challenge. In the final section, we consider the implications of this work for the future of research on the development of emotion regulation.

DEVELOPMENTAL PERSPECTIVES ON EMOTION REGULATION

Contemporary inquiry into emotion regulation has two distinct but overlapping theoretical foundations. The first builds on the study of stress and coping, inquiry into psychological defense processes (based on the psychoanalytic tradition), and functionalist emotions theory. This approach is reflected in contemporary work in personality theory that regards emotion regulation as a core component of personality functioning and an important predictor of psychological adjustment and social competence.

The second approach to emotion regulation also builds on functionalist emotions theory, but within a developmental framework that highlights the biological, constructivist, and relational foundations of emotional growth. Emotion regulation is viewed as developing from multiple influences, including temperamental individuality, significant relationships, and the child's growing understanding of emotion and processes of emotion management. Individual differences in emotion regulation reflect the developing child's adaptation to situational demands and expectations as well as enduring personality organization and are affected by developmental changes in how children construe their emotional experiences and children's emotional goals.

Each approach makes important contributions to the study of emotion regulation. Because ours is a developmental approach, it has important implications for defining emotion regulation, methodology, and understanding individual differences in emotion.

Defining Emotion Regulation

Definitions of emotion regulation are built on broader conceptualizations of emotion. The view that emotions arise from person–environment transactions that are meaningful and motivational because they are relevant to the individual's goals, and that emotions entail interconnected changes in subjective experience, behavior, physiology, and expressions, is a familiar one (see Gross & Thompson, this volume). From a developmental perspective, many of these features of emotion and their interrelationships evolve significantly over the life course. The goals that evoke emotion and children's appraisals of circumstances as relevant to their goals change considerably, of course, as children mature cognitively and emotionally. Young children feel embarrassed when praised effusively only after the second birthday, for example, after a developing sense of self alters the meaning of social praise and motivates efforts to manage the self-consciousness that results (Lagattuta & Thompson, in press). Moreover, the interconnections between emotion components, such as the linkages between subjective experience and facial expressions, become organized developmentally and are affected by social experience (Camras, Oster, Campos, & Bakeman, 2003). A developmental perspective enables emotion researchers to understand that many features of emotional experience are organized and stable in adulthood not necessarily because of their biological foundations but rather because of their origins in multifaceted developmental influences.

Our definition of emotion regulation reflects this developmental approach: *Emotion regulation consists of the extrinsic and intrinsic processes responsible for monitoring, evaluating, and modifying emotional reactions, especially their intensive and temporal features, to accomplish one's goals* (Thompson, 1994). Incorporated within this definition are several assumptions about emotion and emotion regulation (see also Gross & Thompson, this volume).

First, emotion regulation processes target positive as well as negative emotions and can entail diminishing, heightening, or simply maintaining one's current level of emotional arousal. Even young children learn, for example, how to blunt their exuberance when necessary in formal social situations, or how to enhance feelings of sadness to elicit nurturance. Because of this, emotion regulation usually alters the *dynamics* of emotion rather than changing its quality. In other words, individuals alter the intensity, escalation (i.e., latency and rise time), or duration of an emotional response, or speed its recovery, or reduce or enhance the lability or range of emotional responding in particular situations, depending on the individual's goals for that situation (Thompson, 1990). We usually think of emotionally well-regulated people as those who are capable of altering how long, how intensely, or how quickly they feel as they do, rather than transforming the valence of emotion (such as changing anger into happiness).

Second, consistent with a functionalist approach to emotion, strategies of emotion regulation are rarely inherently optimal or maladaptive. Rather, emotion regulation strategies must be evaluated in terms of the individual's goals for the situation. This functionalist orientation is especially important for developmental analysis. A toddler's petulant crying or an adolescent's sullenness may be intuitively interpreted as revealing deficient skills in emotion regulation until one realizes that the toddler's crying causes parents to accede and the adolescent's sullenness causes adults to withdraw, each of which may be the child's goal (even if this goal is not shared by others). A functionalist orientation is also important for understanding emotion regulatory processes relevant to developmental psychopathology. Children with anxiety disorders are typically regarded as deficient in emotion regulation, but their hypervigilance to threatening events, fear-oriented cognitions, and sensitivity to internal visceral cues of anxiety are part of a constellation of self-regulatory strategies for anticipating and avoiding encounters with fear-provoking situations. In light of their temperamental vulnerability and family processes that heighten risk for anxious pathology, these emotion regulatory strategies may be the most adaptive options available to the child (Thompson, 2000). To be sure, the same emotion regulatory strategies that provide immediate relief exact long-term costs that make anxious children vulnerable to continued pathology, and this double-edged sword is typical of emotional regulatory processes for many forms of developmental psychopathology (see Thompson & Calkins, 1996). But understanding emotion regulation for children at risk requires appreciating the emotional goals that the child is seeking to achieve, consistent with a functionalist approach.

Third, a developmental analysis underscores that emotion regulation includes how people monitor and evaluate their emotions as well as modifying them. Indeed, children's developing capacities for emotional self-awareness and for appraising their feelings in light of personal and cultural expectations are core features of developing emotion regulation (Saarni, 1999). This is consistent with the constructivist view that emotion self-regulation emerges in concert with children's developing understanding of emotion and its meaning. During the preschool years, for example, young children proceed from being "emotion situationists" focused only on the external instigators of their feelings to becoming "emotion psychologists" who comprehend the association between emotion and desires, beliefs, memories, and other psychological influences (Thompson & Lagattuta, 2006). With increasing age, children also begin to understand the associations between emotions and personal expectations, standards, and goals (Lagattuta & Thompson, in press). These conceptual advances provide a foundation for growth in children's understanding of strategies for emotion self-regulation and for enacting these strategies with greater competence. Their conceptual growth also interacts with socialization influences by which children appropriate sociocultural and family beliefs about emotion and its regulation.

Methodological Implications

The developmental study of emotion regulation is also distinct in methodology. It is common for studies of emotion regulation in adults or adolescents to rely on respondent self-report, typically through questionnaires, to index individual differences in emotion self-regulation. Infants and young children are not informative reporters, however, and developmental researchers must use other procedures, such as detailed observations of emotional reactions in carefully structured experimental situations, often with convergent behavioral and psychophysiological measures, along with the reports of mothers and other secondary sources concerning the child's emotional qualities. These methods are informative, but behavioral measures (whether of infants or adults) are also complicated by interpretive difficulties, including that (1) behavior that may reflect the influence of emotion regulatory processes is multidetermined, (2) emotional reactions and emotional regulatory influences are not easily distinguished behaviorally, and (3) situational context can have a profound effect on children's emotional reactions (Cole, Martin, & Dennis, 2004; Thompson, 2006). Studying emotion regulation *in vivo* in this manner is thus conceptually and methodologically more difficult than enlisting self-report.

Adding further complexity to the study of emotion regulation is the functionalist requirement of understanding the goals motivating self-regulatory efforts. Although these goals are usually assumed in studies of adults (e.g., diminishing negative affect and enhancing positive emotion), behavioral studies of emotion regulation require carefully designed assessment procedures in which the goals for managing emotion are either implicit or incorporated into the design (e.g., coping with a disappointing gift). In short, developmental research into emotion regulation is not for the fainthearted because of the special methodological challenges it presents.

Individual Differences in Emotion Regulation

Socialization processes are among many influences on the development of individual differences in emotion self-regulation. As profiled in other chapters in this volume, emotion regulation is also influenced by developing neurobiology (especially in the prefrontal cortex), the growth of attentional processes, conceptual advances in emotion understanding, temperamental individuality, and the growth of personality (see Calkins & Hill, this volume; Davidson, Fox, & Kalin, this volume; Eisenberg, Hofer, & Vaughn, this volume; Meerum Terwogt & Stegge, this volume; Rothbart & Sheese, this volume; see also Fox & Calkins, 2003; Thompson, 1994). Socialization processes interact developmentally with these other influences. If young offspring are not buffered from overwhelming stress by parental care, for example, neurohormonal stress systems within the brain can become stress-sensitive in ways that can make offspring biologically vulnerable to enduring problems in stress regulation (Gunnar & Vazquez, 2006).

These complex developmental processes suggest that although psychologists tend to regard "emotion regulation" as if it was a single, coherent personality construct or developmental phenomenon, the growth of emotion regulation is actually based on a multidimensional network of loosely allied developmental processes arising from within and outside the child. Many aspects of psychobiological, conceptual, and socioemotional growth are enfolded into developing capacities to independently manage emotion. Although emotion regulation is often viewed as one component of the general growth of broader self-regulatory capacity, moreover, many of these developmental influences are specific to emotion. The influence of children's developing conceptions of emotion on emotion self-regulation may not, for example, generalize to other forms of self-regulation. Emotion regulation is thus an integrative field of study, but it is also challenging to conceptualize and study, especially in developmental analysis. Moreover, because of these multifaceted developmental processes, individual differences in emotion regulation can arise from surprisingly diverse influences at different stages of growth.

FAMILY INFLUENCES ON DEVELOPING EMOTION REGULATION

It is easy to see the influence of socialization processes when parents soothe an infant or coach young offspring to remain quiet in church. But many social influences are also involved in how children learn to appraise their feelings (and themselves as emotional beings), confront the demands of emotion regulation at home or in other social settings, acquire specific skills for managing their feelings, and represent emotion in psychologically complex ways relevant to self-regulation. Because these socialization processes extend throughout life and mediate cultural and gender differences in emotion management, individuals reach adulthood with skills of emotion self-regulation that have been, to a large extent, socially constructed. Unfortunately, as we shall see, in some family environments these processes contribute to risk for affect-dysregulated psychopathology because they undermine the development of constructive forms of emotion management.

Direct Interventions to Manage Emotion

The most basic form of extrinsic emotion regulation is when someone intervenes directly to alter another's emotions, and this begins early. Virtually from birth, parents and other caregivers strive earnestly to soothe infant distress that may arise from hunger, fatigue, discomfort, or other sources. These interventions usually accomplish their intended purpose, and they also contribute to the emergence of rudimentary behavioral expectations in the baby that predictable parental ministrations will relieve distress. Lamb (1981) argued that such distress–relief sequences are easily learned associations for young infants, and there is experimental evidence for this. By 6 months of age, distressed infants begin quieting in apparent anticipation of the arrival of their mothers when they can hear the adult's approaching footsteps; infants also protest loudly if the adult approaches but does not pick them up to soothe them (Gekoski, Rovee-Coller, & Carulli-Rabinowitz, 1983; Lamb & Malkin, 1986). The learned association between distress, the adult's approach, and subsequent soothing has emotion regulatory consequences because of the infant's anticipatory soothing before the parent's arrival. These findings also suggest that variations in the quality of the adult's responsiveness are likely to influence how readily infants soothe to the adult or to expectations of the adult's approach.

Parents also intervene to manage the feelings of their offspring in emotionally positive contexts. In face-to-face play, beginning when infants are 2–3 months of age, caregivers engage in brief, focused episodes of social interaction with the baby that occur without competing caregiving goals or other demands on either partner. Detailed microanalytic studies show that mothers respond animatedly to maintain the baby in a positive emotional state by mirroring the child's positive emotional expressions and ignoring or responding with surprise to the infant's negative expressions. In one study, maternal modeling and contingent responding of this kind helped to account for gradually increased rates of infant joy and interest during the first year (Malatesta, Culver, Tesman, & Shepard, 1989; Malatesta, Grigoryev, Lamb, Albin, & Culver, 1986). These episodes of face-to-face play are believed to contribute to the growth of rudimentary capacities for self-regulation as the infant learns how to maintain manageable arousal in the context of a supportive or insensitive response by the caregiver (Gianino & Tronick, 1988; see Feldman, Greenbaum, & Yirmiya, 1999, for supportive evidence).

There are other ways that parents intervene directly to manage the emotions of offspring. They distract the child's attention away from potentially frightening or distressing events, assist in solving problems that children find frustrating, and strive to alter the child's interpretation of negatively arousing experiences (e.g., "It's just a game"). They also suggest adaptive ways of responding emotionally, sometimes as alternatives to maladaptive behavior, that facilitate emotion regulation by enabling the child's feelings to be expressed with more constructive, often positive results. Parents might encourage offspring to shout at a peer victimizer rather than hitting, for example, or enlist an adult's assistance rather than fearfully withdraw, or problem-solve rather than dissolve in loud wails. The common parental maxim to toddlers—"use words to say how you feel"—reflects the psychological reality that developing language ability also significantly facilitates young children's capacities to understand, convey, and manage their emotions (Kopp, 1989).

Parents also seek to manage the feelings of offspring by structuring children's experiences proactively to make emotional demands predictable and manageable. They do this by creating daily routines that accord with their knowledge of children's temperamental qualities, activity level, and tolerance for stimulation, scheduling naps and meals, choosing child-care arrangements that are congenial to children's needs and capabilities, and other kinds of "situation selection" (see Gross & Thompson, this volume).

Parents engage in social referencing, in which they provide salient emotional signals, through facial expressions and vocal tone, when young children encounter events that are ambiguous or confusing (Klinnert, Campos, Sorce, Emde, & Svejda, 1983). When encountering a friendly but unfamiliar adult, for example, a mother's reassuring smile can turn a wary 1-year-old into a more sociable baby, and experimental investigations have shown that by the end of the first year, infants regularly use such emotional cues from trusted adults (see Thompson, 2006, for a research review). Social referencing is important not only as a form of distal communication that alters a young child's emotional appraisal of events but also as a social means of imbuing events with emotional meaning that has emotion regulatory consequences for the child, especially when the adult's signals provide reassurance.

What are the effects of these parental interventions? Calkins and Johnson (1998) found that 18-month-olds who became more distressed during frustration tasks had mothers who were independently observed to be more interfering when interacting with their offspring, while children who could use problem solving and distracting during frustration had mothers who had earlier offered greater support, suggestions, and encouragement. In another study, mothers who insisted that their toddlers approach and confront potentially fearful objects in the laboratory had children who exhibited greater stress, as indexed by postsession cortisol levels (Nachmias, Gunnar, Mangelsdorf, Parritz, & Buss, 1996). Little more is known about whether these parental interventions contribute to the development of enduring individual differences in emotion regulatory capacities, and this constitutes an important goal for future study. These findings suggest, however, that the sensitivity with which parents manage children's negative emotions influences the intensity and duration of these reactions and may influence developing emotion self-regulatory capacities through the child's expectation that distress is manageable and of the adult's assistance in managing it.

Additional support for these conclusions derives from studies of emotional development in the young offspring of depressed mothers. Several studies have found that depressed mothers are less responsive and emotionally more negative and subdued during social play with their infants, and as early as 2–3 months their offspring are also observed to show diminished responsiveness and emotional animation with their mothers (Cohn, Campbell, Matias, & Hopkins, 1990; Field, Healy, Goldstein, & Guthertz, 1990; Field et al., 1988). Field and colleagues (1988) found that the 3- to 6-month-old infants of depressed mothers were also more subdued and less animated when interacting with a nondepressed stranger. These findings suggest that sustained early experiences of interacting with a depressed caregiver may undermine healthy emotional functioning and the emergence of behavioral and neurobiological emotion regulatory capacities early in life, especially when maternal depression is chronic. As these children are also exposed to negative, helpless, and denigrating maternal behavior characteristic of depression, it is easy to see why such children are at heightened risk of developing affective disorders of their own (Goodman & Gotlib, 1999).

Direct parental interventions to manage children's emotions decline in frequency in early childhood as young children acquire their own self-regulatory strategies. However, direct interventions remain an important source of extrinsic influence on emotion regulation throughout life and are supplemented by other socialization influences.

Parental Evaluations of Children's Emotions

Emotion regulation can be facilitated or impaired by how others evaluate one's feelings. Sympathetic, constructive responses affirm that one's feelings are justified and provide a resource of social support that aids in coping through the understanding and advice that others can provide. But denigrating, critical, or dismissive responses add stress to the challenges of emotion regulation. This is especially true for negative emotions, when critical or punitive reactions by others contain implicit messages denigrating the appropriateness of the feelings or their expression, the competence of the person feeling this way, or the relationship between the person and the evaluator. Indeed, when others are dismissive, critical, or punitive, it can exacerbate the negative emotions that one is trying to manage (in part by arousing further emotion), as well as diminishing opportunities for acquiring more adaptive modes of emotion regulation or even discussing one's feelings with the other person. Furthermore, emotion self-regulation develops as children internalize the explicit and implicit evaluations of their emotions by significant others and thus begin to evaluate for themselves their feelings in comparable ways. A child who has always been told that "big people don't let things get them down" struggles to manage feelings of sadness with this emotion rule as a continuing influence but without parental support for doing so. Others' evaluations of one's emotions are important throughout life (Thompson, Flood, & Goodvin, 2006), but especially in the early years.

Developmental studies indicate that children cope more adaptively with their emotions in immediate circumstances, and acquire more constructive emotion regulatory capacities, when parents respond acceptingly and supportively to their negative emotional displays. By contrast, outcomes are more negative when parents are denigrating, punitive, or dismissive, or when the child's negative emotions elicit the parent's personal distress (see Denham, 1998; Denham, Bassett, & Wyatt, in press; Eisenberg, Cumberland, & Spinrad, 1998, for reviews). In a socioeconomically disadvantaged sample, for example, mothers who reported exerting more positive control (using warmth and approval) over their sons at age 1½ had children who were observed to manage their negative emotions more constructively (such as by using self-distraction) at age 3½ (Gilliom, Shaw, Beck, Schonberg, & Lukon, 2002; see also Berlin & Cassidy, 2003). Eisenberg, Fabes, and Murphy (1996) found that the mother's self-reported problem-solving responses to their grade-school children's negative emotions were associated with independent reports of their children's constructive coping with problems (such as seeking support, problem solving, and positive thinking), while mothers' punitive and minimizing reactions to children's emotions were negatively associated with children's constructive coping and were instead positively associated with avoidant coping (see also Eisenberg & Fabes, 1994; Eisenberg et al., 1999). Likewise, Denham (1997) reported that preschoolers who described their mothers as providing comfort when they felt badly were rated as more emotionally competent by their teachers (see also Roberts & Strayer, 1987).

These studies indicate that how parents respond supportively or unsupportively to children's emotions, and the behaviors that result, predict children's emotion-related coping in later assessments. Unfortunately, these studies sometimes incorporate a broad range of outcome measures (including empathy, social competence, and cooperativeness) into emotion regulation assessments, although these outcomes are clearly related. Fabes, Leonard, Kupanoff, and Martin (2001) found, for example, that parents who responded harshly (i.e., punitive, minimizing) to their preschoolers' negative emotion expressions had children who expressed more intense negative emotion with peers, and that differences in emotionality were related to preschoolers' social competence. One way that critical parental reactions to children's negative emotions can undermine peer competence, therefore, is how it impairs the development of competent regulation of negative feelings by the child.

In atypical family contexts, critical parental reactions to a child's emotions can even more significantly undermine the development of emotion self-regulation. In some conditions, this phenomenon has been described as "expressed emotion," which is an index of parental attitudes of criticism or emotional overinvolvement in the child's problems that can undermine competent emotional functioning (e.g., Hooley & Richters, 1995). Although expressed emotion has been studied most extensively in clinical studies of schizophrenia, depression, and bipolar disorder because of its relevance to the maintenance or relapse of clinical symptomatology, expressed emotion has also been found in developmental studies to be associated with the onset of conduct problems in children (Caspi et al., 2004) with one study finding expressed emotion to be particularly prevalent in homes with a depressed parent (Rogosch, Cicchetti, & Toth, 2004). In the context of expressed emotion, therefore, critical parental evaluations of a child's emotional behavior can contribute risk for the development of psychopathology involving emotion dysregulation. Risk is enhanced because of how the parent's critical demeanor adds stress, undermines opportunities to learn more adaptive forms of emotion coping, contributes to children's self-perceptions of emotional dysfunction, and creates a more challenging family emotional climate for troubled children.

Emotional Climate of Family Life

The importance of how parents evaluate a child's feelings reflects the broader influence of the emotional conduct of other family members on children's emotions and their efforts to regulate them. The emotional climate of family life makes emotion management easier or more difficult because of the emotional demands that children encounter in the home. As suggested by the research on expressed emotion, when children must cope with frequent, intensive negative emotion from other family members, particularly when it is directed at them, it can overwhelm their capacities for emotion management. The family emotional climate is also relevant to emotion regulation because of the models of emotion regulation to which children are exposed and how the family environment shapes children's developing schemas for emotionality in the world at large (e.g., are emotions threatening? empowering? irrational? uncontrollable?) (Dunsmore & Halberstadt, 1997). Most broadly, capacities for emotion self-regulation are shaped by how children internalize normative expectations for how people typically behave emotionally based on family experiences, and by which they manage their own feelings.

An important facet of the family emotional life is parents' emotional expressiveness (Halberstadt, Crisp, & Eaton, 1999; Halberstadt & Eaton, 2003). A series of studies by Eisenberg and her colleagues has shown that children's social competence is affected by how mothers convey positive or negative feelings in the home—and this association is mediated by differences in children's self-regulatory behavior (Eisenberg et al., 2001; Eisenberg et al., 2003; Valiente, Fabes, Risenberg, & Spinrad, 2004). These findings suggest that a family climate characterized by moderate to high amounts of positive emotion among family members contributes to the growth of emotion regulation, perhaps through the models of skillful emotion self-regulation by other family members and the influence of the child's developing expectations for emotionally appropriate conduct.

With respect to the influence of negative emotional expressiveness in the family, the evidence is not as clear. Several studies report that maternal expressions of negative emotion are negatively associated with children's self-regulation and coping, but others have found a positive association (Eisenberg et al., 1998, 2001, 2003; Valiente et al.,

2004). It is likely that these differential effects are contingent on several considerations. One consideration is whether negative emotions in the family are "negative dominant" (e.g., anger and hostility), which are more likely to elicit the child's fear or defensiveness, or "negative submissive" (e.g., sadness and distress), which are less threatening. Other considerations are whether negative emotions are directed to the child or to another, the frequency and intensity of adult emotional expressions, and the broader circumstances in which emotion is expressed. It is easy to see how emotion regulatory skills might be enhanced (rather than undermined) by a child's exposure to nonhostile negative emotions of moderate intensity in contexts that show that negative feelings can be safely expressed and managed. A more hostile, threatening family emotional environment, however, is more likely to undermine the development of adaptive emotion regulatory capacities.

These hypotheses remain speculative, however, because very little research has distinguished the effects of these variations in negative emotion expressions on the development of emotion regulation, and this constitutes an important future research task. In addition, the role of siblings as a buffer on the emotional climate of the family is virtually unexplored (see, however, Sawyer et al., 2002, for an exception). Furthermore, little is known about how families that are characterized by low levels of both positive and negative emotional expressiveness influence the growth of emotion management in children. Do children acquire greater competence in managing their feelings in such affectively benign environments, or do they instead become oriented toward suppressing emotion entirely, consistent with the conclusion that feelings *should not* be expressed? Much more remains to be learned.

The multifaceted influences of the family emotional climate on the development of emotion regulation are highlighted by the "emotional security hypothesis" of Cummings and Davies to describe the consequences of marital conflict on early emotional growth (Cummings & Davies, 1994; Davies & Cummings, 1994). Marital conflict significantly colors the emotional climate of the family and children's capacities for emotion self-regulation. According to Cummings and Davies, children seek to reestablish the emotional security they have lost by intervening into parental arguments in order to quell disturbance, monitoring parental moods to anticipate the outbreak of arguments, and otherwise striving to manage their emotions in a conflicted home environment. As a consequence, they show heightened sensitivity to parental distress and anger, tend to become overinvolved in their parents' emotional conflicts, have difficulty managing the strong emotions that conflict arouses in them (in a manner resembling the "emotional flooding" described by emotions theorists), and exhibit signs of the early development of internalizing problems. Research derived from this view has found that grade-school children experiencing the most intense marital conflict also exhibited greatest enmeshment in family conflict but also greater efforts to avoid conflict, while also showing greatest signs of internalizing symptomatology (Davies & Forman, 2002; see also Davies, Harold, Goeke-Morey, & Cummings, 2002).

An important influence on the emotional climate of the family—which also affects how parents evaluate and respond to the emotions of offspring—are parental beliefs about emotion and its expression. These include intuitive values about the nature of emotion and its importance (e.g., people should act "from the heart," emotions must be released or they will build up within, or emotions are irrational and should be suppressed or ignored), the importance of expressing one's true feelings, how emotions differ for men and women, the kinds of emotions that should be expressed to family members, and the ways that feelings should be conveyed. Taken together, they can be considered a parent's "meta-emotion philosophy" that shapes the family emotional climate as a continuing influence on how emotions are expressed and perceived in the home.

Gottman, Katz, and Hooven (1997) define a meta-emotion philosophy as "an organized set of feelings and thoughts about one's own emotions and one's child's emotions" (p. 243). It includes an adult's awareness of her or his own emotions, an understanding and acceptance of the child's emotions, and management of the child's feelings (Hooven, Gottman, & Katz, 1995). Based on parental interviews about their philosophy, Gottman and his colleagues distinguish between "emotion coaching" and "emotion dismissing" parenting styles. Emotion-coaching parents are attentive to their own emotions and attend to the child's feelings also and do not believe that feelings should be stifled. They consider the child's emotional expressions as an occasion to validate the child's feelings, and as an opportunity for intimacy and teaching about emotions, expression, and coping. Thus emotion-coaching parents foster the growth of emotion regulation in offspring by offering warm support and specific guidance for managing feelings, such as suggestions about how to cope with distress. Dismissing parents tend to ignore their own emotions or belittle their importance, and they may not constructively attend to their child's feelings either. They view emotions (especially negative ones) as potentially harmful and believe that parents are responsible for promptly subduing negative outbursts in offspring and teaching their children that negative emotions are fleeting and unimportant. Gottman and his colleagues propose that parental meta-emotion philosophy underlies how parents respond to the emotions of their offspring which, in turn, influences the growth of physiological and emotion regulatory capabilities and, through them, children's broader social and emotional competencies.

There has been relatively little research directly testing this provocative formulation. One study found that 5-year-olds with emotion-coaching parents exhibited somewhat better physiological regulation and, at age 8, were rated by their mothers as better in emotion regulation, although the direct association between parental meta-emotion philosophy and children's emotion regulation was untested (Gottman, Katz, & Hooven, 1996; see also Hooven et al., 1995). Another study found that the mother's acceptance of the child's negative emotions combined with low amounts of negative emotional expressiveness in the family was associated with child emotion regulation which, in turn, predicted lower levels of child aggression (Ramsden & Hubbard, 2002). However, the same study failed to confirm an expected association between parental emotion coaching and aggression and only a weak association between parental emotion coaching and child emotion regulation was found. There is thus value to continued examination of the potential influence of parental meta-emotion philosophy as an influence on the family emotional climate.

Parent–Child Conversation and Children's Developing Emotion Representations

Further research on parental beliefs about emotion is valuable because parental beliefs are likely to influence children's developing emotion representations. As noted earlier, developmental changes in emotion regulation are affected by children's explicit and implicit understanding of emotion, including their comprehension of the causes and consequences of their feelings, the suitability of emotional expressions in different social circumstances, the internal indications of emotion (such as increasing heart rate or shortened breath) by which children can monitor their arousal, and specific strategies by which emotions can be managed. These features of emotion understanding enhance emotional self-awareness and enable children to monitor and evaluate their feelings with increasing insight en route to regulating them more effectively. Children's developing conceptions of emotion also begin to incorporate cultural values and gender expectations concerning emotion and its expression.

Young children advance considerably in understanding their emotions, and the content and structure of parent–child conversation is an important contributor to their understanding (see Thompson, 2006, and Thompson & Lagattuta, 2006, for reviews of this research). Consistent with the work of Gottman and his colleagues on parental coaching, these studies indicate that when mothers frequently talk about emotions and do so with greater elaborative detail in everyday conversations, young children develop more sophisticated conceptions of emotion. In one study, for example, the frequency, complexity, and causal orientation of emotion-related conversations between mothers and their 3-year-olds predicted the child's emotion understanding at age 6 (Dunn, Brown, & Beardsall, 1991). Such conversations are important because they offer young children insight into the underlying, invisible psychological processes associated with emotion, such as how feelings can be evoked by satisfied or frustrated desires, accurate or inaccurate expectations, or memories of past events. These insights are difficult for preschoolers to comprehend on their own, and conversations are important also because they provide an avenue for parents to convey their own beliefs about emotion and emotion regulation to offspring. Parents discuss emotions differently with daughters than with sons, for example, using more elaboration and a greater relational focus with daughters (Fivush, 1998), and subcultural and cultural values also guide these emotion-focused conversations (Miller, Fung, & Mintz, 1996; Miller, Potts, Fung, Hoogstra, & Mintz, 1990; Miller & Sperry, 1987).

Parent–child conversations provide a conceptual foundation to the growth of emotion regulation by providing children with the means of understanding how to influence their emotional experience. As conversation contributes to young children's comprehension of the internal constituents of emotional arousal, for example, they also learn that feelings can be altered by redirecting attention, thinking distracting thoughts, altering the physiological dimensions of emotion (e.g., breathing deeply), and leaving or altering the situation as well as by seeking assistance. Children also acquire from such conversations an understanding of the normative expectations for emotion self-management in social situations. Although parents may also directly suggest strategies of emotion management, conversations involving emotional themes also offer young children a conceptual foundation for the construction of their own understanding of emotion regulation.

Little research, however, has been devoted to parent–child conversations about emotion regulation. This is surprising because parents commonly coach offspring about the need to manage their feelings and often suggest specific strategies for doing so, especially when children are in public settings or stressful circumstances (Miller & Green, 1985). In an interesting ethnographic study, Miller and Sperry (1987) described the socialization of anger and aggression by the mothers of three 2½-year-old girls growing up in a lower-income neighborhood in south Baltimore. Consistent with the need for assertiveness and self-defense in this environment, the mothers sought to "toughen" their young daughters by coaching, as well as modeling, reinforcing, and rehearsing specific strategies of anger expression and self-control that were adaptive to their community setting. As a consequence, their daughters developed a rich repertoire of expressive modes for conveying anger but were also capable of regulating its arousal and expression consistently with the rules of the subculture. Further research into how parents socialize emotion regulation in conversational contexts is clearly warranted.

In advancing research on this topic, two further directions should be noted. First, parents and other adults guide the development of emotion regulation through conversational discourse in diverse ways (Thompson, 1990). They can influence children's self-regulation directly by coaching coping strategies, but they also do so by managing information the child receives about potentially upsetting or stressful events (such as describing an anticipated dentist visit as "teeth tickling"). They can enlist feeling rules or emotion scripts that guide the child's assessment of appropriate emotional responding for the situation (e.g., "We don't make a fuss when we're at someone's house"). Parents can also manage the child's emotion by encouraging a conceptual reassessment of the circumstances, such as eliciting sympathy for a physically challenged person of whom the child is afraid or amused. Each of these conversational prompts contributes to emotion regulation by altering the child's cognitive appraisals of the situation to diminish or alter the emotional response (see Gross & Thompson, this volume).

Second, conversations with peers and siblings are also important catalysts to the growth of emotion regulation in childhood. Young children talk about their feelings more frequently with friends and siblings than they do with their mothers, and these conversations also contribute to developing emotional understanding (Brown, Donelan-McCall, & Dunn, 1996; Hughes & Dunn, 1998). As children mature and peer experiences become increasingly important, emotion talk between friends becomes a unique means of affective self-disclosure in close friendships, learning group norms for feeling rules, observing and evaluating examples of emotion self-management in the peer group, and offering and obtaining support for competent emotion self-regulation (Gottman & Parker, 1986). Children need these experiences for learning how emotion self-regulation is different with peers than at home. Indeed, there is reason to believe that many of the skills of emotion self-regulation acquired in family experiences may not generalize well to the peer environment in light of the different norms and emotion scripts pertinent to each setting, and thus peer conversations among friends are uniquely important experiences for acquiring the skills relevant to interactions among agemates. This is another influence on the growth of emotion regulation and merits further research inquiry.

Parent–Child Relationship Quality

When social influences on children are concerned, *what* happens and *who* does it are both important. Most of the socialization influences on emotion regulation discussed in this chapter occur in a relational context, and their influence owes both to the intervention and to the relationship. Indeed, the receptiveness of children to their parents' initiatives derives from their trust in what parents say and do, especially when it concerns emotional experience, and this is why parents are uniquely influential in soothing distress, eliciting pleasure, and otherwise affecting the emotional experience of offspring. For this reason, however, differences in the trust and security of the parent–child relationship have important implications for the development of emotion regulation.

According to Cassidy (1994) and Thompson (1994; Thompson, Laible, & Ontai, 2003), differences in the security of child–parent attachment may be especially significant for the growth of emotion regulation. According to these theorists, young children in secure relationships have mothers who are sensitive to and accepting of their positive and negative feelings, and who are open to talking about intense, disturbing, or confusing feelings with them. Consequently, like the offspring of emotion coaching parents, securely attached children are likely to become more emotionally self-aware, acquire greater emotion understanding, and develop a flexible capacity to manage their emotions appropriate to circumstances. Moreover, the security of the parent–child relationship provides a continuing resource of support on which the child can rely. By contrast, young children in insecure relationships have mothers who are less sensitive and more inconsistently responsive to their feelings, and who are less likely to be comfortable talking with their offspring about difficult emotional experiences. These children are likely to have more limited understanding of emotion and to become more easily emotionally dysregulated, especially in stressful circumstances, because of the lack of support in the parent–child relationship. Children may exhibit emotion dysregulation by displaying heightened, unmodulated levels of negative emotionality or, alternatively, by suppressing the expression of their negative arousal and relying on nonsocial means to regulate their feelings.

There is research evidence in support of this view. In a longitudinal study over the first 3 years, Kochanska (2001) reported that over time, insecurely attached children exhibited progressively greater fear and/or anger, and diminished joy, in standardized assessments compared with secure children. Even by age 1, the mothers of secure infants commented about both positive and negative emotions when interacting with them, while the mothers of insecurely attached infants either remarked rarely about their feelings or commented primarily about negative emotions (Goldberg, MacKay-Soroka, & Rochester, 1994). By early childhood, securely attached preschoolers talk more about emotions in everyday conversations with their mothers, and their mothers are more richly elaborative in their discussions of emotion with them. This may help to explain why secure children are also more advanced in emotion understanding (see Denham, Blair, Schmidt, & DeMulder, 2002; Thompson, 2006; Thompson et al., 2003, for reviews; see also Laible & Thompson, 1998; Raikes & Thompson, 2006). Although there has been relatively little research focused specifically on emotion regulation, there is evidence that children in secure relationships are better at managing negative emotions beginning early in life (see, e.g., Diener, Mangelsdorf, McHale, & Frosch, 2002). Gilliom and his colleagues reported that boys who were securely attached at age 1½ were observed to use more constructive anger-management strategies at age 3½ (Gilliom et al., 2002). In a study of the responses of 18-month-olds to moderate stressors, Nachmias et al. (1996) reported that postsession cortisol elevations were found only for temperamentally inhibited toddlers who were in insecure relationships with their mothers. For inhibited toddlers in secure relationships, the mother's presence helped to buffer the physiological effects of challenging events. Another study reported that by middle childhood, attachment security was significantly associated with children's constructive coping with stress, and the measure of coping mediated the association between attachment and children's peer competence (Contreras, Kerns, Weimer, Gentzler, & Tomich, 2000). Berlin and Cassidy (2003), however, reported no differences by attachment security on a measure of preschoolers' emotional self-control. More research on this topic is warranted.

These findings indicate that the relational context in which emotion regulation develops is important. It is important not only for the specific ways that parents respond to children's feelings but also for the relational support that shapes the growth of emotion self-regulation. An important topic for future research is to explore whether the influence of specific emotion regulatory interventions by parents is mediated by the broader quality of the parent–child relationship (Laible & Thompson, in press). Are children in secure relationships more responsive, for example, to parents' efforts to soothe their distress or coach emotion regulatory strategies? Further research on the association between attachment security, parent–child conversation, and the development of emotion regulation is also warranted. Research of this kind can elucidate how emotional development is colored by the quality of early relationships.

CONCLUSION

In the broadest sense, the research surveyed in this chapter confirms how significantly social influences shape the growth of emotional experience and emotion regulation. Although our review has focused on family influences, it is also apparent (although less intensively studied) that peer influences are important to the growth of emotion regulation, especially in contexts outside the home. Beyond this conclusion, the studies discussed here focus attention on the broader issue of the social construction of emotional life. If it is true that the growth of emotion regulation is shaped by the multifaceted extrinsic influences that we have considered, including the varieties of direct interventions to alter children's emotional experiences, social evaluations and responses to children's feelings, the emotional climate of the family, direct parental coaching of coping strategies, proactive management of emotionally arousing circumstances, the modeling provided by the parent's emotional expressiveness, parent–child conversations that influence children's developing conceptions of emotion and of emotion regulatory processes, and the quality of family relationships, then emotions theory must include a significant role for the socialization of emotion along with the influences of biology, the developing construction of emotional experience, and other processes.

Throughout this discussion, we have also highlighted topics for future research. A general comment is warranted, however, about the need for greater clarity in conceptualizing and assessing emotion regulation in developmental research. As we have noted, measures of emotion regulation and its outcomes have often conflated direct assessments of emotion regulatory processes with its correlates or even substituted the latter for the former. It is common, for example, to find studies of emotion regulation in which regulation assessments combine measures of attentional regulation and cognitive or behavioral self-control with those of emotion management. As a result, it is often unclear what is precisely being measured. Although it is undoubted that emotion regulation shares common variance with measures of attentional, cognitive, and behavioral self-control, these facets of self-regulation also have significant independent sources of variance that make their aggregation in developmental research interpretively problematic. In a similar manner, studies of parental influences on emotion regulation often assess social competence or cooperation as outcomes in children rather than directly measuring emotion regulation. It is unwise to assume that individual differences in emotion regulation are accurately indexed by its positive correlates, partly because these outcomes are multidetermined and may not reflect emotion regulation at all. To be sure, we have noted that differences in emotion self-regulation in children are predictive of differences in social competence and cooperation (although the extent of the prediction varies with age and context), but it is likely that differences in emotion self-regulation also predict children's competence at deception, social manipulation, and other less desirable social outcomes. It is best, therefore, to study emotion regulation directly and enlist further research to clarify the nature of its correlates.

We believe that future progress in developmental research on emotion regulation will benefit from enlisting multiple strategies that each offer a window into this compelling but dauntingly complex developmental process. One essential strategy is, of course, to refine procedures for directly assessing children's management of their feelings, especially in carefully designed experimental contexts in which the child's emotion goals for the situation are straightforward (such as coping with a frustrating task) and specific behaviors can be appraised in relation to this goal (see Cole et al., 2004, for an insightful analysis of relevant methodological approaches). In these contexts, it can be especially valuable to understand children's constructions of their emotional experiences during these episodes through age-appropriate interview probes, because understanding their emotion goals is essential to appropriately interpreting their behavior.

But directly assessing emotion regulation as it occurs is not the only strategy for achieving insight into this developmental process. Another is to deepen understanding of children's comprehension of their emotions, its correlates, and their purposes for managing their feelings. Because their visceral arousal is one of the ways they are aware of emotionality, for example, how much do children know about the association between emotion and enhanced heart rate, "butterflies" in the stomach, and other visceral cues? We have few data with which to answer this question, nor do we know very much about why children seek to control their feelings in everyday circumstances. Because there is reason to believe that children's emotional goals are not necessarily the same as those of adults (Levine, Stein, & Liwag, 1999), it is likely that developmental changes in emotion regulation arise, at least in part, from changes in how children construe their emotional experiences and the needs for emotional self-control. This is a research issue worthy of further attention.

The socialization of emotion regulation involves parents, of course, and another strategy to understanding the growth of emotion regulation focuses on elucidating the socialization processes discussed in this chapter. As we have noted, much more remains to be learned about (1) the manner in which positive and negative emotions are expressed in the family and their influence on children's developing capacities for emotion regulation, (2) parental emotion coaching and emotion-dismissing strategies and their relevance to developing skills at emotion management, (3) how parents talk with their children about emotion and its influence on developing conceptions of emotion and emotion regulation, and (4) the influence of the overall quality of the parent–child relationship on specific processes of emotion socialization. In each of these areas, it is especially important to understand how adults interpret their own emotional experiences as well as the reasons, means, and outcomes of regulating their feelings because these beliefs are likely to influence how they respond to offspring. Adults who believe that it is better not to express one's emotions (whether positive or negative), who have difficulty comprehending why they feel as they do, or who value self-control are likely to approach the socialization of emotion regulation in offspring in very different ways. Much more also remains to be learned about how parents interpret the emotions of their children as they seek to manage and coach emotion regulation skills.

A fourth convergent strategy for future research is to explore other social influences on the development of emotion regulation, especially from peers and siblings. The research discussed in this chapter offers strong suggestions that unique understanding of emotion, and of the requirements for managing one's feelings (especially outside the home), is acquired from children who are closer in age than are parents at home. As children mature, it is likely that they begin to comprehend the distinct emotional rules that apply to home, sibling, and peer contexts, and this probably deepens their skill and flexibility in managing their feelings in unknown ways.

These different but complementary research strategies highlight, of course, the complexity of this developmental phenomenon that warrants study because of its association with our understanding of emotional development, psychological well-being, and social functioning. Understanding the importance of the socialization of emotion regulation confirms that in addition to its biological foundations and connections to personality, emotional development is significantly shaped by children's social experiences.

REFERENCES

Berlin, L. J., & Cassidy, J. (2003). Mothers' self-reported control of their preschool children's emotional expressiveness: A longitudinal study of associations with infant-mother attachment and children's emotion regulation. *Social Development, 12,* 474–495.

Brown, J. R., Donelan-McCall, N., & Dunn, J. (1996). Why talk about mental states?: The significance of children's conversations with friends, siblings, and mothers. *Child Development, 67,* 836–849.

Calkins, S. D., & Hill, A. (2007). Caregiver influences on emerging emotion regulation: Biological and environmental transactions in early development. In J. J. Gross (Ed.), *Handbook of emotion regulation* (pp. 229–248). New York: Guilford Press.

Calkins, S. D., & Johnson, M. C. (1998). Toddler regulation of distress to frustrating events: Temperamental and maternal correlates. *Infant Behavior and Development, 21,* 379–395.

Camras, L. A., Oster, H., Campos, J. J., & Bakeman, R. (2003). Emotional facial expressions in European-American, Japanese, and Chinese infants. In P. Ekman, J. Campos, R. Davidson, & F. de Waal (Eds.), *Emotions inside out: 130 years after Darwin's The Expression of the Emotions in Man and Animals* (pp. 1–17). New York: New York Academy of Sciences.

Caspi, A., Moffitt, T. E., Morgan, J., Rutter, M., Taylor, A., Arseneault, L., et al. (2004). Maternal expressed emotion predicts children's antisocial behavior problems: Using monozygotic-twin differences to identify environmental effects on behavioral development. *Developmental Psychology, 40,* 149–161.

Cassidy, J. (1994). Emotion regulation: Influences of attachment relationships. In N. A. Fox (Ed.), The development of emotion regulation and dysregulation: Biological and behavioral aspects. *Monographs of the Society for Research in Child Development, 59*(2–3, Serial No. 240), 228–249.

Cohn, J., Campbell, S., Matias, R., & Hopkins, J. (1990). Face-to-face interactions of postpartum depressed and nondepressed mother–infant pairs at 2 months. *Developmental Psychology, 26,* 15–23.

Cole, P., Martin, S., & Dennis, T. (2004). Emotion regulation as a scientific construct: Methodological challenges and directions for child development research. *Child Development, 75,* 317–333.

Contreras, J. M., Kerns, K. A., Weimer, B. L., Gentzler, A. L., & Tomich, P. L. (2000). Emotion regulation as a mediator of associations between mother–child attachment and peer relationships in middle childhood. *Journal of Family Psychology, 14,* 111–124.

Cummings, E. M., & Davies, P. T. (1994). Maternal depression and child development. *Journal of Child Psychology and Psychiatry, 35,* 73–112.

Davidson, R. J., Fox, A., & Kalin, N. H. (2007). Neural bases of emotion regulation in nonhuman primates and humans. In J. J. Gross (Ed.), *Handbook of emotion regulation* (pp. 47–68). New York: Guilford Press.

Davies, P., & Cummings, E. (1994). Marital conflict and child adjustment: An emotional security hypothesis. *Psychological Bulletin, 116,* 387–411.

Davies, P. T., & Forman, E. M. (2002). Children's patterns of preserving emotional security in the interparental subsystem. *Child Development, 73,* 1880–1903.

Davies, P. T., Harold, G. T., Goeke-Morey, M. C., & Cummings, E. M. (2002). Child emotional security and interparental conflict. *Monographs of the Society for Research in Child Development, 67*(Serial No. 270).

Denham, S. (1997). "When I have a bad dream mommy holds me": Preschoolers' conceptions of emotions, parental socialization, and emotional competence. *International Journal of Behavioral Development, 20,* 301–319.

Denham, S. (1998). *Emotional development in young children.* New York: Guilford Press.

Denham, S., Bassett, H. H., & Wyatt, T. (in press). The socialization of emotional competence. In J. Grusec & P. Hastings (Eds.), *Handbook of socialization*. New York: Guilford Press.

Denham, S., Blair, K., Schmidt, M., & DeMulder, E. (2002). Compromised emotional competence: Seeds of violence sown early? *American Journal of Orthopsychiatry, 72,* 70–82.

Diener, M. L., Mangelsdorf, S. C., McHale, J. L., & Frosch, C. A. (2002). Infants' behavioral strategies for emotion regulation with father and mothers: Associations with emotional expressions and attachment quality. *Infancy, 3,* 153–174.

Dunn, J., Brown, J., & Beardsall, L. (1991). Family talk about feeling states and children's later understanding of others' emotions. *Developmental Psychology, 27,* 448–455.

Dunsmore, J. C., & Halberstadt, A. G. (1997). How does family emotional expressiveness affect children's schemas. In K. C. Barrett (Ed.), The communication of emotion: Current research from diverse perspectives. *New Directions for Child Development, 77,* 45–68.

Eisenberg, N., Cumberland, A., & Spinrad, T. L. (1998). Parental socialization of emotion. *Psychological Inquiry, 9,* 241–273.

Eisenberg, N., & Fabes, R. (1994). Mothers' reactions to children's negative emotions: Relations to children's temperament and anger behavior. *Merrill-Palmer Quarterly, 40,* 138–156.

Eisenberg, N., Fabes, R. A., & Murphy, B. C. (1996). Parents' reactions to children's negative emotions: Relations to children's social competence and comforting behavior. *Child Development, 67,* 2227–2247.

Eisenberg, N., Fabes, R. A., Shepard, S. A., Guthrie, I. K., Murphy, B. C., & Reiser, M. (1999). Parental reactions to children's negative emotions: Longitudinal relations to quality of children's social functioning. *Child Development, 70,* 513–534.

Eisenberg, N., Gershoff, E. T., Fabes, R. A., Shepard, S. A., Cumberland, A. J., Losoya, S. H., et al. (2001). Mothers' emotional expressivity and children's behavior problems and social competence: Mediation through children's regulation. *Developmental Psychology, 37,* 475–490.

Eisenberg, N., Hofer, C., & Vaughan, J. (2007). Effortful control and its socioemotional consequences. In J. J. Gross (Ed.), *Handbook of emotion regulation* (pp. 287–306). New York: Guilford Press.

Eisenberg, N., Valiente, C., Morris, A. S., Fabes, R. A., Cumberland, A., Reiser, M., et al. (2003). Longitudinal relations among parental emotional expressivity, children's regulation, and quality of socioemotional functioning. *Developmental Psychology, 39,* 3–19.

Fabes, R. A., Leonard, S. A., Kupanoff, K., & Martin, C. L. (2001). Parental coping with children's negative emotions: Relations with children's emotional and social responding. *Child Development, 72,* 907–920.

Feldman, R., Greenbaum, C. W., & Yirmiya, N. (1999). Mother–infant affect synchrony as an antecedent of the emergence of self-control. *Developmental Psychology, 35,* 223–231.

Field, T., Healy, B., Goldstein, S., & Guthertz, M. (1990). Behavior-state matching and synchrony in mother–infant interactions of nondepressed versus depressed dyads. *Developmental Psychology, 26,* 7–14.

Field, T., Healy, B., Goldstein, S., Perry, S., Bendell, D., Schanberg, S., et al. (1988). Infants of depressed mothers show "depressed" behavior even with nondepressed adults. *Child Development, 59,* 1569–1579.

Fivush, R. (1998). Gendered narratives: Elaboration, structure, and emotion in parent–child reminiscing across the preschool years. In C. P. Thompson & D. J. Herrmann (Eds.), *Autobiographical memory: Theoretical and applied perspectives* (pp. 79–103). Mahwah, NJ: Erlbaum.

Fox, N. A., & Calkins, S. D. (2003). The development of self-control of emotion: Intrinsic and extrinsic influences. *Motivation and Emotion, 27,* 7–26.

Gekoski, M., Rovee-Collier, C., & Carulli-Rabinowitz, V. (1983). A longitudinal analysis of inhibition of infant distress: The origins of social expectations? *Infant Behavior and Development, 6,* 339–351.

Gianino, A., & Tronick, E. (1988). The mutual regulation model: The infant's self and interactive regulation and coping and defensive capacities. In T. Field, P. McCabe, & N. Schneiderman (Eds.), *Stress and coping* (Vol. 2, pp. 47–68). Hillsdale, NJ: Erlbaum.

Gilliom, M., Shaw, D. S., Beck, J. E., Schonberg, M. A., & Lukon, J. L. (2002). Anger regulation in disadvantaged preschool boys: Strategies, antecedents, and the development of self-control. *Developmental Psychology, 38,* 222–235.

Goldberg, S., MacKay-Soroka, S., & Rochester, M. (1994). Affect, attachment, and maternal responsiveness. *Infant Behavior and Development, 17,* 335–339.

Goodman, S. H., & Gotlib, I. H. (1999). Risk for psychopathology in the children of depressed mothers: A developmental model for understanding mechanisms of transmission. *Psychological Review, 106*, 458–490.

Gottman, J. M., Katz, L. F., & Hooven, C. (1996). Parental meta-emotion philosophy and the emotional life of families: Theoretical models and preliminary data. *Journal of Family Psychology, 10*, 243–268.

Gottman, J. M., Katz, L. F., & Hooven, C. (1997). *Meta-emotion: How families communicate emotionally.* Mahwah, NJ: Erlbaum.

Gottman, J. M., & Parker, J. (Eds.). (1986). *Conversations of friends: Speculations on affective development.* New York: Cambridge University Press.

Gross, J. J., & Thompson, R. A. (2007). Emotion regulation: Conceptual foundations. In J. J. Gross (Ed.), *Handbook of emotion regulation* (pp. 3–24). New York: Guilford Press.

Gunnar, M., & Vazquez, D. (2006). Stress neurobiology and developmental psychopathology. In D. Cicchetti & D. Cohen (Eds.), *Developmental psychopathology* (2nd ed.). Vol. III. Risk, disorder, and adaptation (pp. 533–577). New York: Wiley.

Halberstadt, A. G., Crisp, V. W., & Eaton, K. L. (1999). Family expressiveness: A retrospective and new directions for research. In P. Philippot & R. S. Feldman (Eds.), *The social context of nonverbal behavior* (pp. 109–155). New York: Cambridge University Press.

Halberstadt, A. G., & Eaton, K. L. (2003). A meta-analysis of family expressiveness and children's emotion expressiveness and understanding. *Marriage and Family Review, 34*, 35–62.

Hooley, J. M., & Richters, J. E. (1995). Expressed emotion: A developmental perspective. In D. Cicchetti & S. Toth (Eds.), *Emotion, cognition, and representation* (pp. 133–166). Rochester, NY: University of Rochester Press.

Hooven, C., Gottman, J. M., & Katz, L. F. (1995). Parental meta-emotion structure predicts family and child outcomes. *Cognition and Emotion, 9*, 229–264.

Hughes, C., & Dunn, J. (1998). Understanding mind and emotion: Longitudinal associations with mental-state talk between young friends. *Developmental Psychology, 34*, 1026–1037.

Klinnert, M., Campos, J., Sorce, J., Emde, R., & Svejda, M. (1983). Emotions as behavior regulators: Social referencing in infancy. In R. Plutchik & H. Kellerman (Eds.), *Emotion: Theory, research, and experience*, Vol. 2. *Emotions in early development* (pp. 57–86). New York: Academic Press.

Kochanska, G. (2001). Emotional development in children with different attachment histories: The first three years. *Child Development, 72*, 474–490.

Kopp, C. B. (1989). Regulation of distress and negative emotions: A developmental review. *Developmental Psychology, 25*, 343–354.

Lagattuta, K., & Thompson, R. A. (in press). The development of self-conscious emotions: Cognitive processes and social influences. In R. W. Robins & J. Tracy (Eds.), *Self-conscious emotions* (2nd ed.). New York: Guilford Press.

Laible, D. J., & Thompson, R. A. (1998). Attachment and emotional understanding in preschool children. *Developmental Psychology, 34*(5), 1038–1045.

Laible, D. J., & Thompson, R. A. (in press). Early socialization: A relational perspective. In J. Grusec & P. Hastings (Eds.), *Handbook of socialization* (rev. ed.). New York: Guilford Press.

Lamb, M. (1981). Developing trust and perceived effectance in infancy. In L. Lipsitt (Ed.), *Advances in infancy research* (Vol. 1, pp. 101–127). New York: Ablex.

Lamb, M., & Malkin, C. (1986). The development of social expectations in distress-relief sequences: A longitudinal study. *International Journal of Behavioral Development, 9*, 235–249.

Levine, L., Stein, N., & Liwag, M. (1999). Remembering children's emotions: Sources of concordant and discordant accounts between parents and children. *Developmental Psychology, 35*, 790–801.

Malatesta, C., Culver, C., Tesman, J., & Shepard, B. (1989). The development of emotion expression during the first two years of life. *Monographs of the Society for Research in Child Development, 54*(1–2, Serial No. 219).

Malatesta, C., Grigoryev, P., Lamb, C., Albin, M., & Culver, C. (1986). Emotion socialization and expressive development in preterm and full-term infants. *Child Development, 57*, 316–330.

Miller, P. J., Fung, H., & Mintz, J. (1996). Self-construction through narrative practices: A Chinese and American comparison of early socialization. *Ethos, 24*(2), 237–280.

Miller, P. J., Potts, R., Fung, H., Hoogstra, L., & Mintz, J. (1990). Narrative practices and the social construction of self in childhood. *American Ethnologist, 17*(2), 292–311.

Miller, P. J., & Sperry, L. (1987). The socialization of anger and aggression. *Merrill-Palmer Quarterly, 33*, 1–31.

Miller, S. M., & Green, M. L. (1985). Coping with stress and frustration: Origins, nature, and development. In M. Lewis & C. Saarni (Eds.), *The socialization of emotions* (pp. 263–314). New York: Plenum Press.

Nachmias, M., Gunnar, M., Mangelsdorf, S., Parritz, R. H., & Buss, K. (1996). Behavioral inhibition and stress reactivity: The moderating role of attachment security. *Child Development, 67*, 508–522.

Raikes, H. A., & Thompson, R. A. (2006). Family emotional climate, attachment security, and young children's emotion understanding in a high-risk sample. *British Journal of Developmental Psychology, 24*, 989–104.

Ramsden, S. R., & Hubbard, J. A. (2002). Family expressiveness and parental emotion coaching: Their role in children's emotion regulation and aggression. *Journal of Abnormal Child Psychology, 30*, 657–667.

Roberts, W., & Strayer, J. (1987). Parents' responses to the emotional distress of their children: Relations with children's competence. *Developmental Psychology, 23*, 415–422.

Rogosch, F., Cicchetti, D., & Toth, S. (2004). Expressed emotion in multiple subsystems of the families of toddlers with depressed mothers. *Development and Psychopathology, 16*, 689–709.

Rothbart, M. K., & Sheese, B. E. (2007). Temperament and emotion regulation. In J. J. Gross (Ed.), *Handbook of emotion regulation* (pp. 331–350). New York: Guilford Press.

Saarni, C. (1999). *The development of emotional competence.* New York: Guilford Press.

Sawyer, K. S., Denham, S., DeMulder, E., Blair, K., Auerbach-Major, S., & Levitas, J. (2002). The contribution of older siblings' reactions to emotions to preschoolers' emotional and social competence. *Marriage and Family Review, 34*, 183–212.

Stegge, H., & Meerum Terwogt, M. (2007). Awareness and regulation of emotion in typical and atypical development. In J. J. Gross (Ed.), *Handbook of emotion regulation* (pp. 269–286). New York: Guilford Press.

Thompson, R. A. (1990). Emotion and self-regulation. In R. A. Thompson (Ed.), *Socioemotional development. Nebraska Symposium on Motivation* (Vol. 36, pp. 383–483). Lincoln: University of Nebraska Press.

Thompson, R. A. (1994). Emotion regulation: A theme in search of definition. In N. A. Fox (Ed.), The development of emotion regulation and dysregulation: Biological and behavioral aspects. *Monographs of the Society for Research in Child Development, 59*(2–3, Serial No. 240), 25–52.

Thompson, R. A. (2000). Childhood anxiety disorders from the perspective of emotion regulation and attachment. In M. W. Vasey & M. R. Dadds (Eds.), *The developmental psychopathology of anxiety* (pp. 160–182). Oxford, UK: Oxford University Press.

Thompson, R. A. (2006). The development of the person: Social understanding, relationships, self, conscience. In W. Damon & R. M. Lerner (Eds.), N. Eisenberg (Vol. Ed.), *Handbook of child psychology* (6th ed.): *Vol. 3. Social, emotional, and personality development* (pp. 24–98). New York: Wiley.

Thompson, R. A., & Calkins, S. (1996). The double-edged sword: Emotional regulation for children at risk. *Development and Psychopathology* [Special Issue on Regulatory Processes], *8*(1), 163–182.

Thompson, R. A., Flood, M. F., & Goodvin, R. (2006). Social support and developmental psychopathology. In D. Cicchetti & D. Cohen (Eds.), *Developmental psychopathology* (2nd ed.): *Vol. III. Risk, disorder, and adaptation* (pp. 1–37). New York: Wiley.

Thompson, R. A., & Lagatutta, K. (2006). Feeling and understanding: Early emotional development. In K. McCartney & D. Phillips (Ed.), *The Blackwell handbook of early childhood development* (pp. 317–337). Oxford, UK: Blackwell.

Thompson, R. A., Laible, D. J., & Ontai, L. L. (2003). Early understanding of emotion, morality, and the self: Developing a working model. In R. V. Kail (Ed.), *Advances in child development and behavior* (Vol. 31, pp. 137–171). San Diego, CA: Academic Press.

Valiente, C., Fabes, R. A., Eisenberg, N., & Spinrad, T. L. (2004). The relations of parental expressivity and support to children's coping with daily stress. *Journal of Family Psychology, 18*, 97–106.

CHAPTER 13

Awareness and Regulation of Emotion in Typical and Atypical Development

HEDY STEGGE
MARK MEERUM TERWOGT

Proficiency in emotion regulation is a developmental achievement. Young children are mainly dependent on the social environment for the successful management of their feeling states. With age, children begin to take a more active role and become skilled at regulating emotions through their own efforts (Denham, 1998). In this learning process, children's increasing ability to reflect on their own and other people's feelings plays an important role. Abstractive reflection is supported by the acquirement of a progressively more explicit and integrated emotion knowledge base that enhances flexibility in children's responses to emotion-eliciting events (Meerum Terwogt & Olthof, 1989; Meerum Terwogt & Stegge, 2002).

In this chapter, we first discuss the core features of the emotion process and argue that the awareness of an emotion stimulates engagement in voluntary regulatory activity. Second, we discuss the critical contribution of explicit emotion knowledge to the process of reflection. Third, the knowledge components that are most crucial to successful regulation are discussed: children's reasoning about the causes of emotion and their knowledge of strategic emotional responding. We then turn to some of the implications of a lack of awareness of emotion for adaptive functioning. Specifically, we discuss awareness and regulation problems in aggressive children and in children with depressive symptoms. Finally, we argue that the social environment should help children acquire a two-level emotion theory in which the autonomous nature of the emotion process is emphasized as well as its status as a to-be-regulated phenomenon.

EMOTION, EMOTION REGULATION, AND EMOTIONAL AWARENESS

Contemporary theories highlight the potentially adaptive and informative value of emotions. Emotions signal the need to change or adjust our behavior in the face of environmental challenges and function to help us realize our short- and long-term intrapersonal and interpersonal needs. Although emotions have proven difficult to define, researchers generally agree on some of their core features. The emotion system can be depicted as a kind of radar and response facility that enables us to quickly *appraise* and *respond to* situations that are relevant to our well-being. (Cole, Martin, & Dennis, 2004; Levenson, 1999; see also Gross & Thompson, this volume). The core of the system consists of an efficient processor that continually matches situations to personal goals. When this primary appraisal process results in a match, an emotion is activated and an attendant response tendency is automatically recruited in order to solve the problem. Harm inflicted on the self, for example, activates the anger system and its associated action tendency: the urge to attack. Similarly, fear is a response to (physical) threat that elicits the tendency to escape from the pertaining danger.

The response package generated by the emotional core system allows for the successful management of prototypical situations that are critical for survival. In the case of imminent danger (a looming car accident or a violent attack), we are able to respond immediately without having to engage in time-consuming thoughts about the best way to react. However, the action programs elicited by the emotional core system are necessarily stereotypical and do not always serve our best interests. Fine-tuning to situational demands is often required, especially when long-term objectives differ from short-term goals and in situations in which other people are involved. Therefore, two-level emotion theories (Levenson, 1999) assume that humans are endowed with a cognitive control system that acts on the activity of the core system in two ways. Cognitive processes may change the appraisal of the input of the system, or they may change response probabilities and thereby influence the actual output of the system. Gross and Thompson (this volume) refer to these different processes as antecedent-focused and response-focused regulation, respectively.

Two-level theories typically distinguish an initial stage of emotion activation and a subsequent stage of emotion regulation. It should be noted, however, that emotion activation involves a continuous process in which both feedback and feed-forward mechanisms are constantly active. As Gross and Thompson (this volume) argue, "regulation occurs in the context of an ongoing stream of emotional stimulation and behavioural responding." People not only influence their emotional responses from the very beginning to the very end but may even try to prevent an emotion being generated in the first place. Emotion regulation seems to be embedded in emotion activation in all phases of the process (Compas, Frankel, & Camras, 2004; see also Frijda, 1986). Although this complicates definitional issues, we follow Gross and Thompson in adopting a two-level approach, because this seems useful for conceptual and analytic purposes. Moreover, neuroscientists suggest that emotion regulation can be studied separately by focusing on one salient aspect of regulatory activity (i.e., cognitive control) (Lewis & Stieben, 2004). In this chapter, our focus is also on cognitive control and, by implication, on voluntary regulatory activity (see also Eisenberg & Spinrad, 2004).

The activation of the basic emotion program along with its corresponding action tendencies usually results in the *experience* of an emotion. In fact, the experience of an emotion is often considered to be its most characteristic feature (cf. Frijda's definition of emotion as a *felt* action tendency). Recent theoretical accounts increasingly emphasize that rather than being a mere epiphenomenon, the *awareness* of an emotion helps people to engage in voluntary controlled action and may thus promote adaptive behavior (e.g., Levenson, 1999; but see LeDoux, 1996, for a different view). In a thoughtful analysis of the content of emotional experience, Lambie and Marcel (2002) argue that there are different ways in which people can be aware of their feelings. They distinguish first-order phenomenal experience from second-order awareness of this experience. Whereas the phenomenological aspect of an emotion state merely refers to "what it's like," second-order awareness refers to thoughts about the experience (including the conscious experience of one's bodily state) and/or to an awareness of the experience *as* a specific emotion (anger, fear, sadness, etc.). In second-order awareness, we focus on *how* we feel, *why* we feel the way we feel, and *what we can do about it.* It is second-order emotional awareness that stimulates voluntary regulatory activity, and the quality and outcome of this appraisal process is dependent on one's general framework of knowledge of emotion (see also Feldman Barrett, Gross, Christensen, & Benvenuto, 2001; Lane & Pollerman, 2002). In the next section, we elaborate on the question of why it is important to study the child's developing conception of the emotion process.

WHY STUDY THE CHILD'S KNOWLEDGE OF EMOTION?

In the early 1980s, researchers such as Paul Harris, Susan Harter, and Carolyn Saarni started to take an explicit interest in children's conception of their own and other people's emotion processes (for an overview of these early studies, see Harris, 1989; Saarni & Harris, 1989). Later on, this type of research linked up with a large body of research on theory of mind. Both research traditions aim to describe children's reasoning about mental phenomena and are concerned with their development as naïve psychologists. Mental state knowledge helps children to adequately explain and predict behavior and in that process emotions play a crucial role.

As has already been argued, emotions are considered to be basically adaptive. They alert the individual to relevant situations and motivate him or her to take action to satisfy the protection of personal concerns (Frijda, 1986). Emotional competence involves the skill of taking full advantage of the potentials of the emotion system (Parrott, 2001). Specifically, it has been defined as the ability to adequately process emotion-laden information, to reflectively regulate emotions, and to access and generate emotional experiences to inform adaptation (Feldman Barrett et al., 2001; Mayer & Salovey, 1997; Salovey, Mayer, & Caruso, 2002). It is the ability to take a reflective, knowledge-based stance toward one's emotions. As Saarni (1999) has put it, emotional competence concerns "the ability to respond emotionally, yet simultaneously and strategically apply knowledge about emotions in interpersonal exchanges" (p. 4).

Conscious reflection on the emotional experience, its eliciting conditions, and the potentials for action enables the child to interrupt the operating emotion program and allows for flexibility. Knowledge critically influences the quality and outcome of this process and is needed for an optimal response to complex situational demands requiring a balance between multiple, often conflicting concerns (Meerum Terwogt & Olthof, 1989). For example, a careful analysis of the emotions of all parties involved in a peer conflict, combined with an insight into the negative interpersonal consequences of anger and aggression, may help the child find a satisfactory way out of this challenging situation by trying to get others to support him or her and protest together against an unjust state of affairs instead of blindly lashing out in anger.

The development of emotional understanding is dependent on the growth of language and cognition. Children develop an increasingly sophisticated conceptual framework for their own emotional experiences. Whenever an emotional situation is encountered, this knowledge base is activated and functions as an internal working model for the online-processing of the information in the prevailing episode. The degree to which the available emotional information can be put to use is dependent on the nature and the complexity of the child's conceptual framework. More differentiated and integrated knowledge helps the child to profit from the informational value of feelings to a greater extent, so that emotions can become a useful guide in the service of adaptive behavior (Arsenio & Lemerise, 2004; Lane & Pollerman, 2002; Lemerise & Arsenio, 2000). Specifically, the ability to sort experiences into discrete emotion categories (or blends of discrete emotion categories) draws the child's attention to strategies that will be useful for dealing with the prevailing event (Niedenthal, Dalle, & Rohman, 2002).

HIGHLIGHTS IN TYPICAL DEVELOPMENT

In the course of development, children learn to make representations of emotional experiences. At first, these representations concern rather fragmented bits of knowledge. A child may learn, for example, that she has to smile upon receiving a present, even if it is something she doesn't particularly like. Similarly, the child may find out that the instruction to "count to 10" when being angry helps him to refrain from responding aggressively to a provocative remark. However, these separate pieces of knowledge become far more powerful in influencing behavior when they are incorporated in more substantial theoretical notions about the emotion process. Smiling, despite being disappointed, may become a useful strategy for dealing with a variety of interpersonal situations as soon as the child understands the display rule behind the parent's instruction: We should be careful in expressing a negative emotion, because we may hurt another person's feelings. Moreover, if a child understands that emotions wane over time (Harris, 1983), that emotions can be expressed in different ways, and that it is often better to think before we act, these principles can be applied flexibly in a wide range of situations involving different emotions. The development of emotional understanding generally involves the transformation from implicit, separate bits of information to an explicit, coherent, and increasingly complex body of knowledge about the emotion process (Lane & Pollerman, 2002; Meerum Terwogt & Olthof, 1989).

Conscious reflection on emotional experiences profits from an introspective attitude on the one hand and the availability of explicit emotion knowledge on the other. We first discuss some of the major age changes in children's tendency to focus on the own inner feeling state. Next we turn to the development of children's knowledge of emotion. Specifically, we focus on those knowledge elements that are crucial for successful input and output regulation: children's understanding of the causes of emotion and their knowledge of strategic emotional responding.

Emotional Awareness:
The Saliency of External versus Internal Cues

Emotional awareness requires an introspective attitude: a child needs to consciously reflect on his or her inner experience in order to be able to identify it as an *emotional* experience. An early interview study by Harris, Olthof, and Meerum Terwogt (1981) has shown that direct questions about emotional awareness ("How do you know that you are happy?") do elicit references to the inner feeling state in 10-year-old children: "I know that I am happy because I *feel* happy." However, 6-year-old children do not seem to appreciate the conscious experience of an inner feeling state as the crucial component. They refer to observable, external elements instead: I know that I'm happy "because it's my birthday," or "because I sing and dance." Similarly, in a series of studies, Flavell and colleagues (Flavell, Green, & Flavell, 1993, 1995) have shown that young children strongly rely on external cues in answering questions about people's mental activity. Preschoolers correctly infer that someone is thinking only when there is clear visible evidence available (i.e., when the person shows a pensive-looking face or is asked to solve a difficult problem). In contrast, they deny that a person is thinking when he or she is merely waiting. Young children were also shown to have only limited awareness of their own mental activity. When asked to reflect on the content of their own consciousness during a waiting period, they deny that they have been thinking. Given the fact that human mental activity can best be characterized as an ongoing "stream of consciousness," this was taken as a sign of young children's limited introspective abilities. Young children's tendency to deny that they have been thinking, even in a situation in which they were presented with something thought provoking, further supports this explanation.

There is reason to assume that children's introspective skills continue to improve during the late elementary school years (Selman, 1981). As a lack of introspection seems to provide a plausible explanation for children's limited knowledge of consciousness and some of the core features of the thinking process, the studies by Flavell and colleagues provide indirect evidence for this claim. It has been shown, for example, that even 6- and 7-year-olds do not always acknowledge that the mind generates a stream of consciousness, and that a sleeping person lacks consciousness and the ability to control mental activity (Flavell, Green, Flavell, & Lin, 1999). Moreover, children's understanding of cognitive cuing was shown to increase gradually between the ages of 5 and 13. With age, children seem to become more aware of the fact that one thought automatically triggers other related thoughts, that people therefore often have unwanted thoughts, and that it is hard to get rid of them (Flavell, Green, & Flavell, 1998).

A study by Casey (1993) on children's responses to an *in vivo* emotion-eliciting situation provides further evidence for their growing introspective skills with age. In this study, children were given positive or negative feedback when playing a game. Their emotional expressions were observed and shortly (95 seconds) after the feedback stimulus, their emotion reports and understanding were obtained in a postgame interview. It was shown that there were stronger relations between emotion expression and report among 12-year-olds than among 7-year-olds, which might reflect older children's greater capacity for self-awareness. When asked how they knew they felt the way they did, both younger and older children referred to stimulus characteristics or distinctive emotion cues (e.g., bodily sensations). Interestingly, older children, but not younger ones, invoked enduring personality characteristics ("I feel good when I have puzzles to solve and do well"), which may indicate that the repeated observation of our own emotional responses contributes to more general self-knowledge in the emotion domain.

Causes of Emotion: What Do I Feel and Why?

At about 2 to 3 years of age, children start to use simple emotion words ("happy," "sad," "mad") in a causal way ("grandma mad," "I wrote on wall"; Bretherton & Beeghly, 1982), thereby demonstrating an early understanding of the link between situation and emotion. In subsequent years, their knowledge about the causes of emotion increases rapidly and is elaborated in a number of ways. First, the capacity for belief–desire reasoning helps the child understand that one and the same situation may evoke different emotions in different people. Second, the tendency to analyze events at greater causal depth promotes children's understanding of multiple and complex emotions.

Beliefs, Desires and Emotion

People do not react to the world as such but to their own mental representation (in terms of mental states like beliefs and desires) of the situation at hand. For quite some time it was assumed that this notion developed between the ages of 3 and 4. However, recent evidence shows that children 15 months of age already acknowledge that people act according to their beliefs, even if these beliefs are false and do not reflect the true state of affairs as known to the child (Onishi & Baillargeon, 2005). Findings such as this give rise to the suggestion that children might have some inborn capacity to use the hypothetical construct of a "mental state" in order to make sense of people's actions. However, innate or not, young children's understanding of how the mind mediates people's behavior becomes more profound over a long period of time as a result of enculturation into the language community (Perner & Ruffman, 2005). Language skills and the presence of knowledgeable others in their direct environment (usually older siblings) tend to speed up theory of mind development (Jenkins & Astington, 1996).

The insight that behavior is mediated by mental states helps children understand why people react differently to one and the same situation: They hold different beliefs and/or desires concerning that situation. The basic theory also helps them to make a plausible guess about what is going on in the black box of other people's minds. Someone who refuses the candy we present may not *like* candies or perhaps *thinks* that this particular candy will not taste good. We can use the information deduced from this specific event in the future (for instance, by not offering candy to this person anymore based on the prediction that he or she probably will refuse again) or seek further information to test your initial hypothesis. For instance, the direct question "Don't you like candy?" might provoke the unexpected answer, "Oh yes, I do, but I have eaten too much candy already today" (i.e., I do not like it at this particular moment).

Belief–desire information not only enables one to predict behavior but can also be used to predict an emotional reaction. At the age of 3, children start to use goal-outcome information to predict or explain a story character's emotional response: getting what we want or avoiding something we don't want results in a positive emotion, whereas not being able to get something we want or getting something we don't want elicits a negative emotion (Stein & Levine, 1989; see also Denham & Kochanoff, 2002). However, it is not until several years later that children are able to adequately apply the more complex belief–desire reasoning to the domain of emotion. Children now realize that it is not so much the actual fulfillment of a desire but rather the person's thoughts about the relation between goal and outcome that determines the emotion. If Ellie likes cola and she *thinks* there is cola in her mug, she will be happy, even if her belief is false because someone has secretly switched its content and replaced it by something Ellie does not like at all. It is not before the age of 6 that children are fully capable of predicting such false belief-based emotions correctly (Harris, Johnson, Hutton, Andrews, & Cooke, 1989). Unlike behavior, the emotional state is still a hypothetical black-box construct. That means that the child's imaginative reasoning has to be extended with an additional step, which makes it more difficult to predict emotions than behaviors (see also Bradmetz & Schneider, 1999).

Multiple and Complex Emotions

Theory-of-mind reasoning enables the child to understand that two people might have a different emotional reaction to a situation, because of different desires and beliefs. Lisa may consider the dog she encounters to be a pleasant playmate, whereas Eric thinks of the same dog as a dangerous animal ready to attack. As a result of these attributions, Lisa most likely will feel happy, whereas Eric will feel afraid. However, different perspectives on one and the same situation are also possible within the same individual. Sam may feel happy because he thinks this particular dog is a friendly one but also may be a bit afraid because he has had a bad experience with another dog recently which causes him to approach this dog more cautiously as well.

Young children, just like everybody else, are at times affected by mixed emotions (Meerum Terwogt, 1987). Nonetheless, when asked open-ended questions about their feelings, they usually report just one of them (Harter, 1983; Meerum Terwogt, Koops, Oosterhoff, & Olthof, 1986). They stop the monitoring process as soon as they have detected this one feeling, because they have conceptual difficulties in accepting the possibility of simultaneous mixed feelings (especially when they are of opposite valence). They hold a one-to-one conception of situation and emotion. A change may be triggered, however, when children encounter situations that challenge this simple conception. If they also feel like laughing, there has to be more to the situation that they appraised as "sad." By the age of 10, a large majority of children have accepted the possibility of different kinds of emotion mixtures. This newly acquired insight stimulates a broader emotion scan. For instance, when we tell these children that their friend was involved in a terrible accident and has broken his leg, they may tell us not just that they feel sad about the broken leg but also that they are happy that nothing worse happened.

The appropriate label for the second feeling in the example above is, of course, "relief," one of the so-called counterfactual emotions. Children's difficulties in understanding this type of emotion is strongly related to the previously described difficulties. In counterfactual emotions, children also have to acknowledge and integrate different representations into their judgment: the actual outcome of the situation and an alternative outcome involving previous expectations (Guttentag & Farrell, 2004). Depending on the content of the second representation, people can experience relief or disappointment in response to the same outcome.

Another group of complex emotions poses the same challenges to children's understanding. Social emotions such as pride and shame depend on the discrepancy between our actual behavior and a conception of how we ought to behave. Again, exactly the same outcome can elicit either pride or shame, depending on whether we fail to meet normative standards or exceed them. As in counterfactual emotions, young children base their judgments in pride- and shame-relevant situations on the actual outcome only. They report being happy if they got what they wanted and sad if not, irrespective of the way they reached this result (Nunner-Winkler & Sodian, 1988). Even though they know the normative standards, they do not seem to take them into account, which suggests that the bottleneck is really the introduction of inner considerations in their reasoning process. Theory-of-mind reasoning alerts children to the relevance of introspective information, but it is only between the ages of 7 to 10 that children get a grasp of counterfactual emotions (Guttentag & Farrell, 2004) as well as complex social emotions (Ferguson & Stegge, 1995; Ferguson, Stegge, & Damhuis, 1991). In this age range, they become increasingly able to base their judgments on the discrepancy between the actual outcome and the presumed reasoning process.

Strategic Emotional Responding: What Can I Do (about It)?

Knowledge about emotion enables children to respond to emotion-eliciting events in a more flexible and less stereotypical way. Preexisting emotion programs can be redirected in order to obtain a more adequate fit with situational demands. In this section, we discuss children's understanding of two major regulation options: exerting control over the outward expression of emotions and exerting control over the inner feeling state.

Regulation of Emotional Expression

Young children not only seem to assume a one-to-one relation between situation and emotion but also start from the assumption of a one-to-one relation between emotion and expression. Nevertheless, quite early in life, they discover that emotional expressions are not always appreciated. In a pioneering study among 6- to 11-year-olds, Saarni (1984) found that children who received a disappointing gift clearly showed their feelings in private but concealed their true feeling with a broad smile (older children) or a transitional half smile (younger children) in the presence of the adult who gave them the present. The same results could even be replicated among 3- to 4-year-old girls (Cole, 1986). Harris (1989) suggests that these very early competencies might be explained by parental indoctrination ("Smile and say thank you") and need not imply that these children already fully appreciate the dissociation between inner experience and outer expression. When asked whether the adult would know how they felt, none of the children in Cole's experiment pointed out that he or she would be misled by the adult's expression, which seems to sustain Harris's conclusion. Thus, the ability to control emotional displays is already there but is probably not yet triggered by children's own evaluation of the situation.

Once children start to monitor their own emotional states, they may sometimes detect a discrepancy between inner feelings and outer expressions. Moreover, in confrontations with older children, parents may not always adapt their facial expressions to their statements. For instance, they might tell their children that they are angry about something without showing it in their face (Dunn & Brown, 1994). This too, might make children attentive to the inner–outer distinction.

The private character of inner processes has to be appreciated before it can be used in a deliberate and strategic way. Theory-of-mind reasoning helps children realize that people tend to use external cues like emotional expressions for inferences about the accompanying inner processes. Therefore, deliberate expressions can be used to mislead observers. Preschoolers begin to show an early understanding of dissemblance

(Banerjee, 1997), but between the ages of 6 and 10, children's understanding in this domain increases significantly. In this age period, they also come to understand the display rules that motivate the hiding of emotion. They now know that either for self-protective reasons (if we reveal our fear, others may call us chicken) or for prosocial reasons (the other person may be hurt by our emotional reaction), it is sometimes better not to show emotion (Gnepp & Hess, 1986; Saarni; 1979).

Social restrictions normally require not much more than the regulation of the outward emotional expression. We are free to feel what we like as long as we do not reveal it. Nonetheless, sometimes "inappropriate feelings" may create additional distress (e.g., feeling guilty about being angry). Indeed, everybody likes to be rid of negative feelings. So for a number of personal reasons, we would like to be able to regulate our subjective feeling state. In the next section, we discuss children's knowledge of strategies to change emotion.

Regulation of Inner Feelings

In an early interview study (Harris et al., 1981), 6-year-old children mainly suggested situational or behavioral changes when asked how they would regulate a negative feeling state, whereas 10-year-olds also acknowledged the potential usefulness of mental manipulations. We may try to modify the actual situation in order to feel better, but it might be equally or sometimes even more effective to change our subjective perception of the situation. The general developmental trend toward a greater emphasis on cognitive strategies of emotion regulation has been replicated in numerous studies since then (see Brenner & Salovey, 1997; Harris, 1989; Meerum Terwogt & Stegge, 1995; Saarni, 1999, for reviews).

The focus of empirical studies on children's reasoning about emotion regulation has been largely confined to the broad distinction between situational/behavioral strategies and cognitive strategies. Insufficient attention has been paid to developments within the extensive domain of cognitive manipulations. In our research, we examined children's perspectives on the usefulness of cognitive strategies in more detail (Meerum Terwogt & Stegge, 1995; Stegge, Meerum Terwogt, Reijntjes, & Van Tijen, 2004). This enabled us to identify an additional step in children's reasoning about effective strategies of emotion regulation. At first, children acquire an insight into the elementary link between thought content and emotion, which we refer to as a "same valence" perspective. Five- and 6-year-old children argue that thinking of something pleasant results in a positive feeling state, whereas thinking of something unpleasant causes negative feelings. Accordingly, they realize that in order to improve a negative feeling state, one has to stop thinking about the negative stimulus and/or to start thinking about something positive instead (see also Harris, 1989). Although very useful for regulation purposes, this conception of the relation between cognition and emotion is limited in that children are still tied to one perspective on reality. A stimulus event is perceived as either positive or negative, and by focusing one's thoughts on it, negative feelings will be diminished or intensified as a result. It is only at the next level that children come to understand the effectiveness of so-called reappraisals: One can take a different perspective on the same stimulus event. A previously valued possession that has been damaged, for example, can be "made" less attractive by mental manipulation in order to feel better. As children acquire a conception of the mind as an interpretative device (Carpendale & Chandler, 1996), they acknowledge the coexistence of different perspectives and are able to apply this knowledge to the domain of emotion regulation. This permits a substantial extension of their coping repertoire. Moreover, because children are now able to weigh the short- and long-term consequences of different strategies simultaneously, their preferences for approach as opposed to avoidance change as well. Whereas young children mainly think that one should keep one's distance from aversive situations, older children increasingly appreciate the usefulness of confrontation. They argue, for example, that paying attention to the negative event and the resulting feeling state will initially intensify the emotion but may also help us to find an optimal solution for the problem by putting it in a different perspective. Positive consequences in the long run may now outweigh anticipated short-term aversive effects in children's decision-making process (Stegge et al., 2004).

To summarize, important changes in children's understanding of emotion take place during the preschool and elementary school period. Children become able to analyze emotional situations in greater detail and gain knowledge of the causes, consequences, and modes of expression of an increasing range of specific emotions. They also learn a lot about the nature of emotion as such. A crucial step in development involves the taking on of a mentalistic perspective on the emotion process. The inclusion of desires, beliefs, and the distinction between inner feeling state and outer expression as central components in children's emotion schemes allows for better explanations and predictions of emotional responses. Increasingly sophisticated cognitive capacities stimulates their knowledge of a broad repertoire of emotion regulation strategies, including (complex) cognitive manipulations. Together with their increasing capacities for introspection, the availability of an extensive emotion knowledge base might be expected to increase the quality of children's secondary appraisal process and help them to use their emotions in the service of adaptation.

However, as explained later, secondary appraisal still involves "hot cognition": The prevailing emotion determines to a certain extent which thoughts come to mind. Conscious thoughts may then act as new input to the process, increase the intensity and duration of the emotion, and result in the actual performance of the emotional behaviors instigated by the primary action tendency (Lambie & Marcel, 2002; Teasdale, 1999). In the next section, we provide two different examples of problematic second-order appraisal processes and their supposed consequences for regulation.

ATYPICAL DEVELOPMENT: A LACK OF AWARENESS OF EMOTION AND DYSFUNCTIONAL EMOTION REGULATION

Second-order appraisal processes in response to an emotional situation resemble general problem solving in many ways. To choose the best response, one has to analyze the situation in order to establish the nature of the problem. The next steps in the process concern goal setting, the generation of strategic options, and the evaluation of these options in terms of personal goals and situational constraints. However, "emotional" problem solving is different from "cold" problem solving in at least two ways.

First, people may or may not become aware of their emotions during the first step. Only if the situation is defined in terms of an emotional problem will emotion regulation goals be explicitly set. Of course, improvement of one's feeling state can be reached by solving the actual problem that gave rise to the emotion. But not all problems are that easily solved without the risk of meeting new problems, and some stressful situations (like the death of a friend) cannot be changed at all. In these cases, so-called secondary (Rothbaum, Weisz, & Snyder, 1982) or emotion-focused strategies (Lazarus & Folkman, 1984) are the best or sometimes even the only option to deal with the problematic situation. Secondary or emotion-focused coping is directly aimed at the improvement of the emotional state. Rather than changing the actual conditions, the person tries to maximize his or her goodness of fit with the conditions as they are.

Second, negative emotions enhance the pressure to find a way out, whether they are acknowledged or not. Consciously or unconsciously, people try to get rid of negative emotions as quickly as possible (Arnold, 1960). As a result "hot" problem solving is often not "rational." The choice for a certain plan of action might be based on an emotionally biased perception of the situation. An incomplete or inaccurate analysis results in a less than optimal evaluation of the situation, in which only a relatively small range of reaction patterns is considered. Again, it is the awareness of an emotional state that may induce deliberate efforts to counter some of these detrimental effects (Meerum Terwogt, 1986).

Many emotional situations involve social situations, and the ways in which emotions are dealt with in these interpersonal encounters play a central role in successful adaptation (Halberstadt, Denham, & Dunsmore, 2001). The functionality of emotional processing in these situations is dependent on the accuracy of the appraisal, the allocation of priorities among multiple goals, and the selection of proper responses (Lemerise & Arsenio, 2000; Parrott, 2001). Online processing is influenced by children's emotion schemas. Individual differences in the quality of this secondary appraisal process in emotion-eliciting events may therefore be due, in part, to the quality of the emotion schemata used.

Although relatively little is known, thus far, about the specific content of children's latent emotion structures, theoretical work and empirical studies in children suffering from internalizing or externalizing symptoms suggest deficits and biases in their reasoning about emotion and emotional situations (i.e., the secondary appraisal process). We discuss these problems next, and argue that these children's difficulties reflect a relative *lack of awareness* of emotion, which interferes with adaptive emotion regulation.

Anger and Aggression

Children with behavior problems are characterized by an anger bias. This may take the form of a sensitivity to anger-related appraisals on the one hand as well as maladaptive responses (i.e., aggression) to anger-eliciting situations on the other (Hubbard et al., 2002; Jenkins & Oatley, 2000). In other words, their problems with anger seem to take the form of inadequate input and output regulation.

Regulation problems may (at least in part) be the result of these children's lack of awareness of their own emotions (Meerum Terwogt, Schene, & Koops, 1990). With anger, people are typically world-focused rather than self-focused (Lambie & Marcel, 2002). Characteristic of the emotion of anger is a feeling that "the world is against you." The chances that an anger-eliciting situation is properly dealt with increase when the emotional state is acknowledged as one of anger. Knowledge of the consequences of anger may then trigger corrective action. In the clinical literature it is argued that anger awareness is limited among adults suffering from an anger disorder (Kassinove, 1995). Similarly, children with behavior problems are described as being focused on the external world and relatively insensitive to internal cues. They tend to attribute their aggressive behavior directly to other people's actions toward the self and fail to acknowledge the role of their own anger as an important factor in eliciting aggression (Shirk, 1988). A study by Casey and Schlosser (1994) is consistent with these clinical observations. These authors showed that children with externalizing disorders were less accurate in reporting their facial displays than nonexternalizers, which might suggest that these children indeed have difficulties in monitoring their own emotional reactions.

Studies conducted within the social information-processing paradigm have extensively examined the way in which mental processes influence children's behavior in social situations. Social information processing is considered to be entirely emotional. According to Dodge (1991) "emotion is the energy level that drives, organizes, amplifies and attenuates cognitive activity and in turn is the experience and expression of this activity" (p. 159). As expected and in line with an account in terms of problematic anger regulation, children with behavior problems differ from normal controls in all of the different processing steps of the sequence: They pay more attention to threatening information, attribute hostile intentions to others, consider instrumental goals more important than relational ones, generate a wider range of aggressive responses, and finally choose to become aggressive more often (Crick & Dodge, 1994). Important for the present argument is the recent finding that secondary appraisal processes in children with externalizing problems seem to be biased to a greater extent under emotional circumstances. After a negative mood induction these children's hostile attribution bias proved to be exacerbated (Dodge & Somberg, 1987; Orobio de Castro, Slot, Bosch, Koops, & Veerman, 2003). Moreover, in a creative study, Troop-Gordon and Asher (2005) showed that when aggressive children encounter obstacles to conflict resolution, they show an *increased* desire to retaliate, whereas nonaggressive children manage to pursue a combination of instrumental and prosocial goals.

These studies suggest that an emotion may trigger conscious thoughts that intensify the emotion and its associated action tendency. Children with externalizing problems seem to adopt an immersed world-focused perspective in their secondary appraisal process and do not seem to take the reflective stance necessary for adequate regulation. In their experience, others *are* adversaries that need to be combatted; they do not seem to realize that a different perspective on the situation can be taken, resulting in different behaviors as well.

Depressive Symptoms

Although depression consists of different classes of symptoms (motivational, cognitive, somatic), it is primarily an *affective* disorder. Its essential feature is sad or depressed affect (American Psychiatric Association, 1994). In an attempt to identify the key mechanism responsible for depressed people's maladaptive (emotional) functioning, depression has been conceptualized as a *failure to regulate* transient negative emotions (Cole & Kaslow, 1988; see Power & Dalgleish, 1997; Teasdale, Segal, & Williams, 1995, for more recent accounts). In this section, we discuss theoretical accounts and empirical evidence pertaining to depressed children's appraisal biases and the response options they endorse in emotion-eliciting events.

In theoretical models of depression, dysfunctional cognitions are assumed to play a causal role. Global negative representations of the self and ruminative thoughts about social rejection, personal inadequacy, and failure are central elements in affect-related schematic mental models (Teasdale, 1996). These cognitive vulnerabilities are shown by adults (Ingram, Miranda, & Segal, 1998) as well as children (Hammen & Rudolph, 1996). The results of empirical studies suggest that these dysfunctional emotion schemes influence the online processing of social information. Children with higher scores on depressive symptoms were shown to process the information provided in a hypothetical social situation in a more negative way (Quiggle, Garber, Panak, & Dodge, 1992). Another study (Reijntjes, Stegge, & Meerum Terwogt, 2006) has shown that children with high levels of depressive symptoms are likely to appraise rejection situations as more emotionally distressing. Moreover, their emotional distress ratings were related to the tendency to have catastrophic thoughts about the event.

Several studies have provided evidence to suggest that children displaying nonclinical depressive symptoms differ in the emotion regulation strategies they anticipate in hypothetical situations. Specifically, depressed children are more likely to endorse cognitive and behavioral avoidance and less likely to advocate active problem-solving strategies and cognitive reappraisals. They also tend to engage in rumination and/or indicate that they stay passive more often. In addition, children higher in depression report lower levels of perceived self-efficacy in solving the problematic situation and expect lower mood improvement from cognitive strategies and active approach (Garber, Baarrladt, & Weiss, 1995; Quiggle et al., 1992; Reijntjes, Stegge, Meerum Terwogt, & Hurkens, in press). Thus, hypothetical situations may activate cognitive biases related to depression.

Importantly, a recent study conducted by our own research group has shown that the same biases in children's reasoning became evident in an actual emotion-eliciting situation (Reijntjes, Stegge, Meerum Terwogt, Telch, & Kamphuis, in press). We examined 9- to 13-year-old children's responses to an *in vivo* manipulation of peer rejection: Children were voted out by their peers when playing an online computer game. Level of depression was associated with self-blame (i.e., a tendency to attribute the rejection experience to internal causes). Children high in depression were also more likely to exaggerate the perceived threat of the rejection experience (i.e., they reported catastrophizing thoughts). On a behavioral level, it was shown that children with higher depression scores are less likely to engage in approach behaviours (gathering information about previous winners and losers of the game; wanting to receive feedback about the reasons for being voted out) and more likely to show passivity.

To summarize, children with elevated depression scores show a tendency to process emotional information in a negative way. Self-blaming thoughts, catastrophizing, and rumination seem to be characteristic responses shown in response to both hypothetical and *in vivo* emotional situations. Depressed children's conscious thoughts in response to emotion-eliciting events will most likely intensify their negative emotions and cause them to avoid the situation or stay passive in order to avoid additional distress. Although direct empirical evidence is lacking, it is plausible that a relative lack of awareness of emotion also plays a role in this case.

Whereas aggressive children's lack of awareness is supposedly due to a strong world focus, depressed children seem to have a different problem. They are self-focused but in an immersed way. Their self-related negative thoughts involve involuntary responses, which are automatically triggered by the presence of a negative emotion-eliciting stimulus. In their intentional coping responses, however, depressed children prefer avoidance to approach. They seem to be motivated to disengage from negative information, including their own feeling state. In depression, involuntary engagement seems to go together with voluntary disengagement (Connor-Smith, Compas, Wadsworth, Thomsen, & Saltzman, 2001). The combination of both tendencies may further enhance a relative lack of awareness of emotion. In depression, the person is overwhelmed by negative feelings and easily identifies with them. The presence of negative affect signifies total failure, immediately triggers a wide range of ruminative thoughts, and prevents a reflective stance in which the prevailing feeling state is focused on directly. Together with their motivated avoidance tendencies, this makes it hard for depressed people to become aware of their negative feelings *as* specific emotions that can be examined and acted on (Teasdale, 1996, 1999).

CONCLUSION:
WHAT CHILDREN NEED TO LEARN ABOUT EMOTION

Emotional competence concerns the ability to make use of the functional qualities of the emotion system for adaptation. The interaction between the emotional core system and the emotional control system is crucial in this respect (Levenson, 1999). Adaptive functioning requires the ability to respond emotionally (i.e., the core system should be given free reign to a certain extent) but also to show proficiency in emotion regulation (i.e., adequate control should be exerted).

As has been argued before, children's ability to put emotions to use is dependent on their knowledge of emotion. We have discussed some of the essential elements that need to become part of the child's knowledge base. In our opinion, the development of an adequate "theory of emotion" requires two levels of knowledge: (1) an understanding of the characteristics of specific emotional core programs, and (2) knowledge of regulatory activity that may impact on one or several of the basic components of these programs. At the first level, knowledge of the most common elicitors of a specific emotion state, its expression, the action tendencies it gives rise to, its impact on bodily reactions, cognition, and the broader social consequences helps children to *identify* this feeling state in themselves and others, and to determine *when* regulation is called for (Meerum Terwogt & Olthof, 1989; Meerum Terwogt, Schene, & Harris, 1986). At the second level, knowledge of different regulation strategies (concerning the expression and/or the experience of the emotion) may help children to decide *how* their goals can best be reached. Of course, this knowledge is critically embedded in the feeling and display rules of the child's social environment (Saarni, 1999).

In their reasoning, children have to incorporate elements referring to the autonomous character of emotion as well as elements relevant for regulation. However, in their naïve theory of emotion they may weigh these two elements to varying degrees. From experience we know that people emphasize different characteristics of the emotion process under different circumstances. A jealous spouse, for example, is likely to claim that "he cannot help himself," whereas a teacher most likely will expect his excited pupils to be able to "calm down." The first person emphasizes the activity of the core system (the autonomous aspect), while the second one calls attention to the potential of the control system. We know that even 6-year-old children sometimes refer to the autonomous character of emotion, and most children also seem to think that emotions can be changed (Harris et al., 1981; Stegge et al., 2004). Knowledge of either element may therefore be expected to show up in children's reasoning in emotional situations (i.e., the secondary appraisal process).

In the previous section we have seen that children's reasoning about each of these two aspects may be limited, especially under emotional circumstances. Their secondary appraisal process is supposedly driven by inadequate emotion schemes and characterized by a relative lack of awareness of emotion. That is, they have difficulties in acknowledging *what* they feel and how this influences their behavior and as a result seem to have different expectations about their coping options as well. In the case of aggression or depression, children's reasoning about emotional situations obviously seems to serve them maladaptively. To a certain extent, however, the same biases may be present in all of us, either because of our developmental level or because of the specific circumstances we find ourselves in.

The ultimate goal of children's emotional learning process is to become skilled at using emotions in the service of adaptive functioning. Scientific theories about the emotion process as well as empirical work on the development of children's reasoning about emotion may provide us with the information necessary to function as capable emotional coaches (Gottman, Katz, & Hooven, 1997). In our opinion, it is essential that the social environment of the child emphasizes both the autonomous character of the emotion process and the fact that emotions can and should be regulated. Children need to learn *when* and *how* to regulate their feelings, and the identification of their own feeling state takes a central role in this process. At a meta-emotive level, the adaptive potential of the emotion system should also be highlighted (see also Greenberg, Kusche, Cook, & Quamma, 1995). This approach has the additional advantage of communicating to children that their feelings are taken seriously and encourages them to do the same.

It is important that children learn to carefully observe their own feelings in order to get a better grasp of the *specific feelings* they experience. Knowledge of the main characteristic of different emotions may provide them with the necessary tools to reach this goal, and a balanced perspective on the general functions and nature of the emotion process may motivate them to actually engage in introspective activity. The child learns that feelings have a phenomenological truth: To be angry *is* to experience the world in a certain way (Lambie & Marcel, 2002). But the child should also learn to take a reflective stance: Emotions are mental states that can be examined and acted on (Teasdale, 1999). To be able to adequately regulate their (sometimes overwhelming) emotions, children need to carefully modulate their attention, so that they will keep the right distance from their emotions. In addition, they need to build a coping template consisting of a wide array of possible means for action. To adequately help children reach these goals, it is crucial that the social environment is sensitive to both the child's developmental level and to specific cognitive or emotional vulnerabilities.

REFERENCES

American Psychiatric Association. (1994). *Diagnostic and statistical manual of mental disorders* (4th ed.). Washington, DC: Author.

Arnold, M. B. (1960). *Emotion and personality* (Vol. 1). New York: Columbia University Press.

Arsenio, W. F., & Lemerise, E. A. (2004). Aggression and moral development: Integrating social information processing and moral domain models. *Child Development, 75,* 987–1002.

Banerjee, M. (1997). Hidden emotions: Preschoolers' knowledge of appearance-reality and emotion display rules. *Social Development, 15,* 107–132.

Bradmetz, J., & Schneider, R. (1999). Is little red riding hood afraid of her grandmother?: Cognitive versus emotional response to a false belief. *British Journal of Developmental Psychology, 17,* 501–514.

Brenner, E. M., & Salovey, P. (1997). Emotion regulation during childhood: Developmental, interpersonal and individual considerations. In P. Salovey & D. J. Sluyter (Eds.), *Emotional development and emotional intelligence* (pp. 168–192). New York: Basic Books.

Bretherton, I., & Beeghly, M. (1982). Talking about internal states of mind: The acquisition of an explicit theory of mind. *Developmental Psychology, 18,* 906–921.

Carpendale, J. I., & Chandler, M. J. (1996). On the distinction between false belief understanding and subscribing to an interpretative theory of mind. *Child Development, 67,* 1686–1706.

Casey, R. (1993). Children's emotional experience: Relations among expression, self-report and understanding. *Developmental Psychology, 29,* 119–129.

Casey, R., & Schlosser, S. (1994). Emotional responses to peer praise in children with and without a diagnosed externalizing disorder. *Merrill–Palmer Quarterly, 40,* 60–81.

Cole, P. M. (1986) Children's spontaneous control of facial expression. *Child Development, 57,* 1309–1321.

Cole, P. M., & Kaslow, N. J. (1988). Interactional and cognitive strategies for affect regulation: Developmental perspective on childhood depression. In L. B. Alloy (Ed.), *Cognitive processes in depression* (pp. 310–345). New York: Guilford Press.

Cole, P. M., Martin, S. E., & Dennis, T. A. (2004). Emotion regulation as a scientific construct: Methodological challenges and directions for child development research. *Child Development, 75,* 317–333.

Compas, J. J., Frankel, C. B., & Camras, L. (2004). On the nature of emotion regulation *Child Development, 75,* 377–394.

Connor-Smith, J. K., Compas, B. E., Wadsworth, M. E., Thomsen, A. H., & Saltzman, H. (2001). Responses to stress in adolescence: Measurement of coping and involuntary stress responses. *Journal of Consulting and Clinical Psychology, 68,* 976–992.

Crick, N. R., & Dodge, K. A. (1994). A review and reformulation of social–information processing mechanisms in children's development. *Psychological Bulletin, 115,* 74–101.

Darwin, C. (1872). *The expression of emotions in man and animals.* London: Murray.

Denham, S. A. (1998). *Emotional development in young children.* New York: Guilford Press.

Denham, S. A., & Kochanoff, A. (2002). Why is she crying: Children's understanding of emotion from preschool to preadolescence. In L. Feldman Barrett & P. Salovey (Eds.), *The wisdom in feeling: Psychological processes in emotional intelligence* (pp. 239–270). New York: Guilford Press.

Dodge, K. A. (1991). Emotion and social information processing. In J. Garber & K. A. Dodge (Eds.), *The development of emotion regulation and dysregulation* (pp. 159–181). Cambridge, UK: Cambridge University Press.

Dodge, K. A., & Somberg, D. R. (1987). Hostile attribution biases among aggressive boys are exacerbated under conditions of threats to the self. *Child Development, 58,* 213–224.

Dunn, J., & Brown, J. (1994). Affect expression in the family, children's understanding of emotions and their interaction with others. *Merrill–Palmer Quarterly, 40,* 120–138.

Eisenberg, N., & Spinrad, T. L. (2004). Emotion-related regulation: Sharpening the definition. *Child Development, 75,* 334–339.

Feldman Barrett, L., Gross, J., Christensen, T. C., & Benvenuto, M. (2001). Knowing what you're feeling and knowing what to do about it: Mapping the relation between emotion differentiation and emotion regulation. *Cognition and Emotion, 15,* 713–724.

Ferguson, T. J., & Stegge, H. (1995). Emotional states and traits in children: The case of guilt and shame. In J. P. Tangney & K. W. Fischer (Eds.), *Self-conscious emotions* (pp. 174–197). New York: Guilford Press.

Ferguson, T. J., Stegge, H., & Damhuis, I. (1991). Children's understanding of guilt and shame. *Child Development, 62,* 827–839.

Flavell, J. H., Green, F. L., & Flavell, E. (1993). Children's understanding of the stream of consciousness. *Child Development, 64,* 387–398.

Flavell, J. H., Green, F. L., & Flavell, E. (1995). Young children's knowledge about thinking. *Monographs of the Society for Research in Child Development, 60*(Serial No. 243).

Flavell, J. H., Green, F. L., & Flavell, E. (1998). The mind has a mind of its own: Developing knowledge about mental uncontrollability. *Cognitive Development, 13,* 127–138.

Flavell, J. H., Green, F. L., Flavell, E., & Lin, N. T. (1999). Development of children's knowledge about unconsciousness. *Child Development, 70,* 396–412.

Frijda, N. (1986) *The emotions.* Cambridge, UK: Cambridge University Press.

Garber, J., Baarladt, N., & Weiss, B. (1995). Affect regulation in depressed and nondepressed children and young adolescents. *Development and Psychopathology, 7,* 93–115.

Gnepp, J., & Hess, D. (1986). Children's understanding of verbal and facial display rules. *Developmental Psychology, 22,* 103–108.

Gottman, J., Katz, L. F., & Hooven, C. (1997). *Meta-emotion.* Hillsdale, NJ: Erlbaum.

Greenberg, M. T., Kusche, C. A., Cook, E. T., & Quamma, J. P. (1995). Promoting emotional competence in school-aged deaf children: The effect of the PATHS curriculum. *Development and Psychopathology, 7,* 117–136.

Gross, J. J., & Thompson, R. A. (2007). Emotion regulation: Conceptual foundations. In J. J. Gross (Ed.), *Handbook of emotion regulation* (pp. 3–24). New York: Guilford Press.

Guttentag, R., & Farrell, J. (2004). Reality compared with its alternatives: Age differences in judgments of regret and relief. *Developmental Psychology, 40,* 764–775.

Halberstadt, A. G., Denham, S. A., & Dunsmore, J. C. (2001). Affective social competence. *Social Development, 10,* 79–119.

Hammen, C., & Rudolph, K. D. (1996). Childhood depression. In E. J. Mash & R. A. Barkley (Eds.), *Child psychopathology* (pp. 153–195). New York: Guilford Press.

Harris, P. L. (1983). Children's understanding of the link between situation and emotion. *Journal of Experimental Child Psychology, 33,* 1–20.

Harris, P. L. (1989). *Children and emotion: The development of psychological understanding.* Oxford, UK: Blackwell.

Harris, P. L., Johnson, C. N., Hutton, D., Andrews, G., & Cooke, T. (1989). Young children's theory of mind and emotion. *Cognition and Emotion, 3,* 379–400.

Harris, P. L., Olthof, T., & Meerum Terwogt, M. (1981). Children's knowledge of emotion. *Journal of Child Psychology and Psychiatry, 22,* 247–261.

Harter, S. (1982). Children's understanding of multiple emotions: A cognitive–developmental approach. In W. F. Overton (Ed.), *The relationship between social and cognitive development* (pp. 147–194). Hillsdale, NJ: Erlbaum.

Hubbard, J. A., Smithmeyer, C. M., Ramsdens, S. R., Parker, E. H., Flanagan, K. D., Dearing, K. F., et al. (2002). Observational, physiological, and self-report measures of children's anger: Relations to reactive versus proactive aggression. *Child Development, 73,* 1101–1118.

Ingram, R. E., Miranda, J., & Segal, Z. V. (1998). *Cognitive vulnerability to depression.* New York: Guilford Press.

Jenkins, J. M., & Astington, J. W. (1996). Cognitive factors and family structure associated with theory of mind development in young children. *Developmental Psychology, 32,* 70–78.

Jenkins, J. M., & Oatley, K. (2000). Psychopathology and short-term emotion: The balance of affects. *Journal of Child Psychology and Psychiatry, 41,* 463–472.

Kassinove, H. (1995). *Anger disorders.* Washington DC: Taylor & Francis.

Lambie, J. A., & Marcel, A. J. (2002). Consciousness and the varieties of emotional experience: A theoretical framework. *Psychological Review, 109,* 219–259.

Lane, R. D., & Pollerman, Z. (2002). Complexity of emotion representations. In L. Feldman Barrett & P. Salovey (Eds.), *The wisdom in feeling: Psychological processes in emotional intelligence* (pp. 271–293). New York: Guilford Press.

Lazarus, R. S., & Folkman, S. (1984). *Stress, appraisal, and coping.* New York: Springer.

LeDoux, J. (1996). *The emotional brain.* London: Weidenfeld & Nicolson.

Lemerise, E. A., & Arsenio, W. F. (2000). An integrated model of emotion processes and cognition in social information processing. *Child Development, 71,* 107–118.

Levenson, R. W. (1999). The intrapersonal functions of emotion. *Cognition and Emotion, 13,* 481–504.

Lewis, M. D., & Stieben, J. (2004). Emotion regulation in the brain: Conceptual issues and directions for developmental research. *Child Development, 75,* 371–376.

Mayer, J. D., & Salovey, P. (1997). What is emotional intelligence?: In P. Salovey & D. Sluyter (Eds.), *Emotional development and emotional intelligence: Implications for educators* (pp. 3–31). New York: Basic Books.

Meerum Terwogt, M. (1986). Affective states and task performance in naive and prompted children. *European Journal of Psychology of Education, 1,* 31–40.

Meerum Terwogt, M. (1987). Children's behavioural reactions in situations with a dual emotional impact. *Psychological Reports, 61,* 1002.

Meerum Terwogt, M., Koops, W., Oosterhoff, T., & Olthof, T. (1986). Development in processing of multiple emotional situations. *Journal of General Psychology, 113,* 109–119.

Meerum Terwogt, M., & Olthof, T. (1989). Awareness and self-regulation of emotion in young children. In C. Saarni & P. L. Harris (Eds.), *Children's understanding of emotion* (pp. 209–239). New York: Cambridge University Press.

Meerum Terwogt, M., Schene, J., & Harris, P. L. (1986). Self-control of emotional reactions by young children. *Journal of Child Psychology and Psychiatry, 27,* 357–366.

Meerum Terwogt, M., Schene, J., & Koops, W. (1990). Concepts of emotion in institutionalized children. *Journal of Child Psychology and Psychiatry, 31,* 1131–1143.

Meerum Terwogt, M., & Stegge, H. (1995). Children's understanding of the strategic control of negative emotions. In J. A. Russell (Ed.), *Everyday conceptions of emotion* (NATO ASI Series) (pp. 373–390). Dordrecht, The Netherlands: Kluwer.

Meerum Terwogt, M., & Stegge, H. (2002). The development of emotional intelligence. In I. M. Goodyer (Ed.), *The depressed child and adolescent* (pp. 24–45). Cambridge, UK: Cambridge University Press.

Niedenthal, P. M., Dalle, N., & Rohman, A. (2002). Emotional response categorization as emotionally intelligent behavior. In L. Feldman Barrett & P. Salovey (Eds.), *The wisdom in feeling: Psychological processes in emotional intelligence* (pp. 167–190). New York: Guilford Press.

Nunner-Winkler, G., & Sodian, B. (1988). Children's understanding of moral emotions. *Child Development, 59,* 1323–1338.

Onishi, K. H., & Baillargeon, R. (2005). Do 15-month-old infants understand false beliefs? *Science, 308,* 255–258.

Orobio de Castro, B., Slot, N. W., Bosch, J. D., Koops, W., & Veerman, J. (2003). Negative feelings exacerbate hostile attributions of intent in highly aggressive boys. *Journal of Clinical Child and Adolescent Psychology, 32,* 56–65.

Parrott, W. G. (2001). Implications of dysfunctional emotions for understanding how emotions function. *Review of General Psychology, 5,* 180–186.

Perner, J., & Ruffman, T. (2005). Infant's insight into the mind: How deep? *Science, 308,* 214–216.

Power, M. J., & Dalgleish, T. (1997). *Cognition and emotion: From order to disorder.* Hove. UK: Psychology Press.

Quiggle, N. L., Garber, J., Panak, W. F., & Dodge, K. A. (1992). Social information processing in aggressive and depressed children. *Child Development, 63,* 1305–1320.

Reijntjes, A. H. A., Stegge, H., Meerum Terwogt, M. (2006). Children's coping with peer rejection: The role of depressive symptoms, social competence and gender. *Infant and Child Development, 15,* 989–107.

Reijntjes, A. H. A., Stegge, H., Meerum Terwogt, M., & Hurkens, E. (in press). The effect of depression on children's reactions to vignette-depicted emotion-eliciting events. *International Journal of Behavioral Development.*

Reijntjes, A. H. A., Stegge, H., Meerum Terwogt, M., Kamphuis, J., & Telch, M. (in press). Children's coping with *in vivo* peer rejection: An experimental investigation. *Journal of Abnormal Child Psychology.*

Rothbaum, F., Weisz, J. R., & Snyder, S. S. (1982). Changing the world and changing the self: A two-process model of perceived control. *Journal of Personality and Social Psychology, 42,* 5–37.

Saarni, C. (1979). Children's understanding of display rules for expressive behavior. *Developmental Psychology, 15,* 424–429.

Saarni, C. (1984). Observing children's use of display rules: Age and sex differences. *Child Development, 55,* 1504–1513.

Saarni, C. (1999). *The development of emotional competence.* New York: Guilford Press.

Saarni, C., & Harris, P. L. (Eds.). (1989). *Children's understanding of emotion.* Cambridge, UK: Cambridge University Press.

Salovey, P., Mayer, J. D., & Caruso, D. (2002). The positive psychology of emotional intelligence. In C. R. Snyder & S. J. Lopez (Eds.), *The handbook of positive psychology* (pp. 159–171). New York: Oxford University Press.

Selman, R. L. (1981). What children understand from intrapsychic processes: The child as a budding personality theorist. In E. K. Shapiro & E. Weber (Eds.), *Cognitive and affective growth: Developmental interaction* (pp. 159–171). Hillsdale, NJ: LEA.

Shirk, S. R. (1988). *Cognitive development and child psychotherapy.* New York: Plenum Press.

Stegge, H., Meerum Terwogt, M., Reijntjes, A. H. A., & Van Tijen, N. (2004). Children's conception of the emotion process: consequences for emotion regulation. In I. Nyklicek, L. Temoshok, & A. Vingerhoets (Eds.), *Emotional expression and health: Advances in theory, assessment and clinical applications* (pp. 240–254). New York: Brunner-Routledge.

Stein, N. L., & Levine, L. J. (1989). The causal organization of emotion knowledge: A developmental study. *Cognition and Emotion, 3,* 343–378.

Teasdale, J. D. (1996). Clinically relevant theory: Integrating clinical insight with cognitive science. In P. M. Salkovskis (Ed.), *Frontiers of cognitive therapy* (pp. 26–47). New York: Guilford Press.

Teasdale, J. D. (1999). Emotional processing and three modes of mind, and the prevention of relapse in depression. *Behaviour Research and Therapy, 37,* S53–S57.

Teasdale, J. D., Segal, Z., & Williams, M. G. (1995). How does cognitive therapy prevent depressive relapse and why should attentional control (mindfulness) training help? *Behaviour Research and Therapy, 33,* 25–39.

Troop-Gordon, W., & Asher, S. R. (2005). Modifications in children's goals when encountering obstacles to conflict resolution. *Child Development, 76,* 568–582.

CHAPTER 14

Effortful Control and Its Socioemotional Consequences

NANCY EISENBERG
CLAIRE HOFER
JULIE VAUGHAN

In 2000, a National Academy of Science committee report, *From Neurons to Neighborhoods*, concluded, "The growth of self-regulation is a cornerstone of early childhood development that cuts across all domains of behavior" (Shonkoff & Phillips, 2000, p. 3). Although the term "self-regulation" was used in a broad sense, much self-regulation involves managing emotional experiences and their expression. In this chapter, we focus on the nature and development of emotion-related regulation, especially effortful control processes, and the role of effortful regulation in children's socioemotional development. First we review definitional issues. Next we outline some central conceptual distinctions, such as between more voluntary aspects of control and more reactive, involuntary control processes. Then we briefly summarize the normative development of emotion-related self-regulation, followed by the review of research illustrating the importance of individual differences in children's emotion-related self-regulatory skills for their socioemotional development. Finally, we discuss some issues and gaps in the research.

CONCEPTUAL ISSUES

Gross and Thompson (this volume) defined emotion as a "person–situation transaction that compels attention, has particular meaning to an individual, and gives rise to a coordinated yet flexible multisystem response to the ongoing personal-situation transaction" (p. 5). Like Gross and Thompson, we believe that emotion has a particular experiential meaning to individuals and is also linked to action tendencies. Defined in this manner, emotions obviously affect the quality of our experience and also provide much of the motivation behind our actions.

There is no consensus on a definition of emotion regulation. As noted by Kopp and Neufeld (2003), definitions of emotion regulation typically focus on the content (i.e., components of emotion regulation), function (i.e., the activities involved in emotion regulation), or the processes (how it happens). For example, Thompson (1994) defined emotion regulation as the "extrinsic and intrinsic processes responsible for monitoring, evaluating, and modifying emotional reactions, especially their intensive and temporal features, to achieve one's goals" (pp. 27–28; see Gross & Thompson, this volume). He discussed various domains for emotion regulation, including neurophysiological responses, attention processes, construals of emotionally arousing events, encoding of internal emotion cues, access to coping resources, regulating the demands of familiar settings, and selecting adaptive response alternatives. Cicchetti, Ganiban, and Barnett (1991) defined emotional regulation as "the intra- and extraorganismic factors by which emotional arousal is redirected, controlled, modulated, and modified to enable an individual to function adaptively in emotionally arousing situations" (p. 15). They include regulating factors from within and outside the organism, but it is unclear if they include the regulation of an emotionally arousing context. Kopp and Neufeld (2003) suggested that "emotion regulation during the early years is a developmental process that represents the deployment of intrinsic and extrinsic processes—at whatever maturity level the young child is at—to (1) manage arousal states for effective biological and social adaptations and (2) achieve individual goals" (p. 360). In this definition, Kopp and Neufeld do not focus on the processes involved in emotion regulation.

Our definition of emotion-related regulation includes many of the elements of others' definitions. In our work, emotion-related self-regulation (henceforth sometimes called emotion-related regulation or emotion regulation for brevity) refers to processes used to manage and change if, when, and how (e.g., how intensely) one experiences emotions and emotion-related motivational and physiological states, as well as how emotions are expressed behaviorally. Thus, emotion-related regulation includes processes used to change one's own emotional state, to prevent or initiate emotion responding (e.g., by selecting or changing situations), to modify the significance of the event for the self, and to modulate the behavioral expression of emotion (e.g., through verbal or nonverbal cues). Like Kopp and Neufield (2003), we believe that emotion-related regulation is used in the service of biological and social adaptation and to achieve individual goals, although it may not always do so. Because it is extremely difficult to differentiate emotionality from its regulation (Gross & Thompson, this volume), it is useful to focus on the processes involved rather than try to define emotion regulation based on the amount of emotion experienced or expressed. Our definition is consistent with Gross and Thompson's (this volume) model in which emotion regulation includes situation selection, situation modification, attentional deployment, cognitive change, and response modulation.

We frequently use the term "emotion-related" regulation because, unlike some investigators, we include in our definition the regulation of behavior associated with emotion as well as the regulation of emotion reactivity. In addition, we prefer this designation because many of the processes frequently involved in emotion-related regulation (e.g., effortful control; see below) are also used for the regulation of other aspects of functioning. Although we acknowledge that emotional control/regulation can be, and often is, externally imposed, especially early in life, we believe it is useful to differentiate between self-regulatory (i.e., internally generated) processes and those processes that the child does not execute (Eisenberg & Spinrad, 2004). Thus, we tend to use the term "regulation" or, better yet, "self-regulation" only for intrinsic regulatory processes, although Gross and Thompson's distinction between extrinsic and intrinsic regulatory processes serves the same purpose.

Effortful Control

Early in the formulation of her theory of temperament, Rothbart (e.g., Rothbart & Derryberry, 1981) proposed that reactivity and the regulation of reactivity (including emotional reactivity) are the two major components of temperament. Rothbart and Bates (2006) define temperament as constitutionally based individual differences in reactivity and self-regulation, in the domains of affect, activity, and attention; consequently, temperament is biologically based albeit affected by the environment. Effortful control, the regulatory component of temperament, is defined as "the efficiency of executive attention, including the ability to inhibit a dominant response and/or to activate a subdominant response, to plan, and to detect errors" (Rothbart & Bates, 2006, p. 129; see Rothbart & Sheese, this volume). It involves the ability to deploy attention willfully (often called attention focusing and shifting and perhaps cognitive distraction) and to willfully inhibit or activate behavior (inhibitory and activational control, respectively), especially when a person prefers not to do so but should to adapt to the context or to achieve a goal. Thus, some executive functioning skills (especially effortful deployment of attention, integrating of information attended to, and planning) are involved in effortful control. These processes can be used to modulate emotional experience and the overt behavioral expression of emotion, as well as to regulate nonemotional behaviors. In our view, effortful control is part of the array of processes or capabilities—part of the bag of tricks—that can be used to manage emotion and its expression in behavior; however, effortful control is not, in itself, necessarily emotion self-regulation because it can be used for other purposes.

The fact that effortful control is effortful or willful does not mean that the individual is always aware that he or she is modulating emotion or behavior. For example, a girl may force herself to attend to an uninteresting task without consciously monitoring what she is doing. A good analogy is climbing steps on a hillside: a person has to inhibit and activate movements when climbing the stairs and visually attend to and assess the size of the steps but may not be actively aware of doing so. However, if the person needs to consciously focus on his or her steps to negotiate a slippery or precarious part of the stairs, he or she can easily do so and modify his or her movements. Some aspects of effortful control may usually be automatic and executed without much conscious awareness in many contexts (Mischel & Ayduk, 2004), even though the individual should be able to shift into an aware mode when needed. Thus, we do not believe that the use of skills involved in effortful control is always, or even usually, highly conscious or effortful/voluntary. One factor that distinguishes effortful regulatory processes from less voluntary reactive processes (see below) is the ease with which they can be effortfully controlled when it is adaptive to move from automatic to effortful status.

Although any particular form of emotion-related regulation is not necessarily good or bad in terms of its consequences, we believe that effortful regulatory processes (including effortful control) are relatively likely to result in adaptive outcomes. This is because they can be applied at will and adapted flexibly to the demands of specific contexts. However, effortful control, like active or engagement coping (Compas, Connor,

Saltzman, Thomsen, & Wadsworth, 2001), may be nonadaptive in some uncontrollable contexts (e.g., when one must deal with medical procedures and/or illness). Individuals also may use effortful control in a manner that is not adaptive; for example, a person may voluntarily persist in focusing his or her attention on a negative event to the extent that is very distressing and undermines adaptive psychological and behavioral functioning. Or effortful control can be used to achieve socially inappropriate goals, such as a youth planning and carrying out a series of well-regulated actions to humiliate a peer or to steal items to impress friends. Moreover, an effortful mode of regulation could be adaptive in the short run but not in the long run, or vice versa. In part, the adaptiveness of effortful control depends on the goals that an individual is striving to achieve.

Control and Regulation: Is Control Always Regulation?

In regard to the issue of the adaptation, like a number of other investigators (e.g., Cole, Michel, & Teti, 1994), we have argued that well-regulated people are not overly controlled or undercontrolled; rather, they can respond flexibly to the varying demands of experience with a range of responses that are socially acceptable but also allow for spontaneity. Well-regulated children can effortfully initiate or inhibit behaviors when appropriate or required to achieve goals but can also be spontaneous (uncontrolled) when control is not needed (Block & Block, 1980). Therefore, optimally regulated people can be flexible in the degree to which they exercise their regulatory capabilities, depending on the circumstances.

Because of the importance of both willfulness and flexibility in effortful control, it is useful to try to differentiate effortful control from less voluntary over- or undercontrolled processes. Control is generally defined in the dictionary as inhibition or restraint. Like Kopp (1982), we view "control" as often less flexible and adaptive than regulation. Sometimes children may appear to be self-regulated, but their inhibition or constraint is relatively involuntary or so automatic that it is difficult to effortfully modulate. An example would be children who have been labeled "behaviorally inhibited." They tend to be wary and overly constrained in novel or stressful situations and have difficulty modulating (e.g., relaxing) their inhibition (Kagan & Fox, 2006). Conversely, the impulse to approach people or inanimate objects in the environment (sometimes called surgency; Rothbart & Bates, 2006) often may be relatively involuntary. For example, individuals may be "pulled" toward rewarding or positive situations or stimuli with relatively little ability to inhibit themselves; such people generally are viewed as impulsive. Although we agree with Gross and Thompson (this volume) that children's emotions are sometimes controlled by processes that are not very voluntary, we find the distinction between effortfully controlled self-regulation and less voluntarily controlled processes involved in modulating emotion useful (see Compas et al., 2001, for a similar distinction when defining coping). In brief, we view effortful control as part of the larger domain of control and have argued that control is most likely to be adaptive if it is effortfully managed and, hence, flexible.

We (e.g., Eisenberg & Morris, 2002) have labeled such overly inhibited and impulsive behavior as two aspects of *reactive control* (i.e., reactive overcontrol and undercontrol), based on the distinction by Rothbart between effortful and reactive temperamental processes. We consider effortful control, not reactive control, to be part of self-regulation. We do not deny that reactive control processes influence affective responding and are involved in the control of both emotions and behavior, but we do not equate having an effect on another system or aspect of functioning with self-regulation.

Rothbart and colleagues (e.g., Derryberry & Rothbart, 1997) have linked what we have labeled "reactive control processes" (e.g., behavioral inhibition and impulsivity) to reactive emotional processes (e.g., fear and desire, hope, or relief, respectively) and their associated motivational systems (defensive and appetitive, respectively). Although we agree that these associations between behavioral inhibition or impulsivity and emotion/motivation exist, we wish to differentiate between emotional reactivity and the aspects of behavior relevant to control that typically are associated with emotion. It is quite possible that children who display behavioral inhibition may not experience fear or anxiety every time they display overly inhibited behavior. Such behavior, although probably originally based on fear or a reaction to novelty (Kagan & Fox, 2006), may become a habitual style of response to novel or potentially stressful contexts (and fear or reactivity to novelty is not necessarily associated with behavioral inhibition). Moreover, highly inhibited children often look controlled (restrained) in their behavior but tend to be prone to fear and anxiety; thus, control of behavior is not the same as control in regard to emotional reactivity. Similarly, impulsive behavior may be linked with both desire/positive affect (e.g., Rothbart, Ahadi, Hershey, & Fisher, 2001) and anger at different times or may not be linked to any clear emotion. Thus, emotion reactivity of a particular sort is not strictly paired with impulsivity, and it is worthwhile to differentiate between impulsivity and emotional reactivity and among associated motivations in specific interactions.

Indeed, overly and undercontrolled behavior are of interest in their own right. Decades ago Jack and Jeanne Block (1980) labeled such behavior as the extremes of ego control and argued that neither extreme was adaptive. In the Blocks' model, ego control—defined as the "threshold or operating characteristic of an individual with regard to the expression or containment of impulses, feelings, and desires" (p. 43)—is regulated by ego resiliency—"the dynamic capacity of an individual to modify his/her modal level of ego-control, in either direction, as a function of the demand characteristics of the environmental context" (p. 48). Thus, ego resiliency is a construct similar to effortful control. Although ego control involves the expression of feelings, it is not synonymous with emotional reactivity. Partly because reactive inhibition and impulsivity have been viewed as high and low levels of ego control, respectively, we use the term "reactive control" to highlight the relative lack of voluntary control (and, thus, flexibility) inherent in both highly inhibited and impulsive behavior.

A disadvantage to invoking the distinction between effortful regulation and reactive control is that it is difficult to categorize some aspects of regulation/control. For example, it is difficult to determine the degree to which young children's self-soothing (e.g., thumb sucking) is voluntary. Similarly, it is difficult to know if the child who is constrained in a new context is regulated (i.e., the constraint is voluntary) or overly controlled (behaviorally inhibited). In our view, a major challenge for the field is differentiating between more effortful and less voluntarily managed inhibition.

Although impulsivity and effortful control are fairly consistently negatively related (Aksan & Kochanska, 2004; Valiente et al., 2003), a finding that supports the distinction between effortful and reactive control, Aksan and Kochanska (2004) reported that behavioral inhibition in young children was positively related to young children's effortful control. However, it actually was children's fearfulness, not their inhibition of behavior in a novel situation, that was associated with effortful control in this study. It is possible, as suggested by Aksan and Kochanska (2004), that the fearfulness associated with a nonimpulsive style facilitates the emerging capacity for voluntary, effortful inhibitory control. However, it is also possible that the relation held because children who are very low in fearfulness tended to be quite impulsive and, thus, had difficulty developing effortful control. That is, fearful children may be similar to average children in effortful control, whereas low fearful children may be unlikely to develop effortful control. Such a finding would be somewhat analogous to the finding that moderate and high levels of impulsivity are equally positively related to ego resiliency in young children whereas low impulsivity is related to low resiliency (Eisenberg, Spinrad, & Morris, 2002). In this case, it was low impulsivity, not high impulsivity, that was most responsible for the relation with resiliency. More research is needed to examine links between effortful control and reactive impulsivity and behavioral inhibition.

In support of the distinction between effortful and less voluntary control, there is evidence suggesting that the neurological bases for reactive control processes differ from those linked with effortful control. The executive attention capacities involved in effortful control appear to be centered primarily in the anterior cingulate gyrus and the lateral prefrontal cortex, parts of the brain associated with relatively high-level processes (Rothbart & Bates, 2006) (see Rothbart & Sheese, this volume; see Davidson, Fox, & Kalin, this volume). In contrast, Pickering and Gray (1999), among others, have argued that approach/avoidance tendencies of these sorts (that seem be less willfully controlled) are anchored in relatively less advanced subcortical systems in the brain rather than in cortical areas (although there are many connections between subcortical and cortical parts of the brain). Also suggestive of different neurological bases of effortful and reactive control, vagal modulation of respiratory driven, high-frequency heart-rate variability has been associated with executive control (i.e., effortful control) on behavioral tasks (and is thus linked to effortful control), whereas passive avoidance, avoidance of punishment, and low-reward dominance (linked to behavior inhibition) have been correlated with sympathetic modulation of heart-rate variability (Mezzacappa, Kindlon, Saul, & Earls, 1998).

THE NORMATIVE DEVELOPMENT OF REGULATION AND EFFORTFUL CONTROL

Children begin to regulate their own emotions and emotion-related behavior in the first few years of life. Developmental psychologists sometimes have discussed the normative development of emotion-related regulation in the context of the emergence of compliance or internalization of adults' commands/values. In influential early work on the topic, Kopp (1982) outlined stages of self-regulation in the early years of life. Children were viewed as moving from simple modulation of arousal and activation of organized patterns of behavior to the ability to flexibly use control processes to delay and behave according to social expectations in the absence of external monitoring in a manner that meets changing situational demands. She outlined the cognitive prerequisites (e.g., intentionality, goal-directed behavior, representational thinking, sense of identity, and strategy production) for each of her five phases. Kopp has emphasized how control is first externally imposed and gradually becomes more self-regulated in the first years of life.

It is generally believed that young infants rely on caregivers to regulate their emotional arousal (e.g., holding the baby while talking to him or her) and, by 6 months of age, are able to actively elicit social assistance from caregivers in regulating their emotion. As an example of a relatively sophisticated *extraorganismic* mode of regulation (i.e., regulation from outside the child), social referencing–the process of the child looking to someone else for information about how to respond to, think about, or feel about some event in the environment—can be observed in infants as young as 6 months of age (see Saarni, Mumme, & Campos, 1998). With development, infants learn how to calm themselves down using both external (sucking a thumb) and internal (looking away from an arousing situation) *intraorganismic* modes of self-regulation strategies. Kopp (1982) suggested that self-soothing and the use of attention are early appearing modes of emotion regulation that are more autonomous and mark the transition from adult-assisted regulation to internal self-regulation. Moreover, with increasing age and experience, children increasingly learn that regulatory strategies are more effective in some situations than in others and that different strategies tend, on average, to be differentially effective in obtaining goals (Eisenberg & Morris, 2002).

A number of researchers have collected data on the use of various modes of early intraorganismic regulation and their development with age. For example, by 6 months of age, infants sometimes reduce their own distress to novelty by looking away from the novel object and by using self-soothing strategies (Crockenberg & Leerkes, 2004). Such behaviors appear to be effective because, in the first year of life, self-soothing (at 5 and 10 months of age) and orienting (at 10 months of age) strategies are associated with lower negativity in frustrating situations (Stifter & Braungart, 1995). Stifter and Braungart (1995) found that self-soothing was the most preferred regulatory strategy at both 5 and 20 months of age. In contrast, Mangelsdorf, Shapiro, and Marzoff (1995) found that (1) 6-month-old infants tended to use gaze aversion as their primary regulatory strategy, (2) 12-month-olds engaged in more self-soothing (e.g., thumb sucking and hair twirling) than 18-month-olds, and (3) 12- and 18-month-old toddlers used more behavioral avoidance and self-distracting strategies than did 6-month-olds. There appears to be a decline in the use of external self-soothing between 24 and 48 months of age, coupled with the emergence of new and more complex use of objects and interactions to regulate emotional state (see Diener & Mangelsdorf, 1999, for a review). By 24 months of age, self-distraction may be the most commonly used and successful regulatory strategy in fearful and frustrative situations (Grolnick, Bridges, & Connell, 1996).

Advances in cognitive, sociocognitive, motor, and language development that occur between the 2 and 5 years of age contribute to the emergence of more sophisticated, diverse, and successful models of self-regulation (Kopp, 1989; Kopp & Neufeld, 2003) such that many children are relatively skilled in managing their impulses by age 4 or 5 (Mischel & Ayduk, 2004; Posner & Rothbart, 2000). For example, the development of an understanding of others' beliefs and desires (i.e., theory of mind) in the preschool years has been linked to behavioral regulation—planning and problem solving (Carlson, Moses, & Claxton, 2004).

Researchers who focused on the development of effortful control processes such as attention shifting and attention focusing (part of executive attention) or the ability to voluntarily inhibit behavior rather than on specific reactions to distress or frustration also have noted developmental changes in their use (Posner & Rothbart, 2000). Eight- to 10-month-olds demonstrate some capacity to focus their attention (Kochanska, Coy, Tjebkes, & Husarek, 1998), and voluntary control of attention increases somewhat between 9 and 18 months of age (Ruff & Rothbart, 1996). Around 12 months of age, infants develop the ability to inhibit predominant responses. For example, Diamond (1991) found that 12-month-olds are able to reach for a target not in their line of sight, which shows that they can coordinate their reaching and vision and attend to both. Moreover, Diamond found that infants were able to inhibit predominant response tendencies when reaching for objects (e.g., move around an object), an ability believed to involve the execution of intentional behavior, planning, and the resistance of more automatic or reactive action tendencies.

According to Posner and Rothbart (2000), a transition in the development of executive attention and the effortful inhibition of behavior can be seen around 30 months of age. Much of the relevant work has been conducted using a Stroop-like task that required toddlers to switch attention and inhibit behavior. Children show significant improvement in performance on such a task between 24 and 30 months of age and often perform with high accuracy by 36 to 38 months of age. Moreover, young children's ability on such tasks has been positively related to adults' ratings of effortful control (Rothbart & Bates, 2006). In addition, with the maturation of attentional mechanisms, the ability to effortfully inhibit motor behavior greatly improves between 22 and 44 months (Kochanska, Murray, & Harlan, 2000; Reed, Pien, & Rothbart, 1984) and is fairly good by 4 years of age (Posner & Rothbart, 2000). Moreover, there appears to be a further increase in the use of internal mental or cognitive regulatory strategies in the school years (Eisenberg & Morris, 2002). Nonetheless, the capacity for effortful control continues to improve in the school years and may even continue to develop at a slower pace into adulthood (Brocki & Bohlin, 2004; Murphy, Eisenberg, Fabes, Shepard, & Guthrie, 1999; Williams, Ponesse, Schachar, Logan, & Tannock, 1999).

THE RELATION OF EFFORTFUL CONTROL TO SOCIOEMOTIONAL DEVELOPMENT

Although there seems to be a normative pattern for the development of self-regulatory skills, there are also individual differences in the development of these skills. In fact, there are stable individual differences in effortful control across time early in life. For example, Kochanska et al. (2000) found that focused attention at 22 months predicts effortful control at 33 and 45 months (Kochanska & Knaack, 2003). The stability of effortful control is even greater after the age of 3 (see Posner & Rothbart, 2000), likely due to deficits and instability in executive attention prior to age 3 (Rothbart & Bates, 2006). Teachers' and parents' reports of aspects of children's effortful control have been found to be relatively stable over 4, or sometimes 6, years during middle childhood (especially for attention focusing and inhibitory control and less so for attention shifting; Eisenberg et al., 2005; Murphy et al., 1999).

If children differ in their regulatory capacities, they are likely to differ in aspects of socioemotional functioning that are predicted to be related to emotion-related self-regulation. Based on the distinction between reactive and effortful control, we (Eisenberg & Morris, 2002; Eisenberg et al., 2005) constructed a heuristic model including three styles of control—overcontrolled, undercontrolled, and optimally controlled—to generate predictions regarding their relations to children's socioemotional adjustment and development.

In this model, highly inhibited or overcontrolled individuals are hypothesized to be high in involuntary reactive control, for example, behaviorally inhibited in novel contexts and rigid and overcontrolled in their expression of emotion; low in impulsivity (reactive undercontrol); average in the ability to effortfully inhibit behavior as needed (inhibitory control); low in effortful attentional regulation (e.g., the abilities to willfully shift and focus attention); and low in the ability to effortfully activate behavior as needed (i.e., activational control). They are expected to be somewhat low in effortful attentional (but perhaps not inhibitory) regulation because shifting or focusing attention can be used to reduce negative emotions such as fear associated with highly inhibited behavior. Because of their inhibition in social situations, such individuals are expected to be prone to internalizing problems (e.g., depression, anxiety, and social withdrawal) and relatively low in social competence, especially if they are also predisposed to experience negative emotions. Moreover, these children may lack the ability to be relaxed and spontaneous in all but very familiar settings, which also could undermine their social attractiveness and peer status (Eisenberg, Fabes, Guthrie, & Reiser, 2000a).

In contrast to overly controlled people, undercontrolled individuals are hypothesized to be low in all types of effortful control, including attentional, inhibitory, and activation control; high in reactive approach tendencies (i.e., impulsive); and low in reactive overcontrol (i.e., low in behavioral inhibition). Individuals with this style of control are predicted to be relatively low in social competence and prone to externalizing behavior problems such as aggression, defiance, and antisocial behaviors (e.g., delinquency).

Finally, optimally regulated individuals are hypothesized to be fairly high in all the various modes of effortful control and, in regard to reactive control, neither overcontrolled nor undercontrolled. These individuals are expected to be well adjusted, socially competent, and resilient when faced with stress and adversity because they typically regulate their behavior in a goal-directed manner in a given context but can also be spontaneous and unconstrained. Accordingly, they are expected to bounce back when stressed, which contributes to better adjustment and social competence.

In brief, in this heuristic model, high levels of effortful control, but not reactive overcontrol, are linked to better adjustment and social competence in children. Moreover, internalizing problems such as anxiety, depression, and social withdrawal are associated with low effortful attentional control, but not level of inhibitory control. We have obtained support for most of these predictions (although a relation between low attentional control and internalizing problems may hold more consistently in younger children). However, these relations are probabilistic; as already noted, high effortful control or regulation may not always be applied in a socially appropriate or adaptive manner.

Social Competence

In a number of studies with preschoolers and older children, emotion-related regulatory capacities have been associated with relatively high levels of social competence. Children's abilities to module their attentional resources are likely to lead to relatively optimal levels of emotional arousal in stressful contexts, accurate information processing linked to understanding the causes of emotion, effective planning, and action suited to the situation. The abilities to effortfully inhibit and activate behavior allow the child to implement or inhibit behaviors as is adaptive in a given context, hence facilitating socially appropriate responses. Consistent with this view, preschoolers who used more attentional strategies (e.g., self-distraction) during a delay task were rated by their teachers as higher in social competence, and peers tended to rate them, compared to peers who used fewer attentional strategies, as popular or average in peer liking rather than as rejected or neglected (Raver, Blackburn, Bancroft, & Torp, 1999; also see Fabes, Martin, Hanish, Anders, & Madden-Derdich, 2003). In addition, adults' reports of attentional control often predicted children's socially appropriate and prosocial behavior at school 2, 4, and 6 years later (Eisenberg et al., 1995, 1997; Murphy, Shepard,

Eisenberg, & Fabes, 2004). In another longitudinal study, young children's lack of regulation (likely indexed by a combination of low effortful control, high reactive undercontrol, and negative emotionality) predicted relatively low social competence in late childhood and adolescence, as well as a relatively low quality of social functioning in adulthood (Caspi, 2000; Caspi, Henry, McGee, Moffitt, & Silva, 1995). In Mischel's (Mischel & Ayduk, 2004) longitudinal study, delay of gratification at age 4 or 5 years, apparently due to attentional regulation, predicted parent-reported social competence in adolescence, as well as socioemotional competencies in adulthood.

Similar relations have been found in other samples in which regulation was first assessed in the school years (see Rothbart & Bates, 2006). For example, Eisenberg et al. (1997) found associations of elementary school children's social status with peers' and teachers' ratings of children's socially appropriate behavior with teachers' and parents' reports of children's attentional control and a behavioral measure of persistence. These relations tended to hold across time and sometimes were stronger for children prone to experience negative emotions (Eisenberg et al., 2000, 2003).

A similar positive relation between effortful control and social competence has been found in other cultures. For example, Eisenberg, Pidada, and Liew (2001) found a positive relation between adult-reported effortful control and Indonesian third graders' peer competence and adult-reported socially appropriate behavior (vs. antisocial behavior); this pattern of findings was replicated 3 years later, especially for boys (Eisenberg, Liew, & Pidada, 2004). Moreover, Chinese children's effortful control has been positively associated with their leadership/sociability (Zhou, Eisenberg, Wang, & Reiser, 2004). Thus, in general, well-regulated children and youth tend to be relatively socially competent.

Social Cognition

Emotion understanding—a sociocognitive skill involved in affective social competence (e.g., Saarni et al., 1998)—involves being able to attend to relevant emotion-laden language and information in one's environment, identify one's own and others' experienced and expressed emotions, understand which emotions are appropriate in different contexts, and recognize the causes and consequence of emotions. Regulation probably is involved in the ability to focus on emotion-relevant environmental cues, which contributes to the development and fine-tuning of emotion understanding. Moreover, children who can avoid emotional overarousal are more likely than emotionally aroused children to focus on relevant information about emotions in social interactions. In support of these ideas, preschoolers' regulation has predicted their understanding of emotion 2 years later (Schultz, Izard, Ackerman, & Youngstrom, 2001), and emotion understanding mediates the relation of regulation to adaptive social behavior (Izard, Schultz, Fine, Youngstrom, & Ackerman, 1999/2000).

Of course, it is also likely that emotion understanding fosters, as well as stems from, emotion-related regulation. Denham and Burton (2003) suggested that emotion understanding gives children labels for their internal feelings, which can then be made conscious. Such conscious emotional awareness allows children to immediately attach feelings with events, which can then facilitate successful and appropriate regulation. Researchers have found that children who are able to understand emotions, communicate about them, and know how to manage emotions are better able to regulate themselves (Denham & Burton, 2003; Kopp, 1989).

Adjustment

In the first 5 years of life and in childhood, better emotion-related self-regulation has been negatively related to negative emotionality, specifically frustration and sadness, and is associated with better emotion-relevant self-regulation (e.g., effortful control; Calkins, Dedmon, Gill, Lomax, & Johnson, 2002; Kochanska & Knaack, 2003; Stifter & Spinrad, 2002; see Eisenberg, Smith, Sadovsky, & Spinrad, 2004, for a review). Thus, it is not surprising that children who are low in effortful control/emotion regulation are more likely than children with higher levels of effortful control/regulation to exhibit problems with adjustment (see Mullin & Hinshaw, this volume).

For example, in a longitudinal study, Kochanska and colleagues found that toddlers who were less compliant at 22, 33, and 45 months had lower levels of effortful control than toddlers who were more compliant (Kochanska & Knaack, 2003) and had higher levels of externalizing problems (Murray & Kochanska, 2002). In another investigation with young children, Calkins and Dedmon (2000) found that 2-year-olds who were rated by their mothers as having more aggressive and destructive behaviors exhibited lower focused attention and more distraction during laboratory tasks compared to children who were rated by their mothers as low in externalizing problems. In addition, Lemery, Essex, and Smider (2002) found that mothers' reports of children's attention focusing and inhibitory control (averaged across 3½ and 4½ years of age) negatively predicted mothers' and fathers' reports of externalizing problems and attention-deficit/hyperactivity disorder at 5½ years of age.

Similarly, many investigators have found negative relations between measures of regulation, including effortful control, and adjustment in children in elementary school and early adolescence (see Caspi, 2000; Eisenberg, Fabes, Guthrie, et al., 2000; Eisenberg, Smith, et al., 2004; Rothbart & Bates, 2006, for reviews). Eisenberg and colleagues (Eisenberg et al., 1995; Eisenberg et al., 1997; Murphy et al., 2004) found that mothers' and fathers' reports of the level of children's externalizing behavior problems in elementary school were occasionally predicted by parents' (but not teachers') reports of attentional control in preschool or kindergarten, and were much more consistently predicted by mothers' (but not teachers') reports of effortful control in elementary school (including across time). In two different longitudinal samples, Eisenberg and colleagues fairly consistently have found negative relations between children's externalizing behaviors at school and teacher-reported, parent-reported, and observed measures of effortful control (including attention focusing and shifting and inhibitory control; Eisenberg, Cumberland, et al., 2001; Valiente et al., 2003). At 2-year (Eisenberg, Guthrie, et al., 2000; Eisenberg, Spinrad, et al., 2004; Eisenberg et al., 2005) and even 4-year (Valiente et al., 2003) follow-ups, effortful control generally provided unique prediction of externalizing behavior, even when controlling for prior levels of regulation and/or externalizing problems. Similarly, school children's externalizing problems have been associated with low delay of gratification (Krueger, Caspi, Moffitt, White, & Stouthamer-Loeber, 1996), with the inability to inhibit behavior upon signal (Oosterlaan, Logan, & Sergeant, 1998), and with children's (as well as parents') reports of children's attention focusing (Lengua, West, & Sandler, 1998).

The association between effortful control and internalizing problems such as social withdrawal, anxiety, and depression is less clear and may be stronger for younger than older children. Mothers' reports of preschoolers' attention focusing and inhibitory control have been modestly, negatively related with children's internalizing problems at 5½ years old, and these relations held even when items that overlapped between the constructs of regulation and internalizing problems were removed from the scales (Lemery et al., 2002). In a study with 9- to 12-year-olds, child- or parent-reported depressive symptoms were correlated with low levels of child- and parent-reported attention focusing (even when controlling for confounded scale items; Lengua et al., 1998). In a different sample (in which some confounded scale items were also removed), young school-age children with internalizing problems were found to be low in adult-rated attentional control but not inhibitory control (Eisenberg, Cumberland, et al., 2001); however, in the 2-year follow-up, neither inhibitory control nor attentional control predicted internalizing problems (Eisenberg et al., 2005). It is not clear why there were discrepancies in the relations across time and studies (see Eisenberg, Cumberland, et al., 2001; Eisenberg et al., 2005, for review of other relevant studies).

In contrast to the aforementioned negative or null relations between effortful control and internalizing problems, Murray and Kochanska (2002) found that mothers rated young children high in effortful control as having more internalizing problems than children who had moderate effortful control. This finding may have occurred because many of the measures of effortful control may have partly assessed reactive control, including low impulsivity and high behavioral inhibition, and behavioral inhibition/low impulsivity is linked to social withdrawal (considered an internalizing symptom; Eisenberg, Cumberland, et al., 2001). Relations between effortful control or regulation and internalizing problems require further study to clarify discrepancies in findings across studies.

Internalization of Parental Rules/Demands and Guilt

Effortful control and related measures of emotion-related regulation or control have also been linked to a variety of measures of moral development, including compliance, internalization of rules, and conscience. Committed compliance is thought to reflect children's wholehearted desire to obey their mothers' commands. When toddlers continue to comply with their mothers' rules when left alone, they are believed to have internalized the rules (e.g., Kochanska, Coy, & Murray, 2001).

Kochanska and colleagues found that toddlers who exhibited more committed compliance were higher in effortful control than their less compliant peers (Kochanska, Murray, & Coy, 1997; Kochanska et al., 2001). In addition, Kochanska et al. (1997) found that effortful control was associated with high levels of conscience during the toddler, preschool, and early school years, and prediction was often across time. Measures of conscience included adults' ratings of children on items assessing the moral self (e.g., concern about others' wrongdoing, apology, and empathy), measures of cheating when an adult was not present, and children's responses to hypothetical moral dilemmas. Kochanska and Knaack (2003) replicated these results and found that effortful control at 22, 33, and 45 months, as well as a composite score of effortful control across three ages, predicted an internalized conscience at 56 months, even after statistically controlling for children's gender and intelligence.

There are few data on the relation between conscience and effortful control in school children. Rothbart, Ahadi, and Hershey (1994) found that parents' reports of children's effortful control were associated with their reports of their 7-year-old children's tendencies to experience guilt. More research is needed to verify and understand the relation of effortful control to conscience and other aspects of moral development in older elementary-school-age children and adolescents.

Empathy/Sympathy and Prosocial Behavior

Eisenberg and colleagues hypothesized that individuals high in effortful emotion-related self-regulation tend to experience sympathy (an other-oriented response to another's emotion or condition) rather than personal distress (i.e., a self-focused, aversive response to another's emotional state or condition). Personal distress is associated with empathic overarousal (possibly due to underregulation), which in turn can lead to a self-focus and self-concerned behavioral response (rather than concern for others; see Eisenberg, Wentzel, & Harris, 1998). Consistent with this premise, relations between effortful control and empathy-related responding have been found in studies with both children and adults. For example, in a study with young school-age children, parents and teachers rated children's effortful control. In addition, children's facial expressions were videotaped while watching an evocative film about a young girl burned during a home fire (and teased by peers for her appearance), and children's reactions to the film were assessed after the film by having them rate their feelings using simple adjectives (Guthrie et al., 1997). Children rated high on effortful regulation exhibited greater facial sadness (but not distress)—presumed to reflect sympathy/empathy—during the film compared to less regulated peers. Children's postfilm reports of sadness and sympathy during the film were also positively related to parents' ratings of effortful control. Conversely, children low in parent-rated effortful regulation were prone to experience personal distress (e.g., anxiety and tension) during the film. Based on these findings, children's emotion regulation might be more predictive of their appropriate emotional responding than the intensity or valence of their response.

Children's effortful control also has been positively related to self- or other-report measures of empathy/sympathy (Valiente et al., 2004; see Eisenberg et al., 1998). In a longitudinal study, a composite of effortful and reactive control (i.e., low impulsivity) predicted sympathy over 2 or 4 years (e.g., Murphy et al., 1999). Similar concurrent relations have been found in studies in which adults reported on their own sympathy and regulation, although sometimes the association was not significant until the effects of individual differences in negative emotionality were controlled (see Eisenberg et al., 1998). In addition, effortful control has been negatively related to children's and adults' reports of personal distress (Eisenberg et al., 1998; Valiente et al., 2004).

Consistent with the empirical relation between effortful control and sympathy, adults' ratings of elementary school children's effortful attentional control and/or a behavioral measure of persistence have been correlated with peers' ratings of prosocial behavior (e.g., Eisenberg et al., 1997), as well as with peers' and teacher reports of pre-schoolers' agreeableness (including niceness, sharing, and helpfulness; Cumberland, Eisenberg, & Reiser, 2004). Thus, people who are skilled at regulating their emotion and behavior are not only more likely to feel concern for them, but also are relatively likely to help others.

CONCLUSIONS AND FUTURE DIRECTIONS

The study of emotion regulation and related processes has progressed tremendously in the last decade. Yet definitional and methodological issues need to be addressed, and examination of relations of emotion-related regulation to other variables generally has not been sufficiently process-oriented. In addition, there are limitations in current methods and gaps in the literature.

In terms of definitional issues, it is clear that there is considerable variation in what various theorists and researchers are labeling as emotion regulation. It might be helpful if the field came to some consensus in regard to important distinctions and ways of labeling them, such as between extrinsic and intrinsic regulation/control and between effortful/voluntary regulation and less voluntary control. Theorists and researchers also need to decide if emotion regulation includes not only regulation of emotions themselves, but also regulation of associated externally manifested behaviors. Coping theorists have spent considerable effort trying to clarify the structure of coping and meaningful distinctions among types of coping (Compas et al., 2001); investigators studying emotion regulation need to commit more effort to delineating critical conceptual distinctions and to testing them with statistical methods such as confirmatory factor analysis (see Eisenberg, Spinrad, et al., 2004).

The Importance of Process

In regard to research on the association of emotion-related regulation to other constructs of developmental importance, findings indicate that children's emotion-related self-regulation, including their effortful control, may be a powerful force in their development. It predicts social competence, as well as problem behaviors. What is less known are the mechanisms through which these effects are likely to be achieved. Although some of the relation between emotion-related self-regulation and developmental outcomes such as adjustment may be due to heredity affecting both variables, environmental and experiential factors likely also play a role. It is obvious that attentional and behavioral regulation facilitate learning, including learning about the social world; children who can concentrate and modulate their behavior are more likely to attend to critical information in their environment. However, additional processes probably mediate the effects of effortful control on developmental outcomes. For example, children who are emotionally well modulated are likely to evoke more positive responses from other people, which would be expected to affect their feelings about other people and themselves (and hence their social behavior and adjustment). If children are exposed to relatively high levels of positive behavior from others in social interactions, they also are more likely to learn constructive ways of interacting with other people and of managing emotion. For example, children who are better regulated are likely to be exposed to more opportunities for learning and for personal development because other people will be more willing to spend time with them and to provide such opportunities. Moreover, children who elicit positive reactions from others are more likely than those who elicit negative reactions to be optimally rather than overly aroused in social interactions. As already noted, this is important because children who are overaroused by negative affect are less likely to attend to critical information outside their own needs and to learn from such information. Thus, the effects of self-regulation (including effortful control) on children's development are likely mediated through cognitive, physiological, and social processes.

Design of Research Studies

Although research designs used to examine emotion-related regulation generally are much more sophisticated than 20 years ago, most of the existing data on the development of emotion-related self-regulation and its relations to children's developmental outcomes are correlational. In a number of studies, longitudinal designs have been used that involve controlling for levels of variables at the first assessment when examining prediction across time (e.g., Eisenberg, Spinrad, et al., 2004; Valiente et al., 2003). Such designs optimize the investigator's ability to draw causal conclusions, yet even with these studies, one cannot actually test causal relations. Experimental studies, especially intervention and prevention trials in which children are randomly assigned to treatment groups, are required to test causal relations. In such studies, parents, teachers, or experimenters could be trained to help children learn regulatory skills. Effects on regulation as well as related developmental outcomes could be assessed. Although interventions sometimes have included procedures designed to foster regulation, they typically have also included procedures to promote other skills (e.g., understanding of emotions) that might account for any effects of the intervention. Moreover, the direct effects of the various treatments on regulation usually have not been directly assessed (rather, outcomes such as adjustment and social competence typically are measured). Thus, strong tests of causal relations between emotion-related self-regulation and developmental outcomes are not available.

Related to this point, experimental designs are needed to clarify the role of socialization in the development of emotion-related self-regulation (and its affect on socioemotional competence). Although we did not review the research on the socialization of emotion-related regulation (including effortful control) in this chapter (see Thompson & Meyer, this volume), there are associations between parental behaviors/practices and children's self-regulation. To assess causal affects of parenting, it would be helpful to use an experimental intervention to train mothers in techniques that might foster children's regulation (e.g., positive expressivity and support or time spend in joint attention and dyadic turn-taking behavior, Raver, 1996; also see Crockenberg & Leerkes, 2004) and to assess the effects of such training on children's emotion-related self- regulation and on those developmental outcomes believed to be influenced by self-regulation.

Genetically informed research designs could also contribute to an understanding of the influences on, and effects of, children's self-regulation. Not only can twin, adoption, or sibling studies be used to assess the role of genetics and environment in self-regulation (see Rothbart & Bates, 2006), but they also can be used to assess environmental influences, especially when genetic influences are held constant. For example, one could examine factors related to differences between identical twins (who are genetically the same) in effortful control.

Much of the research on children's emerging self-regulation/effortful control and developmental correlates has been conducted in North America, and often with predominantly Caucasian, middle-class participants. Although relations between effortful control and developmental outcomes often do not vary by socioeconomic status (e.g., Eisenberg, Spinrad, et al., 2004), this may not always be true, especially if one compares very low socioeconomic children with other children. In addition, there is some evidence that the size of relations among caregiving quality, emotion-related regulation and later outcomes sometimes is greater in high-risk samples (e.g., low-birthweight infants; Raver, 2004). Moreover, although relations between effortful control and developmental outcomes have been found to be similar in fairly diverse cultures, some differences in the socialization correlates have been noted (see Eisenberg, Zhou, Liew, & Champion, 2006). Thus, it cannot be assumed that the causes and consequences of effortful control (or self-regulation more broadly) identified in Western, middle-class samples generalize to other populations.

The Measurement of Emotion-Related Self-Regulation

Measures of children's emotion-related self-regulation require further development and refinement. Behavioral methods of assessing children's regulatory capacities have proliferated in recent years and have proved very useful. However, this is especially true in work with young children; fewer behavioral methods are available for, or used with, adolescents. Indeed, much less research has been conducted on emotion regulation with adolescents than with young children and elementary school children, and there is a need to focus on adolescents.

Physiological methods of assessing emotion-related regulation have not been fully exploited in the existing research. It is possible that some physiological measures tap effortful process; likely candidates are vagal tone and vagal suppression, measures believed to tap physiological regulation (Porges, Doussard-Roosevelt, & Maiti, 1994). It is argued that the fluctuation in heart rate occurring at the frequency of respiration can be used to assess parasympathetic control via the vagal nerve (Huffman et al., 1998; see Rothbart & Bates, 2006). In addition, a drop in vagal tone when one is attending (vagal suppression) is believed to reflect the use of attentional strategies to cope with the environment or respond to stress (Huffman et al., 1998; Rothbart & Bates, 2006). Researchers have used measures of vagal responding primarily with infants, toddlers, and preschoolers and the findings are not highly consistent (see Rothbart & Bates, 2006); nonetheless, a better understanding of such physiological processes, changes in their significance with age, and their measurement would provide conceptual and methodological tools for further exploration of regulatory processes.

Gaps in the Assessment of Emotion-Related Self-Regulation

Finally, there are aspects of emotion-related self-regulation that have received minimal attention. For example, although some behavioral tasks assess both activational control (the ability to willfully activate behavior even when one does not feel like doing so) and inhibitory control, few investigators have examined the development and correlates of activational control per se. In addition, much emotion-related regulation likely is exerted prior to the occurrence of an emotion-eliciting event or before a full-blown emotional reaction through the processes of selecting and changing one's environment or how one's own thinking about events, people, or objects in the environment (see Gross & Thompson, in volume; Eisenberg & Morris, 2002). Despite its obvious importance in everyday life, little is known about such proactive emotion regulation in children. New methods will need to be developed to assess it because few currently exist. Finally, the regulation of positive emotion seldom has been studied, and the regulation of emotion in various contexts—for example, in interactions with peers and teachers or in organized activities (e.g., sports)—has received relatively little attention.

In summary, although the study of children's emotion-related regulation is flourishing, there is much yet to explore and understand. A multimethod approach, influenced by conceptual work in developmental, clinical, personality, social, and neurophysiological psychology is likely to be productive in future attempts to expand our knowledge.

ACKNOWLEDGMENTS

Work on this chapter was supported by Grant No. 2 R01 MH60838 from the National Institute of Mental Health to Nancy Eisenberg and by a Spencer Dissertation Grant (through Arizona State University) to Claire Hofer.

REFERENCES

Aksan, N., & Kochanska, G. (2004). Links between systems of inhibition from infancy to preschool years. *Child Development, 75,* 1477–1490.

Block, J. H., & Block, J. (1980). The role of ego-control and ego-resiliency in the organization of behavior. In W. A. Collins (Ed.), *The Minnesota Symposia on Child Psychology: Vol. 13. Development of cognition, affect, and social relations* (pp. 39–101). Hillsdale, NJ: Erlbaum.

Brocki, K. C., & Bohlin, G. (2004). Executive functions in children aged 6 to 12: A dimensional and developmental study. *Developmental Neuropsychology, 26,* 571–593.

Calkins, S. D., & Dedmon, S. E. (2000). Physiological and behavioral regulation in two-year-old children with aggressive/destructive behavior problems. *Journal of Abnormal Child Psychology, 28,* 103–118.

Calkins, S. D., Dedmon, S. E., Gill, K. L., Lomax, L. E., & Johnson, L. M. (2002). Frustration in infancy: Implications for emotion regulation, physiological processes, and temperament. *Infancy, 3,* 175–197.

Carlson, S. M., Moses, L. J., & Claxton, L. J. (2004). Individual differences in executive functioning and theory of mind: An investigation of inhibitory control and planning ability. *Journal of Experimental Child Psychology, 87,* 299–319.

Caspi, A. (2000). The child is father of the man: Personality continuities from childhood to adulthood. *Journal of Personality and Social Psychology, 78,* 158–172.

Caspi, A., Henry, B., McGee, R. O., Moffitt, T. E., & Silva, P. A. (1995). Temperamental origins of child and adolescent behavior problems: From age three to age fifteen. *Child Development, 66,* 55–68.

Cicchetti, D., Ganiban, J., & Barnett, D. (1991). Contributions from the study of high risk populations to understanding the development of emotion regulation. In K. Dodge & J. Garber (Eds.), *The development of emotion regulation* (pp. 15–48). New York: Cambridge University Press.

Cole, P. M., Michel, M. K., & Teti, L. O. (1994). The development of emotion regulation and dysregulation: A clinical perspective. In N. A. Fox (Ed.), The development of emotion regulation: Biological and behavioral considerations. *Monographs of the Society for Research in Child Development, 59*(2–3, Serial No. 240), 73–100.

Compas, B. E., Connor, J. K., Saltzman, H., Thomsen, A. H., & Wadsworth, M. E. (2001). Coping with stress during childhood and adolescence: Problems, progress, and potential in theory and research. *Psychological Bulletin, 127,* 87–127.

Crockenberg, S. C., & Leerkes, E. M. (2004). Infant and mother behaviors regulate infant reactivity to novelty at 6 months. *Developmental Psychology, 40,* 1123–1132.

Cumberland, A., Eisenberg, N., & Reiser, M. (2004). Relations of young children's agreeableness and resiliency to effortful control and impulsivity. *Social Development, 13,* 191–212.

Davidson, R. J., Fox, A., & Kalin, N. H. (2007). Neural bases of emotion regulation in nonhuman primates and humans. In J. J. Gross (Ed.), *Handbook of emotion regulation* (pp. 47–68). New York: Guilford Press.

Denham, S. A., & Burton, R. (2003). *Social and emotional prevention and intervention programming for preschoolers.* New York: Kluwer-Plenum Press.

Derryberry, D., & Rothbart, M. K. (1997). Reactive and effortful processes in the organization of temperament. *Development and Psychopathology, 9,* 633–652.

Diamond, A. (1991). Neuropsychological insights into the meaning of object concept development. In S. Carey & R. Gelman (Eds.), *The epigenesis of mind: Essays on biology and cognition* (pp. 67–110). Hillsdale, NJ: Erlbaum.

Diener, M. L., & Mangelsdorf, S. C. (1999). Behavioral strategies for emotion regulation in toddlers: Associations with maternal involvement and emotional expressions. *Infant Behavior and Development, 22,* 569–583.

Eisenberg, N., Cumberland, A., Spinrad, T. L., Fabes, R. A., Shepard, S. A., Reiser, M., et al. (2001). The relations of regulation and emotionality to children's externalizing and internalizing problem behavior. *Child Development, 72,* 1112–1134.

Eisenberg, N., Fabes, R. A., Guthrie, I. K., & Reiser, M. (2000). Dispositional emotionality and regulation: Their role in predicting quality of social functioning. *Journal of Personality and Social Psychology, 78,* 136–157.

Eisenberg, N., Fabes, R. A., Murphy, B., Maszk, P., Smith, M., & Karbon, M. (1995). The role of emotionality and regulation in children's social functioning: A longitudinal study. *Child Development, 66,* 1360–1384.

Eisenberg, N., Guthrie, I. K., Fabes, R. A., Shepard, S., Losoya, S., Murphy, B. C., et al. (2000). Prediction of elementary school children's externalizing problem behaviors from attentional and behavioral regulation and negative emotionality. *Child Development, 71,* 1367–1382.

Eisenberg, N., Guthrie, I. K., Fabes, R. A., Reiser, M., Murphy, B. C., Holgren, R., et al. (1997). The relations of regulation and emotionality to resiliency and competent social functioning in elementary school children. *Child Development, 68,* 295–311.

Eisenberg, N., Liew, J., & Pidada, S. (2004). The longitudinal relations of regulation and emotionality to quality of Indonesian children's socioemotional functioning. *Developmental Psychology, 40,* 790–804.

Eisenberg, N., & Morris, A. S. (2002). Children's emotion-related regulation. In R. Kail (Ed.), *Advances in child development and behavior* (Vol. 30, pp. 190–229). Amsterdam: Academic Press.

Eisenberg, N., Pidada, S. U., Liew, J. (2001). The relations of regulation and negative emotionality to Indonesian children's social functioning. *Child Development, 72,* 1747–1763.

Eisenberg, N., Sadovsky, A., Spinrad, T. L., Fabes, R. A., Losoya, S. H., Valiente, C., et al. (2005). The relations of problem behavior status to children's negative emotionality, effortful control, and impulsivity: Concurrent relations and prediction of change. *Developmental Psychology, 41,* 193–211.

Eisenberg, N., Smith, C. L., Sadovsky, A., & Spinrad, T. L. (2004). Effortful control: Relations with emotion regulation, adjustment, and socialization in childhood. In R. F. Baumeister & K. D. Vohs (Eds.), *Handbook of self-regulation: Research, theory, and applications* (pp. 259–282). New York: Guilford Press.

Eisenberg, N., & Spinrad, T. L. (2004). Emotion-related regulation: Sharpening the definition. *Child Development 75,* 334–339.

Eisenberg, N., Spinrad, T. L., Fabes, R. A., Reiser, M., Cumberland, A., Shepard, S. A., et al. (2004). The relations of effortful control and impulsivity to children's resiliency and adjustment. *Child Development, 75,* 25–46.

Eisenberg, N., Spinrad, T. L., & Morris, A. S. (2002). Regulation, resiliency, and quality of social functioning. *Self and Identity, 1,* 121–128.

Eisenberg, N., Valiente, C., Morris, A. S., Fabes, R. A., Cumberland, A., Reiser, M., et al. (2003). Longitudinal relations among parental emotional expressivity, children's regulation, and quality of socioemotional functioning. *Developmental Psychology, 39,* 2–19.

Eisenberg, N., Wentzel, M., & Harris, J. D. (1998). The role of emotionality and regulation in empathy-related responding. *School Psychology Review, 27,* 506–521.

Eisenberg, N., Zhou, Q., Liew, J., & Champion, C. (2006). Emotion, emotion-related regulation, and social functioning. In X. Chen, D. French, & B. Schneider (Eds.), *Peer relationships in cultural context.* Cambridge, UK: Cambridge University Press.

Fabes, R. A., Martin, C. L., Hanish, L. D., Anders, M. C., & Madden-Derdich, D. A. (2003). Early school competence: The roles of sex-segregated play and effortful control. *Developmental Psychology, 39,* 848–858.

Grolnick, W. S., Bridges, L. J., & Connell, J. P. (1996). Emotion regulation in two-year-olds: Strategies and emotional expression in four contexts. *Child Development, 67,* 928–941.

Gross, J. J., & Thompson, R. A. (2007). Emotion regulation: Conceptual foundations. In J. J. Gross (Ed.), *Handbook of emotion regulation* (pp. 3–24). New York: Guilford Press.

Guthrie, I. K., Eisenberg, N., Fabes, R. A., Murphy, B. C., Holmgren, R., Maszk, P., et al. (1997). The relations of regulation and emotionality to children's situational empathy-related responding. *Motivation and Emotion, 21,* 87–108.

Huffman, L. C., Bryan, Y. E., del Carmen, R., Pedersen, F. A., Doussard-Roosevelt, J. A., & Porges, S. W. (1998). Infant temperament and cardiac vagal tone: Assessments at twelve weeks of age. *Child Development, 69,* 624–635.

Izard, C. E., Schultz, D., Fine, S. E., Youngstrom, E., & Ackerman, B. P. (1999/2000). Temperament, cognitive ability, emotion knowledge, an adaptive social behavior. *Imagination, Cognition and Personality, 19,* 305–330.

Kagan, J., & Fox, N. (2006). Biology, culture, and temperamental biases. In N. Eisenberg (Vol. Ed.) & W. Damon & R. M. Lerner (Series Eds), *Social, emotional and personality development: Vol. 3. Handbook of child psychology* (pp. 167–225). New York: Wiley.

Kochanska, G., Coy, K. C., & Murray, K. T. (2001). The development of self-regulation in the first four years of life. *Child Development, 72,* 1091–1111.

Kochanska, G., Coy, K. C., Tjebkes, T. L., & Husarek, S. J. (1998). Individual differences in emotionality in infancy. *Child Development, 69,* 375–390.

Kochanska, G., & Knaack, A. (2003). Effortful control as a personality characteristic of young children: Antecedents, correlates, and consequences. *Journal of Personality, 71,* 1087–1112.

Kochanska, G., Murray, K. T., Coy, K. C. (1997). Inhibitory control as a contributor to conscience in childhood: From toddler to early school age. *Child Development, 68,* 263–277.

Kochanska, G., Murray, K. T., & Harlan, E. T. (2000). Effortful control in early childhood: Continuity and change, antecedents, and implications for social development. *Developmental Psychology, 36,* 220–232.

Kopp, C. B. (1982). Antecedents of self-regulation: A developmental perspective. *Developmental Psychology, 18,* 199–214.

Kopp, C. B. (1989). Regulation of distress and negative emotions: A developmental view. *Developmental Psychology, 25,* 343–354.

Kopp, C. B., & Neufeld, S. J. (2003). Emotional development during infancy. In R. Davidson, K. R. Scherer, & H. H. Goldsmith (Eds.), *Handbook of affective sciences* (pp. 347–374). Oxford, UK: Oxford University Press.

Krueger, R. F., Caspi, A., Moffitt, T. E., White, J., & Stouthamer-Loeber, M. (1996). Delay of gratification, psychopathology, and personality: Is low self-control specific to externalizing problems? *Journal of Personality, 64,* 107–129.

Lemery, K. S., Essex, M. J., & Smider, N. A. (2002). Revealing the relation between temperament and behavior problem symptoms by eliminating measurement confounding: Expert ratings and factor analyses. *Child Development, 73,* 867–882.

Lengua, L. J., West, S. G., & Sandler, I. N. (1998). Temperament as a predictor of symptomatology in children: Addressing contamination of measures. *Child Development, 69,* 164–181.

Mangelsdorf, S. C., Shapiro, J. R., & Marzoff, D. (1995). Developmental and temperamental differences in emotion regulation in infancy. *Child Development, 66,* 1817–1828.

Mezzacappa, E., Kindlon, D., Saul, J. P., & Earls, F. (1998). Executive and motivational control of performance task behavior, and autonomic heart-rate regulation in children: Physiologic validation of two-factor solution inhibitory control. *Journal of Child Psychology and Psychiatry, 39,* 525–531.

Mischel, W., & Ayduk, O. (2004). Willpower in a cognitive-affective processing system: The dynamics of delay of gratification. In R. F. Baumeister & K. D. Vohs (Eds.), *Handbook of self-regulation: Research, theory, and applications* (pp. 99–129). New York: Guilford Press.

Mullin, B. C., & Hinshaw, S. P. (2007). Emotion regulation and externalizing disorders in children and adolescents. In J. J. Gross (Ed.), *Handbook of emotion regulation* (pp. 523–541). New York: Guilford Press.

Murphy, B. C., Eisenberg, N., Fabes, R. A., Shepard, S., & Guthrie, I. K. (1999). Consistency and change in children's emotionality and regulation: A longitudinal study. *Merrill-Palmer Quarterly, 45,* 413–444.

Murphy, B. C., Shepard, S. A., Eisenberg, N., & Fabes, R. A. (2004). Concurrent and across time prediction of young adolescents' social functioning: The role of emotionality and regulation. *Social Development, 13,* 56–86.

Murray, K. T., & Kochanska, G. (2002). Effortful control: Factor structure and relation to externalizing and internalizing behaviors. *Journal of Abnormal Child Psychology, 30,* 503–514.

Oosterlaan, J., Logan, G. D., & Sergeant, J. A. (1998). Response inhibition in AD/HD, CD, and comorbid AD/HD+CD, anxious, and control children: A meta-analysis of studies with the stop task. *Journal of Child Psychology and Psychiatry, 39,* 411–425.

Pickering, A. D., & Gray, J. A. (1999). The neuroscience of personality. In O. P. John & L. A. Pervin (Eds.), *Handbook of personality: Theory and research* (2nd ed., pp. 277–299). New York: Guilford Press.

Porges, S. W., Doussard-Roosevelt, J. A., & Maiti, A. K. (1994). Vagal tone and the physiological regulation of emotion. In N. A. Fox (Ed.), Emotion regulation: Behavioral and biological considerations. *Monographs of the Society for Research in Child Development, 59*(Serial No. 240), 167–186.

Posner, M. I., & Rothbart, M. K. (2000). Developing mechanisms of self-regulation. *Development and Psychopathology, 12,* 427–441.

Raver, C. C. (1996). Relations between social contingency in mother–child interaction and 2–year-olds' social competence. *Developmental Psychology, 32,* 850–859.

Raver, C. C. (2004). Placing emotional self-regulation in sociocultural and socioeconomic contexts. *Child Development, 75*, 346–535.

Raver, C. C., Blackburn, E. K., Bancroft, M., & Torp, N. (1999). Relations between effective emotional self-regulation, attentional control, and low-income preschoolers' social competence with peers. *Early Education and Development, 10*, 333–350.

Reed, M., Pien, D. L., & Rothbart, M. K. (1984). Inhibitory self control in preschool children. *Merrill–Palmer Quarterly, 30*, 131–147.

Rothbart, M. K., Ahadi, S. A., & Hershey, K. L. (1994). Temperament and social behavior in childhood. *Merrill-Palmer Quarterly*, 40, 21–39.

Rothbart, M. K., Ahadi, S. A., Hershey, K. L., & Fisher, P. (2001). Investigations of temperament at three to seven years: The Children's Behavior Questionnaire. *Child Development, 72*, 1394–1408.

Rothbart, M. K., & Bates, J. E. (2006). Temperament. In W. Damon (Series Ed.) & N. Eisenberg (Vol. Ed.), *Handbook of child psychology: Vol. 3. Social, emotional, and personality development* (6th ed., pp. 99–166). New York: Wiley.

Rothbart, M. K., & Derryberry, D. (1981). Development of individual differences in temperament. In M. E. Lamb & A. L. Brown (Eds.), *Advances in developmental psychology* (Vol. 1, pp. 37–86). Hillsdale, NJ: Erlbaum.

Rothbart, M. K., & Sheese, B. E. (2007). Temperament and emotion regulation. In J. J. Gross (Ed.), *Handbook of emotion regulation* (pp. 331–350). New York: Guilford Press.

Ruff, H. A., & Rothbart, M. K. (1996). *Attention in early development: Themes and variations.* New York: Oxford University Press.

Saarni, C., Mumme, D., & Campos, J. (1998). Emotional development: action, communication, and understanding. In W. Damon (Series Ed.) & N. Eisenberg (Vol. Ed.), *Handbook of child psychology: Vol. 3. Social, emotional, and personality development* (pp. 105–176). New York: Wiley.

Schultz, D., Izard, C. E., & Ackerman, B. P., & Youngstrom, E. A. (2001). Emotion knowledge in economically disadvantaged children: Self-regulatory antecedents and relations to social difficulties and withdrawal. *Development and Psychopathology, 13*, 53–67.

Shonkoff, J. P., & Phillips, D. A. (2000). *From neurons to neighborhoods: The science of early childhood development.* Washington, DC: National Academy Press.

Stifter, C. A., & Braungart, J. M. (1995). The regulation of negative reactivity in infancy: Function and development. *Developmental Psychology*, *31*, 448–455.

Stifter, C. A., & Spinrad, T. L. (2002). The effect of excessive crying on the development of emotion regulation. *Infancy, 3*, 133–152.

Thompson, R. A. (1994). Emotional regulation: A theme in search of definition. *Monographs of the Society for Research in Child Development, 59*(Serial No. 240), 25–52.

Thompson, R. A., & Meyer, S. (2007). Socialization of emotion regulation in the family. In J. J. Gross (Ed.), *Handbook of emotion regulation* (pp. 249–268). New York: Guilford Press.

Valiente, C., Eisenberg, N., Fabes, R. A., Shepard, S. A., Cumberland, A., & Losoya, S. H. (2004). Prediction of children's empathy-related responding from their effortful control and parents' expressivity. *Developmental Psychology, 40*, 911–926.

Valiente, C., Eisenberg, N., Smith, C. L., Reiser, M., Fabes, R. A., Losoya, S., et al. (2003). The relations of effortful control and reactive control to children's externalizing problems: A longitudinal assessment. *Journal of Personality, 71*, 1171–1196.

Williams, B. R., Ponesse, J. S., Schachar, R. J., Logan, G. D., & Tannock, R. (1999). Development of inhibitory control across the life span. *Developmental Psychology, 35*, 205–213.

Zhou, Q., Eisenberg, N., Wang, Y., & Reiser, M. (2004). Chinese children's effortful control and dispositional anger/frustration: Relations to parenting styles and children's social functioning. *Developmental Psychology, 40*, 352–366.

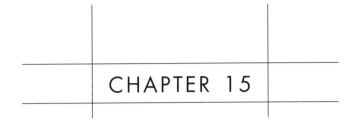

CHAPTER 15

Emotion Regulation and Aging

SUSAN TURK CHARLES
LAURA L. CARSTENSEN

When the 16th-century English coined the term "emotion," they could not have chosen a more appropriate etymological origin. Derived from the Latin word *emovere*, meaning to move or displace, emotions mobilize the body to action. Emotional arousal refers to the activation of multiple physiological systems, affecting neurological, cardiovascular, and endocrine functioning. This mobilization places physical demands on the body, as does the regulation of these experiences. Emotion regulation requires an organism to "undo" heightened arousal and return to homeostasis, or baseline levels of physiological functioning.

Psychologists studying lifespan development of emotional processes observe age-related changes in the regulation of emotions that parallel biological maturation. As children and adolescents acquire and develop the abilities to employ impulse control, gain awareness of themselves and others, and achieve mastery over their environment, they also become increasingly effective at describing and regulating their emotions. Brain maturation and patterns of neurological functioning related to emotional processes continue to develop throughout adolescence (Giedd, 2004) with animal studies showing increases into adulthood (e.g., Cunningham, Bhattacharya, & Benes, 2002). In the latter half of the lifespan, however, the role of biological development in emotional experience and regulation is more difficult to discern. Although aging is related to physiological decrements, these declines may paradoxically aid in emotion regulation. In addition, these changes in motivational goals lead to adaptation to physiological changes that, in turn, maximizes emotional functioning.

The following chapter reviews lifespan developmental findings about emotional experience as well as the cognitive processes we hypothesize are related to age differences in emotion regulation. We first describe the scope of existing literature examining aging, emotion, and emotion regulation and then provide a brief review of this literature. Following, we discuss age differences in the biological processes involved in emotional functioning. Next, we present socioemotional selectivity theory, which posits that motivational goals change across the lifespan such that increasingly greater value is placed on emotional experience with age. After presenting this theory, we review findings suggesting that these motivational shifts lead to differences in social partner preferences, problem-solving strategies, attention, and memory that optimize emotional experience and emotion regulation. We then discuss the importance of individual differences and environmental influences in shaping age-related trajectories of emotional experience. Throughout the chapter we maintain that age-related changes in physiology provide challenges to the aging individual, but individuals adapt to these changes using strategies that maintain and sometimes aid emotion regulation. In conclusion, we offer several future directions in the study of lifespan development of emotional experience and emotion regulation.

THE STUDY OF LIFESPAN DEVELOPMENT OF EMOTIONAL EXPERIENCE AND EMOTION REGULATION

The study of age differences in emotional experience and emotion regulation is relatively new and largely uncharted, and for this reason our chapter covers a diverse set of constructs including affective experience, moods, trait and state affect indices, and coping styles. Few studies examine age differences in regulation of discrete emotions or the enhancement of emotional expression and behavior (cf. Kunzmann, Kupperbusch, & Levenson, 2005). Given the existing literature, we define emotion regulation as low levels of negative affect and high levels of positive affect as opposed to the regulation of discrete emotions (see Gross & Thompson, this volume, for a complete description of emotion regulation). We focus this review on normative aging, a topic which is far from complete yet must be understood completely to comprehend the ramification of diseases, such as dementia and Parkinson's, on emotional functioning. We then discuss cognitive and social processes that are theoretically linked to antecedent emotion regulation strategies, yet we also recognize that future studies need to tie these processes more directly to emotion regulation. Despite the multiple methods of analysis and varied methodology reviewed in this chapter, we maintain that this collection of studies paints a fairly consistent pattern regarding age differences in affective experience. These findings overturn previous stereotypes that once dominated the zeitgeist of emotion and aging, forcing researchers to address how age differences in emotional experience, cognitive processes, and physiological functioning work in concert to yield relatively preserved if not enhanced emotional well-being in later life.

AGE DIFFERENCES IN EMOTIONAL EXPERIENCE

Emotional Well-Being

Emotional experience, like all psychological phenomena, is dependent on physiological functioning. Early theorists relied on their knowledge of biology when positing that emotional well-being and regulation would parallel biological functioning, peaking in the early 20s and declining thereafter (Banham, 1951). So pervasive were these assumptions that few researchers bothered to test these theories, and for many years the portrait of emotion and aging was bolstered more by conjecture than by empiricism (as argued by Schulz, 1985).

Studies examining age differences in emotional experiences have since dispelled the myth of age-related decline. Older age is not associated with high levels of emotional distress (Kobau, Safran, Zack, Moriarty, & Chapman, 2004); for example, reports of subdromal depression—feeling sad, blue, or depressed within the past 30 days—decrease linearly among increasingly older age groups (Kobau et al., 2004). Self-reported negative affect is lower in older adults than in middle-age and younger adults (Lawton, Kleban, Rajagopal, & Dean, 1992), as are rates of anxiety and major depressive disorder (see reviews by Blazer, 2003; Piazza & Charles, 2006). A longitudinal study revealed a steady decline across young, middle, and older adulthood (Charles, Reynolds, & Gatz, 2001). The only caveat to these findings is a slight age-related increase in depressive symptoms documented in some studies, with such increases, though modest relative to depression levels in young adults, more prominent among octogenarians than septogenerians (see reviews by Blazer, 2003; but see Kobau et al., 2004). Notably, however, age increases in negative affect and depression are eliminated once researchers control for functional limitations and chronic illness (e.g., Kunzmann, Little, & Smith, 2000). Life satisfaction (i.e., a global cognitive assessment of the affective quality of life) follows a longitudinal curvilinear trajectory, with increases throughout early and middle adulthood and highest in the 60s, where it then begins to decline (Mroczek & Spiro, 2005). Importantly, however, life satisfaction ratings for the oldest adults included in the study—people in their 80s—equal those of the youngest adults in their 40s. Positive affect, assessed by self-reported experiences from the prior 30 days, is rated higher for older than younger adults (Mroczek & Kolarz, 1998).

One conceivable explanation for the low levels of distress in older adults is that it reflects a serendipitous consequence of reduced physiological reactivity—that is, an inability to experience emotions. However, emotional experience does not appear flattened or diminished. Though older adults report lower frequencies of negative emotions in daily life, there are no age differences in the reported *intensity* of both positive and negative emotions once elicited (Carstensen, Pasupathi, Mayr, & Nesselrode, 2000). In controlled laboratory studies that examine emotions when participants relive emotionally charged events, interact with spouses about highly charged conflicts, or watch film clips to elicit emotions, there is little evidence for age differences (Charles, 2005; Levenson, 2000; Levenson, Carstensen, Friesen, & Ekman, 1991; Tsai, Levenson, & Carstensen, 2000). In fact, when different age groups viewed film clips inducing feelings of sadness and threat related to events that are particularly salient for older people, such as nursing home placement or the onset of illness, subjective ratings of negative emotion were highest among the older adults (Kunzmann & Gruhn, 2005).

Emotional Reactions to Negative Life Events

Studies examining age differences in peoples' reactions to negative events reveal additional advantages for older adults. Compared to younger people, older people report better control over emotions (Gross et al., 1997). Considered on their own, the veracity of subjective reports could be questioned. Yet in a study in which adults ranging from 18 to 94 years old were asked to report the emotions they were experiencing five times a day throughout the course of a week, the probability of continuing to feel a negative emotion from one time point to the next decreased with age (Carstensen et al., 2000).

Researchers have also examined distress differences in response to both minor daily stressors, such as interpersonal arguments (Almeida, 2005), and major life events, including coping with loss of physical health, property, and social ties (Folkman, Lazarus, Pimley, & Novacek, 1987; Lichtenstein, Gatz, Pedersen, & Berg, 1996). Older adults perceive daily stressors as less severe and less threatening than do younger adults (Charles & Almeida, 2005) and report less negative reactivity than younger adults after an interpersonal conflict (Birditt, Fingerman, & Almeida, 2005). When coping with chronic physical health conditions, older age is related to appraising conditions with less blame and hostility (Folkman et al., 1987) and lower feelings of hopelessness in response to chemotherapy treatment (Gil & Gilbar, 2001). These age differences extend to other situations of loss as well: Older adults experienced lower levels of distress than middle-age adults when faced with the damage or complete loss of their homes in a flood (Phifer, 1990), and very old adults reported less stress during spousal bereavement than did their slightly younger counterparts (Lichtenstein et al., 1996).

Reductions in negative affect may be partially influenced by maturational changes through which people develop perspectives on life that help them appraise events in ways that reduce negativity. For example, older adults are less likely to appraise a stressful event as threatening how others perceive them compared to younger adults (Almeida, 2005). Consistent with this premise, older adults are capable of suppressing their emotions (Kunzmann et al., 2005) but engage in this physically and cognitively costly regulation strategy less often than younger adults (John & Gross, 2004).

EMOTIONAL FUNCTIONING WITHIN THE PHYSIOLOGICAL DOMAIN

Emotions are physiological processes, and the first theorists of emotion and aging predicated their statements on age-related biological decline. The findings reviewed preciously have overturned assumptions of greater affective distress with age, and now researchers are studying how age-related changes in biological processes may be related to these emotional experiences. Research on the biology of emotion and aging raises arguably as many questions as answers. Biologists are still differentiating normative processes from disease processes, a task made even more difficult by the vast heterogeneity in rates of declines among individuals as well as within an individual across different organ systems (e.g., Rowe & Kahn, 1997). Despite these challenges, studies of biology are necessary to understand how the aging process influences emotional functioning. Next we describe age differences in three biological systems—brain structure and functioning; cardiovascular function, and neuroendocrine activity—and how these changes may be related to emotional experience.

Brain Structure and Functioning

Studies of brain morphology reveal age-related reductions in brain volume, with small declines prior to age 50 and more substantial linear declines thereafter (DeCarli et al., 2005). Most brains exhibit corticol gliosis, a scarring that appears as a consequence of neuronal cell death (e.g., Beach, Walker, & McGeer, 1989). Existing neurons often show signs of dysfunction; structural abnormalities reveal themselves in neurofibrillary tangles, and demyelination leads to slower reactivity. Although researchers continue to struggle with distinguishing disease processes from normal age-related declines in the aging brain (e.g. Small, Tsai, DeLaPaz, Mayeux, & Stern, 2002), it appears that there are normative reductions in brain volume, which involve reductions in both gray and white matter and synaptic density as well as reductions in neurotransmitter levels (see review by Raz, 2000).

Notably, decline is not uniform across and even within specific brain regions; that is, some areas are more affected than others. The limbic system and the prefrontal cortex are brain regions most critical for emotional processes, and they exhibit very different patterns of decline from each other with age (see Mather, 2004, and Raz, 2000, for comprehensive reviews of age-related change in brain morphology and functioning, and Davidson, Jackson, and Kalin, 2000, and Davidson, Fox, and Kalin, this volume, for neurological substrates of emotional experience). The limbic system, including the hippocampus and amygdala, is a group of interconnected structures located in the midbrain. This area, referred to as the old or paleocortex, is seated below the neocortex and is involved in perceiving, encoding, and recalling emotional stimuli. Within the limbic system, aging is related to declines in some areas and relative stability in others. For example, the amygdala, critical for rapid identification and processing of emotional information, is relatively well maintained with age compared to the prefrontal cortex, and age differences only appear in people age 60 and older (Grieve, Clark, Williams, Peduto, & Gordon, 2005; Mu, Xie, Wen, Weng, & Shuyun, 1999). The hippocampus, an area within the limbic system involved in memory consolidation of both emotional and nonemotional material, exhibits normative age-related declines in the dentate gyrus and subiculum subregions, but not in the entorhinal cortex, an area where decline is clearly observed only among cases with dementia (Small et al., 2002).

In contrast to the limbic system, the prefrontal cortex is associated with pronounced decline. Reductions in synaptic density, dendritic arborization, and increases in neurofibrillary tangles are pervasive in the prefrontal cortex (see review by Raz, 2000; DeCarli et al., 2005). The prefrontal cortex responds more slowly to emotional stimuli than the limbic system (e.g., LeDoux, 2000) and is believed to be responsible for higher-order reasoning about emotional experience and behavior. Located at the foremost region of the frontal lobe and including dorsolateral, orbitofrontal (also called the limbic frontal lobe), and mesial prefrontal subregions, this area is important for executive functions—such as planning, inhibition, and social behavior—as well as emotional processing and emotion-related thoughts and behaviors (see review by Davidson et al., 2000). The importance of the prefrontal cortex for emotional functioning is illustrated in clinical case studies (e.g., Phineas Gage, whose easygoing and restrained personality was dramatically altered after damage to the prefrontal cortex and later characterized by aggressive tendencies and impulsive, uninhibited behavior) (Davidson et al., 2000).

Beyond the Brain: Cardiovascular and Neuroendocrine Functioning

The brain sends messages about emotional stimuli via the peripheral nervous system to activate multiple systems, including both cardiovascular and neuroendocrine processes. Heart rate increases and the epithelial cells lining the vasculature either constrict or dilate in response to an arousing stimulus. Although this overall pattern of reactivity is observed at all ages, reactivity is reduced among older adults (Cacioppo, Berntson, Klein, & Poehlmann, 1997), which likely has a biological basis. For example, epithelial cells increase in rigidity with age (Berdyyeva, Woodward, & Sokolov, 2005), and greater rigidity in the cells lining the vasculature translates to a slower arousal response. In fact, age-related reductions in cardiovascular activity are often more pronounced than age-related changes in other physiological processes (Cacioppo et al., 1997). When people are placed in socially evaluative situations, however, older adults display greater cardiovascular reactivity than do younger adults (Uchino, Holt-Lunstad, Bloor, & Campo, 2005).

The neuroendocrine response portrays a similar story of reactivity with age. The perception of either a real or imagined threat activates a cascading neuroendocrine response along the hypothalamic–pituitary–adrenal (HPA) axis. This system mobilizes the body for action through a series of reactions beginning in the brain and ending with the release of cortisol by the adrenal glands. Although cortisol is a necessary hormone for physiological survival, prolonged elevations of cortisol levels can lead to deleterious physiological effects, including immune dysfunction and glucose intolerance (see review by Sapolsky, this volume).

In both human and animal models, cortisol reactivity in response to psychological and physical stressors is prolonged with age, such that returning to baseline levels takes longer with age (see review by Bjorntorp, 2002; Otte et al., 2005). According to the glucocorticoid cascade hypothesis, this slower recovery of the HPA axis results from an age-related reduction in receptors located in the hippocampus that are responsible for the inhibition of activity along the HPA axis (Sapolsky, Krey, & McEwen, 1986). Thus, inhibitory failures may be related to greater reactivity among older adults, causing a prolonged elevation of cortisol in response to stress among older adults relative to younger adults.

Integrating Physiological Changes and Emotional Experience

Considered along with findings from studies of functional brain imaging (as opposed to studies of brain morphology), a consistent picture begins to emerge across both physiology and experiential data. Brain activation in response to emotional stimuli shifts throughout childhood and into early adulthood toward less activation in the amygdala and greater activation of the prefrontal cortex (Giedd, 2004). Comparing brain activity when people view emotional images, the same age-related shift away from activity in the amygdala and toward activity in prefrontal cortex is found when comparing younger and older adults (Gunning-Dixon et al., 2003). Gunning-Dixon and colleagues commented that the increased reliance on frontal regions was puzzling given that age-related decline is greatest in the prefrontal cortex. Other researchers, however, have explained differences in amygdalar activation in terms of an age-related increase in motivations to regulate emotional experiences (Mather et al., 2004). We know that conscious thought processes reduce amygdalar activation when participants actively strive to regulate negative emotions (Schaefer et al., 2002). Mather et al. (2004) speculate that subconscious changes in motivation also influence activation. Behaviorally, older adults display attentional preferences for positive over negative emotional images (Mather & Carstensen, 2003) and also show heightened amygdalar activity that is greater when viewing positive than negative images (Mather et al., 2004).

The similar intensity for emotional experience discussed earlier (e.g., Carstensen et al., 2000) may also result from activation of different brain regions by age; for older adults, the prefrontal cortex may be largely responsible, but for younger adults, the amygdala may play a greater role in emotional experience. Because the amygdala is involved in the physiological stress response to emotional stimuli (e.g., LeDoux, 2000), this shift from amygdalar to prefrontal cortex activation may be the reason that physiology is attenuated with age even if appraisals of these emotions are similar across age groups. Although neuroendocrinological and cardiovascular response to stress may be prolonged in aging, lower amygdalar activity relative to the prefrontal cortex may slow or decrease the likelihood of activation of the HPA axis in response to stress.

In addition to changes potentially influenced by motivational differences, serendipitous effects of physiological and neurological changes with age should not be dismissed as playing no role in improved regulation. Decreases in synaptic density and neurotransmitters as well as slowed cardiovascular response may at times aid emotion regulation. Older adults exhibit reduced cardiovascular activity in response to relived emotions (Levenson et al., 1991) and to films eliciting happiness (Tsai et al., 2000). Cardiovascular reactivity is also attenuated among older adults when involved in conflicts with their spouses (Levenson, Carstensen, & Gottman, 1994) and when viewing negative pictures (Smith, Hillman, & Duley, 2005). Moreover, cardiac reactivity is lower for older adults when recalling autobiographical memories arousing both negative and positive emotions (Labouvie-Vief, Lumly, Jain, & Heinz, 2003; but see Kunzmann & Gruhn, 2005). Overall, older adults exhibit reduced reactivity, and this reduction has been hypothesized to be one reason why older adults regulate their emotions better than younger adults (Cacciopo et al., 1997; Levenson, 2000).

SOCIOEMOTIONAL SELECTIVITY THEORY

Socioemotional selectivity theory (SST) is a lifespan theory of motivation that offers a conceptual framework to organize and integrate findings noted earlier or into a coherent model of emotional development. SST is grounded fundamentally in the uniquely human ability to monitor time and to adjust time horizons over the life course (see Carstensen, Isaacowitz, & Charles, 1999). At conscious and subconscious levels, this ubiquitous accounting of time guides the relative importance of two constellations of goals that dominate human thought and behavior. One set of goals includes knowledge and information-based goals and is prioritized when time is perceived as expansive. With a long future ahead, accruing knowledge is valued for its potential to inform future pursuits and enable strivings for future payoffs. The other constellation of goals includes those focused on emotions, encompassing motivations to derive meaning in actions, optimize emotional experiences, and invest in activities for their emotional significance. When time is perceived as limited, people will forego knowledge-related goals that are directed for future use and instead focus on more proximal, emotion-related goals. Often these goals conflict and priorities must guide behavior. For example, spending time trying to discover ways to solve problems in a relationship to avoid future conflicts, or foregoing an evening with friends to gather information pertaining to a financial investment, is an example of knowledge-related goals overriding emotion-related goals. Of course, life activities and motivations are difficult to dichotomize, and uniformly defining them as either information related or emotion related paints an overly broad swathe over multiple activities. An emotional goal can contain informational qualities, and information related goals can be emotionally gratifying. The relative importance of emotional and information goals is always present and measured, however, and people direct their attention and energies on goals based on the emotional and informational significance they provide.

Because time perspective is inherently linked to place in the lifespan, growing older is accompanied by an increasing awareness of the ephemeral nature of existence: As a result, emotional goals increase in relative importance to knowledge-related goals as people age. The theory maintains that people become increasingly selective in their choice of social partners as they age to make their social interactions become more emotionally meaningful and satisfying, a strategy of antecedent emotion regulation. The theory also suggests that people allocate more effort to maintaining emotional balance, attempting to improve important relationships, accepting small disagreements as not worth the effort, and using experience-based skills to manage social relationships well. Yet, the theory also maintains that motivational shifts operate at a subconscious level by directing attention to positive and away from negative information. In other words, according to socioemotional selectivity theory, motivational shifts that occur with age result in cognition operating in the service of emotion regulation.

One central postulate of socioemotional selectivity theory was tested in the context of social interaction. New friendships take time to develop, and investing the time necessary to gain information about this person is beneficial when cultivating this friendship for long-term benefits. Close friends and family members offer less new information and new opportunities but more immediate affirmation and emotional connection. Recognizing how different social interactions yield different benefits, Carstensen (1992) interpreted the well-established age-related decline in social interactions as neither an inability by older adults to make new friends (e.g., Maddox, 1963) nor a strategy for older adults to disengage from social interactions (e.g., Cumming & Henry, 1961) but as the result of older adults selectively pruning certain types of social partners from their networks based on their current life goals. Whereas social interactions with close friends and family members would be prioritized and remain a vital part of their life, new friends and acquaintances would not be as highly valued or sought after as people grew older. These patterns of relationships were found in both longitudinal (Carstensen, 1992) and cross-sectional (Lang & Carstensen, 1994) studies. Furthermore, social preferences were related to emotional and informational goals as postulated by SST; older adults weighted emotional goals more heavily in their preferences for social partners, whereas younger adults more heavily weighted the potential for knowledge and future-related possibilities (Fredrickson & Carstensen, 1990; Lang & Carstensen, 2002). Time perspective, defined as how much time people perceived was left in their lives and measured by asking people questions such as the extent that they feel that they have a long future ahead of them, or that time is running out, influenced the weighting of these goals; an open-ended time perspective was related to information and knowledge-related social goals, and a limited time perspective was related to emotion-focused social goals (Lang & Carstensen, 2002).

SOCIAL PARTNERS AND EMOTION REGULATION

SST makes specific predictions regarding how age-related changes in social partner preference and interactions serve emotion regulatory goals. In fact, Carstensen, Gross, and Fung (1997) argued several years ago that age-related improvements in well-being could be accounted for by the antecedent emotion regulation strategy of situation selection (see also Gross & Thompson, this volume), whereby older adults more often avoid socially toxic environments than do younger adults. Older people have smaller and more carefully pruned social networks than younger people do, and they contain relatively larger percentages of emotionally close social partners than younger peoples' networks. Well-known social partners offer interactions that are more predictable and reaffirm the self (Pasupathi, 2001), perhaps explaining why older women report more stable self-descriptions of themselves than do younger women (Charles & Pasupathi, 2003). Younger peoples' networks, by way of contrast, often include many social partners who were not chosen freely but rather are incorporated because of relationships to work or offspring (Lang & Carstensen, 1994; Lansford, Sherman, & Antonucci, 1998). Thus, with age social networks probably become easier to navigate emotionally. Because most strong emotions occur in social contexts, careful selection of social partners is arguably a highly effective strategy.

Because goals influence thoughts and behaviors, socioemotional selectivity posits age-related differences in emotion regulation strategies when faced with interpersonal conflict, such that older adults will engage in strategies aimed at maintaining emotional well-being. As a result, socioemotional selectivity posits that older adults will engage more often in situation modification when interacting with close friend and family members, whereby they will opt for more passive strategies aimed at emotion regulation as opposed to more active strategies aimed at discovering more information about the problem. Findings support this tenet, showing that older adults more often report emotion-focused, passive strategies in response to highly emotional interpersonal conflict situations (Birditt & Fingerman, 2005), but not for problems related to consumer issues or home repairs compared to middle-age adults (Blanchard-Fields, Chen, & Norris, 1997; Blanchard-Fields, Jahnke, & Camp, 1995; Blanchard-Fields, Stein, & Watson, 2004). In contrast, middle-age adults opt for strategies to solve interpersonal problems that focus on problem-solving, a strategy that often includes gathering facts about the problem and sorting out details to find solutions for the dilemmas.

EMOTIONAL EXPERIENCE AND REGULATION BEYOND INTERPERSONAL INTERACTIONS

Emotional Salience

SST posits not only differences in social partner preferences and interactions but also specific patterns of emotional experience as a function of time perspective, and therefore age as well (Carstensen, Fung, & Charles, 2003). The salience of emotional information is posited to increase among successively older age groups and extend beyond the confines of social interactions. In a study examining memory for emotional and nonemotional material, individuals ranging from teenagers to octogenarians read a passage from a novel and were later asked to recall as much of the information that they could (Carstensen & Turk-Charles, 1994). Findings from this incidental memory paradigm indicate that the proportion of emotional information increases linearly as a function of age. In addition, emotional saliency is greater with age when recalling autobiographical information (Alea, Bluck, & Semegon, 2004). Older adults also recall emotional details of prior information more than perceptual details (Johnson, Nolde, & De Leonardis, 1996; Mather, Johnson, & De Leonardis, 1999), and they weight this information more heavily when making confidence ratings for their memory performance (Hashtroudi, Johnson, & Chrosniak, 1990).

Further evidence of greater emotional saliency with age is found in studies examining everyday problem-solving strategies. Older adults weigh the emotional saliency of a problem more strongly before selecting a problem-solving strategy than do younger adults, choosing different strategies for highly emotional situations than low emotional situations (Blanchard-Fields et al., 2004; see review by Blanchard-Fields, 1997). In daily problem-solving situations, older adults prefer both problem-solving and emotion-focused coping strategies and view them as both effective, whereas younger and middle-age adults prefer and perceive problem-solving strategies as most effective (Watson & Blanchard-Fields, 1998). In a problem-solving task in the laboratory, older adults rely more heavily on emotional information whereas younger adults rely on memory and learning (Wood, Busemeyer, Koling, Cox, & Davis, 2005). Despite these very different strategies, both age groups successfully complete the task.

In addition to increased emotional saliency with age, SST posits that emotion regulation will become increasingly valued as time grows shorter (Carstensen et al., 2003). As a consequence, motivations to appraise situations more positively, focus on positive information, and remember this information in ways that optimize well-being grow stronger with age. Older adults are not blind to negative information—they focus on negative information and are able to detect negative information sometimes as well as younger adults (Mather & Knight, 2006), but they are less likely to focus on this information and to recall this information later, using the emotion regulation strategy of attention allocation to focus more on positive than negative stimuli. Negative information is favored over positive information in youth, a bias that shifts in adulthood. This developmental shift in the ratio of positive to negative is referred to as the "positivity effect" (Carstensen & Mikels, 2005; Carstensen, Mikels, & Mather, 2006; Mather & Carstensen, 2005).

Age-Related Advantages of Selective Attention

SST posits that increases in emotional saliency will lead to differences in attention for emotional information, particularly for positive information. According to the theory, older adults will engage in attention allocation toward positive information as an emotion regulation strategy more often than do younger adults. In one study, individuals were placed before a computer screen as two faces, one with a neutral expression and another with either a positive or negative expression, were presented on the left and right of the screen. After this 1-second presentation, a dot flashed on either the left- or right-hand side of the screen and the participant was asked to identify where the dot had appeared (Mather & Carstensen, 2003). Older adults responded more slowly when the dot was placed in the position of the previously viewed negative facial expression and more quickly when the dot followed a positive facial expression. Response time for younger adults was unaffected by the valence of the facial expression. The authors interpreted their findings as an age-related positive bias; older adults, more focused on the positive faces, had faster response times when the dot flashed in the position where they had focused their attention. In another study of more effortful attentional processing, younger and older adults read positive and negative information about two different automobiles and were asked to choose between then. When viewing these options, older adults spent a greater proportion of time on the positive aspects and a lower proportion of their time focused on the negative aspects than did younger adults (Mather, 2006). Other studies of attention, memory, and aging do not display a positivity effect, particularly studies that require rapid automatic processing (see review by Mather & Carstensen, 2005). Researchers posit that this discrepancy in the literature only highlights the motivational aspect driving age differences in effortful processing (Mather & Carstensen, 2005); motivations influence effortful processing more than automatic processing, and age differences for effortful processing suggest greater priority on emotion regulation with age.

These changes in attention cannot be dismissed as simple denial of negative stimuli. In studies published by Hess and colleagues (see review by Hess, 2005), older people show particular sensitivity to negative information about people. When descriptions of prospective social partners are presented and participants are asked to make judgments about them, older adults rely more heavily on the negative information than do younger adults (Hess & Pullen, 1994). Even when positive information about a person is subsequently presented, older peoples' views change little. One could view such judgments as a protective mechanism whereby older adults avoid contact with risky strangers or acquaintances. Interestingly, older adults are least likely to change negative views when characteristics concern a person's morality and more likely to modify views when information pertain to intelligence. For example, older people are unlikely to modify their views of a cheater if told that the person later behaved in an honest manner. In contrast, they are relatively more likely to modify their opinions about a person who first appeared unintelligent but later displayed some degree of intellectual acumen (Hess, Bolstad, Woodburn, & Auman, 1999). Moreover, when older participants are told that they would later share their impressions with another person, thereby making them interpersonally relevant, the information is better remembered (Hess, Rosenberg, & Waters, 2001).

Studies of source memory reveal a consistent pattern, suggesting that attention allocation is motivated by goals directed toward antecedent emotion regulation. When older people are asked to source information related to an interpersonally relevant characteristic (e.g., Was the source honest or dishonest?), they perform better than when asked to source information according to gender (e.g., whether the person who provided the information was male or female) (Rahhal, May, & Hasher, 2002). In fact, when source is focused on an interpersonally relevant characteristic, older people perform as well as younger people. Overall, this pattern of findings suggests that older adults pay attention to information that holds emotional relevance, which in and of itself may aid emotion regulation.

Further Evidence of Memory as an Emotion Regulation Tool

Memory for emotions are related to current emotional states (see review by Levine & Pizarro, 2004). To the extent that memories influence current and future thoughts and behavior, memory is a powerful regulation strategy. Just as older adults selectivity attend to positive emotional stimuli in studies of attention, they also are more likely to attend to memories that are more positive relative to younger adults. Regardless of the exact mechanism, this shift in valence toward positive information with age has been documented in studies examining memory for life events as well as memory for laboratory stimuli. Memories of events become more positive over time in younger people (Field, 1981), but the strength of this effect increases with age (Kennedy, Mather, & Carstensen, 2004). These same age differences hold true for shorter periods of time as well. For example, one study compared daily reports of affective distress reported over the course of the week to an overall week-end evaluation of overall emotional distress among adults ranging from 25 to 74-years-old (Almeida, 1998). Whereas younger adults were more likely to anchor their overall weekly reports on the most stressful day, older adults' retrospective reports were more similar to the average rating across the aggregated 8 days and were thus more positive as well as more accurate as an aggregate measure of well-being.

Laboratory studies underscore the shift toward events being remembered more positively with age. In one study, younger, middle-age, and older adults were shown positive, negative, and neutral images on a computer screen and were later asked to recall and to recognize these previously viewed images from a larger set of images (Charles, Mather, & Carstensen, 2003). Younger adults recalled and recognized a greater proportion of negative images than positive or neutral images, confirming a bias for negative stimuli documented previously among younger adults (see review by Rozin & Royzman, 2001). Older adults displayed no such negative bias, resulting in age differences that were greatest for negative images and least for positive images (Charles et al., 2003). This age-associated shift toward positive emotion was also found in a study examining age differences in recall and recognition for positive, negative, and neutral words and faces (Leigland, Schulz, & Janowsky, 2004).

Benefits of these age-related differences in memory are highlighted in another study where older and younger adults were read both positive and negative qualities of two items (e.g., two homes) and asked to choose one of the two items. After making their selection, they were given a memory task about these two options. Older adults were more likely to have a choice-supportive memory, whereby they remember the positive qualities of the option they chose and the negative qualities of the unselected option (Mather & Johnson, 2000). The authors interpret this memory bias as beneficial for increasing the happiness of a chosen selection and reducing possible "buyer's remorse." In another study in which older and younger adults examined positive and negative features of two choices (two apartments or two health plans), older adults were more accurate at later recognizing the positive feature than the negative features of these options, whereas younger adults correctly recognized positive and negative aspects equally (Mather, Knight, & McCaffrey, 2005).

Physiology, Cognition, and Emotion

Older age is related to changes in memory and attention that serve emotion regulation, yet the biological underpinnings of these processes as well as cognitive studies examining overall memory performance often point to cognitive decline (Craik & McDowd, 1987). Working memory is vital for emotional functioning and planning, as working memory allows an individual to focus on the potential for rewards and enhance goal-seeking behavior (Davidson et al., 2000). Age-related declines are evident in situations requiring working memory. For example, age differences are marked in neuropsychological tasks such as the Stroop test or the Wisconsin Card Sort, tasks that suffer from declines in inhibitory processes (Zacks & Hasher, 1997; Wurm, Labouvie-Vief, Aycock, Rebucal, & Koch, 2004).

Age declines in these inhibitory processes, however, show different patterns according to the emotional qualities of the material. In a study examining automatic processing using the Stroop paradigm, highly arousing emotional stimuli affected the performance of older adults to a relatively greater degree than low arousal information (Wurm et al., 2004). For younger adults, arousal did not predict performance. The authors posited several interpretations for this difference, including higher arousal information having a greater ability to disrupt cognitive performances among people with already low levels of capacity. Another interpretation suggested by the authors, however, is that older adults are more motivated to avoid highly arousing emotional information (Wurm et al., 2004) to improve emotion regulation. This explanation is consistent with self-reports from older adults that highly arousing emotions are experienced less frequently with age (Lawton et al., 1992).

Other inhibitory failures at the physiological level may also relate to memory for emotional material. Researchers have often considered emotional material irrelevant, and the memory of emotional features over other details an example of poor inhibitory processes (Hashtroudi et al., 1990). Benefits may exist, however, in processing this seemingly extraneous information (for a review, see Isaacowitz, Charles, & Cartensen, 2000). In a study of visual motion processing, researchers found that age-related reduced inhibition resulted in older adults outperforming younger adults in tasks requiring motion discrimination of stimuli with high-contrast patterns, a task when inhibition usually impairs performance (Betts, Taylor, Sekuler, & Bennett, 2005). Failure to focus on small perceptual details enabled older adults to make more accurate judgments when examining the object in its entirety. Although researchers studied these effects in visual processing, this phenomenon holds interesting possibilities for processing emotional information. Older adults, compared to younger adults, often describe emotional information in terms of a "bigger picture," recalling and interpreting text using psychological themes and metaphors more than narrative details (Labouvie-Vief & Hakim-Larson, 1989; Adams, Smith, Nyquist, & Perlmutter, 1997) and discussing more evaluative and subjective information when describing their vacations rather than the itinerary (Gould & Dixon, 1993). These age differences have been interpreted as examples of inhibitory failures—failures to inhibit "irrelevant" emotional information—characteristic of aging (Persad, Abeles, Zacks, & Denburg, 2002). The vision researchers likewise saw inhibitory failure as ubiquitously negative, until they recognized advantages for the incorporation of seemingly irrelevant information when adopting a different viewpoint. Perhaps attention paid to multiple aspects of a situation may also hold positive consequences for higher-order emotional processing as well. For example, older adults consider emotions during decision-making tasks to a greater extent than do younger adults (see review by Blanchard-Fields, 1997), so perhaps these inhibitory failures allow older adults to consider a broader range of information, including information previously considered irrelevant.

Age Differences in the Environmental Context of Emotional Experience

SST posits that older adults proactively engage in behaviors directed at situation selection, situation modification, and attention allocation that serve antecedent emotion regulation purposes. Some researchers, however, have argued that greater well-being among older adults may not illustrate the ability to regulate emotions but instead reflect differences in environmental contexts, such that older adults find themselves in situations in which negative experiences occur less frequently (Lawton et al., 1992; see review by Lawton, 2001).

Findings from twin studies provide information on the powerful roles of the environment in shaping emotion-related phenotypes and how the strength of environmental influences may change with age. In behavioral genetic research, environmental influences refer not only to the situation and events completely external to the individual but also to the experiences, cognitive styles, and other internal processes that have developed over time. Researchers have found that both genetic and unique environmental influences are important for emotional experience but that the unique environmental variance for both emotional well-being (Neiss & Almeida, 2004) and the perceived severity of negative events (Charles & Almeida, 2005) is stronger among older than younger adults. The environment—not genes—determines individual differences to a greater extent among older adults than younger adults. In addition, genetic influences on emotional experience exert a weaker role for those with physical health problems and functional limitations, and thus higher prevalence rates of chronic health problems among older adults may play a role in these age-related environmental influences (McGue & Christensen, 2005).

Behavioral genetics research underscores the importance of examining individual variation in human behavior and emotional experience. Older adults represent a heterogeneous group, and the mean differences mentioned throughout this chapter belie the vast differences observed among older adults populations. For example, Charles et al. (2001) found that declines in subjective reports of negative affect did not occur among people scoring high in neuroticism, and Mroczek and Spiro (2005) found that people higher on neuroticism were more likely to show declining life satisfaction in old age. Thus, there may be some personality types for whom emotional experience does not benefit from aging. Other people may vary in their awareness of time left in life, and thus their time perspective may not align with their chronological age. Indeed, terminally old younger adults look more similar to older people than their peers when evaluating potential social partners (Carstensen & Fredrickson, 1998).

Trajectories of physiological reactivity to emotional experiences also reveal different patterns based on environmental context, again displaying the great variability that characterizes old age. For example, a recent study (Traustadottir, Bosch, & Matt, 2005) found that although aging is related to increased cortisol reactivity to a stressor (e.g., Sapolsky et al., 1986), this increased reactivity is only observed among women who perform poorly on a treadmill task. Older women who exercise and are physically in shape, as assessed by maximum oxygen consumption during a treadmill test, do not vary in their HPA reactivity compared to younger women; among younger women, physical fitness had no relationship with cortisol reactivity. Because physical fitness influenced physiological reactivity among older adults but not younger adults, exercise and other health-promoting behaviors may play a stronger role in emotional experience and emotional reactivity with age.

Environmental influences provide pathways in which processes related to emotional experience may be modified both negatively, as in the case of poor health, or positively, as in the cases of exercise. They also, however, influence the context of these emotional experiences. Lazarus (1996) emphasizes the importance of focusing on the changing contexts of coping rather than orthogenetic factors that may have a developmental trajectory. For example, in a study in which he and his colleagues compared adult ages 35–45 years old to those 65–74 years old, they found that the younger adults were predominantly working parents whose daily stressors revolved around work and parental roles (Lazarus, 1996). In contrast, the older sample was comprised predominantly of retired people whose children were grown and no longer living with them. Instead of work and childrearing stressors, older adults discussed problems around their health and ability to carry out functional activities of daily life. When comparing coping responses across the age groups, younger adults rated their stressors as more controllable and used more problem-focused strategies compared to the older adults. In viewing these results, Lazarus interpreted age differences not in terms of developmental process or biological mechanisms but instead as a reflection of having to cope with a different set of issues and life circumstances. Thus, understanding age differences in environmental context, such as social network composition, is vital for understanding age differences in emotional experience.

FUTURE DIRECTIONS AND CONCLUSIONS

Empirical findings amassed over the past 30 years have dramatically changed the landscape of research on emotion and aging. Among healthy adults, emotional experiences and emotion regulation do not decline across the lifespan but instead are well maintained and sometimes show areas of improvement. The previous chapter provides a brief overview of emotional experience and emotion regulation in the context of physiological, cognitive, and social age-related changes. Although findings consistent with the tenets of socioemotional selectivity reveal age differences in processes of attention and appraisal, future studies will need to link these processes directly to emotion regulation. Research in emotion and aging only began in earnest near the end of the 20th century, and studies of discrete emotions and specific emotion regulation strategies are necessary to clearly understand developmental trajectories in emotion regulation. Researchers need to examine response-focused regulation styles and include maintenance, exacerbation, and attenuation of emotional experience in their investigations. For example, attenuated physiological reactivity may paradoxically aid in the downregulation of negative emotions (e.g., Levenson, 2000), but this attenuated arousal may pose a disadvantage to older adults if they need to increase positive emotions.

In addition to understanding age differences in both downregulation and upregulation in emotional experience, researchers must face a number of methodological issues that could potentially confound age differences. First, the arousal of emotional stimuli is important to consider when examining age differences (Wurm et al., 2004), as is the complexity of emotional stimuli (Charles, 2005). Second, age differences in both emotional experience and emotion regulation may vary for discrete emotions. For example, no large study to date has reported increases in levels of anger with age, but several studies find age differences related to increases in reports of sadness (e.g., Gatz, Kasl-Godley, & Karel, 1996). In addition, cognitive tasks have revealed age similarities for some emotional stimuli but age differences in others. For example, older adults performed worse than younger adults on a facial recognition task for the emotions of anger and sadness but equally well when recognizing expressions of fear (Phillips, MacLean, & Allen, 2002). A third methodological issue that frequently arises in lifespan developmental research is the issue of cohort effects. Cross-sectional research points to potentially interesting suggestions of developmental phenomena, but only longitudinal research can confirm developmental processes postulated by socioemotional selectivity theory.

Besides making methodological refinements to existing paradigms, new innovations and findings provide a framework on which to launch future research programs in the area of emotion and aging. For example, functional imaging studies of brain activity have allowed researchers to examine the relations between cognition and brain activation and how experience shapes this relationship. Studies in cognitive neuroscience have the potential to disentangle normative and nonnormal biological-related decline as well as changes that occur as a result of motivational strivings. Understanding these processes will provide further insight into how changes in cognitive appraisals alter the processing of emotional stimuli and how these associations are related to age. A second innovation that will shape the future of psychological science is the growing area of health psychology and new techniques allowing for convenient and affordable assessments of cardiovascular, neuroendocrine, and immunological responses in the laboratory and in daily life. With these studies of physiological stability and reactivity, researchers will be able to examine how cognitions and behaviors are related to the physiological arousal and reactivity accompanying emotional experience.

Finally, psychologists have long recognized the importance of the environment in shaping behavior (see review by Hess, 2005), but relatively few studies have recognized the importance of context when interpreting age differences. Although notable exceptions exist, such as studies examining age differences in social cognition (e.g., Blanchard-Fields et al., 2004; Hess, 2005) and in health-related contexts (e.g., Consedine & Magai, 2006), further studies are needed to understand how similar behaviors or cognitions may have different outcomes according to age-specific contexts. For example, passive emotion regulation strategies may be compensatory strategies in some situations but optimal solutions in others (e.g., Folkman & Moskowitz, 2000). In addition, even when situations are controlled in the laboratory, perceptions are guided by experiences, and these experiences may alter the meaning and interpretation of emotional stimuli. A picture of an operation, for example, may elicit more sadness in older adults but more disgust among younger adults (e.g., Kunzmann et al., 2005). The death of a parent is often speculation for a college student and a reality for an older adult. To this end, the study of emotions and aging is a study of how people's cognitions and behaviors shape, and are shaped by, the interplay between physiological processes and the environment across the lifespan. As a result, researchers need to be sensitive to these changing dynamics.

In conclusion, emotions mobilize people to action. They arouse physiological systems, direct attention, and motivate people to action. Emotions are critical for successful adaptation across the lifespan, but developmental processes alter multiple facets of emotional experience, including cognitive appraisals, behavioral responses, physiological reactivity, and environmental context. Research in emotion and aging has revealed that shifts in cognitive processes can offset physiological declines, such that even though biological functioning peaks relatively early in life, emotional experience remains vital and well maintained into late adulthood.

ACKNOWLEDGMENTS

This work was supported Grant No. R01-AG23845 from the National Institute on Aging to Susan Turk Charles and Grant No. R01-8816 from the National Institute on Aging to Laura L. Carstensen.

REFERENCES

Adams, C., Smith, M. C., Nyquist, L., & Perlmutter, M. (1997). Adult age-group differences in recall for the literal and interpretive meanings of narrative text. *Journal of Gerontology: Psychological Sciences, 52*, P187–P195.

Alea, N., Bluck, S., & Semegon, A. B. (2004). Young and older adults' expression of emotional experience: Do autobiographical narratives tell a different story? *Journal of Adult Development, 11*, 235–250.

Almeida, D. M. (1998, August). Age differences in daily weekly and monthly estimates of psychological distress. In W. Fleeson & D. Mroczek (Chairs), *Intraindividual variability and change processes: New directions in understanding personality*. Symposium presented at the meeting of the American Psychological Association, San Francisco.

Almeida, D. M. (2005). Resilience and vulnerability to daily stressors assessed via diary methods. *Current Directions in Psychological Science, 14*, 64–68.

Banham, K. M. (1951). Senescence and the emotions: A genetic theory. *Journal of Genetic Psychology, 78,* 175–183.

Beach, T. G., Walker, R., & McGeer, E. G. (1989). Lamina-selective A68 immunoreactivity in primary visual cortex of Alzheimer's disease patients. *Brain Research, 501,* 171–174.

Berdyyeva, T. K., Woodworth, C. D., & Sokolov, I. (2005). Human epithelial cells increase their rigidity with ageing *in vitro*: Direct measurements. *Physical Medical Biology, 50,* 81–92.

Betts, L. R., Taylor, C. P., Sekuler, A. B., & Bennett, P. J. (2005). Aging reduces center-surround antagonism in visual motion processing. *Neuron, 45,* 361–366.

Birditt, K. S., & Fingerman, K. L. (2005). Do we get better at picking our battles?: Age group differences in descriptions of behavioral reactions to interpersonal tensions. *Journals of Gerontology: Series B: Psychological Sciences and Social Sciences, 60,* P121–P128.

Birditt, K. S., Fingerman, K. L., & Almeida, D. M. (2005). Age differences in exposure and reactions to interpersonal tensions: A daily diary study. *Psychology and Aging, 20,* 330–340.

Bjorntorp, P. (2002). Alterations in the ageing corticotropic stress-response axis. In Novartis Foundation Symposium (Ed.), *Novartis Foundation Symposium 242–Endocrine facets of ageing* (pp. 46–58). London: Wiley.

Blanchard-Fields, F. (1997). The role of emotion in social cognition across the adult lifespan. In K. W. Schaie, & M. P. Lawton (Eds.), *Annual review of gerontology and geriatrics: Vol. 17. Focus on emotion and adult development* (pp. 238–265). New York: Springer.

Blanchard-Fields, F., Chen, Y., & Norris, L. (1997). Everyday problem solving across the adult lifespan: Influence of domain specificity and cognitive appraisal. *Psychology and Aging, 12,* 684–693.

Blanchard-Fields, F., Jahnke, H. C., & Camp, C. (1995). Age differences in problem-solving style: The role of emotional salience. *Psychology and Aging, 10,* 173–180.

Blanchard-Fields, F., Stein, R., & Watson, T. L. (2004). Age differences in emotion-regulation strategies in handling everyday problems. *Journals of Gerontology: Series B: Psychological Sciences and Social Sciences, 59,* P261–P269.

Blazer, D. G. (2003). Depression in late life: Review and commentary. *Journals of Gerontology: Series A: Biological Sciences and Medical Sciences, 58,* 249–265.

Cacioppo, J. T., Berntson, G. G., Klein, D. J., & Poehlmann, K. M. (1997). Psychophysiology of emotion across the lifespan. In K. W. Schaie, & M. P. Lawton (Eds.), *Annual review of gerontology and geriatrics:: Vol. 17. Focus on emotion and adult development* (pp. 27–74). New York: Springer.

Carstensen, L. L. (1992). Social and emotional patterns in adulthood: Support for socioemotional selectivity theory. *Psychology and Aging, 7,* 331–338.

Carstensen, L. L., & Fredrickson, B. F. (1998). Influence of HIV status and age on cognitive representations of others. *Health Psychology, 17,* 494–503.

Carstensen, L. L., Fung, H., & Charles, S. T. (2003). Socioemotional selectivity theory and emotion regulation in the second half of life. *Motivation and Emotion, 27,* 103–123.

Carstensen, L. L., Gross, J., Fung, H. H. (1997). The social context of emotional experience. In K. W. Schaie & M. P. Lawton (Eds.), *Annual review of gerontology and geriatrics: Vol. 17. Focus on emotion and adult development* (pp. 325–352). New York: Springer.

Carstensen, L. L., Isaacowitz, D. M., Charles, S. T. (1999). Taking time seriously: A theory of socioemotional selectivity. *American Psychologist, 54,* 165–181.

Carstensen, L. L., & Mikels, J. A. (2005). At the intersection of emotion and cognition: Aging and the positivity effect. *Current Directions in Psychological Science, 14,* 117–121.

Carstensen, L. L., Mikels, J. A., & Mather, M. (2006). Aging and the intersection of cognition, motivation and emotion. In J. Birren & K. W. Schaie (Eds.), *Handbook of the psychology of aging* (6th ed., pp. 343–362). San Diego, CA: Academic Press.

Carstensen, L. L., Pasupathi, M., Mayr, U., & Nesselroade, J. R. (2000). Emotional experience in everyday life across the adult lifespan. *Journal of Personality and Social Psychology, 79,* 644–655.

Carstensen, L. L., & Turk-Charles, S. (1994). The salience of emotion across the adult lifespan. *Psychology and Aging, 9,* 259–264.

Charles, S. T. (2005). Viewing injustice: Age differences in emotional experience. *Psychology and Aging, 20,* 159–164.

Charles, S. T., & Almeida, D. M. (2005). *Genetic and environmental influences on the occurrence and perceived severity of daily stressors.* Paper presented at the 35th annual meeting of the Behavior Genetics Association: Hollywood, CA.

Charles, S. T., Mather, M., & Carstensen, L. L. (2003). Aging and emotional memory: The forgettable nature of negative images for older adults. *Journal of Experimental Psychology: General, 132,* 310–324.

Charles, S. T., & Pasupathi, M. (2003). Age-related patterns of variability in self-descriptions: Implications for everyday affective experience. *Psychology and Aging, 18,* 524–536.

Charles, S. T., Reynolds, C. A., & Gatz, M. (2001). Age-related differences and change in positive and negative affect over 23 years. *Journal of Personality and Social Psychology, 80,* 136–151.

Consedine, N. S., & Magai, C. (2006). Emotion development in adulthood: A developmental functionalist review and critique. In C. Hoare (Ed.), *The Oxford handbook of adult development and learning* (pp. 209–244). New York: Oxford University Press.

Craik, F. I., & McDowd, J. M. (1987). Age differences in recall and recognition. *Journal of Experimental Psychology: Learning, Memory, and Cognition, 13,* 474–479.

Cumming, E., & Henry, W. H. (1961). *Growing old: The process of disengagement.* New York: Basic Books.

Cunningham, M. G., Bhattacharyya, S., & Benes, F. M. (2002). Amygdalo-cortical sprouting continues into early adulthood: Implications for the development of normal and abnormal function during adolescence. *Journal Comparative Neurology, 453,* 116–130.

Davidson, R. J., Fox, A., & Kalin, N. H. (2007). Neural bases of emotion regulation in nonhuman primates and humans. In J. J. Gross (Ed.), *Handbook of emotion regulation* (pp. 47–68). New York: Guilford Press.

Davidson, R. J., Jackson, D. C., & Kalin, N. H. (2000). Emotion, plasticity, context, and regulation: Perspectives from affective neuroscience. *Psychological Bulletin. Special Psychology in the 21st Century, 126,* 890–909.

DeCarli, C., Massaro, J., Harvey, D., Hald, J., Tullberg, M., Au, R., et al. (2005). Measures of brain morphology and infarction in the Framingham heart study: Establishing what is normal. *Neurobiology of Aging, 26,* 491–510.

Field, D. (1981). Retrospective reports by healthy intelligent elderly people of personal events of their adult lives. *International Journal of Behavioral Development, 4,* 77–97.

Folkman, S., Lazarus, R. S., Pimley, D., & Novacek, J. (1987). Age differences in stress and coping processes. *Psychology and Aging, 2,* 171–184.

Folkman, S., & Moskowitz, J. T. (2000). Positive affect and the other side of coping. *American Psychologist, 55,* 647–654.

Fredrickson, B. L., & Carstensen, L. L. (1990). Choosing social partners: How age and anticipated endings make people more selective. *Psychology and Aging, 5,* 335–347.

Gatz, M., Kasl-Godley, J. E., & Karel, M. J. (1996). Aging and mental disorders. In J. E. Birren, & K. W. Schaie (Eds.), *Handbook of the psychology of aging* (4th ed., pp. 365–382). San Diego, CA: Academic Press.

Giedd, J. N. (2004). Structural magnetic resonance imaging of the adolescent brain. *Annual Review of the New York Academy of Sciences, 1021,* 77–85.

Gil, S., & Gilbar, O. (2001). Hopelessness among cancer patients. *Journal of Psychosocial Oncology, 19,* 21–33.

Gould, O. N., & Dixon, R. A. (1993). How we spent our vacation: Collaborative storytelling by young and older adults. *Psychology and Aging, 6,* 93–99.

Grieve, S. M., Clark, C. R., Williams, L. M., Peduto, A. J., & Gordon, E. (2005). Preservation of limbic and paralimbic structures in aging. *Human Brain Mapping, 25,* 391–401.

Gross, J. J., Carstensen, L. L., Pasupathi, M., Tsai, J., Götestam Skorpen, C., & Hsu, A. Y. C. (1997). Emotion and aging: Experience, expression, and control. *Psychology and Aging, 12,* 590–599.

Gross, J. J., & Thompson, R. A. (2007). Emotion regulation: Conceptual foundations. In J. J. Gross (Ed.), *Handbook of emotion regulation* (pp. 3–24). New York: Guilford Press.

Gunning-Dixon, F. M., Gur, R. C., Perkins, A. C., Schroeder, L., Turner, T., & Turetsky, B. I. (2003). Aged-related differences in brain activation during emotional face processing. *Neurobiology of Aging, 24,* 285–295.

Hashtroudi, S., Johnson, M. K., & Chrosniak, L. D. (1990). Aging and qualitative characteristics of memories for perceived and imagined complex events. *Psychology and Aging, 5,* 119–126.

Hess, T. M. (2005). Memory and aging in context. *Psychological Bulletin, 131,* 383–406.

Hess, T. M., Bolstad, C. A., Woodburn, S. M., & Auman, C. (1999). Trait diagnosticity versus behavior consistency as determinants of impression change in adulthood. *Psychology and Aging, 14,* 77–89.

Hess, T. M., & Pullen, S. M. (1994). Adult age difference in informational biases during impression formation. *Psychology and Aging, 9*, 237-250.

Hess, T. M., Rosenberg, D. C., & Waters, S. J. (2001). Motivation and representational processes in adulthood: The effects of social accountability and information relevance. *Psychology and Aging, 16*, 629-642.

Isaacowitz, D. M., Charles, S. T., & Carstensen, L. L. (2000). Emotion and cognition. In F. I. M. Craik & T. A. Salthouse (Eds.), *The handbook of aging and cognition* (2nd ed., pp. 593-631). Mahwah, NJ: Erlbaum.

John, O. P., & Gross, J. J. (2004). Healthy and unhealthy emotion regulation: Personality processes, individual differences, and lifespan development. *Journal of Personality. Special Emotions, Personality, and Health, 72*, 1301-1333.

Johnson, M. K., Nolde, S. F., & De Leonardis, D. M. (1996). Emotional focus and source monitoring. *Journal of Memory and Language. Special Illusions of Memory, 35*, 135-156

Kennedy, Q., Mather, M., & Carstensen, L. L. (2004). The role of motivation in the age-related positivity effect in autobiographical memory. *Psychological Science, 15*, 208-214.

Kobau, R., Safran, M. A., Zack, M. M., Moriarty, D. G., & Chapman, D. (2004). Sad, blue, or depressed days, health behaviors and health-related quality of life, Behavioral Risk Factor Surveillance System, 1995-2000. *Health and Quality of Life Outcomes, 2*, 40.

Kunzmann, U., & Grühn, D. (2005). Age differences in emotional reactivity: The sample case of sadness. *Psychology and Aging, 20*, 47-59.

Kunzmann, U., Kupperbusch, C. S., & Levenson, R. W. (2005). Behavioral inhibition and amplification during emotional arousal: A comparison of two age groups. *Psychology and Aging, 20*, 144-158.

Kunzmann, U., Little, T. D., & Smith, J. (2000). Is age-related stability of subjective well-being a paradox?: Cross-sectional and longitudinal evidence from the Berlin aging study. *Psychology and Aging, 15*, 511-526.

Labouvie-Vief, G., & Hakim-Larson, J. (1989). Developmental shifts in adult thought. In S. Hunter & M. Sundel (Eds.), *Midlife myths* (pp. 69-96). Newbury Park, CA: Sage.

Labouvie-Vief, G., Lumley, M. A., Jain, E., & Heinze, H. (2003). Age and gender differences in cardiac reactivity and subjective emotion responses to emotional autobiographical memories. *Emotion, 3*, 115-126.

Lang, F. R., & Carstensen, L. L. (1994). Close emotional relationships in late life: Further support for proactive aging in the social domain. *Psychology and Aging, 9*, 315-324.

Lang, F. R., & Carstensen, L. L. (2002). Time counts: Future time perspective, goals, and social relationships. *Psychology and Aging, 17*, 125-139.

Lansford, J. E., Sherman, A. M., & Antonucci, T. C. (1998). Satisfaction with social networks: An examination of socioemotional selectivity theory across cohorts. *Psychology and Aging, 13*, 544-552.

Lawton, M. P. (2001). Emotion in later life. *Current Directions in Psychological Science, 10*, 120-123.

Lawton, M. P., Kleban, M. H., Rajagopal, D., & Dean, J. (1992). Dimensions of affective experience in three age groups. *Psychology and Aging, 7*, 171-184.

Lazarus, R. S. (1996). The role of coping in the emotions and how coping changes over the life course. In C. Magai & S. H. McFadden (Eds.), *Handbook of emotion, adult development, and aging* (pp. 289-306). San Diego, CA: Academic Press.

LeDoux, J. E. (2000). Emotion circuits in the brain. *Annual Reviews in Neuroscience, 23*, 155-184.

Leigland, L. A., Schulz, L. E., & Janowsky, J. S. (2004). Age related changes in emotional memory. *Neurobiology of Aging, 25*, 1117-1124.

Levenson, R. W. (2000). Expressive, physiological, and subjective changes in emotion across adulthood. In S. H. Qualls & N. Abeles (Eds.), *Psychology and the aging revolution: How we adapt to longer life* (pp. 123-140). Washington, DC: American Psychological Association.

Levenson, R. W., Carstensen, L. L., Friesen, W. V., & Ekman, P. (1991). Emotion, physiology, and expression in old age. *Psychology and Aging, 6*, 28-35.

Levenson, R. W., Carstensen, L. L., & Gottman, J. M. (1994). Influence of age and gender on affect, physiology, and their interrelations: A study of long-term marriages. *Journal of Personality and Social Psychology, 67*, 56-68.

Levine, L. J., & Pizarro, D. A. (2004). Emotion and memory research: A grumpy overview. *Social Cognition, 22*, 530-554.

Lichtenstein, P., Gatz, M., Pedersen, N. L., & Berg, S. (1996). A co-twin-control study of response to widowhood. *Journals of Gerontology: Series B: Psychological Sciences and Social Sciences, 51*, P279–P289.

Maddox, G. L. (1963). Activity and morale: A longitudinal study of selected elderly subjects. *Social Forces, 42*, 195–204.

Mather, M. (2004). Aging and emotional memory. In D. Reisberg, & P. Hertel (Eds.), *Memory and emotion* (pp. 272–307). London: Oxford University Press.

Mather, M. (2006). A review of decision making processes: Weighing the risks and benefits of aging. In L. L. Carstensen & C. R. Hartel (Eds.), *When I'm 64: Committee on Aging Frontiers in Social Psychology, Personality, and Adult Developmental Psychology*. Washington, DC: National Academies Press.

Mather, M., Canli, T., English, T., Whitfield, S., Wais, P., Ochsner, K., et al. (2004). Amygdala responses to emotionally valenced stimuli in older and younger adults. *Psychological Science, 15*, 259–263.

Mather, M., & Carstensen, L. L. (2003). Aging and attentional biases for emotional faces. *Psychological Science, 14*, 409–415.

Mather, M., & Carstensen, L. L. (2005). Aging and motivated cognition: The positivity effect in attention and memory. *Trends in Cognitive Sciences, 9*, 496–502.

Mather, M., & Johnson, M. K. (2000). Choice-supportive source monitoring: Do our decisions seem better to us as we age? *Psychology and Aging, 15*, 596–606.

Mather, M., Johnson, M. K., & De Leonardis, D. M. (1999). Stereotype reliance in source monitoring: Age differences and neuropsychological test correlates. *Cognitive Neuropsychology, 16*, 437–458.

Mather, M., & Knight, M. (2006). Angry faces get noticed quickly: Threat detection is not impaired among older adults. *Journal of Gerontology: Psychological Sciences, 61*, 54–57.

Mather, M., Knight, M., & McCaffrey, M. (2005). The allure of the alignable: Younger and older adults' false memories of choice features. *Journal of Experimental Psychology: General, 134*, 38–51.

McGue, M., & Christensen, K. (2005). *Physical disability and late-life depression: Main and interactive effects.* Paper presented at the 35 annual meeting of the Behavior Genetics Association, Hollywood, CA.

Mroczek, D. K., & Kolarz, C. M. (1998). The effect of age on positive and negative affect: A developmental perspective on happiness. *Journal of Personality and Social Psychology, 75*, 1333–1349.

Mroczek, D. K., & Spiro, A., III. (2005). Change in life satisfaction during adulthood: Findings from the veterans affairs normative aging study. *Journal of Personality and Social Psychology, 88*, 189–202.

Mu, Q., Xie, J., Wen, Z., Weng, Y., & Shuyun, Z. (1999). Quantitative MR study of the hippocampal formation, the amygdala, and the temporal horn of the lateral ventricle in healthy subjects 40 to 90 years of age. *American Journal of Neuroradiology, 20*, 207–211.

Neiss, M., & Almeida, D. M. (2004). Age differences in the heritability of mean and intraindividual variation of psychological distress. *Gerontology, 50*, 22–27.

Otte, C., Hart, S., Neylan, T. C., Marmar, C. R., Yaffe, K., & Mohr, D. C. (2005). A meta-analysis of cortisol response to challenge in human aging: Importance of gender. *Psychoneuroendocrinology, 30*, 80–91.

Pasupathi, M. (2001). The social construction of the personal past and its implications for adult development. *Psychological Bulletin, 127*, 651–672.

Persad, C. C., Abeles, N., Zacks, R. T., & Denburg, N. L. (2002). Inhibitory changes after age 60 and the relationship to measures of attention and memory. *Journals of Gerontology: Series B: Psychological Sciences and Social Sciences, 57*, P223–P232.

Phifer, J. F. (1990). Psychological distress and somatic symptoms after natural disaster: Differential vulnerability among older adults. *Psychology and Aging, 5*, 412–420.

Phillips, L. H., MacLean, R. D., & Allen, R. (2002). Age and the understanding of emotions: Neuropsychological and sociocognitive perspectives. *Journals of Gerontology: Series B: Psychological Sciences and Social Sciences, 57*, 526–P530.

Piazza, J., & Charles, S. T. (2006). Mental health and the baby boomers. In S. K. Whitbourne & S. L. Willis (Eds.), *The baby boomers at midlife: Contemporary perspectives on middle age* (pp. 111–148). Mahwah, NJ: Erlbaum.

Rahhal, T. A., May, C. P., & Hasher, L. (2002). Truth and character: Sources that older adults can remember. *Psychological Science, 13*, 101–105.

Raz, N. (2000). Aging of the brain and its impact on cognitive performance: Integration of structural and functional findings. In F. I. M. Craik & T. A. Salthouse (Eds.), *The handbook of aging and cognition: The handbook of aging and cognition* (2nd ed., pp. 1–90). Mahwah, NJ: Erlbaum.

Rowe, J. W., & Kahn, R. L. (1997). Successful aging. *Gerontologist, 37*, 433–440.

Rozin, P., & Royzman, E. B. (2001). Negativity bias, negativity dominance, and contagion. *Personality Social Psychology Review, 5*, 296–320.

Sapolsky, R. M. (2007). Stress, stress-related disease, and emotion regulation. In J. J. Gross (Ed.), *Handbook of emotion regulation* (pp. 606–615). New York: Guilford Press.

Sapolsky, R. M., Krey, L. C., & McEwen, B. S. (1986). The neuroendocrinology of stress and aging: The glucocorticoid cascade hypothesis. *Endocrinological Review, 7*, 284–301.

Schaefer, S. M., Jackson, D. C., Davidson, R. J., Aguirre, G. K., Kimberg, D. Y., et al. (2002). Modulation of amygdalar activity by the conscious regulation of negative emotion. *Journal of Cognitive Neuroscience, 14*, 913–921.

Schulz, R. (1985). Emotion and affect. In J. E. Birren & K. W. Schaie (Eds.), *Handbook of the psychology of aging* (2nd ed., pp. 531–543). New York: Van Nostrand Reinhold.

Small, S. A., Tsai, W. Y., DeLaPaz, R., Mayeux, R., & Stern, Y. (2002). Imaging hippocampal function across the human lifespan: Is memory decline normal or not? *Annals of Neurology, 51*, 290–295.

Smith, D. P., Hillman, C. H., & Duley, A. R. (2005). Influences of age on emotional reactivity during picture processing. *Journals of Gerontology B: Psychological Sciences and Social Sciences, 60*, P49–P56.

Traustadottir, T., Bosch, P. R., & Matt, K. S. (2005). The HPA axis response to stress in women: Effects of aging and fitness. *Psychoneuroendocrinology, 30*, 392–402.

Tsai, J. L., Levenson, R. W., & Carstensen, L. L. (2000). Autonomic, subjective, and expressive responses to emotional films in older and younger Chinese Americans and European Americans. *Psychology and Aging, 15*, 684–693.

Uchino, B. N., Holt-Lunstad, J., Bloor, L. E., & Campo, R. A. (2005). Aging and cardiovascular reactivity to stress: Longitudinal evidence for changes in stress reactivity. *Psychology and Aging, 20*, 134–143.

Watson, T. L., & Blanchard-Fields, F. (1998). Thinking with your head and your heart: Age differences in everyday problem-solving strategy preferences. *Aging, Neuropsychology, and Cognition, 5*, 225–240.

Wood, S., Busemeyer, J., Koling, A., Cox, C. R., & Davis, H. (2005). Older adults as adaptive decision makers: Evidence from the Iowa gambling task. *Psychology and Aging, 20*, 220–225.

Wurm, L. H., Labouvie-Vief, G., Aycock, J., Rebucal, K. A., & Koch, H. E. (2004). Performance in auditory and visual emotional Stroop tasks: A comparison of older and younger adults. *Psychology and Aging, 19*, 523–535.

Zacks, R., & Hasher, L. (1997). Cognitive gerontology and attentional inhibition: A reply to Burke and McDowd. *Journals of Gerontology: Series B: Psychological Sciences and Social Sciences, 52*, P274–P283.

PART V

PERSONALITY PROCESSES AND INDIVIDUAL DIFFERENCES

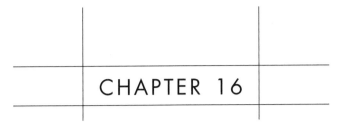

CHAPTER 16

Temperament and Emotion Regulation

MARY K. ROTHBART
BRAD E. SHEESE

Temperament refers to constitutionally based individual differences in emotional reactivity and self-regulation, and understanding these differences is needed for a complete understanding of emotion regulation. Research on links between temperament and emotion regulation has been the subject of several recent reviews (e.g., Eisenberg, Hofer, & Vaughan, this volume; Eisenberg, Smith, Sadovsky, & Spinrad, 2004; Rothbart & Bates, 2006). This chapter complements these reviews by considering how emotion regulation can be conceptualized within a temperament systems framework (Derryberry & Rothbart, 1997; Rothbart & Derryberry, 1981).

Historically, temperament has linked individual differences to the underlying constitution of the person, in both Eastern and Western traditions (Rothbart, 1989). More recently, however, temperament research has focused on individual differences in early development, particularly infancy through early childhood. An assumption has been that differences observed early in life were more likely to reflect biology than those observed later. A related assumption was that the impact of biological influences wanes as children grow older, being largely supplanted by the influence of socialization. Current research, however, suggests that both biological and environmental factors are important throughout development and may have different effects during different periods of the life course (e.g., Jaffee et al., 2005). In addition, biological and environmental factors are intimately linked, and they are not easily considered in isolation (e.g., Newman et al., 2005).

This view of developmental processes has had direct effects on contemporary theories of temperament. While there is still a strong emphasis on biological contributions, temperament is increasingly considered to be a multiply determined outcome of both biological and experiential processes, and temperament research has expanded beyond infancy and early childhood as periods of interest (Rothbart & Posner, 2006).

While concepts of temperament differ somewhat from one theory to another, many core questions and concerns are the same. The earliest research on childhood temperament was concerned with descriptions of infants (Thomas & Chess, 1977). Thomas and Chess identified nine dimensions of temperament based on interview protocols from parents of infants ages 3 to 9 months. These dimensions were: Activity Level, Approach–Withdrawal, Mood, Adaptability, Threshold, Intensity, Distractibility, Attention Span/Persistence, and Rhythmicity. Subsequent research has employed increasingly sophisticated psychometric methods to develop a basic taxonomy of temperament (see review by Rothbart & Bates, 2006) that extends from infancy (Gartstein & Rothbart, 2003) to adulthood (Evans & Rothbart, 2005). In our research, factors of Fear, Frustration, Negative affect, Extraversion/Surgency, Orienting/Perceptual Sensitivity, and Effortful Control have been extracted (Putnam, Ellis, & Rothbart, 2001). Although final consensus on a taxonomy has not been reached, individual differences in emotionality and emotion regulation are basic components of temperament (Bates, 2000; Rothbart & Bates, 2006; Rothbart & Derryberry, 1981).

This chapter describes concepts of emotion and emotion regulation within a temperament systems framework and discusses how these ideas go beyond the usual list of temperament traits (Derryberrry & Rothbart, 1997). We first put forward definitions of temperament, emotion, and emotion regulation. We then introduce a temperament systems approach, place it in relation to other concepts of temperament, and describe interactions among temperament systems. We consider in detail how temperament describes individual differences in the reactivity of emotions, the regulation of one emotional system by another, the regulation of attention by the emotions, and the regulation of emotions and emotion-related behavior by the attention system. We emphasize how regulation is related to individual differences in executive attention, as reflected in the temperamental construct of effortful control. Finally, because temperament itself develops, we describe these systems and their interactions in a developmental context.

DEFINING TEMPERAMENT, EMOTION, AND EMOTION REGULATION

Rothbart and Bates (2006) define temperament as "constitutionally based individual differences in reactivity and self-regulation, in the domains of affect, activity, and attention." The term "constitutional" indicates that temperament is biologically based and influenced over time by heredity, maturation, and experience. "Reactivity" and "self-regulation" are umbrella terms used originally by Rothbart and Derryberry (1981) to broadly organize the temperament domain. *Reactivity* refers to responses to change in the external and internal environment, including a broad range of reactions (e.g., negative affect, motor activity, fear, orienting, and cardiac reactivity). Reactivity is measured in terms of the latency, duration, and intensity of affective, motor, and orienting reactions (Rothbart & Derryberry, 1981).

Because emotional reactions include both action tendencies and the physiological support for these tendencies, all reactive systems contain self-regulatory aspects. Thus, fear can predispose withdrawal, attack, or behavioral inhibition, and positive affectivity can predispose the speed and energy of approach. Orienting early in life is reactive, but when adults present distractors to infants, it has regulative effects on the expression of the infants' emotions (Harman, Rothbart, & Posner, 1997). Later, orienting comes under the control of executive attention. A purer form of *self-regulation* is seen in the executive attentional processes underlying effortful control that can modulate reactivity.

When we first divided temperament into its reactive and self-regulatory components (Rothbart & Derryberry, 1981), we did not recognize the extent to which the reactive emotions and attentional orienting were also self-regulatory. However, when we later considered the emotions and orienting in detail, their self-regulatory aspects became clear. We now realize emotions can be seen as broadly integrative systems that order feeling, thought, and action (LeDoux, 1989). They represent the output of information processing networks assessing the meaning or affective significance of events for the individual. Whereas neural object recognition systems and spatial processing systems address the questions "What is it?" and "Where is it?," emotion-processing networks address the questions "Is it good for me?," "Is it bad for me?," and "What shall I do about it?" These networks have been evolutionarily conserved to allow the organism to deal with environmental and internally generated threat, opportunity, and social affiliation. When we discuss temperamental reactivity, we refer to individual differences in the temporal and intensive patterns of emotional response and ultimately to individual differences in the organization and functioning of emotion-processing networks.

By emotion regulation, we mean the modulation of a given emotional reaction, including its inhibition, activation, or graded modulation. Down- and upregulation refer to general reductions or increases in the activation of emotion-related neural systems. Emotion regulation includes attentional strategies employed through effortful control as well as the modulating effects of other emotions. We do not treat temperament and emotion regulation as distinct entities, nor do we claim that temperament causes emotion regulation, or that emotion regulation causes temperament. In fact, observations that orienting modulates distress and fear opposes extraversion/surgency suggest that when we consider individual differences in temperament, we are dealing with a dynamic balance among emotional and orienting tendencies as well as executive attention. We further recognize that emotion regulation strategies go far beyond temperament, although temperamental characteristics may influence their development.

Gross and Thompson (this volume) note that emotion regulation can refer to either how emotions regulate other responses or how emotions may be regulated. They focus on how emotions are regulated. In assessing temperament, however, we need to understand how one emotion system affects another, and how they affect and are affected by attention. A number of temperament constructs have been proposed that are directly related to emotion regulation, including persistence, soothability, inhibitory control, behavioral inhibition, adaptability, and effortful control. This list also includes constructs thought to reflect failures of regulation, such as impulsivity, negative affectivity, and anger (see Rothbart & Bates, 2006, for a review). Of these constructs, behavioral inhibition is a self-regulatory aspect of the reactive emotion of fear, and effortful control reflects of the efficiency of executive attention (e.g., Eisenberg et al., this volume).

A TEMPERAMENT SYSTEMS APPROACH: EMOTIONAL REACTIVITY

Temperament systems have much in common with theoretical approaches that link temperament directly to underlying biological processes (e.g., Gray, 1991; Posner & Rothbart, 2007a, 2007b; reviews by Rothbart, Derryberry, & Posner, 1994b; Rothbart & Posner, 2006). With recent advances in imaging technology, these approaches have begun to inform research at the psychological and behavioral levels of analysis. Imaging and genetic methods, however, carry their own limitations and conceptual problems, providing an important but not a privileged source of information. For this reason, convergence across multiple levels of analysis is emphasized, with the expectation that behavioral and psychological levels will also inform research on biological substrates.

A key hypothesis of the systems approach is that affect, cognition, and behavior are organized around the goals of the organism (Campos, Barrett, Lamb, Goldsmith, & Stenberg, 1983; Derryberry & Rothbart, 1997). These goals have been evolutionarily conserved in the nervous system but will also be programmed by the person's specific experiences and plans. Affective–motivational systems of emotion evaluate goal-relevant situations and organize goal-appropriate behavior. Based on a review of the literature, Derryberry and Rothbart (1997) described a number of systems that represent emotionally reactive components of temperament. These include systems that support defense and harm–avoidance, approach and appetitive behaviors, and nurturance/affiliation. Here, we concentrate on the first two of these reactive systems, the defense and approach systems.

The Defense System: Fear and Anger

The defense system describes a system of brain networks that serves the goal of avoiding harm by promoting organized responses to immediate and long-term threats (Derryberry & Rothbart, 1997). Portions of the lateral and central amygdala appear to be key neural structures in the functioning of this network (Fox, Henderson, Marshall, Nichols, & Ghera, 2005b). Fear, anxiety, and defensive anger reflect broad alterations in neurological and physiological responding that occur with the activation of defense system. These alterations in processing can be seen in behavioral tendencies to withdraw from active threats and avoid potentially threatening situations (i.e., a "flight" response). When withdrawal from severe threats is blocked, however, the defense system also serves to bias processing to promote defensive aggression (i.e., a "fight" response). Systems analogous to the defense system described by Derryberry and Rothbart are common to many psychobiological approaches to emotion. These include LeDoux's fear system and Gray's Behavioral Inhibition System (see review by Rothbart & Posner, 2006).

Fear and anxiety are aversive states that are commonly associated with various forms of dysfunction and pathology in the clinical literature (Fox et al., 2005b; Rothbart & Posner, 2006). Consequently, it might be expected that individuals exhibiting higher levels of fear would be more prone to pathology than those exhibiting lower levels. The systems approach, however, notes that fear and anxiety are evolutionarily conserved mechanisms to promote potentially adaptive behavior (see also Öhman & Mineka, 2001; Rothbart & Bates, 2006), so that very low levels of fear and anxiety are also problematic. There is a need for some level of fear and anxiety to promote adaptive patterns of responding, while under- or overactivation of the system may promote maladaptive responding. Although all negative emotions contribute to general negative affectivity or stress proneness, we have also found it useful to differentiate anger from fear. Anger tends to be positively related to the approach (surgency/extraversion) system described next, and it is particularly linked to externalizing problems in development (Rothbart & Bates, 2006; Rothbart & Posner, 2006).

The Approach (Surgency/Extraversion) System

An affective–motivational system that serves to modulate approach behaviors is common to most psychobiological approaches to emotion. Examples include Gray's Behavioral Activation System, Depue and Iacono's Behavioral Facilitation System, and Panksepp's Seeking System (see review by Rothbart et al., 1994b). An approach system serves the goal of resource acquisition by promoting organized responses to potential rewards (Derryberry & Rothbart, 1997). Dopaminergic neurons appear to form the core of this network, which also extends to the basolateral amygdala, ventral tegmental area, and the nucleus accumbens. Positive emotional states, such as joy and elation, as well as feelings of eager anticipation, are thought to reflect broad alterations in neurological and physiological responding that occur in activation of the approach. These alterations in processing serve to bias responding toward reward acquisition and can be seen in behavioral tendencies to seek out and approach rewards.

HOW DO EMOTION SYSTEMS REGULATE EACH OTHER?

In situations that present reward along with risk, both the approach and defense systems may become active and compete to influence perceptual processing, physiological arousal, and basic action tendencies. In some networks, there appears to be a localized competition affecting specific cortical and subcortical processes in a winner-take-all process, where the "strongest" system dominates (Norman & Shallice, 1986). However, over time, activation strength may vary, leading to alternation of opposing behaviors or to the appearance of disorganized or inconsistent responding. We have seen the opposing behaviors in infants in our laboratory, who show abrupt alternation between approach-related and withdrawal-related behaviors, including smiling and distress to threatening stimuli.

The effective inhibitory influence of the affective–motivational systems may not be symmetric. Instead, some systems appear to have preferential status in the modulation of responding. Observation of a normative "negativity bias" in humans and other animal species (e.g., Cacioppo & Berntson, 1994) suggests that defense may tend to dominate approach in situations that present both risk and reward. However, while the balance may be usually skewed toward defensive processing, this balance may not characterize every individual. Instead, individuals would be expected to temperamentally differ in the degree to which they exhibit a negativity bias (Ito & Cacioppo, 2005).

Approach versus Fearful Inhibition

Aspects of the approach system, including sociability, positive affect, and approach to novel objects, can be observed by 3 months of age and show stability from 3 to 9 months of age, while also demonstrating normative increases throughout the first year of life (Rothbart, Derryberry, & Hershey, 2000). Late in the first year, some infants also begin to demonstrate fear and strong behavioral inhibition in response to unfamiliar and intense stimuli (Schaffer, 1974; Rothbart, 1988), and fearful behavioral inhibition shows considerable longitudinal stability across childhood and into adolescence (Kagan, 1998). Fearful inhibition developing late in the first year of life allows control of approach. In our longitudinal research, infant fear assessed in the laboratory predicted childhood fear, sadness, and shyness at 7 years (Rothbart et al., 2000). Fear did not predict later frustration/anger and was inversely related to later approach, impulsivity, and aggression. These findings suggest that fear is involved in the self-regulation of both approach and aggressive tendencies (Gray & McNaughton, 1996).

More fearful infants also later showed greater empathy, guilt, and shame in childhood (Rothbart, Ahadi, & Hershey, 1994a). These findings suggested that fear might be involved in the early development of moral motivation, and Kochanska (1997) has found that temperamental fearfulness predicts conscience development in preschoolage children. On the other hand, extreme fear may lead to problems in children's rigid overcontrol of behavior, as reflected in Block's (2002) description of inflexible patterns of response that can limit children's positive experiences. Thus, although temperamental fear and its component behavioral inhibition allows the first major control system over approach, it is a reactive one that can lack flexibility.

A TEMPERAMENT SYSTEMS APPROACH: EFFORTFUL CONTROL AND EXECUTIVE ATTENTION

We now turn to processes underlying the development of effortful control. We devote our major review to this area, because of its importance to behavior and emotional regulation, and because many of the advances in this area are relatively recent. Effortful control is defined as the ability to inhibit a dominant response in order to perform a subdominant response, to plan, and to detect errors (Rothbart & Rueda, 2005). Effortful control initially emerged from factor-analytic work with temperament scales. It is a higher-order factor that includes lower-order scales of attentional focusing, perceptual sensitivity, low-intensity pleasure, and inhibitory control in childhood (Rothbart, Ahadi, Hershey, & Fisher, 2001) and attentional control, inhibitory control and activational control in adulthood (Evans & Rothbart, 2005). We have proposed that effortful control describes individual differences in conscious self-regulatory capacities linked to executive attention and the functioning of the anterior attention system (Posner & Rothbart, 1998; Rothbart et al., 1994b).

Effortful control has been linked to a broad array of external criteria (Rothbart & Bates, 2006). One focus of recent research has linked effortful control to the development of prosocial and antisocial behavior. The direct regulation of negative emotional reactions, such as anger, anxiety, or fear, represents one avenue through which effortful control may be associated with the expression and development of prosocial and antisocial behavior. It has been argued that individuals who exhibit greater degrees of effortful control are better able to regulate the affective responses that promote antisocial behavior (e.g., Kochanska, Murray, & Harlan, 2000). Consistent with this hypothesis, effortful control has been positively linked to empathy and prosocial behavior (Eisenberg et al., this volume; Rothbart & Bates, 2006). Effortful control has also been shown to interact with contextual variables to predict behaviors linked to emotion regulation. For example, early temperament has been shown to interact with parenting practices to predict later behavioral inhibition (Park, Belsky, Putnam, & Conic, 1997), externalizing behavior problems (Bates, Pettit, Dodge, & Ridge, 1998), and conscience development (Kochanska, 1997).

Kochanska et al. (2000) have characterized the construct of effortful control as being "situated at the intersection of the temperament and behavioral regulation literatures" (p. 220). What does effortful control mean for theories of temperament and personality? It means that contrary to earlier theoretical models of temperament emphasizing how people are driven by their positive and negative emotions or level of arousal, we are not always at the mercy of affect. Using effortful control, we can more flexibly approach situations we fear and inhibit actions we desire. The efficiency of control, however, will depend on the strength of the emotional processes against which effort is exerted (Rothbart & Derryberry, 2002). For example, when a child must delay an approach response to an appealing toy, the child with a stronger disposition to approach will require greater effortful control to succeed.

Effortful control can also support the internalization of competence-related goals (e.g., being kind to others and school performance) and their achievement, and is involved in the inhibition of immediate approach with the goal of attaining a larger reward later, in Mischel's research and in Block's (2002) hedonism of the future. Effortful control also allows the activation of behavior that would otherwise not be performed. In general, it allows the person to act "on principle." Effortful control is not itself a basic motivation but, rather, provides the means to effectively satisfying desired ends. It resembles the attentional capacities that underlie Block's (2002) construct of ego resiliency, which supports the ability to flexibly shift levels of control depending on the situation.

The Executive Attention System

Posner and colleagues have identified three attention networks in the brain that serve different functions and have different neural anatomies and neuromodulators (Posner & Fan, 2004b; Rueda, Posner, & Rothbart, 2004). The first two networks control alerting and orienting, respectively. The third, the executive attention network, functions to monitor and resolve conflict and involves the anterior cingulate cortex (ACC) and lateral prefrontal cortex (Rueda et al., 2004b). Dorsal areas of the cingulate have been implicated in the regulation of cognitive processing, while more ventral areas have been implicated in emotional processing (Bush, Luu, & Posner, 2000). In recent research, individual differences in the functioning of the executive attention network have been theoretically and empirically linked to the temperament construct of effortful control (Chang & Burns, 2005; Posner & Rothbart, 2007a; Rothbart & Rueda, 2005).

According to one theory, executive attention, and the ACC in particular, is involved primarily in the monitoring of conflict between potentially competing systems (Botwinick, Braver, Barch, Carter, & Cohen, 2001). There is also evidence that the prefrontal cortex, particularly on the right side, is involved in control through inhibition of the competing systems. This division of labor between the ACC and the prefrontal cortex cannot be the full story, because the ACC is also involved more directly in upregulating emotions, but these ideas suggest divisions of labor between the ACC and the prefrontal cortex in regulation.

The anterior cingulate gyrus, one of the main nodes of the executive attention network, has been linked to specific functions related to self-regulation (see review by Rothbart & Rueda, 2005). These include the monitoring of conflict, control of working memory, regulation of emotion, and response to error. In emotion studies, the cingulate is often seen as part of a network involving the orbital frontal cortex and amygdala that regulates our emotional response to input. Activation of the anterior cingulate is observed when people are asked to control their natural reactions to strong positive (Beauregard, Levesque, & Bourgouin, 2001) and negative (Ochsner, Bunge, Gross, & Gabrieli, 2002) emotions.

Another assessment involving conflict is the spatial conflict task for young children, in which object identity and spatial location of a stimulus are placed in conflict. In this task the child has two response keys, labeled with pictures of stimuli. The stimuli are presented on a computer screen and the child is instructed to press the key corresponding to the picture presented. Conflict trials are those in which the stimulus appears on the side opposite the corresponding key (Gerardi-Caulton, 2000).

Between 30 and 36 months of age, children learn to perform this task, which requires inhibiting the dominant response toward a spatial location in order to make a response based on matching identity (Gerardi-Caulton, 2000; Rothbart, Ellis, Rueda, & Posner, 2003). At 24 months, children are only able to carry out this task when the stimulus is on the same side of the computer screen as the matching response key (the congruent condition), but by 30 months, most children can handle the incongruent trials where the matching target is on the opposite side of the stimulus, although they are slowed (adults are also slowed in this condition). Children with higher performance on spatial conflict have also been rated by their parents as having relatively higher levels of temperamental effortful control and lower levels of negative affect (Rothbart et al., 2003), and children at 30 months who performed well on the spatial conflict task also performed well on an eye movement conflict task that can be used with children even younger than 24 months. Two-year-old children who were unable to complete the spatial conflict task were described by their parents as having lower effortful control and higher negative affectivity on the Children's Behavior Questionnaire (CBQ) measure of temperament (Rothbart, Ahadi, Hershey, & Fisher, 2001). These findings are consistent with the idea that the capacity to engage in rule-based action in conflict situations can support responding to social rules and regulating emotion.

In the Attention Networks Task (ANT) flanker task, the response to a target is in conflict with surrounding stimuli (Rueda et al., 2004a). Both the spatial conflict and flanker tasks have been linked in imaging studies to functioning of the brain's executive attention network (Fan, Flombaum, McCandliss, Thomas, & Posner, 2003) and have been used as model tasks for the functioning of this network (Rothbart & Rueda, 2005). In adolescents and adults, ANT performance has been linked to a number of psychopathologies (see review by Rothbart & Posner, 2006). Using the child ANT (Rueda et al., 2004a), significant improvement in conflict resolution was found up until age 7 but a remarkable similarity in both reaction time and accuracy was found from the age of 7 to adulthood.

Effortful Control in Childhood

Evidence for stability of effortful control has been found in research by Mischel and his colleagues (Shoda, Mischel, & Peake, 1990). Preschoolers were tested on their ability to wait for a delayed treat that was larger than a readily accessible treat. Children better able to delay gratification were found to have better self-control and greater ability to regulate reactions to stress and frustration. Their delay of gratification in seconds also predicted later parent-reported attentiveness, concentration, emotion regulation, and intelligence during adolescence. In follow-up studies when the participants were in their 30s, preschool delay predicted goal setting and self-regulatory abilities (Ayduk et al., 2000), suggesting remarkable continuity in self-regulatory skills.

Effortful control plays an important role in the development of conscience, with greater internalized conscience in children high in effortful control (Kochanska et al., 2000). Both the reactive temperamental control system of behavioral inhibition (part of fear reaction) and the attentionally based system of effortful control appear to regulate the development of socialized thought and behavior, with the influence of fearful inhibition found earlier in development. We have found that children 6–7 years old who were high in effortful control were also high in empathy and guilt/shame and low in aggressiveness (Rothbart et al., 1994a). Effortful control may support empathy by allowing children to attend to the other child's condition instead of focusing only on their own sympathetic distress. Eisenberg, Fabes, Nyman, Bernzweig, and Pinulas (1994) found that 4–6-year-old boys with good attentional control tended to deal with anger by using nonhostile verbal methods rather than overt aggression.

During the toddler and preschool years, development of the executive attention system underlying effortful control allows children greater control of stimulation and response, including the ability to select responses in a conflict situation. Exciting developmental work by Aksan and Kochanska (2004) links behavioral inhibition and effortful control, finding that children who were more fearful and inhibited at 33 months showed more volitional inhibitory control at 45 months. They suggest that more fearful and inhibited children have a greater opportunity to foster their own self-control during their periods of slow approach to novel situations.

HOW DOES EMOTION REGULATE ATTENTION?

As discussed previously, emotional defense and approach systems regulate behavior, thoughts, and other emotions. Activation of defense or approach may also alter attention and the processing of sensory information (LeDoux, 2000; Öhman & Mineka, 2001). Most situations present a number of potential foci for attention, and in situations related to significant consequences for the health and well-being of the individual, selection and attention to specific stimuli may be critically important.

This selection process can be viewed as involving multiple potential targets in competition for attention (Desimone & Duncan, 1995). Orienting of attention can produce a bias toward one or more of these potential targets (Corbetta, Kincade, & Shulman, 2002), and emotion is related to attentional bias. For example, more threatening stimuli have been associated with greater vigilance in a probe detection task (Mogg et al., 2000), threatening stimuli previously paired with an aversive noise are related to increased allocation of attention (Beaver, Mogg, & Bradley, 2005), and presentation of aversive stimuli is associated with increased interference during mathematical problem-solving and line detection tasks (Schimmack, 2005).

The temperament systems approach suggests that the effect of emotions on perceptual processes will vary as the systems develop and will differ across individuals, reflecting each person's pattern of temperamental reactivity. In adults, negative affectivity, neuroticism, and trait anxiety have been related to differential patterns of looking to various kinds of threatening stimuli (e.g., Mogg, Bradley, & Williams, 1995), as well as to altered patterns of attention toward detecting errors (Paulus, Feinsten, Simmons, & Stein, 2004). Neuroticism has also been linked to difficulty in disengaging attention from sources of threat (Derryberry & Reed, 1994, 2002), while Extraversion is related to similar difficulties in disengaging from rewarding stimuli (Derryberry & Reed, 1994).

As noted previously, dorsal areas of the cingulate have been implicated in the regulation of cognitive processing and more ventral areas in emotional processing (Bush et al., 2000). The portion of the ACC related to emotion regulation has a very high level of tonic activity, even at rest (Fox et al., 2005a). There is also evidence of an inhibitory interaction between the more ventral emotion regulation part of the ACC and the more dorsal areas related to cognitive control (Drevets & Raichle, 1998). Recently, a task requiring eye movements away from a stimulus revealed that an early reduction of activity in the ventral part of the ACC related to emotion regulation may be a necessary prerequisite for a correct response (Polli et al., 2005). On error trials, subjects failed to reduce activation of the emotional area. This finding may open the way for more detailed studies of how anxiety interferes with accurate performance.

Initial orienting to threatening or rewarding stimuli is often accompanied by behavioral freezing and muted physiological responding, including cardiac deceleration (Huffman et al., 1998), but the initial orienting phase may be quickly followed by an action phase involving behaviors such as fight or flight that require dramatic changes in metabolic functioning (Bradley, Cuthbert, & Lang, 1999). The modulation of autonomic arousal in preparation for behavioral responding presents another mechanism through which defense and approach systems can influence responding (Porges, 1996), including changes in skin conductance, heart and respiration rate, blood pressure and patterns of blood circulation, potentiation of the startle response, and secretion of cortisol and catecholamines (Bradley, Codispoti, Cuthbert, & Lang, 2001).

A variety of evidence links reactive temperament dimensions to aspects of physiological responding (see Rothbart & Bates, 2006, for a review). For example, heart-rate variability has been linked to low behavioral inhibition (Kagan, 1998) and vagal tone to both high approach and irritability (Beauchaine, 2001). Recent research on cortisol secretion provides strong support for links between reactive aspects of temperament and physiological responses to specific environmental challenges. Donzella, Gunnar, Krueger, and Alwin (2000) found that children who showed cortisol increases following a competitive interaction with an adult were higher in temperamental surgency or approach and lower in effortful control. Dettling, Parker, Lane, Sebanc, and Gunnar (2000) found that for children in poor-quality child care, higher cortisol levels were related to high negative emotionality and low effortful control. The interactions between reactive and regulatory components of temperament predicting cortisol levels are important findings, as is the dependence of the results on context.

HOW DOES ATTENTION REGULATE EMOTION?

The early life of the infant is concerned with the regulation of state, including regulation of distress. Orienting, the selection of information from sensory input, is a major mechanism for this regulation. Caregivers report how they use infant attention to regulate the state of the infant, distracting their infants by bringing their attention to other stimuli. As infants orient, they are often quieted, and their distress appears to diminish.

We have conducted a systematic study of orienting and soothing in 3- to 6-month-old infants (Harman et al., 1997). Infants were first shown a sound and light display that led to distress in about 50% of the infants. These infants strongly oriented to interesting visual and auditory soothing events when they were presented, however, and during their orienting, facial and vocal signs of distress disappeared. Nevertheless, as soon as the orienting stopped (e.g., when the object was removed), the infants' distress returned to almost exactly the levels shown prior to presentation of the distractor. An internal system, which we termed the "distress keeper," appeared to hold a computation of the initial level of distress, so that it returned if the infant's orientation to the novel event was lost. In later studies, we found that infants could be quieted by distraction for as long as 1 minute, without changing the eventual level of distress reached once the orienting ended (Harman et al., 1997).

For young infants, the control of orienting is at first largely in the hands of caregiver presentations. By 4 months, however, infants have gained considerable control over disengaging their gaze from one visual location and moving it to another, and greater orienting skill in the laboratory has been associated with lower parent-reported negative affect and greater soothability (Johnson, Posner, & Rothbart, 1991). Related phenomena appear to be present in preschool and older children and adults, and they provide an important aspect of self-regulation. Adults and adolescents who report themselves as having good ability to focus and shift attention also say they experience less negative affect (Evans & Rothbart, 2005), and negative emotion and effortful control are also inversely related in parent reports of temperament in toddlers and school-age children (Putnam et al., 2001). Indeed, many of the ideas of both modern cognitive therapy and Eastern methods for controlling the mind are based on using attention to reduce the intrusive influence of negative ideation.

We observed a number of changes in emotion regulation across longitudinal observation of infants between 3 and 13 months (Rothbart, Ziaie, & O'Boyle, 1992). First, older infants increasingly looked to their mothers during presentation of arousing stimuli such as masks and unpredictable mechanical toys. Infants' disengagement of attention from arousing stimuli was also related to lower levels of negative affect in the laboratory at 13 months. Stability from 10 to 13 months was found in infants' use of attentional disengagement, mouthing, hand to mouth (e.g., thumb sucking), approach, and withdrawing the hand, suggesting that some of the infants' self-regulation strategies were becoming habitual. Over the period of 3 to 13 months, passive self-soothing decreased and more active approach, attack, and body self-stimulation increased. Infants who showed the greatest distress at 3 months, however, tended to persist in a very early form of regulation, self-soothing. Once a mechanism for emotion regulation develops, it may persist because it has brought relief, even though more sophisticated emotion regulation mechanisms are now available, an important consideration in developmental approaches to clinical problems.

More recent studies have found direct links between infants' self-regulated disengagement of attention and decreases in their concurrent negative affect (Stifter & Braungart, 1995), and there is also support for the idea that early mechanisms for coping with negative emotion may later be transferred to the control of cognition and behavior, as suggested by Posner and Rothbart (1998). Correlations have been found, for example, between infants' use of self-regulation in anger-inducing situations and their preschool ability to delay responses (Calkins & Williford, 2003). In research by Mischel and his colleagues (Sethi, Mischel, Aber, Shoda, & Rodriguez, 2000), toddlers' use of distraction strategies in an arousing situation was also positively related to their later delay of gratification at age 5.

In adults as well as infants, attention may regulate affective–motivational systems by controlling orienting to stimuli. In the previous section we described how the defense and approach systems monitor for goal-relevant stimuli and, once activated, bias orienting toward some targets. Levels of emotional activation are thus maintained or increased until something occurs to interrupt the cycle. One way to interrupt the cycle is to perform actions that remove the stimulus or make the stimulus less relevant, as in the distraction of infants. For example, if a person is afraid of heights, visual cues indicating precipitous drops may initiate a cycle of anxiety and fear. One way to interrupt this cycle is to back away from the ledge. If such an action is not available or is undesirable, a second approach is to "not look down." Information reception can thus be controlled to reduce the activation of the system. This kind of regulation can also be applied to the approach system. Just as one can look away from things that are feared, one can also look away from things that are desired. Consistent with this hypothesis, children who are most able to resist temptation are those most likely to divert their attention away from desired stimuli while waiting for them (e.g., Sethi et al., 2000).

Regulating orienting may not always be sufficient to manage emotional reactions. Not looking at a cookie may reduce the probability we will eat it, but even when we are not looking at it, we still know it is there. Conceptual processing and memory allow us to effectively maintain an internal representation of the stimulus over time. Internal representations may be just as effective, or even more so, in triggering and maintaining the activation of affective systems. Consequently, regulating internal representations becomes an important avenue for the regulation of emotional responding. The same general network involved in control of emotions is also active during the manipulation of internal representations, such as generating word associations (Posner & Raichle, 1994). Because working memory is finite, focusing attention on other representations may lead to the exclusion of "unwanted" representations. The executive attention system serves to monitor and resolve conflict among brain networks and may thus facilitate the manipulation of internal representations by allowing for the selection of one representation over another. We can attempt to control emotional responding by literally thinking about other things, a process that has been referred to as suppression (Gross, 2002). However, as an emotion regulation strategy, suppression may have limited utility and ultimately adverse long-term consequences.

Research on sensory systems has shown that attention can work by increasing activation in an attended sensory system as well as by reducing activation of other systems (Posner & Raichle, 1994). To date, the upregulation of emotions has not been commonly addressed in either theoretical treatments or empirical studies of emotion regulation, although Kieras, Tobin, Graziano, and Rothbart (2005) have found that children higher in inhibitory skills are more likely to be able to smile at the presentation of a disappointing gift, and recent research in our laboratory has linked high executive attention on the child ANT to smiling in this paradigm. Existing evidence also shows links between efforts at upregulation through reappraisal and activation of the prefrontal cortex, including the dorsal anterior cingulate (Ochsner et al., 2004). Executive attention has been related to suppression of inappropriate cognitions as in the Stroop effect (Posner & DiGirolamo, 1998), and similar mechanisms are likely involved in emotional regulation.

Links have also been found between the executive attention network and another strategy for altering representations to promote emotion regulation, reappraisal. Reappraisal involves reinterpreting the meaning or value of a representation (Gross, 2002). Ochsner et al. (2002) found that reappraisal intended to reduce negative emotions led to reduced activity in the amgydala, suggesting that reappraisal changes emotion-related processing. Subsequent research has indicated that prefrontal and anterior cingulate regions are involved in the modulation of emotion processing through reappraisal (Ochsner et al., 2004). Reappraisal may thus present another mechanism through which the executive attention system regulates affective systems in that reappraisal can be construed as a competition among alternate internal representations. The executive attention system facilitates the selection of a secondary representation over the prepotent representation.

Controlling attentional orienting, excluding prepotent representations, and reinterpretation are strategies for reducing activation of reactive systems by altering overt or internal "input" into those systems. A different avenue for regulation concerns altering the "output" associated with the reactive systems. Bidirectional links between the affective–motivational systems and areas of output, such as the autonomic system, allow for feedback loops that can maintain emotional activation states. The executive attention system may enable efforts to modulate different aspects of physiological arousal, including both upregulation and downregulation. Direct manipulation of the aspects of physiological arousal that are under conscious control, such as changes in rates of respiration and body muscle tension, is one possibility. Evidence from imaging studies and animal models indicates that the ACC plays a substantial role in the modulation of autonomic reactivity in response to situational demands (e.g., Critchley et al., 2003). This includes evidence that ACC activation may mediate the link between meditation and breathing exercises and reductions in sympathetic activity (Kubota et al., 2001).

So far, we have primarily considered emotion regulation in terms of the reduction of activation. The defense and approach systems motivate adaptive behavior by inducing emotional states, while the executive attention system allows for the suppression of these reactive systems. However, it is important to note that the same mechanisms through which the executive attention system produces reductions in activation of reactive systems can also be used to produce increases in activation. If we want to induce an affective state we can consciously shift attention to the appropriate affect-inducing stimuli, we can recall affect-inducing representations, or reinterpret neutral representations to promote affective responses. The executive attention system may also allow us to elicit emotional responses by increasing physiological arousal or by producing behaviors that are consistent with the desired emotional state. We now describe a program for training executive attention that may in the future be related to children's emotion regulation.

Training Executive Attention

We have examined conflict performance on the ANT in 4- to 6-year-old children, finding strong improvement in executive attention from age 4 to 6 (Rueda, Rothbart, McCandliss, Saccomanno, & Posner, 2005). We also tested for effects of training attention in children by using computer exercises based on training that improved attention in rhesus monkeys and chimpanzees in their preparation for space flights (Rumbaugh & Washburn, 1995). Both 4- and 6-year-olds showed improvement over 5 days of training in their performance on the ANT and on event-related potentials recorded during ANT performance (Rueda et al., 2005), as well as on IQ measures. These results suggest that attention training can enhance the development of executive attention and may be helpful to children both with and without problems in attention. As yet, generalization of training effects to emotion regulation in children has not been tested, although Rumbaugh and Washburn (1995) anecdotally reported greater emotion regulation in primates who had participated in attention training.

FUTURE RESEARCH DIRECTIONS

In temperament studies involving emotion regulation it has been common to consider only individual differences in components of reactive temperament, such as behavioral inhibition, without considering either regulatory aslpects of temperament, such as effortful control, or the interaction among these components. Studies focusing on only single traits or looking only at main effects may be missing important opportunities for understanding the dynamic contribution of temperament to developmental outcomes. Recent research supports the importance of considering interactions among dimensions of temperament in predicting external criteria. For example, Gunnar, Sebanc, Tout, Donzella, and van Dulmen (2003) found that high levels of surgency (approach) combined with low levels of effortful control were associated with higher cortisol levels and higher peer rejection in childhood (see also reviews by Rothbart & Bates, 2006; Rothbart & Posner, 2006).

When considering interactions among systems, it is also important to consider system goals within the demands of the current context. Depending on context, the systems may act relatively independently, in direct competition, or may complement one another. Without considering the goals of the system it is difficult to predict their relation to particular outcomes a priori. For example, reconsidering fearfulness in terms of the defense system emphasizes that the network serves not only to inhibit behavior in some circumstances but also to motivate avoidance or attack. In contrast, effortful control, considered as an index of individual differences in the functioning of the executive attention system, serves to inhibit and facilitate processing in diverse cognitive and affective networks, with the goal of modulating prepotent responses. In some instances, the goals of the defense and executive attention systems may be congruent. In these instances we would expect both temperamental fearfulness and effortful control to independently contribute to predicting an outcome (e.g., following directions during a fire drill). In other circumstances the goals of the systems may be at odds and we would expect behavioral outcomes to reflect an interaction between the two systems (e.g., in jumping out of an airplane).

More speculatively, interacting temperament systems may exhibit nonlinear relations with outcomes of interest. Consider temperamental contributions to aggression against peers in childhood. Children exhibiting low levels of defense motivation may be more likely to engage in physical aggression because they are less likely to fear their peers or fear disapproval of authority figures. At the opposite end of the spectrum, children higher in behavioral inhibition may be more likely to withdraw from contentious interactions with peers. However, in very threatening situations children higher in fearfulness as part of defense motivation may also be more prone to acts of defensive aggression.

Overall, we would expect a curvilinear relation between defense motivation and physical aggression, with children lower in defense motivation more likely to exhibit aggression in their interactions with their peers, while children higher in defense motivation may more likely to exhibit infrequent but intense bouts of physical aggression.

Children exhibiting low levels of effortful control will also have limited self-regulatory capacities, and their patterns of physical aggression will be more likely to reflect the reactive aspects of their temperaments. Thus, we might only expect links between the reactive systems and aggression for children with moderate to low levels of effortful control. In contrast, children high in effortful control would only be likely to exhibit aggression under circumstances in which aggression was considered socially appropriate or when they were under a great deal of regulatory "load."

The approach adopted here also suggests that it is important to consider how each system contributes to temperament assessments. When we bring a child into the laboratory and attempt to assess effortful control using a variety of game-like tasks, task performance will reflect dynamic interactions among all the systems, not just effortful control. The approach system may respond to engaging activities and rewards; the defense system may respond to the novelty of the lab, the procedures, and the experimenters; and the executive attention system will contribute to task performance, as well as to keeping emotional responses in line with the parent's, experimenter's, and personal expectations. We can try to get direct assessments of one aspect of temperament, but outcomes will almost always reflect a mix of reactive and regulatory processes. Inhibitory control tasks, commonly employed in behavioral assessments of effortful control, present an interesting example of how even very basic assessments may potentially tap into multiple temperament systems. Assessments such as the day/night Stroop task focus on assessing the inhibition of prepotent responses. However, to successfully perform this task, children must also sit still, follow instructions, attend to the stimuli, and activate nonprepotent responses.

Even in the absence of overt feedback or reward from the experimenter, we might expect some variability from participants in their reactive responses to good performance on these tasks. Consistent with this idea, Wolfe and Bell (2004) found that while parent-reported inhibitory control was a significant predictor of performance on inhibitory control lab tasks ($r = .36$), parent-reported approach/anticipation was a better predictor ($r = -.555$). Thus, while inhibitory control as a construct may be properly considered a facet of effortful control, in practice inhibitory control measures may reflect an interaction between the approach and the executive attention systems.

This dynamic view of interacting systems suggests that single-method assessments of temperament may be problematic. When possible, batteries of differentiated assessments should be employed in which the common feature is the temperament characteristic of interest. Multimethod assessment procedures are further complemented by the assessment of multiple traits, particularly when reactive and regulatory components of temperament are being examined. A multitrait approach allows us to better assess individual differences in regulation by controlling for individual differences in reactivity, and vice versa.

CONCLUSIONS

The earliest work on temperament focused on describing individual differences in infancy; subsequent research has explored the structure of temperament across development and sought to link individual temperament constructs to developmental outcomes. We suggest that our understanding of emotion regulation will be advanced if we (1) reconceptualize temperament constructs in terms of affective–motivational and attentional systems, and (2) consider dynamic interactions among these systems. Considering individual differences in emotional reactivity and emotion regulation as core components of temperament represents a first step toward a more dynamic process-oriented view. The second step is to consider reactive and regulative components of temperament together rather than in isolation. Linking temperament to the study of emotion and emotion regulation also provides temperament researchers with a rich empirical base for generating models of temperament development. Advances in understanding the basic processes in emotional reactivity and emotion regulation should inform and enrich research on temperament. At the same time, research on temperament offers a unique perspective for examining emotion and emotion regulation.

REFERENCES

Aksan, N., & Kochanska, G. (2004). Links between systems of inhibition from infancy to preschool years. *Child Development, 75,* 1477–1490.

Ayduk, O., Mendoza-Denton, R., Mischel, W., Downey, G., & Peakeodriguez, M. (2000). Regulating the interpersonal self: Strategic self-regulation for coping with rejection sensitivity. *Journal of Personality and Social Psychology, 79,* 776–792.

Bates, J. E. (2000). Temperament as an emotion construct: Theoretical and practical issues. In M. Lewis & J. M. Haviland-Jones (Eds.), *Handbook of emotions* (2nd ed., pp. 382–396). New York: Guilford Press.

Bates, J. E., Pettit, G. S., Dodge, K. A., & Ridge, B. (1998). The interaction of temperamental resistance to control and restrictive parenting in the development of externalizing behavior. *Developmental Psychology, 34,* 982–995.

Beauchaine, T. (2001). Vagal tone, development, and Gray's motivational theory: Toward an integrated model of autonomic nervous system functioning in psychopathology. *Development and Psychopathology, 13,* 183–214.

Beauregard, M., Levesque, J., & Bourgouin, P. (2001). Neural correlates of conscious self-regulation of emotion. *Journal of Neuroscience, 21,* 165.

Beaver, J. D., Mogg, K., & Bradley, B. P. (2005). Emotional conditioning to masked stimuli and modulation of visuospatial attention. *Emotion, 5,* 67–79.

Block, J. (2002). *Personality as an affect-processing system: Toward an integrative theory.* Mahwah, NJ: Erlbaum.

Botwinick, M. M., Braver, T. S., Barch, D. M., Carter, C. S., & Cohen, J. D. (2001). Conflict monitoring and cognitive control. *Psychological Review, 108,* 624–652.

Bradley, M. M., Codispoti, M., Cuthbert, B. N., & Lang, P. J. (2001). Emotion and motivation: I. Defense and approach reactions in picture processing. *Emotion, 1,* 276–299.

Bradley, M. M., Cuthbert, B. N., & Lang, P. J. (1999). Affect and the startle reflex. In M. E. Dawson, A. Schell, & A. Boehmelt (Eds.), *Startle modification: Implications for neuroscience, cognitive science and clinical science* (pp. 157–183). New York: Cambridge University Press.

Bush, G., Luu, P., & Posner, M. I. (2000). Cognitive and emotional influences in anterior cingulate cortex. *Trends in Cognitive Sciences, 4*(6), 215–222.

Cacioppo, J. T., & Berntson, G. G. (1994). Relationship between attitudes and evaluative space: A critical review, with emphasis on the separability of positive and negative substrates. *Psychological Bulletin, 115,* 401–423.

Calkins, S. D., & Williford, A. P. (2003, April). *Anger regulation in infancy: Consequences and correlates.* Paper presented at the meeting of the Society for Research in Child Development, Tampa, FL.

Campos, J. J., Barrett, K. C., Lamb, M. E., Goldsmith, H. H., & Stenberg, C. (1983). Socioemotional development. In M. W. Haith & J. J. Campos (Eds.), *Handbook of child psychology: Vol. 2. Infancy and developmental psychology* (pp. 783–915). New York: Wiley.

Chang, F., & Burns, B. M. (2005). Attention in preschoolers: Associations with effortful control and motivation. *Child Development, 76,* 247–263.

Corbetta, M., Kincade, J. M., & Shulman, G. L. (2002). Neural systems for visual orienting and their relationships to spatial working memory. *Journal of Cognitive Neuroscience, 14*(3), 508–523.

Critchley, H. D., Mathias, C. J., Josephs, O., O'Doherty, J., Zanini, S., Dewar, B.-K., et al. (2003). Human cingulate cortex and autonomic control: Converging neuroimaging and clinical evidence. *Brain, 126*, 2139–2152.

Derryberry, D., & Reed, M. A. (1994). Temperament and attention: Orienting toward and away from positive and negative signals. *Journal of Personality and Social Psychology, 66*, 1128–1139.

Derryberry, D., & Reed, M. A. (2002). Anxiety-related attentional biases and their regulation by attentional control. *Journal of Abnormal Psychology, 111*, 225–236.

Derryberry, D., & Rothbart, M. K. (1997). Reactive and effortful processes in the organization of temperament. *Developmental Psychopathology, 9*, 633–652.

Desimone, R., & Duncan, J. (1995). Neural mechanisms of selective visual attention. *Annual Review of Neuroscience, 18*, 193–222.

Dettling, A. C., Parker, S., Lane, S. K., Sebanc, A. M., & Gunnar, M. R. (2000). Quality of care and temperament determine whether cortisol levels rise over the day for children in full-day childcare. *Psychoneuroendocrinology, 25*, 819–836.

Donzella, B., Gunnar, M. R., Krueger, W. K., & Alwin, J. (2000). Cortisol and vagal tone response to competitive challenge in preschoolers: Associations with temperament. *Developmental Psychobiology, 37*, 209–220.

Drevets, W. C., & Raichle, M. E. (1998). Reciprocal suppression of regional blood flow during emotional versus higher cognitive processes: Implications for interactions between emotion and cognition. *Cognition and Emotion, 12*, 353–285.

Eisenberg, N., Fabes, R. A., Nyman, M., Bernzweig, J., & Pinulas, A. (1994). The relations of emotionality and regulation to children's anger-related reactions. *Child Development, 65*, 109–128.

Eisenberg, N., Hofer, C., & Vaughan, J. (2007). Effortful control and its socioemotional consequences. In J. J. Gross (Ed.), *Handbook of emotion regulation* (pp. 287–306). New York: Guilford Press

Eisenberg, N., Smith, C. L., Sadovsky, A., & Spinrad, T. L. (2004). Effortful control: Relations with emotion regulation, adjustment, and socialization in childhood. In R. F. Baumeister & K. D. Vohs (Eds.), *Handbook of self-regulation: Research, theory, and applications* (pp. 259–282). New York: Guilford Press.

Evans, D., & Rothbart, M. K. (2005). *Developing a model for adult temperament.* Manuscript submitted for publication.

Fan, J., Flombaum, J. I., McCandliss, B. D., Thomas, K. M., & Posner, M. I. (2003). Cognitive and brain consequences of conflict. *NeuroImage, 18*(1), 42–57.

Fox, M. D., Snyder, A. Z., Vincent, J. L., Corbetta, M., Van Essen, D. C., & Raichle, M. E. (2005a). The human brain is intrinsically organized into dynamic, anticorrelated functional networks. *Proceedings of the National Academy of Sciences, USA, 102*, 9673–9678.

Fox, N. A., Henderson, H. A., Marshall, P. J., Nichols, K. E., & Ghera, M. M. (2005b). Behavioral Inhibition: Linking biology and behavior within a developmental framework. *Annual Review of Psychology, 56*, 235–262.

Gartstein, M. A., & Rothbart, M. K. (2003). Studying infant temperament via the revised Infant Behavior Questionnaire. *Infant Behavior and Development, 26*, 64–86.

Gerardi-Caulton, G. (2000). Sensitivity to spatial conflict and the development of self-regulation in children 24–36 months of age. *Developmental Science, 3*, 397–404.

Gray, J. A. (1991). The neuropsychology of temperament. In J. Strelau & A. Angleitner (Eds.), *Explorations in temperament: International perspectives on theory and measurement* (pp. 105–128). New York: Plenum Press.

Gray, J. A., & McNaughton, N. (1996). *The neuropsychology of anxiety: Reprise.* Paper presented at the Nebraska Symposium on Motivation: Perspectives on anxiety, panic and fear, Lincoln, NE.

Gross, J. J. (2002). Emotion regulation: Affective, cognitive, and social consequences. *Psychophysiology, 39*, 281–291.

Gross, J. J., & Thompson, R. A. (2007). Emotion regulation: Conceptual foundations. In J. J. Gross (Ed.), *Handbook of emotion regulation* (pp. 3–24). New York: Guilford Press

Gunnar, M. R., Sebanc, A. M., Tout, K., Donzella, B., & van Dulmen, M. M. (2003). Peer rejection, temperament, and cortisol activity in preschoolers. *Developmental Psychobiology, 43*, 346–358.

Harman, C., Rothbart, M. K., & Posner, M. I. (1997). Distress and attention interactions in early infancy. *Motivation and Emotion, 21*, 27–43.

Huffman, L. C., Bryan, E. E., del Carmen, R., Pedersen, F. A., Doussard-Roosevelt, J. A., & Porges, S. W.

(1998). Infant temperament and cardiac vagal tone: Assessments at twelve weeks of age. *Child Development, 69*, 624–635.

Ito, T. A., & Cacioppo, J. T. (2005). Variations on a human universal: Individual differences in positivity offset and negativity bias. *Cognition and Emotion, 19*, 1–26.

Jaffee, S. R., Caspi, A., Moffitt, T. E., Dodge, K. A., Rutter, M., Taylor, A., et al. (2005). Nature x Nurture: Genetic vulnerability interacts with physical maltreatment to promote conduct problems. *Development and Psychopathology, 17*, 67–84.

Johnson, M. H., Posner, M. I., & Rothbart, M. K. (1991). Components of visual orienting in early infancy: Contingency learning, anticipatory looking, and disengaging. *Journal of Cognitive Neuroscience, 3*, 335–344.

Kagan, J. (1998). Biology and the child. In W. Damon & N. Eisenberg (Eds.), *Handbook of child psychology: Vol. 3. Social, emotional and personality development* (5th ed., pp. 177–235). New York: Wiley.

Kieras, J. E., Tobin, R. M., Graziano, W. G., & Rothbart, M. K. (2005). You can't always get what you want: Effortful control and children's responses to undesirable gifts. *Psychological Science, 16*, 391–396.

Kochanska, G. (1997). Multiple pathways to conscience for children with different temperaments: From toddlerhood to age 5. *Developmental Psychology, 22*, 228–240.

Kochanska, G., Murray, K. T., & Harlan, E. T. (2000). Effortful control in early childhood: Continuity and change, antecedents, and implications for social development. *Developmental Psychology, 36*, 220–232.

Kubota, Y., Sato, W., Toichi, M., Murai, T., Okada, T., Hayashi, A., et al. (2001). Frontal midline theta is correlated with cardiac autonomic activities during the performance of an attention demanding meditation procedure. *Cognitive Brain Research, 11*, 281–287.

LeDoux, J. E. (1989). Cognitive–emotional interactions in the brain. *Cognition and Emotion, 3*, 267–289.

LeDoux, J. E. (2000). Emotion circuits in the brain. *Annual Review of Neuroscience, 23*, 155–184.

Mogg, K., Bradley, B. P., & Williams, R. (1995). Attentional bias and anxiety and depression: The role of awareness. *British Journal of Clinical Psychology, 34*, 17–36.

Mogg, K., McNamara, J., Powys, M., Rawlinson, H., Seiffer, A., & Bradley, B. P. (2000). Selective attention to threat: A test of two cognitive models of anxiety. *Cognition and Emotion, 14*, 375–399.

Newman, T. K., Syagailo, Y. V., Barr, C. S., Wendland, J. R., Champoux, M., Graessle, M., et al. (2005). Monoamine oxidase A: Gene promoter variation and rearing experience influence aggressive behavior in rhesus monkeys. *Biological Psychiatry, 57*, 167–172.

Norman, D. A., & Shallice, T. (1986). Attention to action: Willed and automatic control of behavior. In G. E. Schwartz & D. Shapiro (Eds.), *Consciousness and self-regulation* (Vol. 4, pp. 1–18). New York: Plenum Press.

Ochsner, K. N., Bunge, S. A., Gross, J. J., & Gabrieli, J. D. E. (2002). Rethinking feelings: An FMRI study of the cognitive regulation of emotion. *Journal of Cognitive Neuroscience, 14*(8), 1215–1229.

Ochsner, K. N., Ray, R. D., Cooper, J. C., Robertson, E. R., Chopra, S., Gabrieli, J. D., et al. (2004). For better or for worse: Neural systems supporting the cognitive down- and up-regulation of negative emotion. *NeuroImage, 23*, 483–499.

Öhman, A., & Mineka, S. (2001). Fears, phobias, and preparedness: Toward an evolved module of fear and fear learning. *Psychological Review, 108*, 483–522.

Park, S. Y., Belsky, J., Putnam, S., & Conic, K. (1997). Infant emotionality, parenting, and 3–year inhibition: Exploring stability and lawful discontinuity in a male sample. *Developmental Psychology, 33*, 218–227.

Paulus, M. P., Feinstein, J. S., Simmons, A., & Stein, M. B. (2004). Anterior cingulate activation in high trait anxious subjects is related to altered error processing during decision making. *Biological Psychiatry, 55*, 1179–1187.

Polli, F. E., Barton, J. J. S., Cain, M. S., Thakker, K. N., Rauch, S. L., & Manoach, D. S. (2005). Rostral and dorsal anterior cingulate cortex make dissociable contributions during antisaccade error commission. *Proceedings of the National Academy of Sciences, USA, 102*, 15700–15705.

Porges, S. W. (1996). Physiological regulation in high-risk infants: A model for assessment and potential intervention. *Development and Psychopathology, 8*, 45–58.

Posner, M. I., & DiGirolamo, G. J. (1998). Executive attention: Conflict, target detection, and cognitive control. In R. I. Parasuraman (Ed.), *The attentive brain* (pp. 401–424). Cambridge, MA: MIT Press.

Posner, M. I., & Fan, J. (in press). Attention as an organ system. In J. Pomerantz (Ed.), *Neurobiology of perception and communication: From synapse to society the IVth De Lange Conference.* Cambridge, UK: Cambridge University Press.

Posner, M. I., & Raichle, M. E. (1994). *Images of mind.* New York: Scientific American Library.

Posner, M. I., & Rothbart, M. K. (1998). Attention, self-regulation and consciousness. *Philosophical Transactions of the Royal Society of London, B, 353,* 1915–1927.

Posner, M. I., & Rothbart, M. K. (2007a). *Educating the human brain.* Washington DC: American Psychological Association Books.

Posner, M. I., & Rothbart, M. K. (2007b). Research on attentional networks as a model for the integration of psychological science. *Annual Review of Psychology.*

Putnam, S. P., Ellis, L. K., & Rothbart, M. K. (2001). The structure of temperament from infancy through adolescence. In A. Eliasz & A. Angleitner (Eds.), *Advances in research on temperament* (pp. 165–182). Lengerich, Germany: Pabst Science.

Rothbart, M. K. (1988). Temperament and the development of inhibited approach. *Child Development, 59,* 1241–1250.

Rothbart, M. K. (1989). Biological processes of temperament. In G. A. Kohnstamm, J. E. Bates, & M. K. Rothbart (Eds.), *Temperament in childhood* (pp. 77–110). Chichester, UK: Wiley.

Rothbart, M. K., Ahadi, S. A., & Hershey, K. L. (1994a). Temperament and social behavior in childhood. *Merrill-Palmer Quarterly, 40,* 21–39.

Rothbart, M. K., Ahadi, S. A., Hershey, K. L., & Fisher, P. (2001). Investigations of temperament at three to seven years: The children's behavior questionnaire. *Child Development, 72*(5), 1394–1408.

Rothbart, M. K., & Bates, J. E. (2006). Temperament in children's development. In W. Damon, R. Lerner, & N. Eisenberg (Eds.), *Handbook of child psychology* (6th ed.): *Vol 3. Social, emotional, and personality development* (pp. 99–166). New York: Wiley.

Rothbart, M. K., & Derryberry, D. (1981). Development of individual differences in temperament. In M. E. Lamb & A. L. Brown (Eds.), *Advances in developmental psychology* (Vol. 1, pp. 37–86). Hillsdale, NJ: Erlbaum.

Rothbart, M. K., & Derryberry, D. (2002). Temperament in children. In C. von Hofsten & L. Backman (Eds.), *Psychology at the turn of the millennium. Vol. 2: Social, developmental, and clinical perspectives* (pp. 17–35). East Sussex, UK: Psychology Press.

Rothbart, M. K., Derryberry, D., & Hershey, K. (2000). Stability of temperament in childhood: Laboratory infant assessment to parent report at seven years. In V. J. Molfese & D. L. Molfese (Eds.), *Temperament and personality development across the life span* (pp. 85–119). Hillsdale, NJ: Erlbaum.

Rothbart, M. K., Derryberry, D., & Posner, M. I. (1994b). A psychobiological approach to the development of temperament. In J. E. Bates & T. D. Wachs (Eds.), *Temperament: Individual differences at the interface of biology and behavior* (pp. 83–116). Washington, DC: American Psychological Association.

Rothbart, M. K., Ellis, L. K., Rueda, M. R., & Posner, M. I. (2003). Developing mechanisms of temperamental effortful control. *Journal of Personality, 71,* 1113–1143.

Rothbart, M. K., & Posner, M. I. (2006). Temperament, attention, and developmental psychopathology. In D. Cicchetti & D. J. Cohen (Eds.), *Developmental psychopathology: Vol. 2. Developmental neuroscience* (2nd ed., pp. 465–501). New York: Wiley.

Rothbart, M. K., & Rueda, M. R. (2005). The development of effortful control. In U. Mayr, E. Awh, & S. W. Keele (Eds.), *Developing individuality in the human brain: A tribute to Michael I. Posner* (pp. 167–188). Washington, DC: American Psychological Association.

Rothbart, M. K., Ziaie, H., & O'Boyle, C. G. (1992). Self-regulation and emotion in infancy. In N. Eisenberg & R. A. Fabes (Eds.), *Emotion and its regulation in early development* (pp. 7–23). San Francisco: Jossey-Bass.

Rueda, M. R., Fan, J., McCandliss, B. D., Halparin, J. D., Gruber, D. B., Lercari, L. P., et al. (2004a). Development of attentional networks in childhood. *Neuropsychologia, 42*(8), 1029–1040.

Rueda, M. R., Posner, M. I., & Rothbart, M. K. (2004b). Attentional control and self-regulation. In R. F. Baumeister & K. D. Vohs (Eds.), *Handbook of self-regulation: Research, theory, and applications* (pp. 283–300). New York: Guilford Press.

Rueda, M. R., Rothbart, M. K., McCandliss, B. D., Saccomanno, L., & Posner, M. I. (2005). Training, maturation, and genetic influences on the development of executive attention. *Proceedings of the National Academy of Sciences, USA, 102*(41), 14931–14936.

Rumbaugh, D. M., & Washburn, D. A. (1995). Attention and memory in relation to learning: A comparative adaptation perspective. In G. R. Lyon & N. A. Krasengor (Eds.), *Attention, memory and executive function* (pp. 199–219). Baltimore: Brookes.

Schaffer, H. R. (1974). Cognitive components of the infant's response to strangeness. In M. Lewis & L. A. Rosenblum (Eds.), *The origins of fear* (pp. 11–24). New York: Wiley.

Schimmack, U. (2005). Attentional interference effects of emotional pictures: Threat, negativity, or arousal? *Emotion, 5,* 55–66.

Sethi, A., Mischel, W., Aber, J. L., Shoda, Y., & Rodriguez, M. L. (2000). The role of strategic attention deployment in development of self-regulation: Predicting preschoolers' delay of gratification from mother-toddler interactions. *Developmental Psychology, 36,* 767–777.

Shoda, Y., Mischel, W., & Peake, P. K. (1990). Predicting adolescent cognitive and self-regulatory competencies from preschool delay of gratification: Identifying diagnostic conditions. *Developmental Psychology, 26,* 978–986.

Stifter, C. A., & Braungart, J. M. (1995). The regulation of negative reactivity in infancy: Function and development. *Developmental Psychology, 31,* 448–455.

Thomas, A., & Chess, S. (1977). *Temperament and development.* New York: Brunner/Mazel.

Wolfe, C. D., & Bell, M. A. (2004). Working memory and inhibitory control in early childhood: Contributions from electrophysiology, temperament, and language. *Developmental Psychobiology, 44,* 68–83.

CHAPTER 17

Individual Differences
in Emotion Regulation

OLIVER P. JOHN
JAMES J. GROSS

Emotions often seem to be forced on us by external events that are outside our control. Take the statement "Talking to Joe makes me so sad!" The speaker indicates that it is Joe who causes her sadness and implies that there is not much she can do about it. Contrary to this intuition, however, people actually exercise considerable influence over the emotions they have. Many different strategies may be used to regulate emotions, and people seem to differ widely in which ones they tend to use. These individual differences in the use of emotion-regulatory strategies are the focus of this chapter.

Our overarching framework is a process model of emotion regulation based on a generally accepted conception of the emotion-generative process (for reviews, see Gross, 1998, 2001; Gross & Thompson, this volume). Briefly put, this conception holds that an emotion begins with an evaluation of emotion cues. When attended to and evaluated in certain ways, emotion cues trigger a coordinated set of response tendencies. Once these response tendencies arise, they may be modulated in various ways. Because emotion unfolds over time, emotion regulation strategies can be differentiated in terms of *when* they have their primary impact on the emotion-generative process. As shown in Figure 17.1, five families of more specific strategies can be located along the timeline of the emotion process (Gross, 1998, 2001).

In particular, *situation selection* refers to avoiding certain people, places, or activities to limit one's exposure to situations likely to generate negative emotion. Once selected, *situation modification* operates to tailor or change a situation to decrease its negative emotional impact. Third, situations have many different aspects, so *attentional deployment* can be used to focus on less negatively valenced aspects of the situation. Once

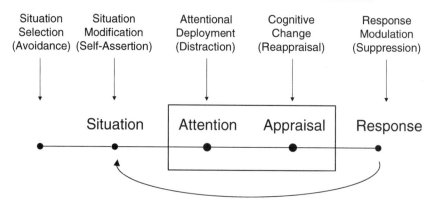

FIGURE 17.1. A process model of emotion regulation. Individual differences in emotion regulation may arise at five points in the emotion-generative process: (1) selection of the situation, (2) modification of the situation, (3) deployment of attention, (4) change of cognitions, and (5) modulation of experiential, behavioral, or physiological responses. Specific instantiations of these five families of regulatory strategies (given in parentheses) may be used for the downregulation of negative emotion, as described in the text.

focused on a particular aspect of the situation, *cognitive change* refers to constructing a more positive meaning out of the many possible meanings that may be attached to that situation. Finally, *response modulation* refers to various kinds of attempts to influence emotion-response tendencies once they already have been elicited. In this chapter, we focus on five particular instances of these strategies that individuals use to achieve the most frequent goal of emotion regulation in everyday life: downregulating (decreasing) emotions that typically have a negative valence, such as anxiety/fear, sadness, and anger (Gross, Richards, & John, 2006). These specific forms of emotion downregulation are indicated in Figure 17.1 in parentheses under each family name.

Our aim in this chapter is to use these five emotion regulation strategies as a conceptual framework to analyze a broad range of constructs selected from three theoretical paradigms: (1) broad personality traits; (2) dynamic approaches including coping styles and adult attachment; and (3) social–cognitive approaches. In trying to achieve this aim, we faced the difficulty that relatively little is known about individual differences in these five specific forms of emotion regulation. For this reason, we have drawn extensively on our own studies (Gross & John, 2003; see also John & Gross, 2004) that have tested whether there are consistent individual differences in the use of reappraisal and suppression and how these naturally occurring individual differences relate to healthy adaptation: the experience of positive and negative emotion, cognition, relationships, and well-being.

These findings, summarized in Figure 17.2, were generally consistent with the temporal assumptions in our process model (see Figure 17.1) and with earlier experimental results. Specifically, we found that reappraisal—which occurs early in the emotion-generative process before emotion-response tendencies have been fully generated—permits the modification of the entire emotional sequence, including the experience of more positive and less negative emotion, without notable physiological, cognitive, or interpersonal costs. By contrast, suppression—which comes relatively late in the emotion-generative process—primarily modifies the behavioral aspect of the emotion-response tendencies, without reducing the experience of negative emotion. Because it comes late in the emotion-generative process, suppression requires the individual to effortfully manage response tendencies as they arise continually, consuming cognitive resources that could otherwise be used for optimal performance in the social contexts in which the emotions arise. Moreover, suppression creates a sense of discrepancy between inner experience and outer expression, leading to negative feelings about the self and alienating the individual from others, impeding the development of emotionally close relationships (John & Gross, 2004).

Because we refer back to these studies throughout this chapter, we note that we measured individual differences in the habitual use of reappraisal and suppression with the Emotion Regulation Questionnaire (ERQ; see Gross & John, 2003, for details). Example items are "I control my emotions *by changing the way I think* about the situation I'm in" for reappraisal, and "I control my emotions *by not expressing them*" for suppression. Note that each of the 10 ERQ items indicates clearly the one emotion-regulatory process it is intended to measure, and nothing else, to avoid any potential confounding by mentioning any positive or negative adjustment consequences. The correlation between the reappraisal and suppression scales was zero in multiple samples, and the two ERQ scales were not related to cognitive ability or social desirability, probably because the items are worded fairly neutrally and do not mention individual differences in adjustment or well-being. More generally, we conceptualize these individual differ-

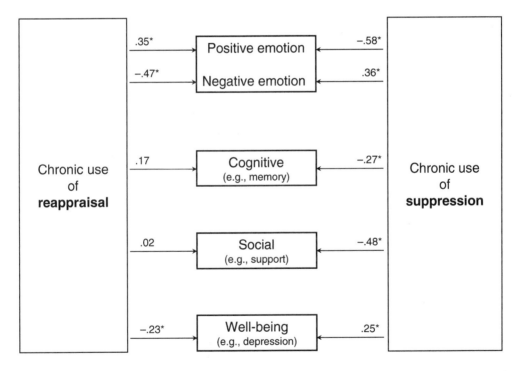

FIGURE 17.2. Summary of previous research (see Gross & John, 2003; John & Gross, 2004) on individual differences in the chronic use of reappraisal and suppression: Differential associations with emotion experience, cognition, relationships, and well-being. Specific correlations in the figure refer to the illustrative variables given in parentheses. For example, use of reappraisal correlated –.23 with depression and use of suppression correlated .25.* $p < .05$.

ences in emotion regulation not as fixed or immutable traits but as socially acquired strategies that are sensitive to individual development, as shown by age-related changes toward a healthier pattern of strategy use from early to middle adulthood (John & Gross, 2004).

For the remaining three emotion regulation strategies, we rely on theoretical argument and careful comparison of the measurement procedures and scales used to operationalize each construct. The conclusions presented here thus reflect our best current (though limited) understandings of constructs and measures; by necessity, they are sometimes speculative. They should therefore be taken not as a definitive roadmap but instead as an initial compilation of where we stand and what needs to be known, a set of ideas and hypotheses that await being put to empirical test. We also wish to emphasize at the outset that we use the five particular kinds of emotion-regulatory strategies in Figure 17.1 as an organizing framework not because we think our model is the only or best one. On the contrary, comparing this model to other constructs in the field will serve to illuminate its limitations and ambiguities. We started with this model because we needed to start somewhere, because even an imperfect model is better than none, and because this model is, in our view, most specifically tied to our core topic—the particular strategies individuals habitually use to regulate their emotions.

LINKS TO GLOBAL PERSONALITY TRAITS

Personality traits are generalized response dispositions that "initiate and guide consistent (equivalent) forms of adaptive and expressive behaviors" (Allport, 1937, p. 295). One should thus expect individual differences in emotion regulation strategies to play an important role in generating the individual differences represented by traits. What traits should we consider here? After decades of research on the "right" number and definition of the most important trait dimensions, the field has converged on a consensual, general taxonomy of personality traits, the "Big Five" personality domains (John, 1990). Rather than replacing all previous systems, this taxonomy serves an integrative function: It can represent the various and diverse systems of personality description within one common framework (John & Srivastava, 1999). It is worth emphasizing that the Big Five are very broad constructs that subsume a wide range of more specific, subordinate constructs, and they are manifested across all response classes, including behavior, emotion, and cognition. They are diverse not only in content but also in terms of underlying processes. We therefore expected each of these broad trait domains to show a particular patterning, or configuration, of associated emotion regulation strategies, rather than any simple one-to-one correspondences between any one trait domain and any one strategy (Table 17.1).

Conscientiousness

Conscientiousness describes *socially prescribed impulse control* that facilitates task- and goal-directed behavior, such as thinking before acting; delaying gratification; following norms and rules; and planning, organizing, and prioritizing tasks (John & Srivastava, 1999). What kinds of emotion-regulation strategies might highly conscientious individuals use? Their characteristic traits (Costa & McCrae, 1992) lead to two straightforward predictions. First, their ability to plan, organize, and think ahead about potential consequences before acting should make it far easier for them to use *situation selection*.

TABLE 17.1. Linking Global Personality Traits to Habitual Use of Emotion Regulation Strategies

Big Five personality trait domains	Five regulation strategies for downregulating negative emotions				
	Situation selection (avoidance)	Situation modification (self-assertion)	Attention deployment (distraction)	Cognitive change (reappraisal)	Response modulation (suppression)
Conscientiousness	+	+	+	0	0
Extraversion	–	+	0	0	–
Neuroticism	(+)	–	–	–	0
Openness	(–)	(+)	+	+	–
Agreeableness	0	–	0	0	(0)

Note. The table entries indicate the sign of the predicted relation between each Big Five personality domain and the habitual use of each emotion regulation strategy: "+" indicates a positive relation, "–" a negative relation, and "0" a prediction of no clearly positive or clearly negative relation. For entries shown in parentheses, such as (+), the prediction was not unequivocal and likely depends on other factors or considerations (see text).

Compared to the more impulsive individuals low in Conscientiousness, they should be able to avoid knowingly entering or getting trapped in situations that cause them negative emotions. For example, the highly conscientious college student who knows she will feel bad about not finishing her class paper on time will decline a social invitation before completing the paper. This prediction fits with findings that conscientious individuals tend to have fewer regrets (Cate, 2006)—by carefully choosing situations that are consistent with their goals and plans, they end up doing fewer things they later come to regret.

Highly conscientious individuals should also use *situation modification* more frequently. When they find themselves in a situation that makes them feel negative emotion and they cannot "unselect" that situation, they would seem likely to do something about it—the situation, interaction partner, or behavior eliciting their negative affect. Whereas individuals low in conscientiousness are likely too disorganized to effectively modify the situation, highly conscientious individuals generally have the competence to function effectively in the world.

Our third regulation strategy, *attention deployment*, should also be related to conscientiousness: Being able to focus on a task and deploy attention to goal-relevant features of the environment is one of the defining features of conscientiousness (e.g., self-discipline, deliberation, and order; Costa & McCrae, 1992) and low levels of conscientiousness have been linked to the attentional deficits so common in attention-deficit/hyperactivity disorder (ADHD) (Nigg et al., 2002). Thus, when situation selection and situation modification are not possible, we expect highly conscientious individuals to use attentional skills, such as distracting themselves from an emotionally negative stimulus by switching their attentional focus to another task, goal, or activity.

Everything else being equal, situation selection should be their most preferred chronic regulatory strategy, followed by situation modification, with attentional strategies such as distraction serving only as an option of last resort. Taken together, these three predictions suggest that on average, highly conscientious individuals will encounter fewer emotionally intense situations, and if they do, will more effectively modify them or focus away from them, thus leading lives that are overall less emotional, more balanced and more predictable, with fewer extreme lows (as well as highs). This conclusion is consistent with findings that conscientiousness is the least emotionally charged of the Big Five domains and least correlated with either positive or negative emotion (e.g., Watson & Clark, 1997; Gross & John, 1998; Shiota, Keltner, & John, 2006). Therefore, we predict no correlations with the habitual use of either of the remaining two strategies (see Table 17.1), not because conscientious individuals lack the capacity for reappraisal or suppression but because they should have relatively little need to use these strategies frequently. Using our ERQ Reappraisal and Suppression scales, we have found small, if any, correlations with conscientiousness (Gross & John, 2003).

Extraversion

Briefly put, extraversion implies an *energetic approach* toward the social and material world and includes traits such as sociability, activity, assertiveness, and positive emotionality (John & Srivastava, 1999). Compared to more introverted individuals, extraverts forcefully pursue their goals (including romantic partners), seek out and achieve positions of influence and leadership, and feel free to express both positive and negative emotions (e.g., Anderson, John, Keltner, & Kring, 2001; Gross & John, 1998; see Pervin & John, 2001, for a review). Given their strong behavioral approach orientation (Carver & White, 1994), deliberate situation selection would seem an unlikely emotion regulation strategy for extraverts; they should approach potentially rewarding situations despite any negative emotion-eliciting potential. In contrast, introverts should try to avoid or withdraw from such situations, as indicated by the negative sign for this link in Table 17.1.

For situation modification, the predicted link in Table 17.1 is positive, whereas for the response modulation strategy of suppression it is negative: extraverts should exert their energy, social skill, and emotion–expressive effort to positively change the situation whereas introverts will be more withdrawn and hold in their feelings and hide them from being observed by others. These predictions are consistent with findings that extraverts are much more likely than introverts to express their emotions, both positive and negative (e.g., Gross & John, 1998), even though in terms of emotion *experience* they differ from introverts only in terms of positive emotion experience (Watson & Clark, 1997; Gross, Sutton, & Kettelar, 1998). More recently, we found that measures of extraversion correlated negatively with ERQ Suppression (Gross & John, 2003).

Table 17.1 indicates no clear predictions for the habitual use of either distraction or reappraisal. Highly extraverted individuals might use physical and other energizing activities (e.g., exercise) to distract themselves from negative emotions in those rare situations when all paths toward active situation modification are blocked, but that would seem a matter of last resort, not a frequent choice. The zero-relation entry in Table 17.1 reflects the nonsignificant correlation we found for extraversion and our ERQ Reappraisal scale.

Neuroticism

Neuroticism contrasts emotional stability and even-temperedness with *negative emotionality*, such as feeling anxious, nervous, sad, and tense. Overall, we expected neuroticism to relate negatively to most of the emotion regulation strategies—that is, everything else being equal, individuals high in neuroticism would make fewer, and less effective, attempts at emotion regulation. In part, this hypothesis derives from the beliefs and attitudes highly neurotic individuals hold regarding emotions: They are less likely to believe that people can change their emotions and more likely to report that their own emotions are very strong and difficult to control (Gross & John, 1998). In turn, this pessimistic assessment of their emotion-regulatory prospects should make it less likely that they will engage in frequent attempts to use any of the regulatory strategies, suggesting a general failure to even attempt regulatory efforts.

For situation modification, for example, we clearly predict a negative link, as individuals high in neuroticism will lack the self-esteem and confidence to assert their needs and enforce specific changes in the situation. Similarly, given their intense negative emotions, highly neurotic individuals are unlikely to have at their disposal the attentional resources needed to effectively distract themselves; on the contrary, research suggests that anxious and depressed individuals ruminate about their negative emotions and thus inadvertently upregulate their negative emotion states (e.g., Nolen-Hoeksema, Parker, & Larson, 1994). For reappraisal, we indeed found a negative correlation with neuroticism (Gross & John, 2003).

Predictions about the link with situation selection are interesting because they illustrate an important complexity. Aware of their predisposition to experience negative emotion, highly neurotic individuals would likely be concerned about negative emotion-eliciting situations and prefer to avoid them, leading us to predict a positive relation. However, in Table 17.1 this prediction appears in parentheses because their concern and worry may not translate into effective action: Highly neurotic individuals may not have the confidence and self-efficacy needed to plan and prepare to effectively avoid negative-emotion contexts. In summary, the pattern of predictions in Table 17.1 suggests that individuals high in neuroticism are likely to fail at downregulating their substantial negative emotion, at least in part because, we suggest, they do not even try to use potentially effective strategies.

Openness to Experience

Openness to Experience (vs. closed-mindedness) is the most cognitive of the Big Five domains and describes the breadth, depth, originality, and complexity of an individual's *mental and experiential life*. In terms of emotion processes, Openness has been shown to relate to aesthetic emotions, such as interest and awe (Shiota et al., 2006), as well as to greater awareness, clarity, and intensity of whatever emotion the individual is feeling at the time (i.e., openness to feelings; cf. Costa & McCrae, 1992; also Buss, 1980).

Which strategies would open individuals use to regulate their emotions? Being open to their own feelings, they accept their emotions as real, important, and generally worth attention and regulation and should thus feel optimistic about the prospect of regulating their emotions. Given their cognitive complexity and imagination, attentional and cognitive-change strategies should be most accessible to them, as shown in Table 17.1. Our ERQ data provided some support for the positive link with reappraisal (Gross & John, 2003), though the size of that correlation was not as large as we expected. We also found some empirical support for the predicted negative relation to suppression (i.e., open individuals value both the reality of their emotions and their behavioral autonomy).

General predictions were hardest to make for situation selection and modification because they seem to depend on the nature of the situation. Consider situation selection: Open individuals are interested in novel and stimulating situations and seem unlikely to avoid an interesting situation just because it has the potential for negative emotion (see also Carstensen & Charles, 1998). In short, Openness is likely to interact with specific situation characteristics in determining the use of these regulatory strategies.

Agreeableness

Agreeableness refers to interpersonal features of personality, contrasting a *prosocial and communal orientation* toward others with mistrust, selfishness, and antagonism and includes traits such as altruism, tender-mindedness, trust, and modesty. As shown in Table 17.1, few general predictions could be made for agreeableness, suggesting that individual differences in the habitual use of emotion regulation were least central to this Big Five domain. We can make one general prediction, namely, regarding situation modification, because highly agreeable individuals are more concerned with others than with the assertion of their self-interest (e.g., altruism and modesty) and do not value having power (Roccas, Sagiv, Schwartz, & Knafo, 2002); thus, we suggest, highly agreeable individuals will forgo forceful attempts to modify the situation to regulate their emotions.

No general predictions can be made for the other regulatory strategies in Figure 17.1 because most effects for agreeableness will depend on the specific interpersonal features of the situation in which regulatory efforts take place. Consider situation selection: To predict whether highly agreeable individuals would seek out or avoid a particular situation, we need to know their attitudes and feelings about the other individuals in the situation. For example, if another person is distressed and in clear need of help, highly agreeable individuals would likely offer assistance, even though helping may expose them to negative emotion themselves. In short, whether highly agreeable individuals use a particular regulation strategy will likely depend on social, rather than emotional, features of the situation.

Indeed, in our ERQ data, Agreeableness was not related to either the Reappraisal or the Suppression scale (Gross & John, 2003). However, despite this lack of overall effects, there may be some important emotion-specific (and context-specific) effects. For example, highly agreeable individuals may be more likely to use suppression to regulate feelings of anger and contempt within a close relationship to avoid confrontations and retain interpersonal harmony. We return to the issue of emotion and context-specific regulation efforts at the end of this chapter.

LINKS TO DYNAMIC APPROACHES

Psychodynamic concepts and ideas remain an active force in work on emotion regulation, in such diverse areas as affect (see Westen & Blagov, this volume), self-esteem (see Baumeister, Geyer, & Tice, this volume), and close relationships (see Shaver & Mikulincer, this volume), but, most important, they provided the starting point for the now vast literature on stress and coping.

Stress and Coping

Researchers interested in stress have conducted extensive research on individual differences in coping styles—the ways individuals attempt to deal with adversity (e.g., Carver & Scheier, 1994; Lazarus & Folkman, 1984; Zeidner & Endler, 1996). In their pioneering work, Folkman and Lazarus (e.g., 1985) emphasized two major functions of coping, namely, "the regulation of distressing emotions and doing something to change for the better the problem causing the distress" (p. 152). This emphasis on regulatory efforts focused on the external problems facing the individual (e.g., a final exam) shows that in some ways the concerns of coping research are broader than those of emotion regulation research (e.g., coping also includes processes such as analyzing the problem in order to understand it better). At the same time, the domain of coping is defined more narrowly because it is limited, by definition, to stressful situations—that is, how the individual deals with potential or actual harms, losses, or threats and with the strong and immediate negative reactions these events arouse in the individual. Thus, the goals, scope, and focus of research on coping and on emotion regulation overlap only partially.

There are also some methodological differences. Much coping research has examined individual differences within the context of a specific stressful encounter and focused on the individual's behavioral and cognitive responses to the stressor. This emphasis on what individuals actually do or try to do in a specific context (as reported on questionnaires or in interviews) contrasts with the global-trait approach discussed earlier which emphasizes what individuals usually do or would typically do.

What, then, are the major dimensions of coping in which individuals differ from each other? Folkman and Lazarus (e.g., 1985, 1988) reasoned that multiple ways of coping could be distinguished but, lacking an established theoretical framework, concluded that they would have to set out to discover the major dimensions of coping empirically. They assembled 68 items they intended to capture a wide variety of behavioral and cognitive coping responses, representing the things people commonly do when they are dealing with stress. Some of these items were inspired by previous theory and literature, including that on defense mechanisms (e.g., wishful thinking, denial), whereas others were added later at the suggestion of subjects in their studies (e.g., prayer). Exploratory factor analyses and rational item selection led initially to six and eventually eight scales assumed to measure distinct ways of coping: *Confrontive, Distancing, Self-Controlling, Seeking Social Support, Accepting Responsibility, Escape-Avoidance, Planful Problem Solving,* and *Positive Reappraisal* (Folkman & Lazarus, 1988), and these eight Ways of Coping quickly became "the most commonly used measure of basic coping responses" (Parker, Endler, & Bagby, 1993, p. 361).

The last of these scales, initially labeled "Emphasizing the Positive" (Folkman & Lazarus, 1985), is of particular interest here, as its name implies a link to the family of emotion regulation strategies we have here called cognitive change (see Figure 17.1), especially to the cognitive reappraisal strategy. Consider the seven items on Folkman and Lazarus's (1988) Positive Reappraisal scale: 20. I was inspired to do something creative; 23. I changed or grew as a person in a good way; 30. I came out of the experience better than I went in; 36. I found new faith; 38. I rediscovered what is important in life; 56. I changed something about myself; and 60. I prayed. While these items indeed describe a person who emphasizes particular positive aspects of a stressful experience, these items serve to illustrate some important differences between their and our approaches. Most of these items do not directly address emotion-regulatory processes, as we have defined them, and certainly do not assess the particular process of changing the meaning or appraisal of an emotion-eliciting event. Instead, these items describe diverse, though generally positive, consequences arising from or after the stressful experience (e.g., I came out of the experience better than I went in), including personal growth, self-transformation, greater creativity, and even spiritual renewal.

This complex item content poses serious issues for research on the correlates and adaptational consequences of using a particular emotion-regulatory strategy. As Lazarus (2000) explained, "The danger of confounding is that measures of coping could contain some of the same variables—for example, distress or psychopathology—as the outcome measure of mental health. Thus, if the antecedent and consequent measures are essentially the same, any correlation between them would represent some degree of tautology" (p. 666). This point underscores the importance of focusing item content specifically on the regulatory process of interest. Indeed, among the items listed earlier, only one (I prayed) would seem to capture a potential emotion-regulatory effort. Yet, the meaning of this item is vague vis-à-vis the particular strategy used: Individuals may indeed pray in order to gain a new perspective or understanding of an emotion-eliciting event, but they may also pray to distract themselves, to share their feelings with a greater power (low suppression), or even to gain the inner strength to modify the situation (see Table 17.2).

Currently, the most commonly used coping measure is the COPE, developed by Carver, Scheier, and Weintraub (1989), which includes 13 short and internally consistent scales measuring coping styles, plus a single item on alcohol/drug use.[1] As shown in Table 17.2, we expected several of the coping styles measured by the COPE scales to show conceptual links to our emotion regulation strategies (the remaining five COPE scales seem to fall largely outside the scope of the emotion regulatory domain).

TABLE 17.2. Linking Dynamic Constructs to Habitual Use of Emotion Regulation Strategies

Dynamic constructs: coping styles and attachment	Five regulation strategies for downregulating negative emotions				
	Situation selection (avoidance)	Situation modification (self-assertion)	Attention deployment (distraction)	Cognitive change (reappraisal)	Response modulation (suppression)
Coping styles (COPE)					
Planning	+	+	(−)	0	0
Active coping	+	+	−	0	0
Seeking social support					
Emotional	0	0	−	0	−
Instrumental	0	0	−	0	−
Positive reinterpretation and growth	0	0	0	+	0
Turning to religion	(+)	0	(+)	(+)	(−)
Focus on and venting of emotion	0	0	−	0	−
Mental disengagement	+	0	+	0	0
Attachment					
Avoidance	(+)	(+)	(+)	0	+

Note. The table entries indicate the sign of the predicted relation between each construct (indicated in the first column) and the habitual use of each emotion regulation strategy: "+" indicates a positive relation, "−" a negative relation, and "0" a prediction of no clearly positive or clearly negative relation. For entries shown in parentheses, such as (+), the prediction was not unequivocal and likely depends on other factors or considerations (see text).

Both the *Active Coping* and *Planning* scales measure anticipatory, active coping efforts and should therefore relate to situation selection and to situation modification. The *Positive Reinterpretation and Growth* scale should relate primarily to cognitive change, especially reappraisal (and to longer-term consequences and adaptations the individual might make later, following the stressful experience). Specifically, the Positive Reinterpretation and Growth scale involves looking for the silver lining in stressful situations and trying to learn from difficult experiences; this scale also measures generally optimistic appraisals and particular longer-term consequences and adaptations the individual might make much later, following the stressful experience, such as learning from experience. Gross and John (2003) found that, as expected, ERQ Reappraisal was correlated with this COPE scale, but its inclusion of long-term consequences that have little to do with the immediate coping or regulatory response makes the scale unnecessarily complex. Indeed, Carver at al. (1989) found that the two explicit growth items had low loadings on this factor (.23 and .19) in one study; in their other study (recollections of coping during a stressful event) this factor broke apart into two separate factors.

Similarly, *Focus on and Venting of Emotions* involves being aware of one's upset and distress and "letting it out." Our analysis suggests that the Focus on and Venting of Emotions scale in the COPE is heterogeneous from an emotion-regulatory perspective: Items such as "I get upset, and am really aware of it" are conceptually related to what we call attention deployment (focusing on the emotion is the conceptual opposite of distraction), whereas items such as "I feel a lot of emotional distress and I find myself expressing those feelings a lot" combines elements of both attention–awareness and expression (i.e., low suppression efforts). Interestingly, Carver et al. assumed that this is a dysfunctional coping style but found its empirical correlates to be complex; for example, Focus/Venting correlated in one study with the functional coping style of social support seeking. In our model, the low-suppression aspect of Focus/Venting scale should be psychologically advantageous whereas its attention deployment aspect (low distraction) should be disadvantageous. Why would seeking social support for emotional reasons correlate with the Focus/Venting scale? Because, we suggest (see Table 17.2), both involve aspects of response modulation linked to low suppression, such as expression and sharing, which we hypothesize to be generally positive emotion-regulatory strategies.

As with the Focus on and Venting of Emotions scale, the two *Seeking Social Support* scales should relate to *less* use of both distraction (i.e., focusing away from one's emotions) and emotional suppression. After all, talking to another person about one's problems requires some sharing and expression of one's feelings (low suppression) and will serve to focus the individual on these emotions rather than distract from them. In contrast, the *Mental Disengagement* scale (coping by turning to work; going to the movies) should relate most to distraction. However, as Carver et al. (1989) noted, these items form a somewhat loose set of diverse activities; moreover, the inclusion of items about sleep and daydreaming suggests a potential link to situation selection because these activities can be performed for reasons other than distraction (e.g., avoiding the stressful situation). The single item on *Drug and Alcohol Use* "in order to think about it less" might also be related to distraction.

As we noted previously in our earlier discussion of using prayer, the *Turning to Religion* scale could serve several of our strategies, as shown in Table 17.2; it will be interesting to study it further to understand the emotion-regulatory processes that may mediate the often positive effects of religiosity on well-being (e.g., having a safe place for expression by sharing feelings with God; or reappraisal, or distraction).

Adult Romantic Attachment

Attachment theory (e.g., Bowlby, 1969/1982; Cassidy & Kobak, 1988) predicts an important link between attachment working models and the use of particular emotion regulation strategies, suggesting that attachment styles originate from the child's need to regulate the anxiety emerging from early relationship patterns with the caregiver. In particular, if the caregiver is consistently unavailable, the child will learn to expect nonresponsive caregiving from others and develop an attachment style that promotes a detachment from, and devaluation of, close attachment figures. This avoidant attachment pattern permits downregulation of the otherwise overwhelming negative affect the child would feel when the caregiver is (again) not available to meet the child's needs; behaviorally, this attachment pattern promotes early independence and self-reliance, an adaptive response given the child's early rearing environment.

In adulthood, the *avoidant attachment pattern* is manifested in feeling uncomfortable with, and actively avoiding, emotionally close relationships; an example item used to assess attachment avoidance in adult romantic relationships is "I get uncomfortable when a romantic partner wants to be very close" (Brennan, Clark, & Shaver, 1998). How do these theoretical considerations relate to the five kinds of emotion regulation strategies in Figure 17.1?

One clear prediction is a link to response-modulation strategies such as suppression: When faced with an emotional situation they cannot avoid or escape, avoidantly attached individuals should be more likely to try to regulate their emotion via expressive suppression than nonavoidant individuals. That is, they would try to not share their emotions with others and to keep their emotions from showing in their expressive behavior. Consistent with this prediction, Gross and John (2003) found the ERQ Suppression scale correlated positively and substantially with two different measures of attachment avoidance. Moreover, individuals chronically using suppression to regulate their emotions felt they had less social support available to them, and their peers agreed that they had less emotionally close relationships, both findings consistent with our analysis of the use of suppression in avoidant attachment.

A second prediction is a link with situation selection. Individuals with an avoidant attachment pattern should be less likely to seek out closeness and comfort from others than less avoidant individuals, especially in stressful or emotionally charged situations. Studies of proximity and social-support seeking (Simpson, Rholes, & Nelligan, 1992; also Fraley, Garner, & Shaver, 2000) have provided evidence for the use of such situation-selection strategies by avoidant individuals. Of course, seeking social support, as noted above in the discussion of that coping strategy in the COPE, involves the anticipation of sharing one's emotion (or distress), something we have just suggested the avoidantly attached individual wants to avoid. More broadly, then, this proposed link with situation selection would seem to apply only to a limited range of situations—avoidantly attached individuals should avoid only those kinds of situations that bring with them social expectations or pressure to share and express their emotions.

A more general point is that attachment theory is focused on one particular domain, behavior in close relationships, and thus addresses emotion regulation only in that domain. Thus, we would expect the first three strategies in our model to be important for avoidant individuals only if the emotion to be regulated is interpersonal in origin or direction. From that follows, clearly, the suppression link explicated previously, as well as more contextually narrow versions of situation selection (e.g., avoiding interpersonal situations that may generate the expression of strong feelings about others and breaking up with a partner who wants to be close), situation modification (e.g., changing the subject in a "relationship-defining" discussion with one's partner), and distraction (e.g., reading a book instead of discussing one's feelings). Finally, reappraisal seems least relevant because it does not involve avoidance of the emotion-eliciting stimulus but a cognitive–transformational effort—to psychologically change the stimulus into something else, rather than simply avoid it (situation selection), remove it (situation modification), or ignore it (distraction). This view is consistent with our findings that ERQ Reappraisal did not correlate with several measures of avoidant attachment or with several measures of social support (Gross & John, 2003).

LINKS TO SOCIAL–COGNITIVE CONSTRUCTS

Social–cognitive theories of personality (Bandura, 1999; Cantor & Zirkel, 1990; Mischel & Shoda, 1999) emphasize that the person is a conscious agent actively construing, and interacting with, the world. They also emphasize that most behavior is learned and needs to be understood with reference to the current goals, concerns, and expectations of the individual as well as the particular social and cultural context. Social–cognitive theories have paid considerable attention to individual differences in the social and cognitive processes that are involved in domains broadly defined as self-control and self-regulation. Although self-control is defined more broadly than the emotion-regulatory processes that are the focus of the present chapter, one would nonetheless expect similarities in the individual-difference constructs considered in the two fields. Social–cognitive theories (Mischel, 1973; Mischel & Shoda, 1999) often highlight individual differences in particular conceptual units, and we focus on three here: outcome expectancies (Optimism), cognitive processes that accompany mood experiences (Meta-Mood constructs), and beliefs (implicit theories about people's ability to change their feelings).

Optimism and Pessimism: Generalized Expectations for Success and Failure

Scheier and Carver's (1985) work on optimism (see Carver & Scheier, 1999, for a review), and their control-theory approach more generally, emphasizes the importance of expectations for coping and for self-regulation more generally: When people expect to succeed, they keep trying and make an even greater effort; when people believe they cannot reach their goal, they withdraw effort or give up completely. This fundamental psychological principle is central to a broad range of theories that, following Rotter (1966), are referred to as expectancy-value theories.

Individual-difference theories built around expectations as the core construct usually postulate that the individual holds some sort of *generalized* expectations, such as Rotter's (1966) concept of internal and external locus control, defined as individual differences in expectations about whether events are under the individual's personal (internal) control (Peterson & Park, this volume).

Scheier and Carver (1985) focused on generalized outcome expectancies and operationalized individual differences in optimism versus pessimism in terms of positive (success) expectancies versus negative (failure) expectancies. Hewing closely to their conceptual definition in terms of global outcomes and generalized expectations, they developed a questionnaire, called the LOT (Life Orientation Test), using a combined rational and factor-analytic approach. The items include direct but general statements about expectations (e.g., In uncertain times, I usually expect the best); some make use of laypeople's intuition about optimism (I am generally optimistic about the future); and another set assesses what might be called optimistic information processing (e.g., I always look on the bright side of things) but also resembles the notion of construing the meaning of future events in more positive terms, not unlike the emotion regulation strategy we have called cognitive reappraisal.

In a series of studies, Scheier and Carver (1992) have shown that relatively more optimistic individuals use different coping methods than more pessimistic individuals, such as more planning and problem-focused coping when the event was controllable, more positive reframing overall, and more acceptance of the situation when the stressor was not controllable; they would try to see the best in bad situations and, over time, try to learn something from them. In contrast, pessimists were more likely to use denial and to distance themselves from the problem, suggesting that greater optimism was generally correlated with a whole range of more functional, effective coping responses and predicted less psychological distress and better adjustment after a stressful event.

On the basis of this theorizing and research, we predict that Optimism should relate to the use of four of our emotion regulation strategies. The predictions are most straightforward to make for reappraisal (some aspects of which are explicitly mentioned in the optimistic information-processing items), suppression (there is little reason for optimists to hide their feelings from others), and situation modification (which we have previously linked conceptually to active coping and planning). Situation selection may turn out to be related but this prediction is complicated: Optimists (like extraverts) may not worry much about, and spend time anticipating, situations that may lead to negative emotions. For distraction, finally, we have no clear prediction, as previous research and theorizing have not highlighted the use of attentional resources among optimists.

Emotional Intelligence:
Meta-Mood Processes of Attention, Clarity, and Repair

Drawing on their social intelligence framework, Salovey, Mayer, Golman, Turvey, and Palfai (1995) adopted a cognitive perspective to understand the reflective processes that accompany many mood states. These "meta-mood" processes capture how individuals reflect on their feelings, including how they monitor, evaluate, and regulate them (Mayer & Gaschke, 1988). Salovey et al. (1995) assumed that emotions serve as an important source of information for the individual, and that individuals differ in how skilled they are at processing this kind of information. Salovey et al. designed the Trait Meta-Mood Scales (TMMS) to measure stable and general attitudes about moods and enduring strategies individuals use to deal with mood experiences. The TMMS measures three constructs: people's tendency to attend to their moods and emotions (attention), to discriminate clearly among them (clarity), and to regulate them (repair), each capturing individual differences "fundamental to the self-regulatory domain of emotional intelligence" (Salovey et al., 1995, p. 147).

Given that the TMMS is focused on individual differences in meta-moods—that is, thoughts and attitudes that accompany ongoing mood experiences—we did not expect any links to our regulatory strategies that occur further "upstream" in the emotion process, prior to the onset of an emotional episode itself, such as situation selection or modification. However, attentional processes, cognitive change, and response modification should be of considerable relevance.

The TMMS Attention scale refers to paying close attention to feelings, accepting feelings, valuing them positively, and letting oneself experience them fully and intensively, using items such as "I believe in acting from the heart" versus "I don't think it's worth paying attention to your emotions or moods" (reversed-scored). As shown in Table 17.3, we expected the Attention scale to relate negatively to the chronic use of the emotion regulation strategies of distraction and suppression. The link to distraction is theoretically interesting because paying close attention to negative mood states has been shown to magnify and intensify the experience of negative affect and the risk for depression (Scheier & Carver, 1977); conversely, in our model distraction is expected to decrease negative emotion experience. Indeed, in one of Salovey et al.'s studies, the Attention scale was related to higher depression scores. Regarding the negative link to suppression, being intensely aware of and paying close attention to one's emotions should interfere with the considerable and ongoing cognitive effort required to effectively suppress one's emotions (Richards & Gross, 2000), and that should be especially true for individuals who experience their emotions intensely. Moreover, individuals scoring high on the Attention scale value their feelings and believe in letting them guide their behavior, quite the opposite to individuals habitually using suppression whose expressive behavior is often inconsistent with their inner feelings and who therefore experience themselves as inauthentic (John & Gross, 2004). Indeed, Attention correlated negatively with our ERQ Suppression scale.

The TMMS Clarity scale assesses being aware of and at ease with one's feelings, as contrasted with a deep and troubling confusion about one's feelings and what they mean. True-scored item examples include "I am usually very clear about my feelings" versus false-scored items such as "I can't make sense out of my feelings" and "My beliefs

TABLE 17.3. Linking Social–Cognitive Constructs to Habitual Use of Emotion Regulation Strategies

Social-cognitive constructs	Five regulation strategies for downregulating negative emotions				
	Situation selection (avoidance)	Situation modification (self-assertion)	Attention deployment (distraction)	Cognitive change (reappraisal)	Response modulation (suppression)
Optimism	(+)	+	0	+	−
Meta–mood processes					
Attention	0	0	−	0	−
Clarity	0	0	−	0	−
Repair	0	0	+	+	−
Incremental theory:					
Emotions can be controlled	(+)	+	+	+	0

Note. The table entries indicate the sign of the predicted relation between each social–cognitive construct and the habitual use of each emotion regulation strategy: "+" indicates a positive relation, "−" a negative relation, and "0" a prediction of no clearly positive or clearly negative relation. For entries shown in parentheses, such as (+), the prediction was not unequivocal and likely depends on other factors or considerations (see text).

and opinions seem to change depending how I feel." We expected a positive relation of Clarity with distraction (the ability to use attentional resources to move away from a negative emotion stimulus, rather than ruminating about it). Moreover, we expected a negative relation to suppression. Similar to our reasoning for the Attention scale, individuals who are clear about and comfortable with their emotions should feel little need to suppress their behavioral expression, and we did indeed find evidence for this negative relation (Gross & John, 2003).

The TMMS Repair scale, finally, assesses attempts to improve negative mood by thinking positively and an optimistic (rather than pessimistic) attitude more generally. Item examples include "Although I am sometimes sad, I have a mostly optimistic outlook" and "No matter how badly I feel, I try to think about pleasant things." As shown in Table 17.3, we expected the Repair scale to relate positively to distraction as well as reappraisal: the explicit mood repair efforts included in the scale involve using thought (1) for focusing on something other (e.g., pleasant things or good thoughts) than the distressing stimulus, thus implicating distraction, and also (2) trying to think differently (e.g., more positively) about the situation, thus implicating reappraisal. In contrast, the use of suppression is hardly an optimistic process, as we have described (Gross & John, 2003), and its habitual use reflects the pessimistic expectation that others cannot be trusted to be shown the "real self." Indeed, we found that the Repair scale was related to ERQ Reappraisal and Suppression.

Implicit Theories: Beliefs about People's Ability to Control Their Emotions

In this chapter, we have argued that people can generally regulate their emotions. However, our individual-difference perspective qualifies that general statement by emphasizing that some individuals do so more than others. But what do the "people in the street" think about this issue? That is, what are people's implicit theories about the degree to which emotions are fixed like an "entity" or malleable so that they can be controlled?

Dweck (e.g., 1999) and her colleagues have studied the beliefs people hold about the malleability of personal attributes: Individuals who hold *entity beliefs* view attributes as fixed and impossible to control, whereas individuals who hold *incremental beliefs* view attributes as malleable and controllable. Whereas most research on implicit theories has focused on intelligence, Tamir, John, Srivastava, and Gross (in press) studied beliefs about emotions. They modified items from the Implicit Theories of Intelligence Scale (Dweck, 1999) to refer to general beliefs about the extent to which emotions are malleable and incremental (e.g., "If they want to, people can change the emotions that they have") or fixed and uncontrollable (e.g., "The truth is, people have very little control over their emotions"). Results showed that these beliefs were internally consistent and, as expected, relatively distinct from implicit theories of intelligence; there were substantial individual differences, with only a small majority (about 60%) favoring the belief that emotions are relatively more malleable than fixed.

These general beliefs should importantly influence the individual's emotion-regulatory efforts. One source of influence involves the self and self-efficacy—after all, individuals who believe that emotions are fixed and cannot be changed will likely apply those beliefs to their own emotions as well. If they have no reason to think regulatory efforts will be successful, individuals would have little perceived competence and confidence in this domain (i.e., emotion regulation efficacy) and, in turn, should expend little effort and energy on implementing emotion regulation strategies. In contrast, individuals who believe emotions are not fixed but can be controlled should have high levels of emotion regulation efficacy and, everything else being equal, use the effective regulatory strategies. As indicated in Table 17.3, this prediction should hold in particular for situation modification, distraction, and reappraisal.

According to this model, beliefs about emotion are at the nexus of a cognitive emotional interface by which cognitive belief structures constrain the emotion-regulatory efforts an individual makes and thus the emotions that result. As predicted, Tamir et al. (in press) found that implicit theories of emotion were indeed related to individuals' sense of efficacy in emotion regulation: Individuals who believed emotions are fixed were less likely to believe that they can actually modify their own emotions whereas individuals who believed emotions are malleable were more likely to believe that they possess the ability to control their emotions. Driven by the belief that change is impossible, entity theorists should be less likely to employ antecedent (i.e., anticipatory) strategies of emotion regulation; Tamir et al. found support for this prediction using the ERQ Cognitive Reappraisal scale: individuals who viewed emotion as more malleable were more likely to report actively modifying their emotions by changing their appraisal of emotion-eliciting events. On the other hand, once an emotional response has been set in motion, individuals should be able to use response-modification strategies, such as expressive suppression, in order to conform to social rules. Regardless of whether individuals believe emotion is fixed or malleable, they may be equally likely to mask their feelings in certain situations; indeed, malleable emotion beliefs were not related to the habitual use of suppression on the ERQ.

This leaves us with our predictions for situation selection and modification. Tamir et al. did not have available measures of the habitual use of these two strategies, but several of their findings seem relevant. First, students holding malleable emotion theories showed better emotional and social adjustment during the difficult transition from high school to college: They experienced less negative and more positive emotion, were less lonely, and had increasing levels of social support from their new college friends. These findings suggest, albeit indirectly, that they selected and modified situations in emotionally and socially advantageous ways. However, mediation analyses showed that the beneficial social consequences of malleable emotion theories could not be attributed to emotion-regulatory self-efficacy. That is, the situation selection and modification effects of emotion theories may involve a different causal pathway, such as beliefs and expectations individuals hold about other people's emotion experience and regulation.

CONCLUSIONS AND FUTURE DIRECTIONS

Our analysis of links between five emotion regulatory processes and previous constructs in the individual-difference literature suggests three major conclusions. First, emotion regulation strategies are ubiquitous in trait, dynamic, and social–cognitive traditions, although they are not necessarily explicitly defined as involving emotion regulation. Second, most existing constructs are broad and conceptually complex, consisting of various mixtures (or conglomerations) of several basic processes that are not explicitly differentiated. Third, this conceptual complexity is also reflected in complex scales and measures of individual differences that impede the interpretation of findings and comparisons among seemingly related constructs. But this review has also highlighted limitations in our model, which we now discuss along with broader issues for future research.

Upregulation and Specific Emotion Effects

This chapter has focused on the downregulation of negative emotions, by far the most common target of emotion regulation efforts (Gross et al., 2006) and clearly a central concern in trait, dynamic, and social–cognitive approaches as well, as shown by the considerable number of conceptual links detailed in our review and Tables 17.1–17.3.

However, although this is a reasonable place to start, there is a lot of work ahead. One concern is that the rubric of "negative emotion" is broad and heterogeneous, and downregulation is not the sole purpose of emotion regulation. For example, individuals high in neuroticism show upregulation of negative emotion in some contexts (Tamir, 2005) as do individuals with a preoccupied or anxious–ambivalent attachment style (Cassidy & Kobak, 1988). In addition, individual differences in the up- or downregulation of positive emotions (e.g., pride, love, joy, and amusement) also bear examination. In our own work (Gross & John, 2003), we have found that individuals who habitually use suppression tend to apply that regulatory strategy to both negative and positive emotions. However, we suspect that such generalization of strategy use across broad swathes of negative and positive emotions is more likely the exception than the rule.

More generally, these considerations about differences among negative and positive emotions raise broader issues about general and emotion-specific aspects of individual differences in strategy use. Future research should examine individual differences in the regulation of specific emotions because there may be important strategy-by-emotion interactions, such that particular emotions are more likely to be regulated by particular strategies (e.g., pride not by reappraisal but by suppression) and that individuals differ in how much they regulate particular emotions using particular strategies (e.g., individuals low in Agreeableness may be less likely to suppress pride).

To make matters even more complex, individuals sometimes try to regulate multiple and at times even conflicting emotions, such as simultaneous feelings of pride about one's own achievement and sadness and concern about the failure of a friend, or both joy and guilt about partaking in some "forbidden pleasure." How individuals integrate such complex instances of emotion regulation is of particular interest to dynamic approaches to personality functioning (e.g., Westen & Blagov, this volume) and an interesting avenue for future research.

Effects of Situational and Cultural Contexts

Another limitation of the present approach arises from another simplification, namely, that we have not explicitly considered the effects of specific contexts. In our discussion of the Big Five trait domains, we noted that some predictions can be made only with reference to specific contexts (e.g., individuals high in Openness should not use situation selection when they find the situation intellectually stimulating, and individuals high in Agreeableness may suppress anger in peer but not work contexts); we noted in the dynamic section that predictions for attachment avoidance apply only in close-relationship contexts that activate the attachment system. Similarly, gender and cultural factors will likely play a role, as work on display rules (Ekman, 1972) has suggested; indeed, everything else being equal, we have found that men use suppression more than women, and individuals with ethnic-minority backgrounds use suppression more than mainstream European-Americans do (Gross & John, 2003).

Unfortunately, the problem with situation- and culture-specific theorizing and empiricism is similar to including emotion-specific effects, namely, the enormous increase in the number of cells that would need to be considered in research designs and measurement. In particular, simultaneous study of all 5 regulatory strategies, 2 regulatory purposes (up and down), and just 10 specific (negative and positive) emotions would already yield 100 potential combinations; further crossing those with several central situational or cultural contexts would make the research task not only unwieldy but unfathomable. Our own strategy has thus been to focus in greater depth on fewer (two) regulatory strategies and on downregulation, but that choice of research strategy should not be mistaken to mean that we underestimate the importance of specific emotion and context effects.

Individual Differences in Frequency of Strategy Use and Self-Perceived Capability

This chapter has also focused on one particular aspect of individual differences in emotion regulation, namely, individual differences in the habitual *frequency* of strategy use (i.e., how likely an individual is to use a particular strategy). Again, that would seem a sensible starting place, but it hardly exhausts all aspects of individual differences. For example, in our discussion of Neuroticism we suggested that individuals high on this trait often wish (or even try) to avoid negative emotion-generative situations but fail to do so effectively, in part because they lack the confidence, or *self-perceived capability* (Bandura, 1999), to use this regulatory strategy. As we noted in our discussion of social–cognitive approaches, people's beliefs and expectancies are central determinants of what they will actually attempt to do. Thus, future research should study both frequency of use and self-perceived capability and compare these two aspects of individual differences in emotion regulation in terms of their correlates and consequences for adaptation.

Implications for Well-Being and Psychopathology

Although our emphasis has been on the normal (or healthy) range of individual variation, we have commented on the effectiveness and adaptive value of the use of particular strategies. In our empirical work (see Figure 17.2), habitual use of reappraisal has been associated with generally healthy adjustment outcomes, and habitual use of suppression has been associated with a general pattern of less healthy outcomes, such as disadvantageous emotion experience, lack of social support, and depressive symptoms (Gross & John, 2002; John & Gross, 2004). One important direction for future research is to consider emotion regulation in the context of samples in which there is more variability in both psychological and physical health status. Moreover, future research needs to define more clearly the boundaries of when individuals overuse a generally effective strategy or apply it in unrealistic ways. For example, at what point does reappraisal cease to be sensible and effective and instead turns into a maladjusted strategy, as implied by defense mechanisms such as intellectualization, rationalization, or even denial?

An important distinction here involves the degree to which emotion-regulatory strategies are used in conscious and controlled ways, or in more automatized ways that operate outside conscious control (Bargh & Williams, this volume; Mauss, Evers, Wilhelm, & Gross, 2006). Clearly, although in our empirical work we have assumed that people can generally observe and report on their emotion-regulatory efforts, most of these efforts are likely executed without much attention or conscious awareness. The distinction between such implicit and explicit forms of emotion regulation, and their likely interaction, is a topic of considerable importance for a more complete understanding of emotion regulation and its possible differentiation from dynamic notions of defense mechanisms (see Westen & Blagov, this volume). This distinction is also likely to play a role in understanding the origin and lifespan development of individual differences in emotion regulation, issues that hold great promise for future research.

ACKNOWLEDGMENTS

Preparation of this chapter was supported by Grant Nos. MH58147 and MH43948 from the National Institute of Mental Health, Grant No. RRF 2005-325 from the Retirement Research Foundation, as well as a Faculty Research Grant from the University of California, Berkeley. We are grateful to Joshua Eng and Maya Tamir for their thoughtful comments on an earlier draft.

NOTE

1. Carver et al.'s (1989) factor analyses showed that the COPE scales defined 11 distinct dimensions, with each factor correspondng to only one scale except for two: Active Coping and Planning jointiy defined one factor, and Seeking Social Support for Instrumental Reasons and for Emotional Reasons jointly formed one overall Social Support factor.

REFERENCES

Allport, G. W. (1937). *Personality: A psychological interpretation.* New York: Holt.
Anderson, C., John, O. P., Keltner, D., & Kring, A. (2001). Who attains social status? Effects of personality and physical attractiveness in social groups. *Journal of Personality and Social Psychology, 81,* 116–132.
Bandura, A. (1999). Social cognitive theory of personality. In L. A. Pervin, & O. P. John (Eds.), *Handbook of personality: Theory and research* (2nd ed., pp. 154–196). New York: Guilford Press.
Bargh, J. A., & Williams, L. E. (2007). The nonconscious regulation of emotion. In J. J. Gross (Ed.), *Handbook of emotion regulation* (pp. 429–445). New York: Guilford Press.
Baumeister, R. F., Zell, A. L., & Tice, D. M. (2007). How emotions facilitate and impair self-regulation. In J. J. Gross (Ed.), *Handbook of emotion regulation* (pp. 408–426). New York: Guilford Press.
Bowlby, J. (1982). *Attachment and loss: Vol. 1. Attachment* (2nd ed.). New York: Basic Books. (Original work published 1969)
Brennan, K. A., Clark, C. L., & Shaver, P. R. (1998). Self-report measurement of adult attachment: An integrative overview. In J. A. Simpson & W. S. Rholes (Eds.), *Attachment theory and close relationships* (pp. 46–76). New York: Guilford Press.
Buss, A. H. (1980). *Self-consciousness and social anxiety.* San Francisco: Freeman.
Cantor, N., & Zirkel, S. (1990). Personality, cognition, and purposive behavior. In L. A. Pervin (Ed.), *Handbook of personality: Theory and research* (pp. 135–164). New York: Guilford Press.
Carstensen, L. L., & Charles, S. T. (1998). Emotion in the second half of life. *Current Directions in Psychological Science, 7,* 144–149.
Carver, C. S., & Scheier, M. F. (1994). Situational coping and coping dispositions in a stressful transaction. *Journal of Personality and Social Psychology, 66,* 184–195.
Carver, C. S., & Scheier, M. F. (1999). Stress, coping, and self-regulatory processes. In L. A. Pervin, & O.

P. John (Eds.), *Handbook of personality: Theory and research* (2nd ed., pp. 553–575). New York: Guilford Press.

Carver, C. S., Scheier, M. F., & Weintraub, J. K. (1989). Assessing coping strategies: A theoretically based approach. *Journal of Personality and Social Psychology, 56,* 267–283.

Carver, C. S., & White, T. L. (1994). Behavioral inhibition, behavioral activation, and affective responses to impending reward and punishment: The BIS/BAS scales. *Journal of Personality and Social Psychology, 67,* 319–333.

Cassidy, J., & Kobak, R. R. (1988). Avoidance and its relationship with other defensive processes. In J. Belsky & T. Nezworski (Eds.), *Clinical implications of attachment* (pp. 300–323). Hillsdale, NJ: Erlbaum.

Cate, R. (2006). *Who is going to be sorry? The role of personality in life regrets.* Unpublished doctoral dissertation, Department of Psychology, University of California, Berkeley.

Costa, P. T., & McCrae, R. R. (1992). *NEO PI-R Professional manual.* Odessa, FL: Psychological Assessment Resources.

Dweck, C. S. (1999). *Self-theories: Their role in motivation, personality, and development.* New York: Psychology Press.

Ekman, P. (1972). Universals and cultural differences in facial expression of emotion. In J. Cole (Ed.), *Nebraska symposium on motivation* (pp. 207–283). Lincoln: University of Nebraska Press.

Folkman, S., & Lazarus, R. S. (1985). If it changes it must be a process: Study of emotion and coping during three stages of a college examination. *Journal of Personality and Social Psychology, 48,* 150–170.

Folkman, S., & Lazarus, R. S. (1988). *Manual for the Ways of Coping Questionnaire.* Palo Alto, CA: Consulting Psychology Press.

Fraley, R. C., Garner, J. P., & Shaver, P. R. (2000). Adult attachment and the defensive regulation of attention and memory: Examining the role of preemptive and postemptive defensive processes. *Journal of Personality and Social Psychology, 79,* 816–826.

Gross, J. J. (1998). The emerging field of emotion regulation: An integrative review. *Review of General Psychology, 2,* 271–299.

Gross, J. J. (2001). Emotion regulation in adulthood: Timing is everything. *Current Directions in Psychological Science, 10,* 214–219.

Gross, J. J., & John, O. P. (1998). Mapping the domain of emotional expressivity: Multi-method evidence for a hierarchical model. *Journal of Personality and Social Psychology, 74,* 170–191.

Gross. J. J., & John, O. P. (2002). Wise emotion regulation. In L. Feldman Barrett & P. Salovey (Eds.), *The wisdom of feelings: Psychological processes in emotional intelligence* (pp. 297–318). New York: Guilford Press.

Gross, J. J., & John, O. P. (2003). Individual differences in two emotion regulation processes: Implications for affect, relationships, and well-being. *Journal of Personality and Social Psychology, 85,* 348–362.

Gross, J. J., Richards, J. M., & John, O. P. (2006). Emotion regulation in everyday life. In D. K. Snyder, J. A. Simpson, & J. N. Hughes (Eds.), *Emotion regulation in couples and families: Pathways to dysfunction and health* (pp. 13–35). Washington, DC: American Psychological Association.

Gross, J. J., Sutton, S. K., & Ketelaar, T. V. (1998). Relations between affect and personality: Support for the affect-level and affective-reactivity views. *Personality and Social Psychology Bulletin, 24,* 279–288.

Gross, J. J., & Thompson, R. A. (2007). Emotion regulation: Conceptual foundations. In J. J. Gross (Ed.), *Handbook of emotion regulation* (pp. 3–24). New York: Guilford Press.

John, O. P. (1990). The "Big Five" factor taxonomy: Dimensions of personality in the natural language and in questionnaires. In L. A. Pervin (Ed.), *Handbook of personality: Theory and research* (pp. 66–100). New York: Guilford Press.

John, O. P., & Gross, J. J. (2004). Healthy and unhealthy emotion regulation strategies: Personality processes, individual differences, and life-span development. *Journal of Personality, 72,* 1301–1333.

John, O. P., & Srivastava, S. (1999). The Big Five trait taxonomy: History, measurement, and theoretical perspectives. In L. A. Pervin & O. P. John (Eds.), *Handbook of personality: Theory and research* (2nd ed., pp. 102–138). New York: Guilford Press.

Lazarus, R. S. (2000). Toward better research on stress and coping. *American Psychologist, 55,* 665–673.

Lazarus, R. S., & Folkman, S. (1984). *Stress, appraisal and coping.* New York: Springer.

Mauss, I. B., Evers, C., Wilhelm, F. H., & Gross, J. J. (2006). How to bite your tongue without blowing your top: Implicit evaluation of emotion regulation predicts affective responding to anger provocation. *Personality and Social Psychology Bulletin, 32,* 589–602.

Mayer, J. D., & Gaschke, Y. N. (1988). The experience and meta-experience of mood. *Journal of Personality and Social Psychology, 55,* 102–111.

Mischel, W. (1973). Toward a cognitive social learning reconceptualization of personality. *Psychological Review, 80,* 252–283.

Mischel, W., & Shoda, Y. (1999). Integrating dispositions and processing dynamics within a unified theory of personality: The cognitive–affective personality system. In L. A. Pervin, & O. P. John (Eds.), *Handbook of personality: Theory and research* (2nd ed., pp. 197–218). New York: Guilford Press.

Nigg, J. T., John, O. P., Blaskey, L., Huang-Pollock, C., Willcutt, E. G., Hinshaw, S. P., et al. (2002). Big Five dimensions and ADHD symptoms: Links between personality traits and clinical symptoms. *Journal of Personality and Social Psychology, 83,* 451–469.

Nolen-Hoeksema, S., Parker, L. E., & Larson, J. (1994). Ruminative coping with depressed mood following loss. *Journal of Personality and Social Psychology, 67,* 92–104.

Parker, J. D. A., Endler, N. S., & Bagby, R. M. (1993). If it changes, it might be unstable: Examining the factor structure of the ways of coping questionnaire. *Psychological Assessment, 5,* 361–368.

Pervin, L. A., & John, O. P. (2001). *Personality: Theory and research* (8th ed.). New York: Wiley.

Peterson, C., & Park, N. (2007). Explanatory style and emotion regulation. In J. J. Gross (Ed.), *Handbook of emotion regulation* (pp. 159–179). New York: Guilford Press.

Richards, J. M., & Gross, J. J. (2000). Emotion regulation and memory: The cognitive costs of keeping one's cool. *Journal of Personality and Social Psychology, 79,* 410–424.

Roccas, S., Sagiv, L., Schwartz, S., & Knafo, A. (2002). The Big Five personality factors and personal values. *Personality and Social Psychology Bulletin, 28,* 789–801.

Rotter, J. B. (1966). Generalized expectancies for internal versus external control of reinforcement. *Psychological Monographs, 80*(1, Whole No. 609).

Salovey, P., Mayer, J. D., Golman, S. L., Turvey, C., & Palfai, T. P. (1995). Emotional attention, clarity, and repair: Exploring emotional intelligence using the trait meta-mood scale. In J. W. Pennebaker (Ed.), *Emotion, disclosure, and health* (pp. 125–154). Washington, DC: American Psychological Association.

Scheier, M. F., & Carver, C. S. (1977). Self-focused attention and the experience of emotion: Attraction, repulsion, elation, and depression. *Journal of Personality and Social Psychology, 35,* 625–636

Scheier, M. F., & Carver, C. S. (1985). Optimism, coping and health: Assessment and implications of generalized outcome expectancies. *Health Psychology, 4,* 219–247.

Scheier, M. F., & Carver, C. S. (1992). Effects of optimism on psychological and physical well-being: Theoretical overview and empirical update. *Cognitive Therapy and Research, 16,* 201–228.

Shaver, P. R., & Mikulincer, M. (2007). Adult attachment strategies and the regulation of emotion. In J. J. Gross (Ed.), *Handbook of emotion regulation* (pp. 446–465). New York: Guilford Press.

Shiota, L., Keltner, D., & John, O. P. (2006). Positive emotion dispositions differentially associated with Big Five personality and attachment style. *Journal of Positive Psychology, 1,* 61–76.

Simpson, J. A., Rholes, W. S., & Nelligan, J. S. (1992). Support seeking and support giving within couples in an anxiety-provoking situation: The role of attachment styles. *Journal of Personality and Social Psychology, 62,* 434–446.

Tamir, M. (2005). Don't worry, be happy? Neuroticism, trait-consistent affect regulation, and performance. *Journal of Personality and Social Psychology, 89,* 449–461.

Tamir, M., John, O. P., Srivastava, S., & Gross, J. J. (in press). Implicit theories of emotion: Affective and social outcomes across a major life transition. *Journal of Personality and Social Psychology.*

Watson, D., & Clark, L. A. (1997). Extraversion and its positive emotional core. In R. Hogan, J. Johnson, & S. Briggs (Eds.), *Handbook of personality psychology* (pp. 767–793). New York: Academic Press.

Westen, D., & Blagov, P. S. (2007). A clinical–empirical model of emotion regulation: From defense and motivated reasoning to emotional constraint satisfaction. In J. J. Gross (Ed.), *Handbook of emotion regulation* (pp. 373–392). New York: Guilford Press.

Zeidner, M., & Endler, N. S. (Eds.). (1996). *Handbook of coping: Theory, research, applications.* New York: Wiley.

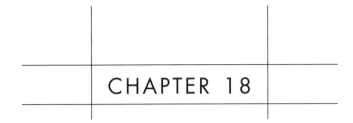

CHAPTER 18

A Clinical–Empirical Model of Emotion Regulation

FROM DEFENSE AND MOTIVATED REASONING TO EMOTIONAL CONSTRAINT SATISFACTION

DREW WESTEN
PAVEL S. BLAGOV

Although the systematic study of emotion regulation is a relatively recent development, one could make a case that much of psychology has long been about emotion regulation. People regulate their emotions through explicit problem solving (which is always directed toward eliminating an aversive state of affairs or creating a more positive one) and explicit coping (e.g., telling oneself "it will be all right"). They also regulate feeling states (including emotions as well as pleasant and unpleasant sensations) through operant conditioning, by which humans and other animals are implicitly drawn toward and away from stimuli that elicit positive and negative feeling states; and via other implicit procedures designed to protect people from negative affect (e.g., denial in the face of an ominous growth on the skin) or elicit positive affect (e.g., focusing on aspects of identity that emphasize our strengths and deemphasize our weaknesses).

Theoretically, researchers could classify emotion regulation strategies in multiple ways, for example, by where in the process of emotional arousal and interpretation they are employed (Gross, this volume), or by the emotions that tend to elicit them (Westen, 1994). One way of doing so of particular relevance from a clinical standpoint is to array these strategies along two axes, defined by the extent to which they are *adaptive* (whether their consequences are ultimately positive, negative, or mixed for the individual and others) and the extent to which they are *conscious* (whether they are largely explicit, and hence involve effortful control, or implicit, and hence are largely inaccessible to consciousness). As illustrated in Figure 18.1, emotion regulation strategies can be

	Explicit	**Implicit**
	I.	II.
Adaptive	Adaptive coping strategies (e.g., reframing) and conscious decision making (e.g., weighing options and their likely emotional consequences)	Adaptive operant conditioning (e.g., reinforcement of prosocial behavior) and relatively "benign" defensive processes (e.g., defensive humor)
Maladaptive	Maladaptive coping strategies (e.g., suppression and rumination) and conscious decision making (e.g., obsessive focus on details)	Maladaptive operant conditioning (e.g., social avoidance) and defensive processes (e.g., externalizing causes of consequences of behavior onto others)
	III.	IV.

FIGURE 18.1. Two axes for classifying emotion regulation strategies (adaptive vs. maladaptive, explicit vs. implicit)

adaptive and explicit (Quadrant I), such as cognitively reframing a negative event when there is no way to change it (see, Gross, 1998); adaptive and implicit (Quadrant II), such as moderate self-serving biases that allow most of us to look in the mirror without needing to smash it; maladaptive and explicit (Quadrant III), such as rumination; or maladaptive and implicit (Quadrant IV), such as narcissistic self-aggrandizement in the face of threatening information about the self.

In this chapter we describe a clinical–empirical model of emotion regulation that defines emotion regulation as the explicit and implicit (conscious and unconscious) procedures people use to try to maximize pleasant and minimize unpleasant feelings, emotions, and moods (Westen, 1985, 1994). We describe the model as clinical–empirical because it emerged from both clinical observation and theory (Bowlby, 1969; A. Freud, 1936; S. Freud, 1933; Sandler, 1987) and from research, much of which was not originally conceptualized in terms of affect regulation (e.g., on obedience to authority or self-serving biases in social psychology) (for a review, see Westen, 1994). (Throughout this chapter we use the terms "emotion" and "affect" as synonyms; hence, we use the terms "emotion regulation" and "affect regulation" as synonyms.) The model was first elaborated in the mid 1980s (Westen, 1985) and has evolved along with advances in a number of domains of psychology (Westen, 1994, 1998a, 1998b, 1999, in press; Westen, Muderrisoglu, Shadler, Fowler, & Koren, 1997; Westen, Weinberger, & Bradley, in press). The model suggests that emotions are evolved response tendencies that reinforce behavioral and mental processes that are pleasurable and select against those that are aversive. This generally leads to adaptive behavior but can also lead to maladaptation, depending on learning environment, temperament, and their interactions (see Westen, 1998a). From this point of view, operant conditioning, psychological defense, and motivated reasoning can be understood as forms of implicit emotion regulation, whereas coping and decision making can be understood as forms explicit emotion regulation.

In this chapter we briefly consider in turn the evolutionary, behavioral, psychodynamic, and cognitive components of this approach to emotion regulation. We then examine the most recent version of the model, which draws on connectionist–inspired models in cognitive science. We argue that much of thought and behavior reflects an equilibration process by which the brain responds simultaneously to *cognitive constraints* that maximize goodness of fit to the data and *emotional constraints* that maximize positive affect and minimize negative affect (and hence "goodness of fit" to emotional pulls).

EVOLUTION AND THE SELECTIVE RETENTION OF ADAPTIVE BEHAVIOR

From an evolutionary perspective, emotions serve an adaptive function by channeling behavior in directions that maximize survival, reproduction, and care for kin and reciprocally altruistic others (see also Plutchik, 2003; Tomkins, 1981). In other words, emotions serve a signaling function that impels humans and other animals to act to regulate (augment or eliminate) them, simultaneously regulating behavior in ways that generally foster adaptation. Affects lead people away from dangerous situations, reinforce sexual behavior, lead them to protect their offspring, guide their choice of mates, and guide their actions with others with whom they have regular social relations, such as friends and coalition partners (e.g., outrage at betrayal, leading to breaking off ties, confronting, etc.). In some cases the adaptive function of emotions (and pleasant or unpleasant sensory states that serve similar functions) is relatively obvious, as when organisms learn to avoid foods previously associated with nausea (Garcia & Koelling, 1966). In other cases, the role of emotion may be less intuitively obvious, as when emotions guide attitudes toward protection of kin of differing degrees of relatedness or differential male and female reproductive strategies, such as sexual jealousy (Buss, Larsen, Westen, & Semmelroth, 1992; Westen, 1985).

From an evolutionary standpoint, variation in the intensity, valence, and specific emotion experienced should all be important in regulating behavior by virtue of motivated efforts at regulating emotion. Intensity of emotion, particularly negative emotion, prioritizes response tendencies at any given moment (an emotional analog, in some respects, to Maslow's [1970] concept of a hierarchy of needs). Valence (positive or negative) leads to approach or avoidance (or, in other cases, fight/flight) (Carver, 2001; Gray, 1990, 2001; Gray, Braiver, & Raichle, 2002). The specific emotion or feeling-state experienced is also important in channeling behavior. For example, self-conscious emotions such as shame and guilt may temper momentary self-interest with the more distal effect of maximizing reciprocal altruism in a broader social context.

Although emotional responses can be seen as a "compass" that leads people toward and away from stimuli or actions that are valuable or threatening, evolved affective mechanisms are also implicated in multiple forms of maladaptation. For example, separation distress is an evolved mechanism that leads children to stay in close proximity to attachment figures. However, problematic caregiving behavior on the part of attachment figures can lead to forms of attachment regulation and dysregulation that produce distress, dysfunction, or vulnerability to negative affects such as anxiety and depression (Cassidy & Mohr, 2001; Fonagy, Target, Gergely, Allen, & Bateman, 2003). Similarly, mate selection or position in status hierarchies can be associated with a range of affects, from excitement, pride, and happiness to anxiety and depression, depending on the outcomes of these processes (e.g., inability to find a mate and low status; see, e.g., Gilbert, Gilbert, & Irons, 2004).

OPERANT CONDITIONING
AND IMPLICIT AFFECTIVE FORECASTING

Skinner directly linked his theory of learning to evolutionary theory, suggesting that the natural selection of behavior by contingencies of reinforcement and punishment is a natural extension of evolutionary mechanisms of natural selection. What he meant was that evolution selected mechanisms that allow humans and other organisms to avoid aversive consequences and attain reinforcing ones. Although Skinner preferred for philosophical reasons not to specify the mechanisms by which this occurs, we argue that the mechanisms are largely implicit and affect regulatory. In other words, the consequences (reinforcing and punishing events) that influence subsequent behavior are largely affective or involve the (usually implicit) anticipation of evaluatively significant events.

Ample evidence suggests a link between feelings and operant conditioning. When a rat is punished with an electric shock each time it pushes a bar, the rat will desist bar pressing. In more mentalistic terms, the rat is motivated to avoid bar pressing by feelings of pain and by fear of the shock. Latane and Schachter (cited in Westen, 1985) found, in fact, that rats injected with epinephrine, which enhances anxious arousal, are substantially superior in avoidance learning to control rats; up to a point (when fear is disorganizing), the more fear, the more avoidance, because fear motivates avoidance. The opposite occurs when rats are administered antianxiety drugs, such as benzodiazepines: When their anxiety is chemically inhibited, they show a correlative difficulty inhibiting punished responses (Gray, 1979).

Neuroimaging studies with humans (e.g., Tabbert, Stark, Kirsch, & Vaitl, 2004) have established the role of the amygdala and the orbitofrontal cortex in the evaluation of conditioned stimuli subsequent to their onset in fear conditioning paradigms. These two structures also seem to have a role in forming and encoding predictive representations or affective expectations in relation to conditioned stimuli (Gottfried, O'Doherty, & Dolan, 2003). Bechara, Damasio, Damasio, and Lee (1999) have shown that damage to the amygdala in humans can lead to a failure to respond physiologically and behaviorally to linkages between stimuli or consequences and behavior, inhibiting aversive conditioning even when the person has an intact hippocampus and hence can *cognitively* anticipate that a given stimulus or behavior will be associated with an aversive feeling-state. Consistent with theoretical descriptions of deficits in psychopathic individuals who may consciously *know* moral rules but have no emotional investment in them (Westen, 1991) and theories of psychopathy that describe a subtype of psychopath low in conditionability and hence unresponsive to punishment (e.g., Lykken, 1995), recent neuroimaging research implicates a neural circuit involving the orbitofrontal cortex, amygdala, and anterior cingulate that fails to produce autonomic reactivity in a fear conditioning paradigm in a subset of psychopaths despite their explicit knowledge of the link between a conditioned stimulus and an unconditioned stimulus (painful pressure) (Birbaumer et al., 2005).

Glimcher, Dorris, and Bayer (2005) have wedded research on operant conditioning, decision making, and psychophysiology to suggest that even saccadic eye movements in humans and monkeys that direct gaze in anticipation of the presence or absence of stimuli are under control of reward contingencies. Glimcher and colleagues have shown that such eye movements, represented and controlled cortically by neurons at the intersection of the sensory and motor cortices, make implicit "decisions" based on the likely consequences or "expected utility" of reinforcing stimuli. They have shown that dopamine neurons are responsible for such affective "calculations" for reinforcing stimuli and predict that serotonin neurons will similarly be implicated with aversive stimuli.

One way to think about operant conditioning is to consider it an implicit form of affective forecasting. Affective forecasting refers to people's predictions about what they will feel in the future under various circumstances (e.g., if their favored team lost the Super Bowl or a romantic relationship ended) (e.g., Gilbert & Ebert, 2002). Social psychologists have discovered that people's conscious or explicit forecasting is often quite inaccurate, in large part because they fail to factor in their own coping and defensive processes that are likely to allow them to reframe and rationalize. It may well be that the affective forecasts implicit in operant conditioning, whereby humans and other animals essentially predict future outcomes based on past outcomes, are more accurate. Implicit affective forecasting relies less on the accuracy of people's causal theories about themselves and more on the regularities of their emotional responses to particular experiences registered in the brain.

THE PSYCHODYNAMICS OF CONFLICT, DEFENSE, AND COMPROMISE

From a psychodynamic perspective, mental processes, like behaviors, can also be conditioned or selectively retained by their experienced utility in regulating affect. The concept of defense in psychodynamic theory (e.g., Freud, 1936; Vaillant, 1977) represents what was probably the first theory of emotion regulation, although it took a number of years for theorists to link defensive processes specifically to regulation of positive and negative emotional states (Westen, 1985). Bowlby (1969) explicitly linked defense to emotion regulation in describing the attachment system, proposing a cybernetic model by which separation from an attachment figure leads to a negative affective signal (distress), which in turn elicits behavior intended to restore proximity. A number of theorists from different perspectives later extended this way of thinking to other emotions and to stress and coping (Carver & Scheier, 2000; Greenberg, Rice, & Elliott, 1996; Westen, 1985). Psychodynamic theorists have argued, further, that people's judgments and decisions, views of themselves and others, and psychological symptoms can often be understood in terms of simultaneous efforts to regulate multiple emotional–motivational "pulls," some explicit and others implicit and some conflicting and some converging, leading to compromise solutions (Brenner, 1982; Westen, 1985, 1998b, 1999).

A host of studies support the psychodynamic concept of defenses that not only operate outside awareness but can be triggered by events and affective processes automatically and unconsciously (see Baumeister, Dale, & Sommer, 1998; Westen, 1998b). Vaillant (1977; Vaillant & McCullough, 1998) has shown that individual differences in defenses can be scored reliably using a Q-sort procedure, arranged according to levels of adaptiveness, from grossly maladaptive (e.g., blatant denial and externalizing blame onto others) to highly adaptive (e.g., humor, which often includes defensive elements). Defenses scored this way have predictable correlates, both longitudinally and cross-sectionally (e.g., measures of psychological health/sickness, substance abuse problems decades later, and mortality).

Westen and colleagues (1997) developed a Q-sort instrument specifically for assessing individual differences in emotion regulation that addresses both explicit coping strategies and implicit defenses from interviews or clinical hours. Like the Q-sort procedure used by Vaillant to assess defenses, this measure is intended for use by clinically experienced observers, reflecting the assumption that implicit procedures for regulating emotion are, by definition, like other implicit processes, not readily accessible to individuals' conscious awareness. A recent normative study using a random sample of 181 adult patients treated by a random sample of doctoral-level clinicians in North America (Heim & Westen, unpublished data) identified five emotion regulation factors: externalizing strategies (e.g., "Tends to blame others for own mistakes or misdeeds"), emotional avoidance (e.g., "Can think of upsetting ideas or memories but does not feel the attendant emotion"), reality-focused coping (e.g., "Tends to respond flexibly to challenging or stressful situations"), internalizing strategies (e.g., Tends to feel bad or unworthy instead of feeling appropriately angry at others"), and disorganized strategies (e.g., "Behaves in manifestly self-destructive ways when upset; e.g., fast driving, wrist cutting.") The scales predict a range of variables, from general adaptive functioning (e.g., capacity to enter into and maintain meaningful relationships and ability to hold a good job) to specific forms of psychopathology such as borderline personality disorder (Zittel et al., 2006).

One of the most important empirical demonstrations of the concept of defense or emotion regulation outside awareness is research by Shedler and colleagues on a phenomenon they call "illusory mental health." In a seminal set of studies, Shedler, Mayman, and Manis (1993) identified participants who reported minimal distress and symptomatology on self-report questionnaires but whose early memories (narrative descriptions) were rated clinically as showing signs of psychological disturbance. The investigators divided participants into high and low on mental health as assessed by the two methods. They were particularly interested in participants who *reported* that they were psychologically healthy and nondistressed but whose early memories suggested otherwise. While undergoing a mildly stressful task (e.g., reading aloud and providing projective stories), participants who viewed themselves as healthy but showed implicit distress in their early memories were significantly more reactive on a measure of cardiac reactivity related to heart disease than participants who were either low or high on both explicit and implicit distress. They also showed more indirect signs of anxiety (such as stammering, sighing, and avoiding the content of the stimulus) while simultaneously declaring themselves to be the *least* anxious during these tasks. A subsequent study found that illusory mental health (low self-reported distress/high implicit distress) predicted the number of visits students made to the health center over the next year (Cousineau & Shedler, in press). Strikingly, self-reported distress, stress, and life events all predicted *reported* visits to the doctor, but none predicted either actual visits or visits that led to a referral from the nurse to a doctor. In other words, the same people who deny their distress also "forget" their illnesses. Similar findings have emerged in research on "repressive coping style," characterized by a tendency to avoid feeling emotions as a way of managing distress (Weinberger, 1990).

Research on adult attachment has established links between emotion regulation and insecure attachment styles that resemble the results of studies on illusory mental health and regressive coping. Unlike adults with secure attachment styles, who speak freely and openly about their relationships with their parents, individuals with an avoidant attachment style tends to dismiss the importance of attachment relationships, to be less comfortable with physical affection, and to have difficult giving specific examples of interactions with child or adult attachment figures, particularly negative experiences (see Main & Goldwyn, 1985; Main, Kaplan, & Cassidy, 1985). Avoidant adults, like avoidant infants, are hypothesized to shut off or deactivate attachment-related feelings, rather than turn them on (as secure people do), as a way of coping with distress. Dozier and Kobak (1992) monitored electrodermal response while participants were asked to recall memories involving separation, rejection, and threat from their parents. Individuals who used avoidant, deactivating strategies showed increased physiological reactivity during the task and had more difficulty generating specific negative memories. Shaver and Mikulincer (this volume) have explored emotion regulation from an attachment perspective in dozens of studies and have begun tracking the neural correlates of, for example, deactivating strategies (Gillath, Bunge, Shaver, & Mikulincer, 2004).

A host of other social–psychological investigations can be understood as documenting defensive processes as well (Westen, 1994). Of particular relevance is research on self-serving biases (Beer & Robins, 1996; Dunning, 1999) and their extreme version, narcissism (Rhodewalt & Eddings, 2002). For example, people whose views of themselves are overly favorable relative to independent observers or peer informants show numerous psychological and social difficulties, both longitudinally and cross-sectionally (Colvin, Block, & Funder, 1995). Although clinical research on narcissistic personality disorder is relatively rare because of problems in measurement (namely, that narcissistic people do not tend to admit their problems when asked; see Westen, 1997), Russ, Bradley, Shedler, and Westen (2006) have recently documented in a large clinical sample a long-hypothesized clinical distinction between grandiose narcissism, characterized by genuinely inflated views of self and a need-gratifying approach toward other people and relationships, and fragile narcissism, characterized by explicit grandiosity paired with implicit or alternating explicit feelings of inadequacy or self-loathing (see also related social–psychological research by Rhodewalt & Eddings, 2002, and Rhodewalt & Morf, 1998).

Terror management theory, based on Becker's (1973) notion that people use cultural world views to protect themselves from focusing on their own mortality, has demonstrated defensive processes in dozens of studies. Greenberg, Solomon, Pyszczynski, and their colleagues (Greenberg et al., 2003) have demonstrated in dozens of studies that making people peripherally aware of their mortality (e.g., by having them complete a "mortality salience questionnaire" or through subliminal priming) leads them to respond defensively in a number of ways, even though they have no awareness of either the affect that triggered their responses or its effects on their conscious decisions or behavior. In a recent study (Pyszczynski et al., in press), the investigators asked Iranian college students about the desirability of suicide bombing. Participants exposed to a mortality salience condition prior to completing the ratings reported far more favorable attitudes toward suicide bombers than those in the control condition and were substantially more likely to endorse the possibility of becoming a suicide bomber themselves.

The field of political psychology has seen a sustained interest in motivational bases of political beliefs and ideology for over half a century. According to Jost, Glaser, Kruglanski, and Sulloway (2003), political conservatism (characterized by resistance to change and acceptance of inequality) is best understood as a multiply determined outcome serving to regulate epistemic and existential needs. It can reduce the discomfort associated with uncertainty and ambivalence and therefore appeals to people whose epistemic needs include intolerance of ambiguity, need for closure, and low openness to experience. Longitudinal data using observer reports on the personality of a random cohort of children followed up prospectively suggest that those who identified as "conservative" or "very conservative" at age 23 tended to be indecisive, fearful, inhibited, rigid and overcontrolled in nursery school (Block & Block, in press).

A second psychodynamic proposition of particular relevance to a general theory of emotion regulation reflects the emphasis (which now seems quite contemporary) on parallel processing. Freud (1900/1913) and subsequent theorists emphasized that people do not typically process one thought, feeling, or emotion at a time. Rather, they process multiple experiences simultaneously, and the adaptive and maladaptive solutions at which they arrive—including their conscious judgments and beliefs, as well as symptoms—often reflect a process of unconscious conflict and compromise. The concept of "compromise formation" refers to the process whereby the brain settles into a compromise solution in the face of multiple, often competing motives, such as the desire to satisfy particular wishes, to maintain self-esteem, to behave morally, to escape unpleasant emotions, and to perceive reality accurately (Brenner, 1982; Westen, 1985, 1999). For example, during the Clinton–Lewinsky scandal, when Henry Hyde, the President's chief accuser in the House of Representatives, was confronted with his own history of marital infidelity, he construed an affair that occurred in his 40s as a "youthful indiscretion." Doing so allowed him to continue to pursue his desire to impeach the President while simultaneously allowing himself to feel (and appear) moral in admitting (rather than denying) the action. In reality, of course, the President was of similar age when he committed his "youthful indiscretion" in the Oval Office.

Empirical research has begun to document compromises of this sort experimentally. Of particular interest are studies placing people in conflict between accuracy and self-enhancement motives—that is, between seeing themselves the way they are and seeing themselves the way they would like to be. In one study, extraverts misled to believe that extraversion is not good for academic success altered their belief that they were *quite* as extroverted as they had believed earlier but did not come to see themselves as introverts (see Kunda, 1990). In another study, 80% of college students asked to recall their high school grades distorted their recollections in a positive direction; however, their errors were not random (Bahrick, Hall, & Berger, 1996). Percent accurate recall declined in linear fashion as students recalled As, Bs, Cs, and Ds (i.e., the students rarely misremembered their As). For our present purposes, perhaps the most interesting finding was that Ds were as likely to be remembered as Bs and Cs as they were as Ds, but they were virtually never misremembered as As—again suggesting a compromise between accuracy and self-enhancement. In the political–legal realm, Newman, Duff, Schnopp-Wyatt, Brock, and Hoffman (1997) found that the extent to which black women believed O.J. Simpson was guilty of killing his wife depended on the extent to which they identified with being black or being female—two competing pulls (the former for acquittal, the latter, conviction). Later, we describe a series of political studies directly designed to test a model of compromise formation integrated with contemporary connectionist models in cognitive science.

COPING AND DECISION MAKING

From a cognitive perspective, affect regulation mechanisms can be conceptualized as a form of procedural knowledge that can either be explicit (coping) or implicit (defense). Cognitive theorists have often conflated the procedural/declarative distinction with the implicit/explicit distinction (Westen, 2000; Westen et al., in press), creating a confusion between *type of knowledge* (how-to knowledge, which is procedural, and declarative knowledge, which has content) and *the way that knowledge is expressed* (explicitly, through conscious awareness, or implicitly, without conscious control). Declarative knowledge (representations of facts or events) can be either explicit (as when a person remembers a recent event) or implicit (as in semantic priming). Procedural knowledge (representations of internal or external actions) can be either explicit (e.g., conscious decision making, coping skills, or deliberate attempts to remember or forget) or implicit (e.g., skills such as reading facial emotions, responses learned through operant conditioning, and defenses against unpleasant feelings).

Building on stress and coping theories (Lazarus, 1993), Westen (1985) noted that procedures for regulating emotions can operate by changing distressing realities directly (acting on the world behaviorally), altering goals, altering the way one perceives the situation (e.g., reframing), or controlling the emotion directly (e.g., suppression or consuming alcohol). Addressing the conceptual overlap between coping and emotion regulation, Gross (2002, this volume) systematized research on different emotion regulation strategies used in coping, suggesting that regulation can take place in five ways, depending on the stage in the eliciting of the emotional response. Four strategies are antecedent to the emotional experience: (1) selecting the situation, (2) modifying the situation, (3) deploying attention, and (4) altering cognitions. The fifth is response-focused and involves attempts to modulate behavioral, physiological, or experiential aspects of the emotion once it has already occurred. In Gross's review of the literature, antecedent-oriented strategies tended to correlate with more positive emotional outcomes, whereas response-oriented strategies (particularly suppression) reduced both negative and positive emotional experience.

Researchers have begun exploring the neural basis of explicit emotion regulation strategies. Schaefer and colleagues (2002) observed that asking participants to attend to and maintain (as opposed to passively experience) their emotional responses to negative images during functional magnetic resonance imaging (fMRI) scanning led to increased activity in the amygdala. Ochsner, Bunge, Gross, and Gabrieli (2002) asked 15 women to attend to negative or neutral pictures during (fMRI) scanning. In some cases, the participants received instructions to make an effort to reinterpret the negative pictures so that they would not feel negative. The latter instructions led to a lessening of the subjective experience of negative emotion, heightening of activations in the dorsolateral prefrontal cortex (indicative of working memory and cognitive control), and a decrease in activations in the amygdala and medial orbitofrontal cortex (indicative of reduction in negative affect). Below we describe the first study of *implicit* affect regulation, which found a very different but theoretically predictable pattern of activations.

Aside from the use of coping strategies, decision making can be understood as a form of explicit emotion regulation. It is worth noting, of course, that dissociations of implicit and explicit processes only occur in the laboratory. In everyday life, implicit processes have an enormous impact on decision making—and indeed, provide the associative "scaffolding" for it—just as they do in conscious coping. As we argued many years ago (Westen, 1985), decision theories have always had hidden affective components, particularly in the "utility" or "expected utility" terms of expectancy-value theories (theories that suggest that decision making is in large measure a joint function of the utility of a given option weighted by its probability). Thus, every decision is simultaneously an act of emotion regulation, as the goal of any decision is to minimize current or future negative affect states and maximize positive one.

Despite a traditional divide between researchers who study decision making and those who study emotion, an emerging trend in decision research examines the influences of anticipated and remembered mood and affect on decisions (Schwartz, 2000).

Mellers (Mellers & McGraw, 2001) has argued that emotion may motivate decision-making processes that traditionally have been examined through the lens of "cold" cognition. Her theory predicts that a person evaluating the likelihood of desirable or undesirable consequences of each of two choice options will settle for the option that will likely offer the highest average amount of pleasure. She emphasizes that people anticipate elation or disappointment from the choice they make and regret or rejoicing from the option they forsook. Mellers' theory shares some similarities with expected utility theory but may improve predictive validity (Mellers & McGraw, 2001). One difference, similar to the psychodynamic concept of compromise formation but focusing more on conscious cognition, is that the theory takes into account multiple affective pulls on the overall emotional meaning of an anticipated outcome.

Other researchers have begun to explore the "hidden" affect term in decision-making theories. For example, Blanchette and Richards (2004) asked participants to consider simple conditional ("If p, then q") statements that were either neutral ("If one eats a sandwich, then he is eating cheese") or emotional ("If someone is friendly, then he is loved"). Participants made more logical errors in response to the emotional statements. Researchers in the field of behavioral economics (who have traditionally emphasized rational economic decisions and bounded rationality models in which affect tends to play an ancillary role) have begun to incorporate emotional factors in their models as well. For example, Slovic, Finucane, Peters, and MacGregor (2002) used the term "affect heuristic" to denote people's tendency to make automatic evaluations of the valence of a stimulus (how good or bad it feels), and contrast these evaluations with more traditional analytical decision making (see also Finucane et al., 2000).

Perhaps the best known advocate of the role of emotion in decision making is the neurologist Antonio Damasio (1994). Arguing against a dualistic view of the mind that pits passion and reason against each other, Damasio suggests instead that the capacity for rational cognitive judgments evolved to augment evolutionarily older evaluative and motivational processes. The emotional systems of simpler organisms are decision-making systems that initiate approach or avoidance, fight or flight, and so forth, and the neural circuits activated during complex human decision making in the prefrontal cortex do not function independently of these more primitive systems. For example, Damasio described cases of patients with brain damage who had intact intellectual functioning but were incapable of completing essential life tasks because their frontal lobes were unable to integrate cognitive planning with motivation. One of us recently examined a similar patient of average intelligence who reports a sincere desire to work and achieve but is unable to use that motivation to instigate the kinds of planning required to complete vocational tasks.

Thus far we have been describing emotional outcomes or anticipated outcomes as the motivational forces that pull people toward and push people away from particular decisions. Another emotional influence on judgment and decision making occurs in a phenomenon frequently described as *motivated reasoning*, whereby people draw emotionally biased conclusions (e.g., Jost et al., 2000, 2003; Kunda, 1990). In one sense, the term "motivated reasoning" is a misnomer because, as suggested above, *pace* Descartes, all reasoning is essentially motivated by "passions," ranging from interest to excitement and fear (see Marcus, 2002). However, the phenomenon is now well documented and is essentially an extension of the psychodynamic concept of defense, whereby people twist their beliefs to fit what they would like to believe.

For example, Mahoney (1977) demonstrated experimentally years ago motivational biases in journal manuscript reviewing. He found that scientists identified many more methodological limitations in studies that refuted rather than supported their preexisting beliefs even though the methods sections were actually identical. Ditto and colleagues (Ditto, Munro, Apanovitch, & Lockhart, 2003; Ditto, Scepansky, Munro, Apanovitch, & Lockhart, 1998) have produced similar findings, in both science and everyday life. Ditto and colleagues have shown across a number of domains that people engaged in motivated reasoning often generate more cognitions, as they challenge what they read or hear or develop rationalizations to explain away discrepant information.

Although described in different terms (e.g., partisan bias), some of the most extensive research on motivated reason has come from political science and political psychology (Lord, Ross, & Lepper, 1979; McGraw, Fischle, Stenner, & Lodge, 1996; Taber & Lodge, 2006). For decades researchers have documented the influence of partisan preferences on the way people assimilate, refuse to assimilate, or distort information about candidates and policies (e.g., Campbell, Converse, Miller, & Stokes, 1960; Goren, 2002; Green, Palmquist, & Schickler, 2004; Kinder, 1978). Studies have shown that people's judgments of who won presidential debates are strongly biased toward people's predebate emotional preferences (e.g., Bothwell & Brigham, 1983). In a study of voting behavior in a simulated presidential campaign, Redlawsk (2002) found that participants took longer time to process emotional information incongruent within their emotionally charged biases toward the candidate. Paradoxically, incongruent information only *increased* their support of the candidate they already liked.

COGNITIVE AND EMOTIONAL CONSTRAINT SATISFACTION

We are now ready to offer an integrated account of implicit and explicit emotion regulation processes as they play out in reasoning, decision making, coping, defense, and conditioning. According to the model, the same processes of approach and avoidance that evolved to lead humans and other animals toward and away from desirable and threatening stimuli or situations *also* provide motivation toward and away from desirable and threatening *beliefs*. These evolved processes can generate both adaptive and maladaptive ways of regulating emotions. To the extent that a cognitive distortion or defensive judgment leads to increased positive affect or reduction of distress, it will be reinforced (i.e., used again in the future). And to the extent that most judgments and decisions have multiple affective entailments, they are likely to bear the imprint of these multiple entailments, processed at different levels of awareness.

For much of the last decade, we have attempted to focus empirically and theoretically on the complex but commonplace situation in which people must solve multiple affective "equations" simultaneously, reaching solutions that simultaneously regulate multiple motives and emotions while simultaneously attending to the available data. The most recent version of the model draws on the broad spectrum of models inspired by connectionist or neural network models in cognitive science that were originally designed to model the processes through which people perceive, categorize, remember, and make inferences in relatively "cold" cognitive situations (Rumelhart, McClelland, & PDP Research Group, 1986; Smith, 1998). These models have several distinctive features.

First, they assume that a serial processing mechanism that allows conscious processing (via working memory) is superimposed on a largely parallel processing cognitive architecture, in which most information processing occurs outside awareness, in parallel. Second, they view representations not as "located" in any particular part of the brain but as distributed throughout a network of neural units, each of which attends to some part of the representation. Third, they view knowledge as residing in connection weights that index the extent to which two nodes on a neural network are associatively linked through their repeated coactivation. These weights can be positive or negative, such that activation of one node in a network can either facilitate or inhibit nodes associatively linked to it (just as neurons can be excitatory or inhibitory). Fourth, they offer an equilibration model of cognition involving parallel constraint satisfaction, in which the brain simultaneously and unconsciously processes multiple features of a stimulus or situation (called constraints, because they constrain the conclusions that can be drawn) and draws the best tentative conclusion it can based on the available data. Finally, they rely on the metaphor of mind as brain, rather than mind as computer, and are increasingly moving from metaphor to a combination of computational modeling and brain mapping (Wagar & Thagard, 2004).

Connectionist and related models are increasingly drawing the attention of psychologists interested in affectively relevant phenomena such as first impressions, prejudice, cognitive dissonance, attitude shifts, and emotional processes in psychotherapy (e.g., Caspar, 1998; Kunda & Thagard, 1996; Read, Vanman, & Miller, 1997; Spellman, Ullman, & Holyoak, 1993). To account for the emotional biases of jurors in the 1995 trial of O. J. Simpson, for example, Thagard (2003) introduced *evaluation units* into connectionist networks and argued that judgments reflect an effort to attain both explanatory coherence (making the most sense of the data) and what he calls emotional coherence (which combines explanatory coherence with emotional valence).

In the latest version of our model, we have extended such models to include two kinds of constraints: cognitive constraints (imposed by data and their logical entailments) and emotional constraints (imposed by emotional associations and anticipated emotions). Just as information provides constraints on the equilibrated solutions people reach—by spreading activation to networks (and ultimately conclusions) that make sense of the "gestalt" of available data and spreading inhibition to alternatives that make less sense of the totality of the data—feelings and emotion-laden goals provide constraints on the equilibrated solutions people reach by spreading activation to the neural networks or units that lead people toward desired conclusions and inhibiting those that increase the likelihood of undesired ones. Thus, the brain equilibrates to solutions designed not only to maximize goodness of fit to the data but also to maximize positive and minimize negative affect.

This model suggests a continuity between goal-driven decision making (and hence adaptive behavior) and emotion-driven cognitive distortions (Westen, 1985, 1994). Contemporary views of motivation, rooted in research with both human and nonhuman animals, emphasize approach and avoidance systems motivated by positive and negative affect (Carver, 2001; Davidson, Jackson, & Kalin, 2000; Gray, 1990). Our model suggests that, in a symbolic species such as ours, the same processes of approach and avoidance, motivated by affect or anticipated affect, apply to the judgments people reach, the way they see themselves, and other conscious beliefs and decision, such that people will approach and avoid *ideas or representations* based on their emotional consequences. What makes matters particularly complex is that at the same time people are trying to make decisions that "optimize" anticipated emotional consequences, both their consideration of the options and the judgments they ultimately reach regarding choices among alternatives may be compromised by emotion-driven distortions.

We have tested this model using political events, because in politics people have often cross-cutting emotional constraints, many people share similar constraints (feelings toward the parties, candidates, and issues), and we can measure these constraints and examine the ways they interact with cognitive constraints at a given moment to produce equilibrated solutions (political judgments and decisions). We have conducted a series of studies to test this model across several years in United States politics, during the impeachment of Bill Clinton, the disputed presidential election of 2000, and the discovery of torture by the United States at Abu Ghraib prison in Iraq (Westen, Blagov, Feit, Arkowitz, & Thagard, 2005a). In these studies, we collected data from community samples, assessing emotional constraints and assessing or manipulating cognitive constraints to predict judgments that most decision theories would explain in more "cold" cognitive terms.

These studies yielded two primary findings. First, the data supported the model, finding that people's political judgments reflect the simultaneous satisfaction of multiple cognitive and emotional constraints. Second, in high-stakes, emotion-laden political situations, emotional constraints generally overwhelm even relatively strong cognitive constraints—that is, regulation of emotion takes priority over data and logic.

For example, in three studies conducted from early to late in the events that led to the impeachment of Bill Clinton, we assessed cognitive and emotional constraints in predicting judgments about whether the President likely groped Kathleen Willey in the Oval Office (Study 1), whether he lied to the grand jury investigating the case (Study 2), and whether his actions constituted an impeachable offense as defined by the Constitution (Study 3). We hypothesized that people's judgments (e.g., in Study 3, about the extent to which lying about sex to a grand jury constitutes "high crimes and misdemeanors" and hence provides adequate grounds for impeachment and removal from office) would reflect some combination of cognitive constraints (what participants knew about Clinton and the scandal) and affective constraints (what they felt about the Democratic and Republican parties, Clinton, infidelity, and feminism). We assessed cognitive constraints by asking participants 10 factual questions about Clinton's life that would indicate long-standing knowledge about his political and personal history and 10 factual questions about the scandal. We assessed emotional constraints by asking multiple questions about participants' gut-level feelings toward the Democrats and Republicans, Clinton, infidelity, and feminism, which we predicted would provide overlapping but in many cases competing emotional constraints on judgment.

As predicted, participants' judgments in all three studies reflected an equilibration process, rendering their actions predictable by a linear combination of their feelings toward the parties, Clinton, infidelity, and feminism (which each set of emotional constraints contributing significantly after holding the others constant) and constraints imposed by their knowledge. However, the emotional constraints swamped cognition in all three studies. For example, we could predict people' judgments about whether the President's actions crossed the Constitutional threshold for impeachment from cognitive and emotional constraints measured prospectively (6 to 9 months earlier) with remarkable accuracy (88% of the time) using the full model. However, we could predict the same judgments with 85% accuracy when we deleted cognitive constraints from the model, including only emotional constraints. People's knowledge about the scandal placed a statistically significant but practically insignificant constraint on people's judgments longitudinally, with virtually nothing left to be accounted for once people's emotional–motivational "pulls" were modeled, even given measurement error.

Similar findings emerged in a study assessing people's judgments about the relative validity of manual versus machine ballot counts in the disputed presidential election of 2000. We could predict 83.6% of people's judgments about the relative validity of manual and machine counts using the full model, including emotional constraints (feelings about the two parties and the two candidates) and cognitive constraints (knowledge about exit polling, etc., as well as an experimental manipulation). Eliminating cognitive constraints from the model (i.e., including only emotional constraints) left us able to make accurate predictions 83.0% of the time. Thagard (2003; Westen et al., 2005a) has successfully modeled these processes computationally using his HOTCO 2 (hot cognition) program, which is a program for modeling connectionist processes that builds in emotional constraints.

We obtained similar findings in an experiment in which we manipulated cognitive constraints in an alleged case of abuse at Abu Ghraib in 2004. Participants (again, people in the community completing a questionnaire) had to make a decision about whether a particular soldier should be given the right to subpoena senior civilian officials, given his defense that he had been informed that the Geneva Conventions on the treatment of prisoners of war had been suspended by the U.S. government. To manipulate cognitive constraints, we placed participants in one of four conditions, varying the amount of evidence for the soldier's claim that he had been informed that his actions were no longer governed by the Geneva Conventions and hence that torture was permissible. The experimental manipulation had a small, marginally significant effect, but this was once again dwarfed by emotion constraints—in this case, feelings toward the Democrats and Republics, the U.S. military, and human rights as a goal of U.S. foreign policy.

The only study thus far in which we have found a more substantial impact of cognitive constraints is a study recently completed in which we predicted people's beliefs about the state of the national economy from an objective set of economic indicators (e.g., gross domestic product and unemployment), their personal finances, and their feelings toward the political parties (Westen, Kelley, & Abramowitz, 2005b). In this study, we used data from the National Election Studies, a database of surveys conducted over several decades which have retained a number of questions over many elections and hence allows researchers to test hypotheses with a sample of several thousand voters over many years. Once again, supporting the model, cognitive constraints (objective economic indicators) and emotional constraints (partisan feelings) jointly predicted people's judgments in a relatively "cold" cognitive domain (the state of the economy). Although the impact of cognitive constraints was larger in this study than in the political crises examined in the prior five studies, once again emotional constraints had a stronger impact on people's judgments.

In a final study, designed to examine the neural circuits involved as people implicitly regulate their emotions by drawing emotionally biased conclusions, we used functional neuroimaging (fMRI) to study a sample of 30 partisan Democrats and Republicans during the 3 months prior to the U.S. presidential election of 2004 (Westen, Kilts, Blagov, Harenski, & Hamann, in press). We presented participants with 18 sets of stimuli, 6 each regarding President Bush, his challenger Senator John Kerry, and neutral male control figures. For each set of stimuli, participants first read a statement from the target (e.g., Bush), followed by a second statement documenting a clear contradiction between the target's words and deeds that would be threatening to a partisan (suggesting that the candidate was lying or pandering). Next, participants read a slide asking them to consider the discrepancy, followed by a slide asking them to rate the extent to which the target's words and deeds were contradictory. Finally, they were presented with an exculpatory statement that could explain away the apparent contradiction and asked to reconsider and again to rate the extent to which the target's words and deeds were contradictory. (We included the exculpatory evidence and subsequent statements and ratings so that we could subtract neural processes activated during the conditions of interest from those activated by similar conditions intended not to provoke emotionally biased judgments or motivated reasoning.)

Participants' ratings of the extent to which the first and second statements were contradictory strongly supported emotional constraint satisfaction, with partisans denying obvious contradictions for their own candidate that they had no difficulty detecting in the opposing candidate or in politically neutral controls (also included for purposes of subtraction for contrast analyses using the neuroimaging data). Whereas Democrats and Republicans showed no behavioral or neural differences in response to apparent contradictions for the politically neutral control targets, Democrats responded to Kerry as Republicans responded to Bush when reasoning about contradictions from their own candidates. While weighing evidence suggesting contradictions for their own candidate, partisans showed expected activations throughout the orbitofrontal cortex, indicating affective processing and presumably affect regulation, as well as lateral orbital and insular cortex activations suggesting the experience of negative affect. They also showed amygdala activation, which habituated over the course of the experiment. Partisans also showed large activations in the anterior cingulate, including its ventral emotional, regions, suggesting emotion processing and conflict monitoring.

After apparently having found a way to resolve the contradiction, while asked to consider the contradiction, circuits indicative of distress become inactive. Partisans also showed a large activation in the ventral striatum and nucleus accumbens, suggesting reward. The data support the operant conditioning of a defensive response, associating the participant's "revisionist" account of the data with reduction of negative affect (negative reinforcement) and the experience of positive affect (positive reinforcement).

It is interesting to compare these results to those obtained in studies of explicit emotion regulation, as when Ochsner and colleagues (2002) asked 15 women to attend to negative or neutral pictures during fMRI scanning and in one condition (in a within-subject design) instructed them to make an effort to reframe the pictures cognitively so that they would not feel so negative. The latter instructions led not only to a lessening of the subjective experience of negative emotion but to a reduction in activations in the amygdala and medial orbitofrontal cortex, indicative of the same kind of reduction of negative affect as in our study. However, consistent with the use of explicit rather than implicit emotion regulation strategies, reframing activated dorsolateral prefrontal circuits indicative of effortful control, whereas dorsolateral circuits were not differentially activated during implicit affect regulation in our study. Such studies provide preliminary evidencing suggesting that implicit and explicit emotion regulation may involve different neural mechanisms, although they likely share some mechanisms, such as those mediated by the anterior cingulate and some medial frontal circuits involved in conflict monitoring and emotion regulation more generally.

IMPLICATIONS AND FUTURE DIRECTIONS

The model of emotion regulation we have been developing is clearly a work in progress. Although the model was originally developed with psychopathology and individual differences in mind, we have only begun to explore its links to different forms of psychopathology and to treatment (see Thompson-Brenner & Westen, 2005). From the standpoint of understanding the neural circuits involved in implicit emotion regulation, we are also in the beginning stages of this research, and several important tasks remain. It will be important to see if the findings of our preliminary fMRI study replicate not only within the political realm but in other domains in which such processes occur, such as self-serving biases, narcissism, and biases in judgment that occur as scientists evaluate data inconsistent with theories or hypotheses in which they are emotionally invested (Ditto & Lopez, 1992; Klaczynski & Narasimham, 1998; Kuhn, 1962; Mahoney, 1977).

ACKNOWLEDGMENTS

Preparation of this chapter was supported in part by Grant Nos. MH62377 and MH62378 from the National Institute of Mental Health.

REFERENCES

Bahrick, H., Hall, L. K., & Berger, S. A. (1996). Accuracy and distortion in memory for high school grades. *Psychological Science, 7,* 265–271.

Baumeister, R., Dale, K., & Sommer, K. (1998). Freudian defense mechanisms and empirical findings in modern social psychology: Reaction formation, projection, displacement, undoing, isolation, sublimation, and denial. *Journal of Personality, 66,* 1081–1124.

Bechara, A., Damasio, H., Damasio, A. R., & Lee, G. P. (1999). Different contributions of the human amygdala and ventromedial prefrontal cortex to decision-making. *Journal of Neuroscience, 19*(13), 5473–5481.

Becker, E. (1973). *The denial of death.* New York: Free Press.

Beer, J. S., & Robins, R. W. (1996, June). *Consequences of self-enhancement bias: A longitudinal study.* Poster presented at the American Psychological Society, San Francisco.

Birbaumer, N., Veit, R., Lotze, M., Erb, M., Hermann, C., Grodd, W., et al. (2005). Deficient fear conditioning in psychopathy: A functional magnetic resonance imaging study. *Archives of General Psychiatry, 62,* 799–805.

Blanchette, I., & Richards, A. (2004). Reasoning about emotional and neutral materials: Is logic affected by emotion? *Psychological Science, 15*(11), 745–752.

Block, J., & Block, J. H. (in press). Nursery school personality and political orientation two decades later. *Journal of Research in Personality.*

Bothwell, R. K., & Brigham, J. C. (1983). Selective evaluation and recall during the 1980 Reagan–Carter debate. *Journal of Applied Social Psychology, 13,* 427–442.

Bowlby, J. (1969). *Attachment* (Vol. 1). New York: Basic Books.

Brenner, C. (1982). *The mind in conflict.* New York: International Universities Press.

Buss, D. M., Larsen, R. J., Westen, D., & Semmelroth, J. (1992). Sex differences in jealousy: Evolution, physiology, and psychology. *Psychological Science, 3,* 251–255.

Campbell, A., Converse, P. E., Miller, W. E., & Stokes, D. E. (1960). *The American voter.* Oxford, UK: Wiley.

Carver, C. S. (2001). Affect and the functional bases of behavior: On the dimensional structure of affective experience. *Personality and Social Psychology Review, 5,* 345–356.

Carver, C. S., & Scheier, M. F. (2000). Origins and functions of positive and negative affect: A control-process view. In E. T. Higgins & A. W. Kruglanski (Eds.), *Motivational science: Social and personality perspectives* (pp. 256–272). New York: Psychology Press.

Caspar, F. (1998). A connectionist view of psychotherapy. In D. J. Stein & J. Ludik (Eds.), *Neural networks and psychopathology: Connectionist models in practice and research.* Cambridge, UK: Cambridge University Press.

Cassidy, J., & Mohr, J. J. (2001). Unsolvable fear, trauma, and psychopathology: Theory, research, and clinical considerations related to disorganized attachment across the life span. *Clinical Psychology: Science and Practice, 8,* 275–298.

Colvin, R., Block, J., & Funder, D. (1995). Overly positive self-evaluations and personality: Negative implications for mental health. *Journal of Personality and Social Psychology, 68*, 1152–1162.

Cousineau, T. M., & Shedler, J. (in press). Implicit versus explicit mental health measures as predictors of physical illness: A view through the lens of the early memory index. *Journal of Nervous and Mental Disease.*

Damasio, A. R. (1994). *Descartes' error: Emotion, reason, and the human brain.* New York: Grosset/Putnam.

Davidson, R. J., Jackson, D. C., & Kalin, N. H. (2000). Emotion, plasticity, context, and regulation: Perspectives from affective neuroscience. *Psychological Bulletin, 126*, 890–909.

Ditto, P. H., & Lopez, D. F. (1992). Motivated skepticism: Use of differential decision criteria for preferred and nonpreferred conclusions. *Journal of Personality and Social Psychology, 63*(4), 568–584.

Ditto, P. H., Munro, G. D., Apanovitch, A. M., Scepansky, J. A., & Lockhart, L. K. (2003). Spontaneous skepticism: The interplay of motivation and expectation in responses to favorable and unfavorable medical diagnoses. *Personality and Social Psychology Bulletin, 29*(9), 1120–1132.

Ditto, P. H., Scepansky, J. A., Munro, G. D., Apanovitch, A. M., & Lockhart, L. K. (1998). Motivated sensitivity to preference-inconsistent information. *Journal of Personality and Social Psychology, 75*(1), 53–69.

Dozier, M., & Kobak, R. R. (1992). Psychophysiology in attachment interviews: Converging evidence for deactivating strategies. *Child Development, 63*(6), 1473–1480.

Dunning, D. (1999). A newer look: Motivated social cognition and the schematic representation of social concepts. *Psychological Inquiry, 10*, 1–11.

Finucane, M. L., Alhakami, A., Slovic, P., & Johnson, S. M. (2000). The affect heuristic in judgments of risk and benefits. *Journal of Behavioral Decision Making, 13*, 1–17.

Fonagy, P., Target, M., Gergely, G., Allen, J. G., & Bateman, A. (2003). The developmental roots of borderline personality disorder in early attachment relationships: A theory and some evidence. *Psychoanalytic Inquiry, 23*, 412–459.

Freud, A. (1936). *The ego and the mechanisms of defense.* New York: International Universities Press.

Freud, S. (1900/1913). *The interpretation of dreams* (A. A. Brill, Trans.). New York: Macmillan.

Freud, S. (1953). New introductory lectures on psycho-analysis. In J. Strachey (Ed. and Trans.), *The standard edition of the complete psychological works of Sigmund Freud* (Vol. 22, pp. 3–128). London: Hogarth Press. (Original work published 1933)

Garcia, J., & Koelling, R. A. (1966). Relation of cue to consequence in avoidance learning. *Psychonomic Science, 4*(3), 123–124.

Gilbert, D. T., & Ebert, J. E. J. (2002). Decisions and revisions: The affective forecasting of changeable outcomes. *Journal of Personality and Social Psychology, 82*(4), 503–514.

Gilbert, P., Gilbert, J., & Irons, C. (2004). Life events, entrapments, and arrested anger in depression. *Journal of Affective Disorders, 79*, 149–160.

Gillath, O., Bunge, S. A., Shaver, P. R., & Mikulincer, M. (2004, October). *Attachment and the regulation of negative emotions: An fMRI exploration.* Paper presented at the Symposium on Emotion Regulation: Pathways to Health and Dysfunction, Fort Worth, TX.

Glimcher, P. W., Dorris, M. C., & Bayer, H. M. (2005). Physiological utility theory and the neuroeconomics of choice. *Games and Economic Behavior, 52*(2), 213–256.

Goren, P. (2002). Character weakness, partisan bias, and presidential evaluation. *American Journal of Political Science, 46*, 627–641.

Gottfried, J. A., O'Doherty, J., & Dolan, R. J. (2003). Encoding predictive reward value in human amygdala and orbitofrontal cortex. *Science, 301*(5636), 1104–1107.

Gray, J. A. (1979). Anxiety and the brain: Not by neurochemistry alone. *Psychological Medicine, 9*(4), 605–609.

Gray, J. A. (1990). Brain systems that mediate both emotion and cognition. *Cognition and Emotion, 4*, 269–288.

Gray, J. A. (2001). Emotional modulation of cognitive control: Approach–withdrawal states double-dissociate spatial from verbal two-back task performance. *Journal of Experimental Psychology: General, 130*, 436–452.

Gray, J. A., Braver, T. S., & Raichle, M. E. (2002). Integration of emotion and cognition in the lateral prefrontal cortex. *Proceedings of the National Academy of Sciences, USA, 99*(6), 4115–4120.

Green, D., Palmquist, B., & Schickler, E. (2004). *Partisan hearts and minds: Political parties and the social identities of voters.* New Haven: Yale University Press.

Greenberg, J., Martens, A., Jonas, E., Eisenstadt, D., Pyszczynski, T., & Solomon, S. (2003). Psychological defense in anticipation of anxiety: Eliminating the potential for anxiety eliminates the effect of mortality salience on worldview defense. *Psychological Science, 14*(5), 516–519.

Greenberg, L. S., Rice, L. N., & Elliott, R. K. (1996). *Facilitating emotional change: The moment-by-moment process*. New York: Guilford Press.

Gross, J. (1998). The emerging filed of emotion regulation: An integrative review. *Review of General Psychology, 2*(3), 271–299.

Gross, J. (2002). Emotion regulation: Affective, cognitive, and social consequences. *Psychophysiology, 39*, 281–291.

Jost, J. T., Glaser, J., Kruglanski, A. W., & Sulloway, F. J. (2000). Exceptions that prove the rule—Using a theory of motivated social cognition to account for ideological incongruities and political anomalies: Reply to Greenberg and Jonas (2003). *Psychological Bulletin, 129*(3), 383–393.

Jost, J. T., Glaser, J., Kruglanski, A. W., & Sulloway, F. J. (2003). Political conservatism as motivated social cognition. *Psychological Bulletin, 129*(3), 339–375.

Kinder, D. R. (1978). Political person perception: The asymmetrical influence of sentiment and choice on perceptions of presidential candidates. *Journal of Personality and Social Psychology, 36*(8), 859–871.

Klaczynski, P., & Narasimham, G. (1998). Development of scientific reasoning biases: Cognitive versus ego-protective explanations. *Developmental Psychology, 34*, 175–187.

Kuhn, T. (1962). *The structure of scientific revolutions*. Chicago: University of Chicago Press.

Kunda, Z. (1990). The case for motivated reasoning. *Psychological Bulletin, 108*, 480–498.

Kunda, Z., & Thagard, P. (1996). Forming impressions from stereotypes, traits, and behaviors: A parallel-constraint-satisfaction theory. *Psychological Review, 103*, 284–308.

Lazarus, R. S. (1993). From psychological stress to the emotions: A history of changing outlooks. *Annual Review of Psychology, 44*(1–21).

Lord, C. G., Ross, L., & Lepper, M. R. (1979). Biased assimilation and attitude polarization: The effects of prior theories on subsequently considered evidence. *Journal of Personality and Social Psychology, 37*, 2098–2109.

Lykken, D. T. (1995). *The antisocial personalities*. Hillsdale, NJ: Erlbaum.

Mahoney, M. J. (1977). Reflections on the cognitive-learning trend in psychotherapy. *American Psychologist, 32*, 5–13.

Main, M., & Goldwyn, R. (1985). *Adult attachment classification system*. Unpublished manuscript, University of California, Berkeley.

Main, M., Kaplan, N., & Cassidy, J. (1985). Security in infancy, childhood, and adulthood: A move to the level of representation. *Monographs of the Society for Research in Child Development, 50*(1–2), 66–104.

Marcus, G. (2002). *The sentimental citizen: Emotion in democratic politics*. Philadelphia: PennPress.

Maslow, A. H. (1970). *Motivation and personality* (2nd ed.). New York: Harper & Row.

McGraw, K. M., Fischle, M., Stenner, K., & Lodge, M. (1996). What's in a word?: Bias in trait descriptions of political leaders. *Political Behavior, 18*, 263–287.

Mellers, B. A., & McGraw, P. A. (2001). Anticipated emotions as guides to choice. *Current Directions in Psychological Science, 10*(6), 210–214.

Newman, L. S., Duff, K., Schnopp-Wyatt, N., Brock, B., & Hoffman, Y. (1997). Reactions to the O. J. Simpson verdict: "Mindless tribalism" or motivated inference processes? *Journal of Social Issues, 53*(3), 547–562.

Ochsner, K. N., Bunge, S. A., Gross, J., & Gabrieli, J. D. E. (2002). Rethinking feelings: An fMRI study of the cognitive regulation of emotion. *Journal of Cognitive Neuroscience, 14*(8), 1215–1229.

Plutchik, R. (2003). *Emotions and life: Perspectives from psychology, biology, and evolution*. Washington, DC: American Psychological Association.

Pyszczynski, T., Abdollahi, A., Solomon, S., Greenberg, J., Cohen, F., & Weise, D. (in press). Mortality salience, martyrdom, and military might: The Great Satan versus the Axis of Evil. *Personality and Social Psychology Bulletin*.

Read, S. J., Vanman, E. J., & Miller, L. C. (1997). Connectionism, parallel constraint satisfaction processes, and gestalt principles: (Re)introducing cognitive dynamics to social psychology. *Personality and Social Psychology Review, 1*, 93–133.

Redlawsk, D. P. (2002). Hot cognition or cool consideration?: Testing the effects of motivated reasoning on political decision making. *Journal of Politics, 64*, 1021–1044.

Rhodewalt, F., & Eddings, S. K. (2002). Narcissus reflects: Memory distortion in response to ego-relevant feedback among high- and low-narcissistic men. *Journal of Research in Personality, 36*(2), 97–116.

Rhodewalt, F., & Morf, C. C. (1998). On self-aggrandizement and anger: A temporal analysis of narcissism and affective reactions to success and failure. *Journal of Personality and Social Psychology, 74,* 672–685.

Rumelhart, D. E., McClelland, J. L., & PDP Research Group. (1986). *Parallel distributed processing: Explorations in the microstructure of cognition: Vol 1. Foundations.* Cambridge, MA: MIT Press.

Russ, E., Bradley, R., Shedler, J., & Westen, D. (2006). *Refining the narcissistic diagnosis: Identifying defining criteria, subtypes, and endophenotypes.* Unpublished manuscript, Emory University.

Sandler, J. (1987). *From safety to superego: Selected papers of Joseph Sandler.* New York: Guilford Press.

Schaefer, S. M., Jackson, D. C., Davidson, R. J., Aguirre, G. K., Kimberg, D. Y., & Thompson-Schill, S. L. (2002). Modulation of amygdalar activity by the conscious regulation of negative emotion. *Journal of Cognitive Neuroscience, 14*(6), 912–921.

Schwartz, N. (2000). Emotion, cognition, and decision making. *Cognition and Emotion, 14*(4), 433–440.

Shaver, P. R., & Mikulincer, M. (2007). Adult attachment strategies and the regulation of emotion. In J. J. Gross (Ed.), *Handbook of emotion regulation* (pp. 446–465). New York: Guilford Press.

Shedler, J., Mayman, M., & Manis, M. (1993). The illusion of mental health. *American Psychology, 48,* 1117–1131.

Singer, T., Seymor, B., O'Doherty, J., Kaube, H., Dolan, R. J., & Frith, C. D. (2004). Empathy for pain involves the affective but not sensory components of pain. *Science, 303*(4661), 1157–1162.

Slovic, P., Finucane, M. L., Peters, E., & MacGregor, D. G. (2002). Rational actors or rational fools: Implications of the affect heuristics for behavioral economics. *Journal of Socio-Economics, 31,* 329–342.

Smith, E. R. (1998). Mental representation and memory. In D. T. Gilbert, S. T. Fiske, & G. Lindzey (Eds.), *Handbook of social psychology* (Vol. 1, pp. 391–445). New York: McGraw-Hill.

Spellman, B. A., Ullman, J. B., & Holyoak, K. J. (1993). A coherence model of cognitive consistency: Dynamics of attitude change during the persian gulf war. *Journal of Social Issues, 49,* 147–165.

Tabbert, K., Stark, R., Kirsch, P., & Vaitl, D. (2004). Hemodynamic responses of the amygdala, orbitofrontal cortex, and the visual cortex during a fear conditioning paradigm. *International Journal of Psychophysiology, 57,* 15–23.

Taber, C. S., & Lodge, M. (2006). Motivated skepticism in the evaluation of political beliefs. *American Journal of Political Science, 50,* 755–769.

Thagard, P. (2003). Why wasn't O. J. convicted?: Emotional coherence in legal inference. *Cognition and Emotion, 17,* 361–385.

Thompson-Brenner, H., & Westen, D. (2005). Personality subtypes in eating disorders: Validation of a classification in a naturalistic sample. *British Journal of Psychiatry, 186,* 516–524.

Tomkins, S. S. (1981). The quest for primary motives: Biography and autobiography of an idea. *Journal of Personality and Social Psychology, 41,* 306–329.

Vaillant, G. (1977). *Adaptation to life.* Boston: Little, Brown.

Vaillant, G., & McCullough, L. (1998). The role of ego mechanisms of defense in the diagnosis of personality disorders. In J. W. Barron (Ed.), *Making diagnosis meaningful: Enhancing evaluation and treatment of psychological disorders* (pp. 139–158). Washington, DC: American Psychological Association.

Wagar, B. M., & Thagard, P. (2004). Spiking Phineas Gage: A neurocomputational theory of cognitive-affective integration in decision making. *Psychological Review, 111*(1), 67–79.

Weinberger, D. A. (1990). The construct validity of the repressive coping style. In J. L. Singer (Ed.), *Repression and dissociation: Implications for personality theory, psychopathology, and health* (pp. 337–386). Chicago: University of Chicago Press.

Westen, D. (1985). *Self and society: Narcissism, collectivism, and the development of morals.* New York: Cambridge University Press.

Westen, D. (1991). Social cognition and object relations. *Psychological Bulletin, 109*(3), 429–455.

Westen, D. (1994). Toward an integrative model of affect regulation: Applications to social–psychological research. *Journal of Personality, 62*(4), 641–667.

Westen, D. (1997). Divergences between clinical and research methods for assessing personality disorders: Implications for research and the evolution of Axis II. *American Journal of Psychiatry, 154,* 895–903.

Westen, D. (1998a). Affect regulation and psychopathology: Applications to depression and borderline personality disorder. In W. Flack & J. Laird (Eds.), *Affect and psychopathology* (pp. 394–406). New York: Oxford University Press.

Westen, D. (1998b). The scientific legacy of Sigmund Freud: Toward a psychodynamically informed psychological science. *Psychological Bulletin, 124,* 333–371.

Westen, D. (1999). Psychodynamic theory and technique in relation to research on cognition and emotion: Mutual implications. In T. Dalgleish & M. Power (Eds.), *Handbook of cognition and emotion* (pp. 727–746). New York: Wiley.

Westen, D. (2000). Commentary: Implicit and emotional processes in cognitive-behavioral therapy. *Clinical Psychology–Science and Practice, 7,* 386–390.

Westen, D. (in press). *The political brain: The science of the mind and the art of getting elected.* New York: Public Affairs.

Westen, D., Blagov, P., Feit, A., Arkowitz, J., & Thagard, P. (2005a). *When reason and passion collide: Cognitive and emotional constraint satisfaction in high-stakes political decision making.* Submitted manuscript.

Westen, D., Kelley, M., & Abramowitz, A. (2005b). *Is GDP in the eyes of the beholder?: Cognitive and emotional constraint satisfaction in voters' perceptions of the economy.* Unpublished manuscript, Emory University.

Westen, D., Kilts, C., Blagov, P., Harenski, K., & Hamann, S. (in press). The neural basis of motivated reasoning: An fMRI study of emotional constraints on political judgment during the U.S. Presidential election of 2004. *Journal of Cognitive Neuroscience.*

Westen, D., Muderrisoglu, S., Shedler, J., Fowler, C., & Koren, D. (1997). Affect regulation and affective experience: Individual differences, group differences, and measurement using a Q-sort procedure. *Journal of Consulting and Clinical Psychology, 65*(3), 429–439.

Westen, D., Weinberger, J., & Bradley, R. (in press). Motivation, decision making, and consciousness: From psychodynamics to subliminal priming and emotional constraint satisfaction. In M. Moscovitch & P. D. Zelazo (Eds.), *Cambridge handbook of consciousness.* Cambridge, UK: Cambridge University Press.

Zittel, C., Bradley, R., & Westen, D. (2006). Affect regulation in borderline personality disorder. *Journal of Nervous and Mental Disease, 194,* 69–77.

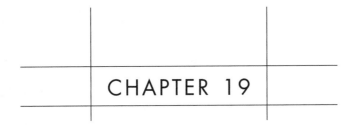

CHAPTER 19

Intelligent Emotion Regulation

IS KNOWLEDGE POWER?

TANJA WRANIK
LISA FELDMAN BARRETT
PETER SALOVEY

John worked overtime on the advertising proposal for his firm's latest client and finally went home at 11:30 P.M., tired but satisfied. The next day, Nick, the senior consultant, started the meeting by presenting John's ideas as his own. John felt the blood rush to his face, trembled, and had a strong urge to shout. But his boss was sitting at the end of the table, and an important client was in the room as well. John did not yell. He sat quietly, and waited for the presentation to finish. He decided to talk with Nick about the situation later.

Most people would probably agree that several skills are necessary for managing and regulating emotional life, and that individuals differ markedly in their proficiency with this skill set. In our opening example, John's decision not to yell was rooted in skills that allowed him to understand his reaction quickly and efficiently and to know how his expressive behavior would be judged by others. Within the blink of an eye, John had to perceive his reaction as an emotional state (perhaps he perceived it as anger, or fear), anticipate how others might judge his reaction, know what to do to adjust his expressive behavior, and execute the chosen course of action (in our example, to inhibit the impulse to yell in favor of meeting some other goal). Because John appeared to master the situation consistently with his goal, we would say that he regulated his emotional episode in an "emotionally intelligent" manner (Salovey & Mayer, 1990).

In this chapter, we use the emotional intelligence (EI) framework originally proposed by Salovey and Mayer (1990; modified by Mayer & Salovey, 1997) to stimulate a discussion of the processes that allowed John to regulate his emotional response effectively. In doing so, we demonstrate that EI provides fertile scientific grounds for understanding how people shape their emotional episodes to a specific situation, for a desired purpose, within a particular context.

EMOTIONAL INTELLIGENCE

Salovey and Mayer (1990; Mayer & Salovey, 1997) proposed the concept of emotional intelligence as an interrelated set of skills that allow an individual to perceive, understand, use, and regulate emotional episodes in an efficient and adaptive manner, thereby allowing effective dealings with the environment. They defined EI to include four major skill sets or "branches" that are related to functionally effective behaviors in young adults (Brackett, Mayer, & Warner, 2004), the quality of social interactions (Lopes et al., 2004; Lopes, Salovey, Côté, & Beers, 2005), perceived quality of social relationships (Lopes, Salovey, & Straus, 2003), and job-related variables such as leadership potential (Lopes, Grewal, Kadis, Gall, & Salovey, in press).

First, EI involves accurately perceiving emotional episodes in others and in the self (*Branch 1: Perception of Emotion*). Most people automatically and effortlessly perceive emotional episodes in others by viewing a set of facial behaviors, vocal cues, or bodily movements (e.g., Ekman & Friesen, 1975; Johnstone, Van Reekum, & Scherer, 2001; Nowicki & Mitchell, 1998). However, there are also strong individual differences in the ability to infer emotional cues from the face and the voice (Baum & Nowicki, 1998; Nowicki & Duke, 1994; Petti, Voelker, Shore, & Hayman-Abello, 2003). Furthermore, people vary widely in the precision or granularity (complexity) with which they automatically and effortlessly perceive their own experience of emotion (Barrett, 1998, 2004; Feldman, 1995).

Second, EI involves using emotion-related information to facilitate thought and make better decisions (*Branch 2: Using Emotion to Facilitate Thought*). This set of skills involves the ability to use emotional information to focus attention on important information in the environment (e.g., Mandler, 1984), resolve control dilemmas (Gray, Schaefer, Braver, & Most, 2005), guide momentary judgments (Clore & Parrott, 1991; Damasio, 1994; Schwarz, 1990; Schwarz & Clore, 1983, 1996), and predict future behavior and outcomes (e.g., Gilbert, Pinel, Wilson, Blumberg, & Wheatley, 1998). Some people appear better able to harness the mental sets generated by different emotional experiences and use them to focus on various kinds of problems, such as inductive or deductive reasoning (Isen, 1987; Schwarz, 1990; Palfai & Salovey, 1993).

Third, EI involves the capacity to understand what emotions are and how they work (*Branch 3: Understanding Emotion or Emotion Knowledge*). This encompasses language and propositional thought and reflects the capacity to analyze emotions, appreciate their probable trends over time, and understand their outcomes (e.g., Frijda, 1988; Lane, Quinlan, Schwartz, Walker, & Zeitlin, 1990; Roseman, 1984). It includes a broad understanding of the emotional lexicon (e.g., Barrett, 2004) and draws on conceptual knowledge about emotion (Barrett, 2006). This branch is strongly influenced by development and is therefore expected to progress with age and experience (Lewis, 2000).

Finally, EI involves efficient emotion regulation in both self and others (*Branch 4: Managing Emotion*). It includes the ability to maintain awareness of emotion-related events, even when they are unpleasant, as well as the ability to solve emotion-laden problems in the most effective manner possible. Although the emotional management branch refers to two domains of skill, managing emotions in the self and managing emotions in other people, research has focused mainly on how individual variation in managing one's own emotional episodes produces better interpersonal outcomes.

The fourth branch of EI, managing emotion, most obviously demonstrates a link between emotionally intelligent skill sets and effective emotion regulation. In John's case, this may mean that he has the ability to inhibit his desire to yell and to control his trembling. Yet to be truly effective, John must have other skills available to him. For example, John's emotion regulation would be facilitated by his ability to perceive and give meaning to his own reaction quickly and effortlessly (Branch 1). In addition, he apparently believed that yelling in front of his boss and the client would not be appropriate, knew that he could control this affective behavior, and planned on talking to Nick at a later time to resolve the problem that triggered his affective response. As a result, the skills associated with understanding emotion (Branch 3) and knowing what behaviors are most appropriate for a chosen goal or situation (Branch 2), as well as actually having the skills to manage the emotions as planned (Branch 4), are all evident in our example. In other words, an individual must tap into his or her skills within all four branches of EI to generate emotion regulation strategies that will allow him or her to adapt to the diverse challenges of the social world in an emotionally intelligent manner.

Although skills from all four branches of EI are important, it may be that skills for understanding emotion (Branch 3) are at the heart of intelligent regulation, influencing the other branches and acting as the driving force. In particular, individual differences in the knowledge of emotion expressions and emotion situations are related to positive social behaviors such as empathy, prosocial behaviors, and peer status in children (for a review, see Denham, 1998). In addition, there appears to be a reciprocal relationship between social competence and specific verbal skills (McCabe & Meller, 2004). For example, labeling of emotional expressions at ages 3 and 4 predicts aggressive behavior in subsequent years (Denham et al., 2002). Yet, correlations between emotion knowledge and cognitive ability are moderate, suggesting that factors other than cognitive ability play a role in explaining individual differences in children's emotion knowledge (Bennett, Bandersky, & Lewis, 2005). Beyond the normal developmental maturation of emotion knowledge there are individual differences that are acquired though childhood and influence emotion regulation in adulthood (Saarni, 1999). This understudied link between emotion knowledge (Branch 3) and emotion regulation (Branch 4) is the major focus of this chapter.

EMOTION KNOWLEDGE AND EMOTION REGULATION

When is a particular emotion regulation behavior "intelligent" and how can emotion knowledge help individuals to use more intelligent emotion regulation strategies? First, we need to consider how individuals acquire emotion knowledge and what this emotion knowledge entails. As defined by Gross and Thompson (this volume), an emotion can be understood as some combination of physiological activation, facial and vocal expressions, and actions that individuals try to understand. Typically, children first learn to identify and appreciate basic emotion categories such as *anger, fear,* and *happiness,* and they acquire these categories in an incremental sequence (Widen & Russell, 2003). Part of what a child learns to do is identify facial cues associated with these basic emotion categories and retrieve verbal labels in memory associated with the facial behaviors (Russell & Widen, 2002a, 2002b; Widen & Russell, 2004). Emotion situation knowledge allows a child to infer and anticipate emotions of others and of the self from social cues (Ackermann & Izard, 2004). However, although many adults categorize their feeling-state, or the state of someone else, as belonging to one or more specific categories, such as *fear, anger, sadness,* many other types of descriptions and labels are also used (Scherer, Wranik, Sangsue, Tran, & Scherer, 2004). Indeed, adults have rich and complex affective lives, and emotion vocabulary and conceptual knowledge about emotion in most languages and cultures mirrors this complexity (Averill, 1975; Wierzbicka, 2005).

Acquiring Emotion Knowledge

One way to understand the variety and depth of emotion language and related emotion knowledge is to consider how abstract knowledge is stored and processed. For example, Barsalou (1999) suggests that the conceptual system is strongly linked to perception and that knowledge about abstract concepts (such as concepts for emotion) is stored as perceptual symbols. These perceptual symbols are dynamic and changeable (not fixed), componential (not holistic) and need not represent prototypical exemplars (such as a single prototypical instance of anger). Moreover, the symbol formation process to acquire complex emotion knowledge is multimodal, including all sensory modalities as well as proprioception and interoception.

More specifically, individuals acquire knowledge about a concept such as anger from at least three sources (Barsalou, 1999; Mandler, 1975). First, anger involves a series of evaluations or appraisals of the situation. Second, anger involves a set of physiological sensations that are perceived to some degree (e.g., heart racing and tenseness). Finally, anger often involves behavioral responses and action tendencies (Frijda, 1986). Each time an adult labels a child's behavior with an emotion term, or a child observes the emotion term being used to label someone else's behavior, the child extracts information about that instance, including the psychological situation and interoceptive environment in which the label was used, the behavioral responses that correspond to the label in that context, as well as the regulation strategies that worked and those that did not. All this new information is integrated with past information associated with the same category that is stored in memory. In addition, because emotions are dynamic processes involving numerous sensorimotor components (e.g., physiological activation and facial and vocal behaviors), the child acquires a host of exemplars of what different emotions "feel like" and "look like" and stores these as fuzzy categories. Whether these categories are linked to core affect (Russell, 2003), to core themes (Lazarus, 1991), or to particular underlying appraisal processes (Scherer 2001; Smith & Ellsworth, 1985) is still a matter of debate and warrants further examination.

In this way, multisensory perception and conceptual knowledge about emotions are closely interrelated. As a result, conceptual knowledge influences the way the emotional world is perceived. Conceptual knowledge shapes perception for colors (Roberson, Davies, & Davidoff, 2000) and people (Gilbert, 1998); it seems reasonable that it also helps shape emotion perception (Barrett, 2006). To date, most of the empirical evidence suggesting this relationship comes from face perception. For example, supplying individuals with verbal information about faces improves facial recognition, and learning to group faces into separate categories improves discrimination of different facial expressions (Gauthier, James, Curby, & Tarr, 2003). Furthermore, interfering with the processing of emotion words interferes with emotion perception (Lindquist, Barrett, Bliss-Moreau, & Russell, 2006). Thus, individuals with complex emotion knowledge will perceive and adapt to a variety of emotional signals or feelings and will probably generate more suitable plans for regulation, whereas those with less complex knowledge may be comparatively limited.

Although children's ability to distinguish between abstract perceptual cues increases with their linguistic development (Yoshida & Smith, 2005), the influence of conceptual emotion knowledge on emotion regulation is probably not limited to lexical ability. Recent research suggests that using an action-related concept (such as an emotion concept) may be separate from naming that concept (Tranel, Kemmerer, Adolphs, Damasio, & Damasio, 2003). Thus, John may "know" not to let his anger show in front of his boss but may not be able to describe the emotion he experienced or why he behaved in a particular way. This is consistent with the research on visual processing which has identified separate processing streams for conscious perception (the ventral stream) and action (the dorsal stream; Faw, 2004). Given that multisensory pathways are involved in conceptual knowledge formation, regulation action tendencies are probably stored as complicated "if . . . then . . . " rule packets, much like the rules described in the area of personality by Mischel and his colleagues (e.g., Mischel, 2004; Mischel & Shoda, 1995). These "rules" will influence emotional behaviors just as primed category knowledge can influence behaviors and actions outside conscious awareness. For example, when the concept "old" is activated, college-age participants walk slower, and when the concept "African American" is activated, European American participants act more aggressively (Bargh, Chen, & Burrows, 1996). Thus, when "injustice" is activated, the concept anger may be activated. When the concept "anger" is activated, specific action tendencies may automatically follow under different situational or contextual cues unless the individual has elaborate emotion knowledge structures that can react quickly to changes and modify behaviors accordingly.

Components of Emotion Knowledge

Knowledge is stored as components and not as holistic exemplars (Barsalou, 1999). Thus, complexity of emotion knowledge can be assessed by examining the underlying components, such as cognitive appraisal processes. A cognitive appraisal perspective suggests that the way a particular individual will interpret a specific event will influence and reflect the experience of emotion (e.g., Arnold, 1960; Frijda, 1986; Lazarus, 1968; Roseman, 1991; Scherer, 1984, 2001; Smith & Ellsworth, 1985). In particular, appraisals reflect the conceptual knowledge (both conscious and unconscious) an individual has about the self, the context, and emotions in general, and at the self-reported level, they reflect the explicit knowledge he or she is willing or able to report. For example, appraisals reflect which situations and events an individual considers to be personally relevant, based on current goals and motivations, or personality factors (Smith & Pope, 1992), beliefs about who (self or other) caused a specific event (Weiner, 1986), and how much control one has to do something to change the event (Lazarus & Folkman, 1984). Evaluations also reflect the relative weight an individual places on personal and cultural norms within specific contexts (Scherer, 2001). These subjective evaluations are thought to occur very rapidly, at conscious and unconscious levels, and can essentially lead to as many different affective experiences as there are combinations of cognitive appraisal outcomes (Ellsworth & Scherer, 2003; for a detailed account of appraisal theory, see Scherer, Schorr, & Johnstone, 2001). It is also widely held that there are distinct relations between certain configurations of evaluations and specific emotion categories. For example, fear/anxiety is thought to be associated with evaluating the situation as threatening; sadness with helplessness in an undesirable situation where there is little or no hope of improvement; anger with blaming someone else for an undesirable situation; and guilt with blaming oneself (Smith & Lazarus, 1993).

Emotion Knowledge Influences Regulation

A better understanding of how appraisals fit into the overall conceptual emotion system would be helpful in understanding the role that emotion knowledge plays in successful emotion regulation. Indeed, adults within a given culture, and between cultures to a certain extent, share fundamental agreements in content and structure of their emotions (Russell & Fehr, 1994; Scherer, 1997; Scherer & Wallbott, 1994; Shweder, 1993; cf. Barrett, 2006). Measuring the extent to which people know these prototypes may be, in and of itself, an aptitude that constitutes an important cultural competence that may predict intelligent emotion regulation. However, there are also individual differences and levels of complexity that underlie an emotion concept such as *anger,* and one should not assume that the use of similar terms, evaluations, or expressions reflects similar experiences or rules about their management.

Wranik (2005; Wranik & Scherer, 2006) examined cognitive appraisals and emotion labels in a stressful interactive task. Although anger was a frequently reported emotion, the responses on the appraisal questions indicated that participants were reporting at least two distinct forms of anger—anger at the self and anger at the collaborative partner. Because anger is usually considered to be an other-directed emotion (Averill, 1982; Lazarus, 1991), the emotion label "anger" could easily lead to the erroneous conclusion that those reporting anger in this situation are angry with the interaction partner.

Knowledge of both emotion categories and associated appraisal processes therefore provides a richer understanding of the emotional experience, which should in turn influence which regulation strategies are considered appropriate in a particular situation. For example, if an individual is angry with a colleague, the most effective emotion regulation strategy may be to question why he or she is blaming this person for a particular action and then to focus regulation energy on acquiring additional information. In our example, John realized that the relationships with his boss and the client were important, and that the situation merited careful examination before jumping to conclusions. However, if an individual is angry at the self for mistakes found in an important proposal, then the most effective strategy may be to focus regulation energy on correcting these mistakes and devising strategies to avoid similar mistakes in the future. In other words, intelligent emotion regulation will be related to underlying appraisal processes, conceptual knowledge about specific evaluations and emotions, and the functional utility of different regulation strategies for personal and social goals. If individuals have a less elaborate knowledge system, they may find themselves resorting to simple rules such as "if I feel angry . . . then I suppress all expression of this emotion when I am in public."

More generally, knowledge about emotion, shaped by prior experiences and culture, will influence how emotional episodes unfold. For example, John apparently comes from an individualistic society (such as the United States or Western Europe), where people expect to receive personal credit for hard work. John's emotional reaction therefore reflects both the evaluation that Nick has violated an important norm (taking credit for someone else's work) and the assumption that Nick shares the same values and therefore should have known better than to take credit for his work. We can therefore imagine that John evaluated Nick's behavior as goal obstructive, unjust, and intentional (Averill, 1982; Lazarus, 1991), and that he categorized the psychological event as anger. Most likely, many of us who share John's cultural heritage would also categorize the emotional episode as anger and applaud his ability to inhibit the urge to yell in this particular situation. But what if this situation had taken place in a culture in which individual achievement is less important and where senior partners always present the ideas of their younger colleagues to clients? In this cultural context, John's angry feeling would probably be considered narcissistic and unnecessary and not as emotionally intelligent. Moreover, if he is aware of these cultural norms, John probably would not expect credit for his work, would evaluate Nick's behavior as normal and nonrelevant, and may experience no emotion at all. Or else, John might be proud that his idea was being presented to the client.

Now imagine that John has just started working in East Asia, and that our opening example reflects John's first client meeting in a new environment. Emotion knowledge skills will help determine if John "intelligently" perceives, understands, and regulates his emotion in at least three ways. First, if John correctly perceives that he is having an emotional episode in response to Nick's behavior, then he can consider strategies to minimize the overt physical behaviors until he has decided on a plan of action. Second, if John knows that emotional episodes are generated from his perception and meaning analysis of a particular situation, then he can quickly question if he correctly perceived and evaluated the event and search for missing clues and alternative explanations. Third, the more complex his emotion knowledge, the more alternative explanations he can generate and the more likely he will be able to question his perception and evaluation of emotional events in the future. Of course, most individuals are not aware of their conceptual knowledge about emotion until forced to acknowledge or modify it (e.g., when living or traveling in a country where emotion rules and feeling rules are different, or in therapy). These processes may therefore be relatively unconscious and, if they function, will not be questioned. However, the more complex John's knowledge of emotion, the more likely he can rapidly adjust perception and ensuing interpretation of events to accommodate a variety of novel situations.

Expanding the Process Model of Emotion Regulation

Examining how this conceptual knowledge of emotion influences emotional responding expands Gross's (1998) process model of emotion regulation. There is now considerable evidence to suggest that antecedent strategies provide more effective regulation outcomes than response-focused strategies. Suppression (as a response-focused strategy) decreases positive emotion experience, impairs memory for social information, and compromises social functioning, whereas reappraisal (as an antecedent-focused strategy) has none of these effects (John & Gross, 2004). Furthermore, there are general and systematic differences in the chronic use of antecedent-focused strategies for emotion regulation (Gross & John, 2003). Individuals using cognitive reappraisal strategies are more "intelligent" regulators than suppressors in the situations examined. As a next step, it could be useful to understand how successful reappraisers wield emotion knowledge during emotion perception and regulation.

Although much of the empirical work is yet to be done, there is general support for the idea that elaborate knowledge about emotion is related to better emotion regulation in adults. For example, a series of studies by Philippot and his colleagues (Philippot, Baeyens, Douilliez, & Francart, 2004) suggests that processing emotional information at a general level results in more intense emotional feelings and arousal than does elaborating it on a specific level, and that voluntarily focusing on specific personal emotional information induces less emotional arousal than does thinking about the same information at a general level. In other words, more specific and targeted knowledge positively influences both the generation and regulation of emotion. Similarly, there is evidence that participants with greater ability to differentiate between negative emotional states report a wider range of regulation strategies (Barrett, Gross, Christensen, & Benvenuto, 2001).

More recently, two experience-sampling studies have indicated that representing negative emotion episodes in a highly differentiated manner facilitated targeted emotion regulation (using a set of emotion regulation strategies consistently), whereas representing positive emotion episodes in a highly differentiated manner facilitated exploratory emotion regulation (using emotion regulation strategies variably) (Tugade, Barrett, & Gross, 2006). These findings suggest that the way individuals represent their emotions shapes the way they regulate them. Finally, sophisticated conceptual knowledge of emotions is related to social adaptation. In particular, individuals who describe themselves as having higher emotional complexity, defined as having emotional experiences that are broad in range and well differentiated, are more attentive to their feelings, are more open to new experiences, are more emphatic toward others, and show greater interpersonal adaptability (Kang & Shaver, 2004).

Practical Implications

If more complex conceptual knowledge of emotion leads to a broader repertoire of regulation strategies, then this also has consequences for training and therapeutic intervention. For example, interventions could teach individuals about social norms related to specific emotion categories as well as educate them concerning the underlying evaluations and the impact these may be having on their emotional lives and regulation efforts. In particular, stable individual differences can influence perception and interpretation of events in a relatively consistent manner and may explain why some people generally experience emotions more frequently or intensely, or experience certain types of emotions under specific conditions (Van Reekum & Scherer, 1997). For example, an impatient person chronically may overestimate the urgency of situations, or a perfectionistic individual the importance of particular events. In both cases, these individuals may be faced with many more opportunities to experience emotions that they will then have to regulate effectively. The more elaborate the knowledge about emotion categories and underlying appraisal processes, the more likely the individual will learn to quickly reappraise a situation on specific evaluative criteria before an emotion episode becomes problematic or else to recover by focusing on those appraisals and elements of an event or the self that may matter most for the emotional episode. Thus, perfectionistic individuals can learn to question the importance they attach to many events and adopt strategies to reappraise situations effectively tailored to fit within their overall conceptual knowledge system. Although increased knowledge and understanding of emotions will not necessarily mean that a person can put it into practice, it is probably a first and necessary step.

ABILITY AND EMOTION REGULATION

Thus far, we have argued that emotion regulation can be understood within a broad definition of EI. We have argued that understanding emotion, and using that knowledge to perceive and shape emotional episodes, is an important yet understudied contribution to effective emotion regulation. In this final section, we focus on the premise that effective regulation is not only based on what we know but also on our ability to use what we know (cf. Barrett & Gross, 2001; Barrett, Tugade, & Engle, 2004). Indeed, John may know that he should not yell at his boss; however, if he is a very impulsive person he may not be able to inhibit his desire to do so (Whiteside & Lynam, 2001). Or else, he may be particularly stressed or tired and therefore not have the necessary resources to regulate his emotion within this particular situation (Vohs, Baumeister, & Ciarocco, 2005). Finally, some individuals may be especially challenged to regulate emotions effectively, because cognitive skills in the form of working-memory capacity (WMC) may play an important role.

WMC is best characterized as the ability to control attention during controlled information processing (Barrett et al., 2004). Controlled processing is not necessarily explicit, conscious, or deliberate processing but, instead can be characterized as goal-directed or top-down, conceptual processing (Barrett et al., 2004; Barrett, Ochsner, & Gross, in press). Complex mental processes and social behavior may operate without conscious awareness (cf. Bargh & Ferguson, 2000), but they rarely occur without the control of attention, especially in social situations. Control of attention is necessary for deliberate activation of knowledge, maintenance or enhancement of already activated knowledge, and suppression of unwanted knowledge. Control of attention may also be implicated in the ability to acquire complex and flexible conceptual representations and provide the cognitive muscle to motivate controlled processing that shapes bottom-up, automatic forms of processing (Barrett et al., 2004).

People differ in their ability to control attention and therefore in their ability to engage in all forms of controlled processing, particularly in circumstances in which there is interference or distraction. Individuals higher in WMC can be thought of as motivated tacticians who have multiple information-processing strategies available to them and can select among them on the basis of goals, motives, and the constraints of the environment (Barrett et al., 2004). A motivated tactician, like a person with a large WMC, should have the resources to bring controlled attention to bear on goal-relevant information processing (and all that it implies about managing activation levels of relevant and irrelevant knowledge structures). Individuals lower in WMC can be thought of as cognitive misers who have severely limited attentional resources and as a result adopt strategies that simplify the need for controlled attention (Barrett et al., 2004). Although they may have an array of goals or motives, they do not have the attentional resources to maintain goal-relevant processing in the face of complex situations, such that they end up emphasizing efficiency over any other processing goal.

Individual differences in WMC contribute to proficiency in a wide range of real-world cognitive activities, such as reading and language comprehension, storytelling, following directions, and problem solving (for a review, see Barrett et al., 2004). Significantly, WMC is also strongly related to measures of fluid intelligence, defined by Cattell (1943) as the ability to reason, solve novel problems, and adapt to new situations (Conway, Cowan, Bunting, Therriault, & Minkoff, 2002; Engle, Tuholski, Laughlin, & Conway, 1999; Kyllonen & Christal, 1990). Some consider WMC to be the main processing component that supports fluid intelligence (Kyllonen, 1996).

Working-Memory Capacity and Emotion Regulation

WMC may be related to intelligent emotion regulation in several ways. First, individuals high in WMC may have a greater wealth of exemplar-based information available to them because they may learn more from their prior experience. For example, a rule-based processing system encodes information as exemplars, creating a situated representation of how or when an episodic event occurred, thereby leaving an enduring source memory trace that can be retrieved at a later time (Lee-Sammons & Whitney, 1991). As a result, it is possible that those high in WMC may develop a richer conceptual system for emotion than do those lower in WMC, providing the basis for more flexible and precise evaluations and conceptualizations. In other words, they will have more complex representations of what different emotions "look like" and "feel like."

Second, individuals higher in WMC may have greater resources to bring conceptual emotion knowledge to bear during antecedent forms of emotion regulation that involve shaping an emotional episode. Individuals low in WMC will probably not have sufficient control of their attentional resources to attempt controlled processing. Their emotional episode will therefore often be the direct result of whatever conceptual emotion knowledge is evoked by bottom-up automatic processing. Thus, they are more likely to use the simple "if I feel angry . . . then I suppress all expression of this emotion when I am in public" rules already discussed, even if they know that other strategies may be more useful. In contrast, those higher in WMC will have the attentional resources to engage in controlled processing and to generate emotional episodes in more strategic and flexible manner. Of course, under conditions of extreme cognitive load, such as very stressful situations, this advantage would disappear. And it is also possible that individuals lower in WMC may fare better in situations that call for quick action when those higher in WMC may engage in unnecessary top-down attentional control, such as excessive rumination.

Third, individuals higher in WMC may be better able to implement effortful control during response-focused emotion regulation and inhibit unwanted but strong behavioral or cognitive responses when they desire to do so. These differences would be most apparent under cognitive load, such as during an emotional episode that emerges in a complex social situation like the one described at the beginning of the chapter. Individuals who are low in WMC may show "functional modularity" to their emotional episodes, such that processing constraints make emotional responses appear more modular and cognitively inflexible than those with higher WMC (see Barrett et al., 2004, for a more detailed discussion). As a result, these individuals will have difficulties reappraising events that triggered an emotional episode, to rapidly imagine alternative hypotheses that explain the behaviors of other persons, or to come up with different regulation strategies for various goals. Thus, if John has low WMC, he may engage in some form of verbal protest during the meeting with the client and his boss and not immediately understand the implications of his actions until it is too late. He may "know" that he should not allow his anger to show under these conditions (e.g., such as when asked on a questionnaire) but may not have the cognitive resources to disentangle the "emotion module" once it is triggered.

Finally, WMC may assist in the ability to resist the attentional capture from negative information and may influence the ability to suppress previously learned affective associations. As a consequence, individuals higher in WMC may have affective systems that are perturbed less often, resulting in fewer events to regulate in the first place.

CONCLUSION

The EI model (Mayer & Salovey, 1997; Salovey & Mayer, 1990) can be seen as an organizing framework for understanding individual differences in effective emotional transactions within a social world. Our goal with this chapter was to use the EI framework as a starting point to open up new lines of inquiry into the scientific understanding of effective emotion regulation. Within this framework, emotion regulation is both a component of EI (e.g., Branch 4) as well as a complex set of abilities anchored within the entire emotion process. However, it may be that skills related to emotion knowledge (Branch 3) are center stage for predicting intelligent emotion regulation and the royal road for interventions when regulation is less than optimal. In particular, conceptual knowledge is used to support perception and action (Branch 1) and will help an individual to decide when and how to regulate (Branch 2). What we know about emotions, ourselves, and our social world will determine what we perceive, if and why we chose to regulate, and the strategies we ultimately employ.

Of course, we are not suggesting that individuals need to be certified emotion psychologists to be emotionally intelligent regulators. The implicit knowledge learned through prior experiences and social interactions allow most of us to function relatively well. In addition, actual performance in emotion regulation is a combination of skills and motivation. Some individuals will be more challenged than others in their regulation attempts because they lack important cognitive resources, are blessed with highly reactive or anxious temperaments, or did not have the kinds of social interactions that foster the conceptual knowledge required. However, we are hopeful that many can improve their emotion regulation skills by learning more about emotions and by putting new knowledge into practice.

ACKNOWLEDGMENTS

We would like to thank the three anonymous reviewers for their helpful comments and suggestions. Preparation of this chapter was supported by Grant No. NIMH K02 MH001981 from the National Cancer Institute to Lisa Feldman Barrett, Grant No. R01 CA68427 from the National Cancer Institute to Peter Salovey, and a postdoctoral fellowship grant awarded by the Swiss National Science Foundation to Tanja Wranik.

REFERENCES

Ackerman, B. P., & Izard, C. (2004). Emotion cognition in children and adolescents: Introduction to the special issue. *Journal of Experimental Child Psychology, 84,* 271–275.

Arnold, M. (1960). *Emotion and personality.* New York: Columbia University Press.

Averill, J. R. (1975). A semantic atlas of emotion concepts. *Catalog of Selected Documents in Psychology, 5,* 33–65.

Averill, J. R. (1982). *Anger and aggression: An essay on emotion.* New York: Springer.

Bargh, J. A., Chen, M., & Burrows, L. (1996). Automaticity of social behavior: Direct effects of trait construct and stereotype activation on action. *Journal of Personality and Social Psychology, 71,* 230–244.

Bargh, J. A., & Ferguson, M. J. (2000). Beyond behaviorism: On the automaticity of higher mental processes. *Psychological Bulletin, 126,* 925–945.

Barrett, L. F. (1998). Discrete emotions or dimensions? The role of valence focus and arousal focus. *Cognition and Emotion, 12,* 579–599.

Barrett, L. F. (2004). Feelings or words? Understanding the content in self-report ratings of experienced emotion. *Journal of Personality and Social Psychology, 87,* 266–281.

Barrett, L. F. (2006). Solving the emotion paradox: Categorization and the experience of emotion. *Personality and Social Psychology Review, 10,* 20–46.

Barrett, L. F., & Gross, J. J. (2001). Emotional intelligence: A process model of emotion representation and regulation. In T. J. Mayne & G. A. Bonanno (Eds.), *Emotions: Current issues and future directions: Emotions and social behavior* (pp. 286–310). New York: Guilford Press.

Barrett, L. F., Gross, J., Christensen, T. C., & Benvenuto, M. (2001). Knowing what you're feeling and knowing what to do about it: Mapping the relation between emotion differentiation and emotion regulation. *Cognition and Emotion, 15,* 713–724.

Barrett, L. F., Ochsner, K. N., & Gross, J. J. (in press). On the automaticity of emotion. In J. Bargh (Ed.), *Social psychology and the unconscious: The automaticity of higher mental processes.* New York: Psychology Press.

Barrett, L. F., Tugade, M. M., & Engle, R. W. (2004). Individual differences in working memory capacity and dual-process theories of the mind. *Psychological Bulletin, 130,* 553–573.

Barsalou, L. W. (1999). Perceptual symbol systems. *Behavioral and Brain Sciences, 22,* 577–660.

Baum, K. M., & Nowicki, S. (1998). Perception of emotion: Measuring decoding accuracy of adult prosodic cues varying in intensity. *Journal of Nonverbal Behavior, 22,* 89–107.

Bennett, D. S., Bandersky, M., & Lewis, M. (2005). Antecedents of emotion knowledge: Predictors of individual differences in young children. *Cognition and Emotion, 19,* 375–396.

Brackett, M. A., Mayer, J. D., & Warner, R. M. (2004). Emotional intelligence and its relation to everyday behavior. *Personality and Individual Differences, 36,* 1387–1402.

Cattell, R. B. (1943). The measurement of adult intelligence. *Psychological Bulletin, 40,* 153–193.

Clore, G. L., & Parrott, W. G. (1991). Moods and their vicissitudes: Thoughts and feelings as information. In J. P. Forgas (Ed.), *Emotion and social judgment* (pp. 107–123). Oxford, UK: Pergamon Press.

Conway, A. R., Cowan, N., Bunting, M. F., Therriault, D. J., & Minkoff, S. R. (2002). A latent variable analysis of working memory capacity, short-term memory capacity, processing speed, and general fluid intelligence. *Intelligence, 30,* 163–184.

Damasio, A. R. (1994). *Descartes' error: Emotion, reason, and the human brain.* New York: Avon Books.

Denham, S. A. (1998). *Emotional development in young children.* New York: Guilford Press.

Denham, S. A., Caverly, S., Schmidt, M., Blair, K., DeMulder, E., Caal, S., et al. (2002). Preschool understanding of emotions: Contributions to classroom anger and aggression. *Journal of Child Psychology and Psychiatry, 43,* 901–916.

Ekman, P., & Friesen, W. V. (1975). *Unmasking the face: A guide to recognizing the emotions from facial cues.* Englewood Cliffs, NJ: Prentice Hall.

Ellsworth, P. C., & Scherer, K. R. (2003). Appraisal processes in emotion. In R. J. Davidson, K. R. Scherer, & H. H. Goldsmith (Eds.), *Handbook of affective sciences* (pp. 572–595). Oxford, UK: Oxford University Press.

Engle, R. W., Tuholski, S. W., Laughlin, J. E., & Conway, A. R. (1999). Working memory, short-term memory, and general fluid intelligence: A latent variable approach. *Journal of Experimental Psychology: General, 128,* 309–331.

Faw, B. (2004). Sight unseen: Exploration of conscious and unconscious vision. *Journal of Consciousness Studies, 11,* 92–94

Feldman, L. A. (1995). Valence focus and arousal focus: Individual differences in the structure of affective experience. *Journal of Personality and Social Psychology, 69,* 153–166.

Frijda, N. H. (1986). *The emotions.* New York: Cambridge University Press.

Frijda, N. H. (1988). The laws of emotion. *American Psychologist, 43,* 349–358.

Gauthier, I., James, T. W., Curby, K. M., & Tarr, M. J. (2003). The influence of conceptual knowledge on visual discriminations. *Cognitive Neuropsychology, 20,* 507–523.

Gilbert, D. T. (1998). Ordinary personology. In D. T. Gilbert, S. T. Fiske, & G. Lindzey (Eds.), *The handbook of social psychology* (4th ed., pp. 37–51). New York: McGraw Hill.

Gilbert, D. T., Pinel, E. C., Wilson, T. D., Blumberg, S. J., & Wheatley, T. P. (1998). Immune neglect: A source of durability bias in affective forecasting. *Journal of Personality and Social Psychology, 75,* 617–636.

Gray, J. R., Schaefer, A., Braver, T. S., & Most, S. B. (2005). Affect and the resolution of cognitive control dilemmas. In L. F. Barrett, P. M. Niedenthal, & P. Winkielman (Eds.), *Emotion and consciousness* (pp. 67–94). New York: Guilford Press.

Gross, J. J. (1998). The emerging field of emotion regulation: An integrative review. *Review of General Psychology, 2,* 271–299.

Gross, J. J., & John, O. P. (2003). Individual differences in two emotion regulation processes: Implications for affect, relationships, and well-being. *Journal of Personality and Social Psychology, 85,* 348–362.

Gross, J. J., & Thompson, R. A. (2007). Emotion regulation: Conceptual foundations. In J. J. Gross (Ed.), *Handbook of emotion regulation* (pp. 3–24). New York: Guilford Press.

Isen, A. M. (1987). Positive affect, cognitive processes, and social behavior. In L. Berkowitz (Ed.), *Advances in experimental social psychology* (Vol. 20, pp. 203–253). New York: Academic Press.

John, O. P., & Gross, J. J. (2004). Healthy and unhealthy emotion regulation: Personality processes, individual differences, and life span development. *Journal of Personality, 72,* 1301–1333.

Johnstone, T., Van Reekum, C., & Scherer, K. R. (2001). Vocal expression correlates of appraisal processes. In K. R. Scherer, A. Schorr, & T. Johnstone (Eds.), *Appraisal processes in emotion: Theory, methods, research* (pp. 271–284). New York: Oxford University Press.

Kang, S. M., & Shaver, P. R. (2004). Individual differences in emotional complexity: Their psychological implications. *Journal of Personality, 72,* 687–726.

Kyllonen, P. C. (1996). Is working memory capacity Spearman's g? In I. Dennis & P. Tapsfield (Eds.), *Human abilities: Their nature and measurement* (pp. 49–75). Hillsdale, NJ: Erlbaum.

Kyllonen, P. C., & Christal, R. E. (1990). Reasoning abilities is (little more than) working memory capacity? *Intelligence, 14,* 389–433.

Lane, R. D., Quinlan, D. M., Schwartz, G. E., Walker, P. A., & Zeitlin, S. B. (1990). The levels of emotional awareness scale: A cognitive–developmental measure of emotion. *Journal of Personality Assessment, 55,* 124–134.

Lazarus, R. S. (1968). Emotions and adaptations: Conceptual and empirical relations. *Nebraska Symposium on Motivation, 16,* 175–266.

Lazarus, R. S. (1991). *Emotion and adaptation.* New York: Oxford University Press.

Lazarus, R. S., & Folkman, S. (1984). *Stress, appraisal and coping.* New York: Springer.

Lee-Sammons, W. H., & Whitney, P. (1991). Reading perspectives and memory for text: An individual differences analysis. *Journal of Experimental Psychology: Learning, Memory, and Cognition, 17,* 1074–1081.

Lewis, M. (2000). The emergency of human emotions. In M. Lewis & J. M. Haviland-Jones (Eds.), *Handbook of emotions* (2nd ed., pp. 265–280). New York: Guilford Press.

Linquist, K., Barrett, L. F., Bliss-Moreau, E., & Russell, J. A. (2006). Language and the perception of emotion, *Emotion, 6,* 125–138.

Lopes, P. N., Brackett, M. A., Nezlek, J. B., Schuetz, A., Sellin, I., & Salovey, P. (2004). Emotional intelligence and social interaction. *Personality and Social Psychology Bulletin, 8,* 1018–1034.

Lopes, P. N., Grewal, D., Kadis, J., Gall, M., & Salovey, P. (in press). Evidence that emotional intelligence is related to job performance and affect and attitudes at work. *Psicothema.*

Lopes, P. N., Salovey, P., Côté, S., & Beers, M. (2005). Emotion regulation abilities and the quality of social interaction. *Emotion, 5,* 2005.

Lopes, P. N., Salovey, P., & Straus, R. (2003). Emotional intelligence, personality, and the perceived quality of social relationships. *Personality and Individual Differences, 35,* 641–659.

Mandler, G. (1975). *Mind and emotion.* New York: Wiley.

Mandler, G. (1984). *Mind and body: The psychology of emotion and stress.* New York: Norton.

Mayer, J. D., & Salovey, P. (1997). What is emotional intelligence? In P. Salovey, & D. Sluyter (Eds.), *Emotional development and emotional intelligence: Educational implications* (pp. 3–31). New York: Basic Books.

McCabe, P. C., & Meller, P. J. (2004). The relationship between language and social competence: How language impairment affects social growth. *Psychology in the Schools, 41,* 313–321.

Mischel, W. (2004). Toward an integrative science of the person. *Annual Review of Psychology, 55,* 1–22.

Mischel, W., & Shoda, Y. (1995). A cognitive–affective system theory of personality: Reconceptualizing situations, dispositions, dynamics, and invariance in personality structure. *Psychological Review, 102,* 246–268.

Nowicki, S., & Duke, M. (1994). Individual differences in the nonverbal communication of affect: The diagnostic Analysis of Nonverbal Accuracy Scale. Special Issue: Development of nonverbal behavior: II. Social development and nonverbal behavior. *Journal of Nonverbal Behavior, 18,* 9–35.

Nowicki, S. J., & Mitchell, J. (1998). Accuracy in identifying affect in child and adult faces and voices and social competence in preschool children. *Genetic, Social, and General Psychology Monographs, 124,* 39–59.

Palfai, T. P., & Salovey, P. (1993). The influence of depressed and elated mood on deductive and inductive reasoning. *Imagination, Cognition, and Personality, 13,* 57–71.

Petti, V. L., Voelker, S. L., Shore, D. L., & Hayman-Abello, S. E. (2003). Perception of nonverbal emotion cues by children with nonverbal learning disabilities. *Journal of Developmental Disabilities, 15,* 23–36.

Philippot, P., Baeyens, C., Douilliez, C., & Francart, B. (2004). Cognitive regulation of emotion: Application to clinical disorders. In P. Philippot & R. S. Feldman (Eds.), *The regulation of emotion* (pp. 71–97). Mahwah, NJ: Erlbaum.

Roberson, D., Davies, I., & Davidoff, J. (2000). Color categories are not universal: Replications and new evidence from a stone-age culture. *Journal of Experimental Psychology: General, 129,* 369–398.

Roseman, I. (1984). Cognitive determinants of emotions: A structural theory. In P. Shaver (Ed.), *Review of personality and social psychology: Vol. 5. Emotions, relationships, and health* (pp. 11–36). Beverly Hills, CA: Sage.

Roseman, I. J. (1991). Appraisal determinants of discrete emotions. *Cognition and Emotion, 5,* 161–200.

Russell, J. A. (2003). Core affect and the psychological construction of emotion. *Psychological Review, 110,* 145–172

Russell, J. A., & Fehr, B. (1994). Fuzzy concepts in a fuzzy hierarchy: Varieties of anger. *Journal of Personality and Social Psychology, 67,* 186–205.

Russell, J. A., & Widen, S. C. (2002a). Words versus faces in evoking preschool children's knowledge of the causes of emotions. *International Journal of Behavioral Development, 26,* 97–103.

Russell, J. A., & Widen, S. C. (2002b). A label superiority effect in children's categorization of facial expressions. *Social Development, 11,* 30–52.

Saarni, C. (1999). *The development of emotional competence.* New York: Guilford Press.

Salovey, P., & Mayer, J. D. (1990). Emotional intelligence. *Imagination, Cognition and Personality, 9,* 185–211.

Scherer, K. R. (1984). On the nature and function of emotion: A component process approach. In K. R. Scherer & P. Ekman (Eds.), *Approaches to emotion* (pp. 293–317). Hillsdale, NJ: Lawrence Erlbaum.

Scherer, K. R. (1997). The role of culture in appraisal. *Journal of Personality and Social Psychology, 73,* 902–922.

Scherer, K. R. (2001). Appraisal considered as a process of multi-level sequential checking. In K. R. Scherer, A. Schorr, & T. Johnstone (Eds.), *Appraisal processes in emotion: Theory, methods, research* (pp. 92–120). New York: Oxford University Press.

Scherer, K. R., Schorr, A., & Johnstone T. (Eds.). (2001). *Appraisal processes in emotion: Theory, methods, research.* New York: Oxford University Press.

Scherer, K. R., & Wallbott, H. G. (1994). Evidence for universality and cultural variation of differential emotion response patterning. *Journal of Personality and Social Psychology, 66,* 310–328.

Scherer, K. R., Wranik, T., Sangsue, J., Tran, V., & Scherer, U. (2004). Emotions in everyday life: Probability of occurrence, risk factors, appraisal, and reaction patterns. *Social Science Information, 43,* 499–570.

Schwarz, N. (1990). Feelings as information: Informational and motivational functions of affective states. In R. Sorrentino & E. T. Higgins (Eds.), *Handbook of motivation and cognition* (Vol. 2, pp. 527–561). New York: Guilford Press.

Schwarz, N., & Clore, G. L. (1983). Mood, misattribution, and judgments of well-being: Informative and directive functions of affective states. *Journal of Personality and Social Psychology, 45,* 513–523.

Schwarz, N., & Clore, G. (1996). Feelings and phenomenal experiences. In E. T. Higgins & A. W. Kruglanski (Eds.), *Social psychology: Handbook of basic principles* (pp. 433–465). New York: Guilford Press.

Shweder, R. A. (1993). The cultural psychology of the emotions. In M. Lewis & J. M. Haviland (Eds.), *Handbook of emotions* (pp. 417–431). New York: Guilford Press.

Smith, C. A., & Ellsworth, P. C. (1985). Patterns of cognitive appraisal in emotion. *Journal of Personality and Social Psychology, 48,* 813–838.

Smith, C. A., & Lazarus, R. S. (1993). Appraisal components, core relational themes, and the emotions. *Cognition and Emotion, 7,* 233–269.

Smith, C. A., & Pope, L. K. (1992). Appraisal and emotion: The interactional contribution of dispositional and situational factors. In M. S. Clark (Ed.), *Review of personality and social psychology, Volume 14: Emotions and social behavior* (pp. 32–62). Newbury Park, CA: Sage.

Tranel, D., Kemmerer, D., Adolphs, R., Damasio, H., & Damasio, A. R. (2003). Neural correlates of conceptual knowledge for actions. *Cognitive Neuropsychology, 20,* 409–432.

Tugade, M. M., Barrett, L. F., & Gross, J. J. (2006). *Matters of feeling precisely: Emotional granularity and emotion regulation*. Manuscript in preparation, Vassar College.

Van Reekum, C. A., & Scherer, K. R. (1997). Levels of processing in emotion-antecedent appraisal. In G. Matthews (Ed.), *Cognitive science perspectives on personality and emotion* (pp. 259–300). New York: Elsevier.

Vohs, K. D., Baumeister, R. F., & Ciarocco, N. J. (2005). Self-regulation and self-presentation: Regulatory resource depletion impairs impression management and effortful self-presentation depletes regulatory resources. *Journal of Personality and Social Psychology, 88*, 632–657.

Weiner, B. (1986). *An attributional theory of motivation and emotion.* New York: Springer.

Whiteside, S. P., & Lynam, D. R. (2001). The five factor model and impulsivity: Using a structural model of personality to understand impulsivity. *Personality and Individual Differences, 30*, 669–689.

Widen, S. C., & Russell, J. A. (2003). A closer look at preschoolers' freely produced labels for facial expressions. *Developmental Psychology, 39*, 114–128.

Widen, S. C., & Russell, J. A. (2004). The relative power of an emotion's facial expression, label, and behavioral consequence to evoke preschoolers' knowledge of its cause. *Cognitive Development, 19*, 111–125.

Wierzbicka, A. (2005). Empirical universals of language as a basis for the study of other human universals and as a tool for exploring cross-cultural differences. *Ethos, 33*, 256–291.

Wranik, T. (2005). *Personality under stress, who get's angry and why?: Individual differences in appraisal and emotion.* Unpublished doctoral dissertation, University of Geneva, Switzerland.

Wranik, T., & Scherer, K. R. (2006). *The dark side of optimism: Blaming others for failure.* Unpublished manuscript.

Yoshida, H., & Smith, L. B. (2005). Linguistic cues enhance the learning of perceptual cues. *Psychological Science, 16*, 90–95.

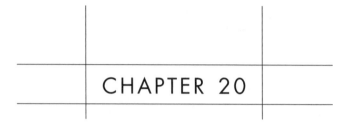

CHAPTER 20

How Emotions Facilitate and Impair Self-Regulation

ROY F. BAUMEISTER
ANNE L. ZELL
DIANNE M. TICE

Bugs, trees, and snakes may thrive and prosper without much in the way of either self-regulation or emotion, but human life is quite different. Probably few days go by without either emotion or self-regulation. Indeed, both emotion and self-regulation may be essential to effective human functioning, at least in the complex cultural worlds in which most people live. It is possible to study emotion or self-regulation separately, but in daily experience they are often interconnected. But how?

Most chapters in this volume focus on the self-regulation of emotion, which is to say the effects of self-regulatory processes on emotion. In this chapter, the perspective is reversed, and we look at the effects of mood and emotion on self-regulation. We use "emotion" as a general term that includes discrete emotions, mood, and affect (see Gross & Thompson, this volume). Furthermore, we consider emotion regulation to be one specific type of self-regulation (Tice & Bratslavsky, 2000). The differences between the self-regulation of emotion and the effects of emotion on self-regulation are perhaps not as fully opposite as they may seem at first blush, but they do raise very different questions and emphases.

The most familiar and important issue in this connection is the negative impact that emotional distress has on self-regulation. The main part of this chapter covers research indicating that unpleasant emotional states tend to cause self-regulation to break down. There is no single causal mechanism for this, and in fact there may be quite a few different causal pathways leading from emotional distress to self-regulation failure.

On the other hand, emotion is not uniformly bad for self-regulation. Hence the final part of this chapter seeks to provide some balance by noting some ways in which emotion (both positive and negative) has been shown to improve self-regulatory functioning.

HOW DISTRESS[1] IMPAIRS SELF-REGULATION

Along with clinicians, lawyers, parents, and indeed the general public, researchers have long observed that self-control appears to deteriorate when people are experiencing acute states of unpleasant emotion. Even the traditional folk concept of counting to 10 before saying anything when one is angry implies that intense emotion can cause people to say or do things that they will later regret, and these are presumably things from which the person would normally refrain. Likewise, common stereotypes suggest that when people are upset, they are more likely than otherwise to break their diets, indulge in substance abuse, or perform other behaviors that they would regulate (successfully) under other circumstances.

Ample research findings have confirmed that emotional distress undermines self-regulation. Anxiety, depression, and other bad feelings lead people (especially overweight people and dieters) to eat more than they usually would (Greeno & Wing, 1994; Heatherton & Polivy, 1992; Logue, 1993; Slochower & Kaplan, 1980). Cigarette smoking increases when people are distressed or upset (Ashton & Stepney, 1982; Schachter et al., 1977), and people who are trying to quit are more likely to relapse when they are emotionally upset (Brownell, Marlatt, Lichtenstein, & Wilson, 1986). Alcohol use and abuse also are stimulated by emotional distress, partly because people believe that drinking alcohol will counteract anxiety and improve one's emotional state (Sayette, 1993; Stockwell, 1985). Efforts to quit drinking are sometimes undermined and defeated by emotional distress (Hull, Young, & Jouriles, 1986; Pickens, Hatsukami, Spicer, & Svikis, 1985). There is some evidence that gambling and compulsive shopping, both of which defeat the self-regulation of money expenditure, are more common in response to emotional distress (O'Guinn & Faber, 1987; Peck, 1986). Last, delay of gratification appears to suffer when people are in a sad mood or other unpleasant emotional state (Fry, 1975; Mischel, Ebbesen, & Zeiss, 1973; Underwood, Moore, & Rosenhan, 1973; Wertheim & Schwartz, 1983).

Reviews of the literature on self-defeating behavior likewise have repeatedly concluded that emotional distress is a common theme and contributing factor to a wide range of self-defeating behaviors (e.g., Baumeister, 1997; Baumeister & Scher, 1988). Self-defeating behavior reflects a failure to guide one's behavior toward desired, beneficial outcomes, and as such self-regulation failure is often central to it (Baumeister, 1997).

Put another way, few experts would dispute the idea that emotional distress can interfere with effective self-regulation. Specifying the precise mechanism by which emotions have that effect, however, is difficult. Most likely there are multiple pathways. This section considers several.

Shifting Priorities

Most likely evolution gave human beings their exceptionally powerful capacity for self-regulation because it would bring them benefits in various ways, especially in terms of long-range outcomes. Self-regulation confers the capacity to seek delayed rather than immediate gratifications (Mischel, 1974, 1996). Foregoing short-term temptations to pursue distal goals of longevity, fitness, thinness, education, wealth, and other options has enabled humans to make their lives happy and comfortable in ways most animals cannot even imagine.

To accomplish these long-term beneficial outcomes, much of self-regulation is specifically geared toward foregoing the pleasures of short-term temptations. Therein lies the seeds of a possible problem, however. Sometimes—and perhaps especially when people are feeling acutely bad, as during emotional distress—people want to feel good right now, or as soon as possible.

There is thus a basic and recurring conflict between many self-regulatory programs and the goal of escaping from emotional distress. Or, to put this another way, there is a basic conflict between emotion and mood regulation (here, defined as the common effort to escape from bad emotions and moods and/or enter good emotions and moods) and other forms of self-regulation. Thus, one aspect of self-regulation—emotion regulation—may sometimes demand precedence over other aspects of self-regulation, to their detriment. Many behaviors are regulated because they feel good and therefore tempt the person to indulge in them to a degree that can be costly in the long run. During emotional distress, however, the long run may seem to matter less, whereas the acute bad feelings in the present moment stimulate the desire to make them stop. Short-term but costly pleasures therefore grow more appealing to the emotionally upset person.

From this reasoning, several of us developed the hypothesis that emotional distress would cause self-regulation failure—because the distraught individual is trying to make him- or herself feel better (Tice, Bratslavsky, & Baumeister, 2001). The key to testing this was to show that people in such emotional states would fail to self-regulate if they thought indulgence might make them feel better, whereas they would not fail at self-regulation if there were no corresponding expectation of mood repair. To accomplish this, we adapted a procedure developed by Manucia, Baumann, and Cialdini (1984) informally known as the *mood-freezing manipulation*. Those authors sought to show that sadness leads to helping because people believe that helping will cure their sadness. They gave some participants a pill and told them that one side effect of the pill was that their current emotional state would be impervious to change for about an hour. Sad people would therefore remain sad for that period, regardless of what they did. Sure enough, Manucia et al. (1984) found that sad people who had taken the mood-freezing pill did not help. Other sad participants, however, who believed their moods were alterable, did increase their helping, suggesting that people were helping in order to improve mood.

Our first study explored the familiar notion that emotional distress causes people to eat fattening and unhealthy (but tasty) food. We induced either a happy or sad mood in people by having them engage in a guided imagery exercise, following the procedure developed by Wenzlaff, Wegner, and Roper (1988) in which people imagine themselves either saving a child's life or accidentally causing a child's death in a traffic accident. Then they participated in an ostensible taste test in which they were to rate cookies, pretzels, and cheese crackers. For our mood-freezing manipulation, we did not use a mood-freezing pill per se in this study. Rather, we relied on the simple expedient of telling some participants the truth. The experimenter in the mood-freezing condition explained that many people believe that eating good-tasting foods will make them feel better but research has clearly shown this belief to be false. She concluded, "Whatever mood you are in right now, you are very likely to stay in the same mood throughout the experiment." In the control condition no such instructions were given. The food tasting and rating task was a sham, and in reality the main measure was how much people ate.

Consistent with the standard view that emotional distress impairs self-regulation, sad participants in the control condition ate more than happy participants. (There was also evidence from a separate survey that students in that population recognized such foods as unhealthy and normally sought to restrain how much of them they ate.) In the mood-freeze condition, however, sad participants did not eat more than happy participants. In fact, sad participants in the mood-freeze condition ate the least of all four conditions. The implication is that sad people eat junk food in the expectation of feeling better. When that expectation is removed, sad people do not eat. Sad people's eating less than happy people in the mood-freeze condition may be strong evidence of their shifted priorities leading to lack of interest in anything that they do not think will make them feel better immediately.

A similar conclusion emerged from two further studies. One of them involved delay of gratification, using a resource management game. This game was developed by Knapp and Clark (1991) as a classic commons dilemma demonstration to simulate the problem of managing fish stock: The short-term gain is to harvest as many fish as possible to maximize immediate profits, but long-term gains are maximized by harvesting slowly so that the fish will replenish themselves (because only the fish left alive will reproduce). Knapp and Clark showed that sad participants depleted the fish stock rapidly via premature harvesting, thus confirming that sadness leads to self-regulation failure. We replicated their finding but added a mood-freeze condition using an ostensibly mood-freezing candle with an aromatherapy cover story, and it eliminated the effect, especially among people who were chronic mood regulators (Catanzaro & Mearns, 1990). Thus, seeking immediate gratification when sad fits the priority shift pattern described, in which emotional distress shifts one's priorities from long-term goals to feeling better immediately. Sad people want to feel good now, and so they indulge in immediate temptations (and especially if they are mood regulators). But if the prospect of escaping from sadness is removed, then sad people do not shift toward seeking immediate gratification.

Procrastination was the focus of our third study. Procrastination is an important and sometimes costly form of self-regulation failure (Ferrari, Johnson, & McCown, 1995; Flett, Hewitt, & Martin, 1995; Shouwenburg, 1995; Tice & Baumeister, 1997). One reason procrastination occurs is that working on tasks requires the person to forego the pleasures and temptations of the moment in order to concentrate on distant deadlines and the sometimes dull or aversive steps toward them. People who feel bad may be more swayed by such temptations and the immediate promise of pleasure. We found that sad participants in the control (no-mood-freeze) condition procrastinated on an upcoming laboratory test, preferring to play video games and read magazines instead of studying. They did not embrace all time wasters, however: When the distracting tasks were dull (e.g., reading out-of-date technical journals or playing with preschool-level puzzles), they worked on the task the same as most other participants. In the mood-freeze condition, however, even the pleasant distractors failed to tempt sad participants away from studying for the test. Thus, sad people procrastinate when they expect that doing so will make them feel better, and only then.

These studies undermine the view that emotion directly causes many behaviors. Rather, the behavioral effects of these emotions are strategic: They are guided by the anticipation of change in emotional state. If sadness directly caused self-regulation to fail, it would have done so even in the mood-freeze conditions. But it did not. Instead, sad people only yielded to temptations and failed at self-regulation when they had reason to expect that these indulgences would make them feel better.

The broader implication is that emotional distress shifts one's priority and focus away from the distal goals that underpin most self-regulatory efforts. Instead, sad people focus on feeling better in the short run. Apparently they are often willing to sacrifice some of their progress toward long-term goals in order to escape from their aversive emotional state.

Ignoring Relevant Information

A widely cited fact about the influence of emotion on decision is its insensitivity to probabilities. That is, emotional processes react strongly to the size of relevant outcomes, but they react weakly to comparable shifts in the probabilities. Loewenstein, Weber, Hsee, and Welch (2001) illustrated this point by noting that one can feel quite differently about winning $10,000 versus $10 million—although both would be positive events, the latter would alter one's life in sweeping ways that the former cannot. In contrast, the difference in odds between 1 in 10,000 and 1 in 10 million (such as one's chances of winning either sum) scarcely registers on one's emotional system.

Early evidence for the insensitivity of emotion to probabilistic outcomes was provided by Monat, Averill, and Lazarus (1972). They showed that when people anticipated a possible electric shock at a particular moment, their arousal levels increased as that moment approached (and decreased afterward). The probability of getting the shock did not alter the degree of arousal (unless it was zero). Thus, the body's arousal and emotional system responded to threat without registering the likelihood of a bad outcome.

Some emotions can cause people to ignore relevant information, in ways that contribute to self-defeating behavior and failures at self-regulation, as shown by Leith and Baumeister (1996). This investigation was designed to investigate the link between emotional distress and self-defeating behavior, and the central hypothesis was that distress would cause people to take foolish risks. (This was intended to replace previous, largely discredited theories about the impact of emotion on self-defeating behavior, such as the view that guilt makes people desire to suffer.) Participants chose between two lotteries, one of which contained a small chance at a large reward—and an expected gain that was substantially worse than the other lottery. Across a series of studies, participants in good or neutral moods generally made the sensible choice of the lottery with the better expected gain, but participants who were in aversive emotional states characterized by high-arousal states—especially anger and embarrassment—shifted toward favoring the high-risk, high-payoff lottery. Thus, emotional distress led to foolish risk taking. Consistent with this finding, research by Lerner and Keltner (2000, 2001) suggests that different negatively valenced emotions, such as fear and anger, may produce distinct effects on people's tendency to make risky choices.

In one study, Leith and Baumeister (1996) sought to undo the effect of emotional distress. Their initial theory had been that people in bad moods reappraise the outcomes based on having less to lose (because of already feeling bad) and more to gain, but multiple measures across several studies had failed to provide any support for that. Instead, then, they thought that perhaps emotional distress caused people to cut short their processing of relevant information, as suggested by some prior research on stress (Keinan, 1987). Hence they added a condition in which they instructed angry participants to pause for a minute and list the pros and cons of each lottery before choosing. These participants chose the play-it-safe lottery, just like neutral and happy participants.

The implication is that emotional distress caused people to attend only to the magnitude of the possible outcome and to ignore the odds. Hence when people were upset, they selected the option with the best possible outcome, even though that option carried a 98% of a bad outcome. A failure to regulate one's attention and cognitive processes to incorporate all the relevant information mediated between the unpleasant emotional state and the self-defeating outcome.

Escaping Self-Awareness

One of the landmark events in the evolution of self-regulation theory was the publication of *Attention and Self-Regulation* (Carver & Scheier, 1981). Carver and Scheier had been known as self-awareness researchers, indeed gradually taking leadership roles in an area that had rapidly burgeoned during the 1970s. Everyone expected that their book would be essentially a summary of self-awareness, but they chose to leave self-awareness out of the title. Their point was to suggest a functional purpose for human self-awareness. Specifically, they proposed that people attend to themselves for the purpose of regulating their responses.

Although the field may have been slow to catch on, the links between self-awareness and self-regulation have continued to be verified in subsequent work. Indeed, it is quite hard to regulate any behavior without paying some attention to it (see Baumeister, Heatherton, & Tice, 1994a, for review). As Carver and Scheier (1981, 1982) pointed out, self-awareness is typically more than simply directing attention to some feature of the self or inner state. Rather, it almost invariably contains comparison to some standard, whereas earlier self-awareness research had treated the comparison to standards as either a quaint coincidence or a distraction, Carver and Scheier proposed that the standards were central to what self-awareness was meant to accomplish. Self-regulation is a process of altering oneself to meet various standards, and so necessarily it relied on careful comparison of one's current actual state with the goal or standard. This is often useful and adaptive, and we shall return to the point later, in our discussion of the positive influence of emotion on self-regulation.

For now, the relevant point is that emotional distress can be linked to unpleasant self-awareness, and so it could motivate people to reduce or escape from self-awareness—which, in turn, would likely impair self-regulation. The negative effect of emotional distress on self-regulation could thus be a side effect of the effort to escape self-awareness.

Self-awareness is not easy to stop. Indeed, directing attention away from the self is itself a form of self-regulation, and as such it requires conscious supervision. Thus, paradoxically, the effort to stop attending to oneself could stimulate attending to oneself, because the monitoring system would regularly check to see "Have I stopped being aware of myself?" only to find that the very act of checking thwarts the goal.

To resolve that problem, Baumeister (1988, 1989, 1990, 1991) proposed that the mind often responds with cognitive deconstruction, which is to say a shift in self-awareness toward more concrete and hence less meaningful aspects of the self. Thus, sexual masochists escape from meaningful self-awareness by instead becoming aware of themselves as merely physical bodies experiencing intense sensations such as pain, or occasionally by being aware of themselves doing things incompatible with their normal identities (e.g., performing humiliating or degrading acts). In parallel fashion, the presuicidal process is often set in motion by some event that depicts the self in a very negative lights, such as being responsible for some failure or calamity, and this experience evokes a very negative view of self that is fraught with emotional distress. To combat it, the presuicidal person often shifts into such a deconstructed state, marked by narrow focus on the immediate present, immersion or self-distraction in mechanical activities, and emotional numbness (Baumeister, 1990). It is the inability to sustain this numb state that prompts the person to move on to attempting suicide. If the person could remain feeling numb amid a relatively meaningless set of activities, there would be no need for the suicide attempt. Unfortunately, each attempt to resume meaningful thought and active engagement in life brings back the awareness of the damaged identity and the associated emotional distress.

The link to self-regulation failure has perhaps best been documented in connection with binge eating (see Heatherton & Baumeister, 1991). Binge eating is both a form of self-defeating behavior (in that it normally occurs amid attempts to lose weight by restricting one's caloric intake and thwarts that goal) and a form of self-regulation failure (in that it involves losing control of precisely the behavior, namely, eating, that the person otherwise regulates carefully).

What leads to an eating binge? Aversive self-awareness has been implicated in multiple ways as a cause (for review, see Heatherton & Baumeister, 1991). Women with bulimia and other binge-eating tendencies typically have negative evaluations of their bodies (Cash & Brown, 1987; Garner, Garfinkel, & Bonato, 1987; Powers, Schulman, Gleghorn, & Prange, 1987; Williamson, 1990), and they also show low self-esteem generally (Eldredge, Wilson, & Whaley, 1990; Garner, Olmstead, Polivy, & Garfinkel, 1984; Gross & Rosen, 1988). They are also prone to high self-awareness (Blanchard & Frost, 1983; Heatherton & Baumeister, 1991). This appears to be specific to public self-awareness, in the sense that dieters and binge eaters are heavily concerned with how others think of them and may even overestimate the extent to which other people focus evaluative attention on them (Bauer & Anderson, 1989; Garfinkel & Garner, 1982; Johnson & Connors, 1987; Weisberg, Norman, & Herzog, 1987). They do not normally show elevated attention to their own inner states, feelings, and processes. Indeed, if anything, they are exceptionally insensitive and unresponsive to these inner aspects of self (Garfinkel & Garner, 1982; Heatherton, Polivy, & Herman, 1989). One likely reason for this is that chronic dieting is in part a process of training oneself to ignore inner signals of hunger and desire for food.

Laboratory manipulations that alter self-awareness often affect eating and in ways consistent with the view that people may eat heavily as part of an attempt to escape self-awareness. Dieters eat more after their self-esteem is threatened, such as after being told they failed at a problem-solving task (Baucom & Aiken, 1981; Heatherton, Herman, & Polivy, 1991; Ruderman, 1985). Manipulations that both increase self-awareness and convey threat to esteem, such as telling dieters that they will have to give a speech or otherwise perform in front of an evaluative audience, lead to increases in eating (Heatherton et al., 1991; Herman, Polivy, Lank, & Heatherton, 1987). In such cases, the person is presumably trying to escape from aversive self-awareness. When people are self-aware without threat, eating is typically reduced. For example, when people believe they are being watched while eating, they eat less (Herman, Roth, & Polivy, 2003).

A full test of the model was conducted by Heatherton, Polivy, Herman, and Baumeister (1993). Dieters and nondieters were first given either a success or a failure experience. Then some were distracted from self by having them watch an intriguing film, while others were kept self-aware with a mirror. Dieters who experienced failure but then could escape from self-awareness by watching the distracting film ate relatively large amounts. Dieters who were kept in a state of self-awareness (unable to escape it) ate relatively little. Nondieters were less affected by these manipulations. These results fit the pattern that self-awareness sustains self-regulation, whereas escaping from self-awareness seems to sweep away these inner restraints.

The relevance of self-awareness to regulating eating was demonstrated in an important study by Polivy (1976). In her study, participants were first exposed to a "preload" manipulation that induced some dieters to eat more than they normally would, thereby breaking their diets, while others kept within normal limits. After this, all were invited to eat as many tiny sandwiches as they wanted. The key measure was a surprise recall test, in which participants were asked to report or estimate how many they had eaten. Most participants, including nondieters and the dieters whose diets had not been violated, were quite accurate. In contrast, dieters who had broken their diets during the preload were wildly inaccurate. Thus, apparently, once people broke their diet, they stopped monitoring, and this lack of keeping track was associated with greater eating.

Similar conclusions emerge from research on alcohol consumption. Research by Hull and his colleagues (see Hull, 1981, for review) has shown that people consume alcohol in order to escape from aversive self-awareness and that alcohol does effectively reduce awareness of self. Although traditional work has assumed that stress is one cause of alcohol abuse, Hull (1981) reviewed evidence that this relationship has often been overstated and oversimplified, because not all stresses lead to increased alcohol consumption. For example, a death in the family is almost universally rated as among the most stressful events that people experience, but it does not normally lead to increased alcohol use or abuse. Only stresses that reflect badly on the self lead to alcohol abuse. Thus, apparently, people turn to alcohol in order to escape from aversive self-awareness.

An important study of alcoholic relapse confirmed the importance of escape from self-awareness (Hull et al., 1986). Patients nearly at the end of an alcoholism detoxification program filled out measures of self-awareness and life events. The highest rates of relapse were found among people who were chronically high in self-focus and whose life events were principally negative. This pattern is presumably the one most likely to engender an aversive self-awareness, prompting the individual to return to alcohol for solace and escape. High self-awareness is not aversive when life is going well, and in fact relapse rates among highly self-aware people with predominantly favorable life events were exceptionally low.

It is certainly no coincidence that alcohol abuse has been linked to binge eating. Polivy and Herman (1976; Polivy, 1976) found that dieters ate more after consuming alcohol than after drinking nonalcoholic drinks. (These were not the so-called expectancy effects, because participants who were falsely told that their drinks contained alcohol did not eat more than controls.) Apparently, alcohol reduces self-awareness, thereby impairing one's ability to monitor one's behavior and contributing to failure at self-regulation. In fact, Abraham and Beaumont (1982) found that nearly half their sample of bulimics reported that alcohol consumption led to their eating binges (see also Williamson, 1990).

More broadly, alcohol has been associated with many patterns of failure at self-regulation (for review, see Baumeister et al., 1994a; also Steele & Southwick, 1985). When intoxicated, people perform many acts that they otherwise would restrain. They spend more, boast more, fight more, and the like.

Converging evidence comes from recent studies on social exclusion and rejection. Based on the hypothesis that people are driven by a fundamental and powerful need to belong (Baumeister & Leary, 1995), some of us began investigating how people would respond to social rejection. We anticipated that rejection and other forms of social exclusion (e.g., hearing that one is likely to end up alone in life) would precipitate emotional distress. Indeed, almost everyone who hears about this work assumes that people would feel sadness, anxiety, depression, or other forms of upset when told that no one in their group had selected them as a potential partner, or that their personality profile forecast a lonely future. However, most participants who experience these manipulations report no emotion and instead seem almost numb (e.g., Twenge, Baumeister, Tice, & Stucke, 2001). But they show a broad range of socially undesirable and even antisocial behaviors. How can these be explained?

We propose that the incipient emotional distress causes people to avoid self-awareness, and this facilitates escape into the numb state of cognitive deconstruction— but at some cost to self-regulation. Twenge, Catanese, and Baumeister (2003) found ample signs of the deconstructed state among socially excluded participants. They reported that time moved slowly, were lethargic on tasks, and engaged in less meaningful thought. In one study, they systematically chose chairs facing away from a mirror instead of ones facing toward the mirror, which is an important indication of evading self-awareness (because mirrors direct attention to the self).

And self-regulation? Recent work has confirmed that rejected people self-regulate less effectively than others (Baumeister, DeWall, Ciarocco, & Twenge, 2005). Across several studies, they ate more cookies and snack foods, consumed less of a healthy but bad-tasting beverage that the experimenter exhorted them to drink, and performed worse than others on a dichotic listening (attention control task). The loss of self-awareness appears to have been an important contributing factor: When participants were seated in front of a mirror and therefore unable to escape from self, they performed as well as controls on the dichotic listening task.

In sum, some of the effects of emotional distress on self-regulation may be connected with aversive self-awareness. Events that make the self look bad and feel bad about itself bring unpleasant emotional states along with an unpleasant awareness of self. People may seek to escape from self-awareness partly because escaping from it may help keep the emotional distress at bay (as in our studies on social exclusion). Unfortunately, however, self-awareness is an important and integral part of effective self-regulation. Escaping from self-awareness therefore handicaps efforts at self-regulation and can produce self-regulation failure.

EMOTION AS AID IN SELF-REGULATION

The preceding sections have established beyond doubt that emotion (especially high-arousal emotional distress) can impair self-regulation. But that is only part of the story. There are various signs that emotion can sometimes benefit self-regulation too.

Indeed, the view that the effects of emotion are mainly negative, even just in terms of effects on self-regulation, seems implausible from an evolutionary standpoint. As already suggested, self-regulation is one of the crucial and distinctive adaptations of human evolution, and effective self-regulation is an important key to success in the sort of cultural societies that humans began to form very early in their prehistory (see Baumeister, 2005). If emotion mainly functioned to impair and undermine self-regulation, emotion would essentially be a backward force against evolutionary progress. Under those circumstances, one might have expected natural selection to favor humans with ever smaller and weaker emotional repertoires. Such individuals would have competed effectively against their more emotional peers, by virtue of superior self-regulation. The fact is that evolution has preserved human emotion in its often powerful and wide-ranging operations, even if the processes and functions of emotion may have changed somewhat.

One landmark in the shift toward a more positive and constructive view of emotion was *Descartes' Error* (Damasio, 1992), which presented insights and conclusions from Damasio's research program examining the effects of brain damage that left cognitive functioning intact but stifled emotional responses. These individuals did not resemble the wise, prudent, rational individuals one might have expected from the view of emotion as essentially a backward, animalistic response that mainly prompts people to do foolish and dangerous things in the heat of passion. Rather, their lives were often severely compromised and sometimes marked by seemingly self-defeating patterns. They also showed costly streaks of impulsive action and a failure to learn from their experiences and mistakes.

Although cynical critics may suggest that it would be unrealistic to expect brain damage to produce broad benefits to psychological functioning, these results do suggest that the loss of emotional responsivity does more harm than good, and they suggest that emotions may play a vital if not immediately obvious role in supporting effective self-regulation. In this section, we indicate several ways that emotion may benefit self-regulation (see Fredrickson, 1998, for more complete summaries of the positive emotions).

Signaling Discrepancies

An influential paper by Higgins (1987) proposed that people experience emotional reactions activated by perceiving discrepancies between the way they are and the way the would like to be or ought to be. Indeed, Higgins went on to propose that different patterns of emotional response are linked to discrepancies from the *ideal self* and discrepancies from the *ought self*. Perceiving that one falls short of one's ideals leads to low-arousal negative emotions such as sadness and disappointment. In contrast, perceiving oneself as falling short of one's "ought" standards (or the ought standards held about the self by others, such as one's parents' expectations for how one should behave) gives rise to high-arousal negative emotions, such as anxiety and guilt.

Although Higgins's initial goal was to link self-construals to emotional reactions, he soon elaborated this into a self-regulation theory (e.g., Higgins, 1996). Negative emotional states give rise to attempts to resolve the discrepancies to escape from the negative affective states. In this, he built on the analyses by Carver and Scheier (1981, 1982) who also emphasized that people feel aversive emotional states when they focus on how aspects of self fall short of relevant standards.

The most distinctive feature of Higgins's approach has been the specificity of emotional reactions—that is, the hypothesis that different emotions arise from different discrepancies. This work has come under some criticism, including failures to replicate (e.g., Tangney, Niedenthal, Covert, & Barlow, 1998), but it continues to excite interest over its theoretical implications. The alternative, after all, is to propose that all negative emotions are essentially interchangeable in their contribution to self-regulation in that all they accomplish is to make the person acutely aware that falling short of standards is bad. Future work may establish whether self-regulation does benefit from the extensive differentiation of human emotion.

Thus, falling short of standards produces negative affect. What about meeting standards, such as reaching goals? The consensus across a broad range of theorists is that positive emotions stem from such positive outcomes. Indeed, the view that reaching goals causes positive emotion is almost a truism in the research literature on goal striving (e.g., Gollwitzer & Bargh, 1996; also Locke & Kristof, 1996). Apart from goals, reaching and surpassing other standards can likewise give rise to favorable emotions. Social comparison against others can make one feel good if one comes up superior (Festinger, 1954; Wills, 1981).

In sum, both positive and negative emotions may serve important signal functions in self-regulation. It is possible to view the feedback loop and its comparisons against standards as a purely cognitive and instrumental function, which would more or less correspond to how it operates in a room thermostat or guided missile. In humans, however, the feedback loop does not appear to be quite so dispassionate, and people feel good or bad depending on how they compare themselves against relevant standards. The thermostat example may suggest that emotion is not absolutely necessary for all feedback loop and self-regulating systems, but emotion is an integral part of the human self-regulating system.

Signaling Progress toward Goals

We have already noted that people feel good when they reach their goals and feel bad when they attend to how they have failed or fallen short. This characterization does, however, have one implication that seems incompatible with many observations. If people only felt good when they reached their goals and felt bad the rest of the time, they would presumably be quite unhappy most of the time, because successful goal achievement is at best an occasional and intermittent experience. If most of life is characterized by goal striving, then people spend most of their lives in a state of negative discrepancy—which would suggest they would be unhappy most of the time. But most research on happiness suggests that, on the contrary, people are generally happy much of the time (e.g., Argyle, 1987).

An elegant and instructive solution was proposed by Carver and Scheier (1990). They dramatically extended the role of positive affect in a way that made it much more plausible that people could spend large portions of daily life feeling good. In their account, positive emotion does not merely recognize goal achievement—it also recognizes progress toward goals and standards.

This important revision adopts a dynamic rather than static view, and as such it seems more appropriate to ongoing processes of self-regulation. A student whose goal is to graduate from college may spend 4 or 5 years in a state of not having reached that goal, but that does not condemn the student to feeling bad all that time. In contrast, the goal may actually foster positive emotions all along, at least whenever the student can feel satisfied with having made some progress toward the goal and being approximately on schedule. Negative affect would mainly arise on occasions on which the progress toward the goal is recognized as being blocked or too slow, such as when the student has to drop some courses, thereby losing some credits and necessitating extra semester to reach the goal.

Facilitating Attending to Relevant Information

Earlier we noted evidence that emotional distress can lead people to ignore relevant information, thus impairing their decision making. Research on the effects of positive emotion on decision making has yielded mixed results. However, one interpretation of the findings is that positive affect tends to facilitate self-regulation by encouraging people to attend to relevant information, even if that information is negative (Aspinwall, 1998). Furthermore, evidence from neurological studies suggests that emotion in general may help people to pay attention to negative future consequences of their actions, improving their decision making (Bechara, 2003, 2004; but see also Shiv, Loewenstein, Bechara, Damasio, & Damasio, 2005).

Recharging a Depleted System

Building on Frederickson's (1998) "broaden and build" view of positive emotions, Tice, Baumeister, Shmueli, and Muraven (in press) conducted four experiments to demonstrate that positive emotions can recharge a depleted self-regulatory system. When people engage in any act of self-control, they may become depleted and have less self-control left for subsequent acts of self-regulation (Baumeister, Bratslavsky, Muraven, & Tice, 1998). But what recharges the system? If engaging in self-control can cause people to become depleted, is there any means of regaining self-control strength and recharging the system? There are probably multiple ways of recharging the system, and Tice et al. (2005) focused on the role of positive emotion as a means to increase self-control after depletion. In four experiments, they depleted people in a variety of ways, such as by having people suppress thoughts, learn a habit and then break it, or resist temptation to eat cookies. Depleted people were less able to engage in subsequent self-control efforts unless they were given a positive mood manipulation. Depleted people who were put in a positive mood were able to exert as much self-control on a task as were people who were not depleted. Thus, these studies suggest that one way in which emotions can affect self-control is by recharging a depleted system, to counteract the ego depletion effects of engaging in self-control. Engaging in self-control can deplete self-control strength, leading to poorer subsequent self-regulation, but positive emotions can recharge the system and increase self-control in depleted people.

Broader Context: Emotion as Feedback System

The preceding sections have suggested some important ways that emotion may serve self-regulation, such as by signaling discrepancies and recording progress (or lack of progress) in self-regulatory functions. A broader context has been proposed by Baumeister, Vohs, DeWall, and Zhang (2006), which depicts emotion as chiefly a feedback system. That approach takes issue with the widespread assumption that the main function of emotion is to cause behavior directly. Conscious emotion in particular may often be too slow to be useful as an online guide for immediate behavior. Indeed, in many cases emotional reactions develop only after the crisis or stimulating event has passed. What is the utility of feeling emotion after the fact? There are two possible and important answers.

First, retrospective emotion may facilitate learning. As Baumeister (2005) has proposed, as soon as a robot or computer finished dealing with one situation, it would turn its cognitive processing to the next event, and if humans were simply animals with computer brains, they might show the same pattern. But in a complex social world defined by language and culture, most events are susceptible to multiple interpretations. In the heat of a crisis, it may be difficult for a person to review all possible interpretations and select the right one, and thus sometimes people do the wrong thing. Learning from one's experiences and mistakes may, however, require some rumination about these different possible meanings and interpretations. A marital argument about an off-color joke that offended a neighbor at a dinner party could, for example, support multiple lessons: Don't tell jokes; don't go to dinner parties; don't tell jokes to that particular neighbor; don't socialize with the spouse; don't tell off-color jokes in general, or that particular joke, to anyone; or even, get a new spouse. Some review of the event with various counterfactual mental simulations seems necessary to learn a useful lesson to prevent a repeat spat while not making overly drastic changes to one's life. There is some evidence that negative emotional states automatically stimulate counterfactual thinking (e.g., Roese, 1997). This pattern seems well designed to promote adaptive and beneficial learning.

Second, behavior may be guided by anticipated emotion. If full-blown emotion often arrives too late to change the course of events, the anticipation of emotion could still play a central role in guiding actions. Converging evidence from multiple sources has suggested that people often make choices and decisions based on anticipated emotional outcomes (e.g., Mellers, Schwartz, & Ritov, 1999), such as avoiding regret (for a summary, see Schwarz, 2000). Although the anticipation of possible regret can occasionally produce deviations from optimal decision making (Anderson, 2003; Krueger, Wirtz, & Miller, 2005), by and large the influence of anticipated emotion is likely to be highly beneficial.

The view of behavior as pursuing emotion rather than caused by emotion can put a more positive spin on the findings from the mood-freezing studies (reviewed earlier). Those findings (e.g., Tice et al., 2001; also Bushman, Baumeister, & Phillips, 2001) suggest that emotion does not directly cause behavior, but rather people make choices and perform actions that they expect will produce desirable emotional states. In those particular studies, decisions were compromised by the urgently felt drive to repair an acutely bad mood, but if people generally behave to bring themselves good moods, self-regulation is likely to benefit in most cases. This optimistic appraisal is especially plausible in light of the Carver and Scheier (1990) findings, which say that progress toward self-regulatory goals will yield positive emotions. Hence a main recipe for feeling good is to regulate one's behavior effectively in general.

This view also helps resolve one of the paradoxes of emotion theory, namely, the influence of guilt. Guilt has acquired a terrible reputation as senseless self-torture, and many pop psychologists cater to the widespread view that getting rid of guilt altogether would be a great boon to humankind. Yet guilt-prone people generally live well-adjusted lives and are valued members of society, whereas individuals who are immune to guilt (psychopaths) create havoc by exploiting and victimizing other people with indifferent impunity (Baumeister, 1997, 2005; Hare, 1993). Interpersonal analyses of guilt suggest that it is a powerful factor for improving interpersonal relations (Baumeister, Stillwell, & Heatherton, 1994).

Is it really necessary to torture oneself with guilt in order to be a good person? No. On the contrary, it is possible to be a highly effective, well-adjusted person who is a good relationship partner and a conscientious member of society without (hardly) ever feeling much in the way of guilt. Anticipated emotion is the key. A person with a well-developed sense of guilt can presumably anticipate which actions will lead to guilt and then avoid those actions. At most, an occasional experience of guilt, followed by scrupulous counterfactual analysis that will reveal what one did wrong and how the guilt could have been avoided, may be enough to train the system to anticipate guilt and subsequently guide behavior to avoid making similar mistakes in the future.

Some evidence that guilt functions in this way was provided by Baumeister et al. (1995), who obtained narrative accounts of transgressions that did versus did not make the person feel guilty. Although the two sets of transgressions were broadly similar in many ways, one strong difference was that the guilty accounts were much more likely to contain a "moral" or lesson that the person had articulated, which indicates that episodes involving guilt seem to be encoded spontaneously together with conclusions about what one did wrong. They were also more likely than the other accounts to contain explicit statements that the person changed his or her behavior subsequently. Guilt thus seems to serve the first function we noted previously, namely, helping people consolidate the lessons from their misadventures, as well as the second function, which is changing behavior to avoid more episodes of guilt.

The emphasis on anticipated emotion as benefiting self-regulation puts a somewhat novel spin on the phenomenon of affective forecasting (Wilson & Gilbert, 2003). That pattern of work has shown that people typically overestimate the duration of future emotions, and it has been characterized as fallacy or shortcoming in human information processing, such as "immune neglect" (the failure to recognize the power of one's resources for recovering from misfortune). However, the overestimation of future emotion may also be highly adaptive, because in a sense it may be more useful to anticipate strong emotion than actually to feel it. Once the event is over, the emotion serves mainly to stimulate some rumination and counterfactual analysis. There is little need to go on feeling miserable for months. But anticipating that one might feel miserable for months may be crucial to enable the person to avoid making the mistake in the first place. (Overestimation in that way may help offset temporal discounting—that is, the tendency for future outcomes to have less impact on present decisions than they rationally deserve.)

CONCLUSION

This chapter has sought to appraise the impact of emotion on self-regulatory processes generally. We have presented both positive and negative effects.

On the negative side, it is well established that current emotional distress can impair self-regulation, and we suggested several mechanisms by which this may occur. People who feel emotional distress typically assign high priority to feeling better immediately, and the quest for good feelings may often entail subverting one's ongoing efforts at self-regulation (as when the dieter indulges in an eating binge in the hope of escaping from depressed feelings). Emotional states also compromise information processing, so that bad decisions may be made, such as ignoring probabilities of possible outcomes and failing to think through the potentially costly ramifications of a contemplated act. In addition, unpleasant emotions are sometimes linked to feeling bad about oneself, and thus people may seek to deconstruct or avoid self-awareness in order to reduce those emotional states—but when self-awareness is reduced, self-regulation is often compromised, insofar as monitoring oneself and one's actions is integral to effective self-regulation.

On the positive side, we think that emotion is typically vital for effective self-regulation, and this view gains some support from evidence that people who lack normal emotional responsivity suffer from several patterns indicating poor self-regulation. Emotion appears to be important to signal both success and failure at self-regulation, not merely in terms of final outcomes but also in terms of progress toward goals. Emotion can also prompt self-regulation to begin by accentuating that one's current behavior or attainments fall short of relevant standards. Emotion can stimulate learning from mistakes, and anticipated emotion can guide behavior and decision making, including encouraging people to self-regulate effectively.

There is no reason to assume that either of these lists is exhaustive. Emotion may benefit and impair self-regulation in additional ways, and further research is eagerly awaited to shed light on such processes. As just one example, research might profitably investigate whether positive emotions can have as adverse an effect on self-regulation as negative emotions have been shown to do. Recent news events have repeatedly shown celebrations over sports victories to end in tragedy, including extensive property destruction, alcohol abuse, and sometimes interpersonal violence, suggesting that positive emotion can sweep aside the normal restraints that promote civilized behavior.

The promise is considerable. Ultimately, self-regulation and emotion are two of the most ubiquitous and powerful operations in the human psyche, and neither is likely to be fully effective without the other. On the contrary, the two are deeply and multiply intertwined.

ACKNOWLEDGMENTS

Support for the preparation of this chapter was provided by Grant No. MH65559 from the National Institute of Mental Health.

NOTE

1. We use "distress" as an umbrella term to refer to unpleasant, upsetting, or negative moods or emotions.

REFERENCES

Abraham, S. F., & Beaumont, P. J. (1982). How patients describe bulimia or binge eating. *Psychological Medicine, 12,* 625–635.

Anderson, C. J. (2003). The psychology of doing nothing: Forms of decision avoidance result from reason and emotion. *Psychological Bulletin, 129,* 139–166.

Argyle, M. (1987). *The psychology of happiness.* New York: Methuen.

Ashton, H., & Stepney, R. (1982). *Smoking: Psychology and pharmacology.* London: Tavistock.

Aspinwall, L. G. (1998). Rethinking the role of positive affect in self-regulation. *Motivation and Emotion, 22,* 1–32.

Baucom, D. H., & Aiken, P. A. (1981). Effect of depressed mood on eating among obese and nonobese dieting persons. *Journal of Personality and Social Psychology, 41,* 577–585.

Bauer, B. G., & Anderson, W. P. (1989). Bulimic beliefs: Food for thought. *Journal of Counseling and Development, 67,* 416–419.

Baumeister, R. F. (1988). Masochism as escape from self. *Journal of Sex Research, 25,* 28–59.

Baumeister, R. F. (1989). *Masochism and the self.* Hillsdale, NJ: Erlbaum.

Baumeister, R. F. (1990). Suicide as escape from self. *Psychological Review, 97,* 90–113.

Baumeister, R. F. (1991). *Escaping the self: Alcoholism, spirituality, masochism, and other flights from the burden of selfhood.* New York: Basic Books.

Baumeister, R. F. (1997). *Evil: Inside human violence and cruelty.* New York: Freeman.

Baumeister, R. F. (2005). *The cultural animal: Human nature, meaning, and social life.* London: Oxford University Press.

Baumeister, R. F., Bratslavsky, E., Muraven, M., & Tice, D. M. (1998). Ego depletion: Is the active self a limited resource? *Journal of Personality and Social Psychology, 74,* 1252–1265.

Baumeister, R. F., DeWall, C. N., Ciarocco, N. J., & Twenge, J. M. (2005). Social exclusion impairs self-regulation. *Journal of Personality and Social Psychology, 88,* 589–604.

Baumeister, R. F., Heatherton, T. F., & Tice, D. M. (1994a). *Losing control: How and why people fail at self-regulation.* San Diego, CA: Academic Press.

Baumeister, R. F., & Leary, M. R. (1995). The need to belong: Desire for interpersonal attachments as a fundamental human motivation. *Psychological Bulletin, 117,* 497–529.

Baumeister, R. F., & Scher, S. J. (1988). Self-defeating behavior patterns among normal individuals: Review and analysis of common self-destructive tendencies. *Psychological Bulletin, 108,* 3–22.

Baumeister, R. F., Stillwell, A. M., & Heatherton, T. F. (1995). Personal narratives about guilt: Role in action control and interpersonal relationships. *Basic and Applied Social Psychology, 17,* 173–198.

Baumeister, R. F., Vohs, K. D., DeWall, C. N., & Zhang, L. (2006). *How emotion shapes behavior: Feedback, anticipation, and reflection, rather than direct causation.* Manuscript under review.

Bechara, A. (2003). Risky business: Emotion, decision-making, and addiction. *Journal of Gambling Studies, 19,* 23–51.

Bechara, A. (2004). The role of emotion in decision-making: Evidence from neurological patients with orbitofrontal damage. *Brain and Cognition, 55,* 30–40.

Blanchard, F. A., & Frost, R. O. (1983). Two factors of restraint: Concern for dieting and weight fluctuation. *Behavior Research and Therapy, 21,* 259–267.

Brownell, K. D., Marlatt, G. A., Lichtenstein, E., & Wilson, G. T. (1986). Understanding and preventing relapse. *American Psychologist, 41,* 765–782.

Bushman, B. J., Baumeister, R. F., & Phillips, C. M. (2001). Do people aggress to improve mood? Catharsis beliefs, affect regulation opportunity, and aggressive responding. *Journal of Personality and Social Psychology, 81,* 17–32.

Carver, C. S., & Scheier, M. F. (1981). *Attention and self-regulation: A control-theory approach to human behavior.* New York: Springer-Verlag.

Carver, C. S., & Scheier, M. F. (1982). Control theory: A useful conceptual framework for personality—Social, clinical, and health psychology. *Psychological Bulletin, 92,* 111–135.

Carver, C. S., & Scheier, M. F. (1990). Origins and functions of positive and negative affect: A control-process view. *Psychological Review, 97,* 19–35.

Cash, T. F., & Brown, T. A. (1987). Body image in anorexia nervosa and bulimia nervosa: A review of the literature. *Special Behavioral and Cognitive-Behavioral Treatment of Anorexia Nervosa and Bulimia Nervosa, 11,* 487–521.

Catanzaro, S. J., & Means, J. (1990). Measuring generalized expectancies for negative mood regulation: Initial scale development and implications. *Journal of Personality Assessment, 54,* 546–563.

Damasio, A. R. (1992). *Descartes' error: Emotion, reason, and the human brain.* New York: Putnam.

Eldredge, K., Wilson, G. T., & Whaley, A. (1990). Failure, self-evaluation, and feeling fat in women. *International Journal of Eating Disorders, 9,* 37–50.

Ferrari, J. R., Johnson, J. L., & McCown, W. G. (1995). *Procrastination and task avoidance: Theory, research, and treatment.* New York: Plenum Press.

Festinger, L. (1954). A theory of social comparison processes. *Human Relations, 7,* 117–140.

Flett, G. L., Hewitt, P. L., & Martin, T. R. (1995). Dimensions of perfectionism and procrastination. In J. R. Ferari, J. L. Johsons, & W. G. McCown (Eds.), *Procrastination and task avoidance: Theory, research, and treatment* (pp. 113–136). New York: Plenum Press.

Fredrickson, B. L. (1998). What good are positive emotions? *Review of General Psychology, 2,* 300–319.

Fry, P. S. (1975). Affect and resistance to temptation. *Developmental Psychology, 11,* 466–472.

Garfinkel, P. E., & Garner, D. M. (1982). *Anorexia nervosa: A multidimensional perspective.* New York: Brunner/Mazel.

Garner, D. M., Garfinkel, P. E., & Bonato, D. P. (1987). Body image measurement in eating disorders. *Advances in Psychosomatic Medicine, 17,* 119–133.

Garner, D. M., Olmsted, M. P., Polivy, J., & Garfinkel, P. E. (1984). Comparison between weight-preoccupied women and anorexia nervosa. *Psychosomatic Medicine, 46,* 255–266.

Gollwitzer, P. M., & Bargh, J. A. (Eds.). (1996). *The psychology of action: Linking cognition and motivation to behavior.* New York: Guilford Press.

Green, J. D., Sedikides, C., Saltzberg, J. A., Wood, J. V., & Forzano, L.-A. B. (2003). Happy mood decreases self-focused attention. *British Journal of Social Psychology, 42,* 147–157.

Greeno, C. G., & Wing, R. R. (1994). Stress-induced eating. *Psychological Bulletin, 115,* 444–464.

Gross, J., & Rosen, J. C. (1988). Bulimia in adolescents: Prevalence and psychosocial correlates. *International Journal of Eating Disorders, 7,* 51–61.

Gross, J. J., & Thompson, R. A. (2007). Emotion regulation: Conceptual foundations. In J. J. Gross (Ed.), *Handbook of emotion regulation* (pp. 3–24). New York: Guilford Press.

Hare, R. D. (1993). *Without conscience: The disturbing world of the psychopaths among us*. New York: Simon and Schuster/Pocket.

Heatherton, T. F., & Baumeister, R. F. (1991). Binge eating as escape from self-awareness. *Psychological Bulletin, 110*, 86–108.

Heatherton, T. F., Herman, C. P., & Polivy, J. (1991). Effects of physical threat and ego threat on eating. *Journal of Personality and Social Psychology, 60*, 138–143.

Heatherton, T. F., & Polivy, J. (1992). Chronic dieting and eating disorders: A spiral model. In J. Crowther, S. Hobfall, M. Stephens, & D. Tennenbaum (Eds.), *The etiology of bulimia: The individual and familial context* (pp. 133–155). Washington, DC: Hemisphere.

Heatherton, T. F., Polivy, J., & Herman, C. P. (1989). Restraint and internal responsiveness: Effects of placebo manipulations of hunger state on eating. *Journal of Abnormal Psychology, 98*, 89–92.

Heatherton, T. F., Polivy, J., Herman, C. P., & Baumeister, R. F. (1993). Self-awareness, task failure, and disinhibition: How attentional focus affects eating. *Journal of Personality, 61*, 49–61.

Herman, C. P., Polivy, J., Lank, C. N., & Heatherton, T. F. (1987). Anxiety, hunger, and eating behavior. *Journal of Abnormal Psychology, 96*, 264–269.

Herman, C. P., Roth, D. A., & Polivy, J. (2003). Effects of the presence of others on food intake: A normative interpretation. *Psychological Bulletin, 129*, 873–886.

Higgins, E. T. (1987). Self-discrepancy: A theory relating self and affect. *Psychological Review, 94*, 319–340.

Higgins, E. T. (1996). The "self digest": Self-knowledge serving self-regulatory functions. *Journal of Personality and Social Psychology, 71*, 1062–1083.

Hull, J. G. (1981). A self-awareness model of the causes and effects of alcohol consumption. *Journal of Abnormal Psychology, 90*, 586–600.

Hull, J. G., Young, R. D., & Jouriles, E. (1986). Applications of the self-awareness model of alcohol consumption: Predicting patterns of use and abuse. *Journal of Personality and Social Psychology, 51*, 790–796.

Johnson, C., & Connors, M. E. (1987). *The etiology and treatment of bulimia nervosa: A biopsychosocial perspective*. New York: Basic Books.

Keinan, G. (1987). Decision making under stress: Scanning of alternatives under controllable and uncontrollable threats. *Journal of Personality and Social Psychology, 52*, 639–644.

Knapp, A., & Clark, M. S. (1991). Some detrimental effects of negative mood on individuals' ability to solve resource dilemmas. *Personality and Social Psychology Bulletin, 17*, 678–688.

Krueger, J., Wirtz, D., & Miller, D. T. (2005). Counterfactual thinking and the first instinct fallacy. *Journal of Personality and Social Psychology, 88*, 725–735.

Leith, K. P., & Baumeister, R. F. (1996). Why do bad moods increase self-defeating behavior? Emotion, risk-taking, and self-regulation. *Journal of Personality and Social Psychology, 71*, 1250–1267.

Lerner, J. S., & Keltner, D. (2000). Beyond valence: Toward a model of emotion-specific influences on judgment and choice. *Cognition and Emotion, 14*, 473–493.

Lerner, J. S., & Keltner, D. (2001). Fear, anger, and risk. *Journal of Personality and Social Psychology, 81*, 146–159.

Locke, E. A., & Kristof, A. L. (1996). Volitional choices in the goal achievement process. In P. M. Gollwitzer & J. A. Bargh (Eds.), *The psychology of action: Linking cognition and motivation to behavior* (pp. 365–384). New York: Guilford Press.

Loewenstein, G. F., Weber, E. U., Hsee, C. K., & Welch, N. (2001). Risk as feelings. *Psychological Bulletin, 127*, 267–286.

Logue, A. W. (1993). *The psychology of eating and drinking: An introduction* (2nd ed.). New York: Freeman.

Manucia, G. K., Baumann, D. J., & Cialdini, R. B. (1984). Mood influences on helping: Direct effects of side effects? *Journal of Personality and Social Psychology, 46*, 357–364.

Martin, L. L., Ward, D. W., Achee, J. W., & Wyer, R. S. (1993). Mood as input: People have to interpret the motivational implications of their moods. *Journal of Personality and Social Psychology, 64*, 317–326.

Mellers, B., Schwartz, A., & Ritov, I. (1999). Emotion-based choice. *Journal of Experimental Psychology: General, 128*, 332–345.

Mischel, W. (1974). Processes in delay of gratification. In L. Berkowitz (Ed.), *Advances in experimental social psychology* (Vol. 7, pp. 249–292). San Diego, CA: Academic Press.

Mischel, W. (1996). From good intentions to willpower. In P. Gollwitzer & J. Bargh (Eds.), *The psychology of action* (pp. 197–218). New York: Guilford Press.

Mischel, W., Ebbesen, E. B., & Zeiss, A. R. (1973). Selective attention to the self: Situational and dispositional determinants. *Journal of Personality and Social Psychology, 27*, 129–142.

Monat, A., Averill, J. R., & Lazarus, R. S. (1972). Anticipatory stress and coping reactions under various conditions of uncertainty. *Journal of Personality and Social Psychology, 24*, 237–253.

O'Guinn, T. C., & Faber, R. J. (1987). Compulsive buying: A phenomenological exploration. *Journal of Consumer Research, 16*, 147–157.

Peck, C. P. (1986). Risk-taking behavior and compulsive gambling. *American Psychologist, 41*, 461–465.

Pickens, R. W., Hatsukami, D. K., Spicer, J. W., & Svikis, D. S. (1985). Relapse by alcohol abusers. *Alcoholism: Clinical and Experimental Research, 9*, 244–247.

Polivy, J. (1976). Caloric perception and regulation of intake in restrained and unrestrained subjects. *Dissertation Abstracts International, 36*, 3620–3621.

Polivy, J., & Herman, C. P. (1976). The effects of alcohol on eating behavior: Disinhibition or sedation. *Addictive Behaviors, 1*, 121–125.

Powers, P. S., Schulman, R. G., Gleghorn, A. A., & Prange, M. E. (1987). Perceptual and cognitive abnormalities in bulimia. *American Journal of Psychiatry, 144*, 1456–1460.

Roese, N. J. (1997). Counterfactual thinking. *Psychological Bulletin, 121*, 133–148.

Ruderman, A. J. (1985). Dysphoric mood and overeating: A test of restraint theory's disinhibition hypothesis. *Journal of Abnormal Psychology, 94*, 78–85.

Sayette, M. A. (1993). An appraisal–disruption model of alcohol's effectiveness on stress responses in social drinkers. *Psychological Bulletin, 114*, 459–476.

Schachter, S., Silverstein, B., Kozlowski, L. T., Perlick, D., Herman, C. P., & Liebling, B. (1977). Studies of the interaction of psychological and pharmacological determinants of smoking. *Journal of Experimental Psychology: General, 106*, 3–40.

Schwarz, N. (2000). Emotion, cognition, and decision making. *Cognition and Emotion, 14*, 433–440.

Shiv, B., Loewenstein, G., Bechara, A., Damasio, H., & Damasio, A. R. (2005). Investment behavior and the negative side of emotion. *Psychological Science, 16*, 435–439.

Shouwenburg, H. C. (1995). Academic procrastination: Theoretical notions, measurement, and research. In J. R. Ferrari, J. L. Johnson, & W. G. McCown (Eds.), *Procrastination and task avoidance: Theory, research, and treatment* (pp. 71–96). New York: Plenum Press.

Slochower, J., & Kaplan, S. P. (1980). Anxiety, perceived control, and eating in obese and normal weight persons. *Appetite, 1*, 75–83.

Steele, C. M., & Southwick, L. (1985). Alcohol and social behavior I: The psychology of drunken excess. *Journal of Personality and Social Psychology, 48*, 18–34.

Stockwell, T. (1985). Stress and alcohol. *Stress Medicine, 1*, 209–215.

Tangney, J. P., Niedenthal, P. M., Covert, M. V., & Barlow, D. H. (1998). Are shame and guilt related to distinct self-discrepancies? A test of Higgins's (1987) hypotheses. *Journal of Personality and Social Psychology, 75*, 256–268.

Tice, D. M., & Baumeister, R. F. (1997). Longitudinal study of procrastination, performance, stress, and health: The costs and benefits of dawdling. *Psychological Science, 8*, 454–458.

Tice, D. M., Baumeister, R. F., Shmueli, D., & Muraven, M. (in press). Replenishing the self: Effects of positive affect on performance and persistence following ego depletion. *Journal of Experimental Social Psychology*.

Tice, D. M., & Bratslavsky, E. (2000). Giving in to feel good: The place of emotion regulation in the context of general self-control. *Psychological Inquiry, 11*, 149–159.

Tice, D. M., Bratslavsky, E., & Baumeister, R. F. (2001). Emotional distress regulation takes precedence over impulse control: If you feel bad, Do it! *Journal of Personality and Social Psychology, 80*, 53–67

Twenge, J. M., Baumeister, R. F., Tice, D. M., & Stucke, T. S. (2001). If you can't join them, beat them: Effects of social exclusion on aggressive behavior. *Journal of Personality and Social Psychology, 81*, 1058–1069.

Twenge, J. M., Catanese, K. R., & Baumeister, R. F. (2003). Social exclusion and the deconstructive state: Time perception, meaninglessness, lethargy, lack of emotion, and self-awareness. *Journal of Personality and Social Psychology, 85*(3), 409–423.

Underwood, B., Moore, B. S., & Rosenhan, D. L. (1973). Affect and self-gratification. *Developmental Psychology, 8,* 209–214.

Weisberg, L. J., Norman, D. K., & Herzog, D. B. (1987). Personality functioning in normal weight bulimia. *International Journal of Eating Disorders, 6,* 615–631.

Wenzlaff, R. M., Wegner, D. M., & Roper, D. W. (1988). Depression and mental control: The resurgence of unwanted negative thoughts. *Journal of Personality and Social Psychology, 55,* 882–892.

Wertheim, E. H., & Schwartz, J. C. (1983). Depression, guilt, and self-management of pleasant and unpleasant events. *Journal of Personality and Social Psychology, 45,* 884–889.

Williamson, D.A. (1990). *Assessment of eating disorders: Obesity, anorexia, and bulimia nervosa.* New York: Pergamon Press.

Wills, T. A. (1981). Downward comparison principles in social psychology. *Psychological Bulletin, 90,* 245–271.

Wilson, T. D., & Gilbert, D. T. (2003). Affective forecasting. In M. Zanna (Ed.), *Advances in experimental social psychology* (Vol. 35, pp. 345–411). New York: Elsevier.

PART VI

SOCIAL APPROACHES

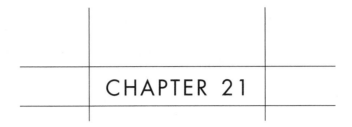

CHAPTER 21

The Nonconscious Regulation of Emotion

JOHN A. BARGH
LAWRENCE E. WILLIAMS

Emotions have long been recognized as powerful influences on human judgments and behavior, yet their function or purpose in our lives has been debated throughout intellectual history. Plato considered emotions, and affective reactions in general, to be "foolish counselors"; two millenia later leading philosophers such as Descartes continued to view emotions as afflictions that biased and obscured thought and decisions. But then came Darwin (1872), who compellingly argued for the functional and adaptive nature of emotional expression across species, followed a century later by scientific psychology, which eventually took Darwin's cue and began the experimental study of the interplay between emotion, cognition, and behavior. (For a contemporary version of Darwin's evolutionary argument, see Haidt, 2001.)

The behaviorist O. H. Mowrer (1960) was one of the first to note the important function emotions played in learning, especially in providing a "safe" internal preview or simulation of the potential consequences of the actual behavior. Herbert Simon (1967), early on in his pioneering work on human cognition and problem solving, called attention to the important role played by motivation and emotion, describing them as necessary and essential controls over cognitive processes. Motivational controls, Simon argued, were needed to prioritize the organism's activities and to provide stopping rules for goal pursuits, such as how to know when to move on from one goal to another; emotional controls were needed to provide interrupts or signals that something needs attention right now and it cannot just wait in the to-do queue. In this view, emotions are important signals about the current state of the world—to paraphrase John Lennon, emotions are what happen to us when we are busy pursuing other plans.

Carver and Scheier's (1981) seminal model of self-regulation gave emotions a formal and prominent place in the process of goal pursuit—lack of sufficient progress toward a desired goal was posited to generate negative emotions (dissatisfaction, anxiety) that gave a further prod to effort toward the goal; positive emotions (see also Carver, 2004) were said to signal that sufficient progress has been made toward the goal such that it is now safe to disengage from that goal for a time in order to pursue other important goals. In other words, progress at a goal (or lack of it) produces positive (or negative) affect, which in turn influences rate of action toward the goal. Affect or emotion in their model is a *signal* to the regulatory system to either increase or decrease effort. And similarly, but at a more chronic, lifelong level of goal pursuit, Higgins's (1987) self-discrepancy theory makes predictions of specific emotional responses to events which call to mind the gap between one's present state and one's long-term self-goals.

More recently, cognitive neuroscience researchers such as Damasio (1996), LeDoux (1996), Davidson and Irwin (1999), and Gray (2004) have documented how emotional processing is involved as a moderator or guide in all sorts of cognitive processes, such that impairment of such processing (as through stroke or other brain damage) has a profound negative impact on decision making, personality, and life quality. This domain of research too has confirmed the intimate relations between emotional and cognitive processes, such that the neural circuitry that supports affect and that which supports cognition appear to be highly interconnected.

As emotions are meant to signal us, as well as guide and shape cognitive processing, we must learn how to manage and deal with these interruptions to our ongoing goal pursuits if we want them to be successful, and not be continually distracted from them. Precisely because emotions have this capability to interrupt our ongoing goal pursuits, they inevitably create attentional and response *conflicts* that must be resolved (see McClure et al., this volume; Morsella, 2005; Oettingen, Grant, Smith, Skinner, & Gollwitzer, in press). Regulation of emotions is thus needed whenever there is a conflict between the responses suggested by the emotion and those called for by one's current goals.

NONCONSCIOUS SELF-REGULATION MECHANISMS

To date, most emotion regulation research has focused on intentional, conscious forms of regulation (Gross, 1999; see Jackson et al., 2003). However, there have been significant advances recently in the study of nonconscious forms of self-regulation (see review in Fitzsimons & Bargh, 2004), which have revealed several self-regulatory mechanisms that operate independently of conscious control. For instance, automatic evaluative processes operate immediately and unintentionally to encode nearly all incoming stimuli in terms of positive or negative valence (see Duckworth, Bargh, Garcia, & Chaiken, 2002), with this initial screening having important "downstream" consequences for approach versus avoidant behavioral predispositions (Chen & Bargh, 1999) as well as biasing further judgments in the direction of the initial, automatically supplied evaluation (Ferguson, Bargh, & Nayak, 2005). As do all nonconscious forms of self-regulation, these automatic evaluative processes keep the person adaptively tied to his or her current environment while conscious attention and thought might be elsewhere (e.g., focused on the person's current goal pursuits).

A second form of nonconscious self-regulation is afforded by automatic linkages between perceptual and behavioral representations such that perceiving another person's behavior creates the tendency to behave the same way oneself—again without intending to or being aware of this influence. This mechanism, alternatively known as the perception–behavior link within social psychology (Dijksterhuis & Bargh, 2001) and the "mirror neuron" effect in social–cognitive neuroscience (e.g., Gallese, Fadiga, Fogassi, & Rizzolatti, 1996; see also Decety & Sommerville, 2003; Frith & Wolpert, 2004), connects us to each other through a brain mechanism designed to facilitate imitation and mimicry. Research has shown that we tend to imitate the posture, facial expressions, and bodily gestures of those with whom we interact, without intending to or being aware of doing so (Chartrand & Bargh, 1999, Study 1), and that in return such mimicry automatically fosters feelings of closeness and empathic understanding between the interaction partners (Chartrand & Bargh, 1999, Studies 2 and 3; also Lakin & Chartrand, 2003). Again, as a default mechanism or process while the conscious mind is elsewhere, the perception–behavior link keeps us on the same page with our interaction partners and help us to respond in an appropriate manner (i.e., similarly to the others we are with at the moment).

But the most relevant form of nonconscious self-regulation for current purposes is *nonconscious goal pursuit* (Bargh & Gollwitzer, 1994). According to the *automotive model* of nonconscious goal pursuit (Bargh, 1990), emotion regulation goals—like all goals—correspond to mental representations (see also Kruglanski, 1996). These are presumed to contain information as to when and how to pursue the goal, how likely one is to succeed, the value of that goal, and so on. More important for present purposes, goals as mental representations can develop automatic associations with other representations, to the extent they are active in the mind at the same time (see Hebb, 1949). Thus, if an individual chooses to pursue the same goal (e.g., to enjoy oneself) each time he or she is in a particular situation (e.g., the classroom) eventually the representations of the situation and of the goal would become automatically associated, so that activation of the former automatically causes the activation of the latter. Because representations of common situations become activated automatically themselves when we merely enter and perceive that situation, the goal too will become active at that time and begin operation, but without the person's conscious choice or knowledge.

Several studies have now shown that goals of various types and levels of abstraction can be nonconsciously activated (i.e., primed) to then guide information processing and social judgment (Chartrand & Bargh, 1996, 2002; Moskowitz, Gollwitzer, Wasel, & Schaal, 1999; Sassenberg & Moskowitz, 2004), verbal task performance (Bargh, Gollwitzer, Lee-Chai, Barndollar, & Troetschel, 2001; Fitzsimons & Bargh, 2003), and interpersonal helping and cooperation (Bargh et al., 2001, Study 2; Fitzsimons & Bargh, 2003). One pillar of support for nonconscious emotion regulation, therefore, comes from existing evidence in support of this model of nonconscious goal pursuit. For example, unobtrusively priming participants with stimuli closely related to the goal of achievement causes them to outperform control groups on a variety of verbal tasks, and subliminal priming of the goal of cooperation caused participants to make a greater number of cooperative responses in a "commons dilemma" situation (Bargh et al., 2001, Study 2).

Critically, across these and similar experiments, the same outcomes are obtained when the goal is primed and operates nonconsciously as when participants are given the goal explicitly through task instructions (see Bargh, 2005; Chartrand & Bargh,

2004; Fitzsimons & Bargh, 2004, for reviews). Moreover, in none of these experiments are participants aware of either the activation of the goal or their pursuit of it, as indicated by systematic questioning during debriefing (as well as the frequently subliminal nature of the priming manipulation itself).

THE *A PRIORI* CASE FOR NONCONSCIOUS EMOTION REGULATION

Given that these nonconscious self-regulatory mechanisms have been established in the case of other external environmental influences, it is likely that emotions—powerful and persistent influences that they are—are also subject to nonconscious forms of regulation. It would be odd indeed if emotions constituted the one form of external influence that was *not* subject to nonconscious control. After all, they are meant to distract one from currently active goal pursuits and they can often engulf one's phenomenal field (Loewenstein & Lerner, 2002), and so we are quite frequently presented with occasions in which we need to control emotional influences if we are to stay on track and accomplish our situational objectives. And, in fact, there is evidence that infants begin to use emotion regulation strategies (such as attentional disengagement) as early as 3 months of age (Calkins, 2004; Calkins & Hill, this volume; Posner & Rothbart, 1998). Thus the sheer frequency alone of these regulatory attempts over the course of one's (early) life should culminate in their automation, according to basic, established principles of skill acquisition (see Bargh, 1996; Bargh & Chartrand, 1999).

Jackson et al. (2003) have recently called for the development of models and research methods to study the more automatic forms of emotion regulation, to complement the historical (and current) emphasis on conscious or voluntary forms. They also provide some of the early data in support of nonconscious emotion regulation: In their study, individual differences in the resting activation levels of the prefrontal cortex predicted the duration of negative affect caused by disturbing photographs, as measured by eye-blink startle magnitude, even though there were no explicit instructions to regulate emotion given to participants in this study. Ochsner, Bunge, Gross, and Gabrieli (2002) had previously shown that the same regions of the prefrontal cortex became active during conscious, intentional emotion regulation. Thus, chronic levels of activation in these regions, as measured by Jackson et al. (2003), seem to correspond to chronic—perhaps "automatic" (as the authors concluded)—emotion regulation tendencies, because participants engaged in them without being told to do so.[1]

The concept of *automaticity* is a complex one with multiple defining features (see Bargh, 1989, 1994; Moors & de Houwer, 2006; Wegner & Bargh, 1998) and cautionary tales can be told against invoking it prematurely (see Fiske, 1989, and Bargh, 1999, in the case of automatic stereotyping research). Automatic processes are characterized by their *unintentional,* relatively *effortless* (i.e., *efficient;* minimal attentional resources required) and *uncontrollable* nature and operation *outside awareness*; conscious processes are generally *intentional, controllable, effortful,* and the person is *aware* of engaging in them (see Bargh, 1994). However, these defining qualities of an automatic or conscious process do not always co-occur in an all-or-none fashion—some of the classic examples of automatic processes such as typing or driving an automobile (for experienced typists and drivers) nonetheless require an intention to be engaged in, and while stereotyping another person might well be unintentional, it is not uncontrollable (see Devine, 1989; Fiske, 1989). Thus, it is problematic to conclude that a process is automatic (conscious) merely because it does not possess one of the features of a conscious (automatic) process.

Because of the problems inherent in the unitary concepts of automatic and conscious processing, researchers interested in automatic emotion regulation might wish to focus instead on the particular quality(ies) of most interest to them. For example, in the highly researched domain of automatic stereotyping and prejudice, the feature of special interest seems to be *intentionality*: Most research is directed at the question of whether people stereotype others even though they do not intend to do so (and perhaps even have strong intentions *not* to do so?). But to researchers of the attitude–behavior relation, it is the *efficiency* or effortlessness of how attitudes become activated by relevant stimuli that is the dimension of most interest (Fazio, Sanbonmatsu, Powell, & Kardes, 1986). Separate research methods have been developed for each of these component features (see Bargh & Chartrand, 2000; also Bargh, 2006) and some of these should prove useful to emotion researchers.

At the same time, the study of automatic emotion regulation is unlikely to be a repeat or merely a matter of applying what is already known about automaticity from cognitive or social psychology. Some of the hard-earned knowledge gained from the study of automaticity in social cognition will transfer to emotion regulation but some will not, and we would wager that emotion researchers will discover some new forms or domains of automatic and nonconscious phenomena that are unique to the case of emotion processing—just as some of the cognitive psychology research on automatic processes transferred to social psychological phenomena (e.g., stereotyping and attitude activation) but entirely new forms were discovered as well (e.g., nonconscious sources of affect, the perception–behavior link, and nonconscious goal pursuit). The past and ongoing research on automaticity in social cognition and self-regulation will likely be informative, even directive, to emotion researchers, but that research is unlikely to map perfectly onto the key concerns and phenomena of emotion research. We eagerly await the new discoveries to be made by researchers of nonconscious emotion regulatory processes in the years ahead.

GENERAL FORMS OF EMOTION REGULATION

As emotions serve important adaptive functions for the human organism, emotion regulation, if it is also to be adaptive and useful, should not be just a blanket, unconditional affair of suppressing or attenuating one's emotional reactions in all cases. Emotions are signals as to the state of the world and our place in it; it would make no sense to have an interrupt or override system that we routinely ignored. Moreover, true flexibility in responding, and adaptation to one's environment, do not always entail overriding impulses or environmentally triggered influences—to do so would be just as rigid as to always *act* on them (Gray, Shaefer, Braver, & Most, 2005). Indeed, some recent attention-based models of self-regulation have moved away from the idealization of top-down control over external influences, to a more balanced approach—one in which, "for any given context, there is an ideal balance in the allocation of top-down attention, such that an individual's goals are met but can be *flexibly modified by new information*" (MacCoon, Wallach, & Newman, 2005, p. 439; emphasis added).

True adaptation, in other words, does not only mean being able to pursue purposes independently of what is going on in the current environment (i.e., escaping stimulus control, as some models of self-regulation would have it; e.g., Mischel & Ayduk,

2004), it also means being open to and taking advantage of the unexpected opportunities that arise. As the neuropsychologist Barkley (2004) put it, the field of mental health "tends to view impulsiveness as a problem or deficit, yet for most species that have a nervous system that learns from contingencies of reinforcement, there actually is no 'problem' of impulsiveness—it is their default state. The 'problem' posed by impulsiveness is relatively unique to humans" (p. 5).

What the existing research shows is that while there are a few general rules of emotion regulation, successful emotion regulation strategies vary as a function of one's current goals and purposes. That is, emotions tend to be regulated on the basis of whether they facilitate versus interfere with our particular ongoing goal pursuits.

Maintaining Stability and Equilibrium

One such general principle is that we need to manage our manifest variability in the eyes of others—to be seen as steady, predictable, and not likely to act suddenly, spontaneously, and unpredictably. In Tetlock's (2002) terms, we are accountable to others in our group on whom we rely for support and aid in pursuing our important life outcomes (many of which require the cooperation if not participation of others), and thus we need to manage their impression of us. Unpredictable = danger, and being *seen* as dangerous is also very dangerous to the person him- or herself. So we need to be "regular," to set within boundaries the range of reactions we might safely and reasonably have in a given situation.

Social or group *norms* serve this purpose by providing these guidelines for us within many situations. Certain emotions are appropriate in certain settings but not others; as Barker and Wright (1955) reminded us, the average person behaves very differently in a library, say, than at a football game (see also Aarts & Dijksterhuis, 2003). And to fit in and be accepted by our fellow group members, we need to respond in a similar fashion as they do to the same external events—for example, if we were grouchy or upset after the home team won, or if we were seemingly not concerned over a threat to the community or group, these would signal that our goals are not the same as the others', and this would threaten our standing within our group. Conversely, as research has shown, having the same emotional expressions or reactions as do the others in our group naturally and automatically strengthens the empathic bond between members (Chartrand & Bargh, 1999; Lakin & Chartrand, 2003).

This tendency to maintain a steady state or equilibrium, or *homeostasis,* is also emphasized in the cybernetic self-regulation model of Carver and Scheier (1981). Given this overarching goal of maintaining a steady state, emotional responses represent a break in equilibrium that should, according to the theory, automatically provoke emotion-regulatory responses.

Forgas and Ciarrochi (2002) have also argued specifically for the existence of automatic emotional homeostatic mechanisms. In their studies, either a good or a bad mood was first induced in participants, who were then asked to generate open-ended responses (e.g., complete word fragments, describe a typical male or female) that were coded for their positivity or negativity. The usual or default mood-congruency effect was shown at first in these free responses, but over time there was a spontaneous shift to mood-incongruent responses. Thus, those in a good mood shifted over time to generate negative instead of positive completions; those in a bad mood shifted over time from negative to more positive completions. Forgas and

Ciarrochi (2002) concluded that people automatically correct for mood-congruency effects over time by shifting to mood-incongruent retrieval, "apparently in an attempt to manage their moods".

Larsen and Prizmic (2005) also posit a general "equilibrium-seeking" emotion regulation goal; according to these authors we generally want "to limit the residual impact of lingering emotions and moods on subsequent behavior and experience" (p. 41) such that we not only seek escape from our bad moods but also often seek to downplay our good moods, especially under circumstances in which it might interfere with our current purposes. One such circumstance is when we expect to interact with another person, especially a stranger: Erber, Wegner, and Therriault (1996) found that people tend to regulate their mood to be neutral in preparation for social interaction, even downplaying their good moods in order to attain this neutral state.

Recently, Jostmann, Koole, van der Wulp, and Fockenberg (2005) have argued that preparation for action in general has the natural, automatic effect of moderating emotional experience. In their model, the personality trait of *action orientation* (a basic orientation toward action and change; as contrasted with *state orientation*) is associated with a tendency to regulate and moderate affective influences. In their studies, they obtained the usual or default affective priming effect on mood (using subliminal emotional faces) but only for state-orientation participants. Action-oriented participants, on the other hand, showed the same tendency toward reestablishing equilibrium as in the Forgas and Ciarrochi (2002) and Erber et al. (1996) studies—with the most negative affect following presentation of happy faces and the most positive affect after the presentation of angry faces.

Koole and Jostmann (2004) argue that such "intuitive affect regulation" serves to facilitate volitional action and higher-order goal pursuits. Note here the similarity of emotion regulation effects obtained for the chronic individual difference of action orientation in the Jostmann et al. (2005) studies and those found for the stable and chronic individual differences in resting prefrontal activation state in the Jackson et al. (2003) study described earlier. In both cases, the "chronic" participants regulated emotions more than did other participants, without being told to do so explicitly by the experimenter, and apparently without awareness of having tried to do so. These findings are consistent with what we would expect if these groups of participants had developed, over frequent use, automatic or nonconscious emotion regulation skills.[2]

However, we do not know from these observed personality differences in regulation success or *outcome* what the responsible regulatory *process* was—how, exactly, did the action-oriented or equilibrium-seeking individual accomplish the regulation? Most likely, they used one of the following strategies (but in an automated fashion) that have been identified in the case of conscious self-regulation.

SPECIFIC (CONSCIOUS) EMOTION REGULATION STRATEGIES

Emotion-regulation researchers have identified several conscious and strategic emotion-control strategies that are commonly used by people, with varying degrees of success, in order to regulate their emotional experience (see Loewenstein, this volume). Here we consider the potential of these for developing into nonconscious emotion regulation mechanisms, based on the principles of skill acquisition (essentially, frequent and consistent use over time in the same situation).

Gross (1999; Ochsner & Gross, 2004; this volume) has identified a variety of such strategies or goals that people select for purposes of moderating their emotional experience. Here we first briefly describe these strategies and then consider the possibility that these strategies could come to operate nonconsciously as well, given frequent and consistent choice of that strategy upon experience of a particular emotion (and also, perhaps, upon particular emotional or affective inputs in the absence of conscious experience of them; see Winkielman, Berridge, & Wilbarger, 2005).

Response modulation strategies involve either decreasing or suppressing emotional responses, or increasing or enhancing them, depending on how appropriate and helpful (vs. inappropriate and detrimental) the emotion is for one's current situation and purposes. For example, if at a funeral one remembers a funny story involving the dearly departed, one would most likely suppress the emotional response. Similarly, there are situations in which the enhancement of an emotional response is necessary. For example, hurricane victims waiting days for rescue workers to arrive may use their feelings of frustration and despair to enhance their visible outrage and anger in order to better gain empathy and needed assistance from others.

Attentional deployment strategies modify or redirect the focus of conscious attention in order to modify their emotions; a classic example is a small child covering his eyes during a scary stretch of a Harry Potter movie. This of course helps by cutting off the stimulus input that is driving an unwanted emotion. Distraction is another common attention deployment strategy, in which one shifts one's attention to something else in the environment or to an effortful internal mental operation (such as counting to 10 when angry).

Cognitive transformation or *reappraisal* involves recategorization of the situation or event that is producing the emotion so that its meaning or emotional significance is changed. The sports pages provide us with a real-life example of this strategy, as employed by Carlos Beltran of the New York Mets baseball team. Asked how he dealt with the intense booing and heckling visited on him by fans of his former team, the Houston Astros, he replied "I can't let it influence my play. I tried to look at it a different way. When they booed me, I tried to think they do it because they care about me. I tried to make it a positive and not a negative."

Other emotion regulation strategies that have been described in the literature are less cognitive and more behavioral in nature, such as *situation selection*, which involves seeking out or avoiding situations that one knows tends to produce certain emotional reactions (e.g., not playing music associated with a failed relationship), and *mood repair*, in which one deliberately does something fun or enjoyable, or stress-reducing such as exercising. But note that these behavioral strategies can become automated just as can the regulating cognitive processes, following the same principle of frequent and consistent use over time (Bargh & Chartrand, 1999).

These emotion regulation goals should be capable of nonconscious activation and operation to the extent the individual has employed them routinely, in a frequent and consistent manner, whenever he or she is in the given situation. Although there is little evidence yet as to whether these particular strategies do come to operate in individuals in an automatic fashion to successfully regulate emotions, this is a fledgling research area and we would not be surprised to see such evidence accumulate in the research journals over the next 5 to 10 years. For one thing, evidence does already exist that one form of emotion regulation—reappraisal of one's situation using social comparison processes (Gross, 1999)—indeed becomes able to operate in a nonconscious fashion. People engage in both upward and downward social comparison with others in order to manage their moods and their sense of self-worth and well-being (e.g., Aspinwall & Taylor, 1993); this strategic selection (upward vs. downward) of standards against which to compare oneself clearly constitutes an act of *reappraisal* of one's standing relative to others.

Spencer, Fein, Wolfe, Fong, and Dunn (1998) demonstrated that people tend to counter threats to their self-esteem by automatically denigrating outgroup members—those who belong to social groupings other than one's own. Their studies made use of a paradigm developed by Gilbert and Hixon (1991), in which a load on the participant's attentional capacity (via a secondary task) was found to eliminate the commonly found automatic stereotyping effect. Spencer et al. first replicated these findings, but then in an extension of the paradigm gave participants failure feedback (thus threatening their self-esteem) prior to the main task. Under these conditions, the automatic stereotyping effect reemerged, even though the person was operating under the same attentional load that Gilbert and Hixon had shown sufficient to knock out the stereotyping effect. The authors concluded that the automatic goal to restore positive feelings about oneself was so strong and efficient in operation that it was capable of overcoming the shortage of attentional resources to then denigrate minority groups (i.e., downward social comparison processes), thereby repairing their mood—despite the participants' lack of awareness that they were stereotyping anyone at all.

Some of the best early evidence for the existence of automatic emotion regulation capabilities comes from a new study by Zemack-Ruger, Bettman, and Fitzsimons (2005). These researchers subliminally primed words related either to guilt or to sadness and then assessed whether behaviors or goal pursuits appropriate for those particular emotional states were set in motion by the primes. Across four experiments, these behavioral and motivational effects were obtained—for example, guilt-primed participants showed higher self-control than those primed with sad emotion—despite no differences between conditions in consciously made ratings of emotional experience. Without the participant knowing it, then, nonconscious activation of the emotion representation triggered a nonconsciously operating goal appropriate to deal with that emotion—exactly what is called for by our hypothesis of nonconscious emotion regulation.

POTENTIAL FOR NONCONSCIOUS OPERATION

For each of the conscious emotion regulation strategies, the assumed causal sequence runs as follows: (1) the person experiences and becomes aware of the emotional state; (2) based on situational constraints as to appropriateness or advisability of expressing that emotion, as well as considerations of whether the emotion would be helpful versus harmful to one's current goal pursuits (i.e., the person's *lay theory* regarding the probable effect of the emotion on the goal pursuit; see Wilson & Brekke, 1994), the person decides whether to attempt to regulate his or her emotional state—and if so, how exactly to go about doing so; and finally (3) the person intentionally pursues that regulatory goal or strategy. These strategies would be expected to develop into nonconscious emotion regulation processes if the same strategy was chosen and pursued given the same emotional situation (i.e., the same emotion–situation complex, such as feeling anxious during the closing minutes of a college entrance exam, or experiencing elation at drawing a very winnable poker hand). With sufficient attempts at regulation, the consistently chosen regulation goal would come to be activated automatically upon the experience of that emotion in that context (see Bargh & Chartrand, 1999).

One straightforward method for testing whether these emotion regulation strategies might operate nonconsciously would be to attempt to subtly and unobtrusively prime those goals, and then present participants with relevant emotional stimuli or emotion-producing situations (see Bargh & Chartrand, 2000, for standard and easy-to-use priming methods, such as the popular "scrambled sentence test"). Goal priming has been one of the more successful research strategies thus far in the study of nonconscious self-regulation. Subliminal versions of priming manipulations can also be used later on in the research program in order to help rule out demand issues (i.e., concerns that the priming manipulation was perhaps too strong and thus telegraphed, consciously, the experimental hypothesis to the participants). If such priming of emotion regulation goals is successful in producing the same or similar effects as when the goal is pursued consciously (as through explicit experimental instructions), as research has shown is true of nonconscious self-regulatory goals in nonemotional domains, this would indicate that these goals are capable of becoming activated and then operating independently of conscious intention and guidance.

Note, however, that people often do not appreciate the actual emotional influences on their judgments, decisions, and behavior, and this lack of recognition would necessarily stand in the way of the development of a useful, successful nonconscious emotion regulation process in that case (see Wilson & Brekke, 1994). There are many strong influences on us that we do not appreciate as such (e.g., social influence attempts by authority figures, as in cognitive dissonance research), and others that concern us overmuch (e.g., subliminal advertising); thus, in order to successfully regulate our emotions we need a correct theory of the direction (facilitative vs. interfering) and strength of their effects (Wilson & Brekke, 1994). Often, however, we do not have this.

For example, Lerner, Small, and Loewenstein (2004) have demonstrated carryover effects of induced emotional states on subsequent pricing and purchasing behavior. In their paradigm, participants are induced to experience a certain emotion in the first part of the experimental session, and then its subsequent effects on judgment are assessed in what participants believe to be an unrelated experiment. These studies have shown that approach-related emotions (e.g., anger) cause participants to be willing thereafter to pay more than usual for an object (pen, coffee mug) that they do not have, and to charge more for an object they do, but participants who have recently experienced avoidance or withdrawal-related emotions (e.g., disgust) are not willing to pay much for the object and require significantly less in return to give it up. Participants in these studies typically show no awareness of how the emotion they consciously felt previously might have influenced their economic decisions, making it unlikely that these biasing effects of recent emotional experience will be successfully regulated, even by conscious regulatory attempts—much less by eventual nonconscious emotion regulation skills. As they used to say of Bob Feller's fastball, "You can't hit what you can't see."

Development of Emotion Regulation Skills

Given the importance of frequent and consistent experience in the development of nonconscious goal pursuit capabilities, we should look to the developmental literature to see how young children deal with emotions and emotional stimuli. This literature shows that from early infancy onward, each of us gets plenty of practice at regulating our emotional states, with such skills beginning to develop as early as infancy. Posner and Rothbart (1998), using brain imaging techniques to study the development of executive attention networks, found that the earliest type of regulation ability that developed in infants in response to distress was attention allocation, such as distraction, which emerges during the first year of life (see also Rothbart & Sheese, this volume). Other lines of research also support the conclusion that infants begin using attentional strategies of engagement and disengagement from the emotion-producing stimulus at 3–6 months of age, and these continue as important regulatory strategies during the preschool years (Calkins, 2004).

Self-control abilities, on the other hand, take significantly longer to develop. In their review, Posner and Rothbart (1998) concluded that successful inhibitory control does not begin to develop in children until about 3 years of age. Yet here too these skills of response inhibition and emotion suppression do emerge and become highly practiced during the preschool years, so that they become easier and less effortful—that is, increasingly automated and potentially nonconscious. Thus the basic skills necessary for nonconscious emotion regulation begin to emerge relatively early in life and would be expected to attain nonconscious operation capability by young adulthood, if not before.

Regulatory Success as a Determinant of Nonconscious Operation

As we have noted, the frequency with which a given regulatory strategy is employed is an important determinant of whether that strategy will become automated. But frequency of use is not the entire story. Although researchers have delineated the different strategies people tend to use, they also note that these strategies are not equally effective in achieving the desired aims. For example, Gross (1999) and Larsen and Prizmic (2005) have concluded from available experimental evidence that reappraisal works better than suppression or distraction at reducing emotional intensity. According to Ochsner and Gross (2004), suppression might mask the observable manifestations of emotion (such as in one's facial expression), but it does not reduce the emotional experience itself (indeed, it increases physiological responding); reappraisal, on the other hand, is effective at attenuating both the behavioral responses and the underlying emotional experience.

Does the relative success of an emotion regulation strategy matter to whether it develops into an automatic or nonconscious form of emotion regulation? There are sound theoretical and good empirical reasons that, independently of frequency of use, relative success of the regulatory strategy should also be important in the development of automatic or nonconscious emotion regulation strategies. First of all, success at a goal attempt is known to increase subsequent strength of that goal or motivation, whereas failure decreases motivational strength (e.g., Bandura, 1977; Heckhausen, 1991). Moreover, relevant to the present thesis of nonconscious emotion regulation capabilities, these same effects on subsequent motivational strength following success or failure have now been obtained when the goal was pursued nonconsciously (Chartrand & Bargh, 2002). Consistent with these ideas, Ochsner and Gross (2004), in their review of emotion regulation strategies, concluded that reappraisal is both the most successful and the most frequently used strategy.

Moreover, recent research suggests that success might have its effect on goal strength through increasing the positive affect associated with the goal representation itself; in other words, the *incentive value* of the goal. Custers and Aarts (2005) used subliminal affective conditioning to implicitly link various goals with positive affect; doing so influenced how hard participants worked on the task (incentives) as well as their desire to complete the tasks. Thus, nonconsciously produced positive affect—such as that resulting from a successful act of goal pursuit—may well play a key role in the development of nonconscious emotion regulation abilities through automatically increasing the motivational strength of the emotion regulation goal.

Consistent with this prediction, Mauss, Evers, Wilhelm, and Gross (2006) have recently shown that a participant's implicit attitude toward emotion regulation itself (which can be considered as the incentive value of the goal of emotion regulation for that individual) was related both to how well the person could regulate his or her emotions in the experimental session and to how effortful the person found the attempt. The more positive the implicit affect associated with the goal of emotion regulation, the better and more automatically (efficiently; less effortfully) that goal operated for the individual.

Different Emotions, Different Strategies

It is likely that different emotions will have different strategies effective for regulating them (see Larsen & Prizmic, 2005), and thus different nonconscious regulation mechanisms associated with them. After all, different emotions serve different functions or purposes for us (Haidt, 2001; Loewenstein & Lerner, 2002), and thus it would follow that different regulatory strategies will be effective on them in turn. For example, disgust-related reactions make us tend to turn away and withdraw from the stimulus, but one can easily imagine doctors and disaster-relief workers having to develop suppression or reappraisal strategies to push on through this tendency in order to accomplish their objectives; these same folks might not regulate anger at all, as it has approach and energization qualities that might be useful under such circumstances (see Loewenstein & Lerner, 2002). The findings of Zemack-Ruger et al. (2005) discussed previously are also consistent with this reasoning; in their study subliminally presented guilt-related stimuli automatically triggered a self-control regulatory goal in their participants, whereas stimuli related to sadness did not.

CONCLUSIONS: THE POTENTIAL BENEFITS OF NONCONSCIOUS EMOTION REGULATION

The word "regulation" comes from the Latin *regula* or "rule"; thus, according to Webster's dictionary (Merriam-Webster, 2002) to regulate means "to govern or direct according to rule," or "to bring order, method, or uniformity to"—that is, to make regular. To make a process automatic upon certain conditions is the pinnacle of regularity; whenever condition X arises, goal or behavior Y is engaged. Automatic processes are much more consistent and reliable than conscious processes, for several reasons, and so nonconscious emotion regulation has the potential to be more effective than conscious regulation over the long term. Across several major domains of social psychological research—attitudes and persuasion, stereotyping and prejudice, and causal attribution—it has been shown that conscious goals are not pursued unless the person has both the motivation as well as the ability to do so. Often, the person is distracted or cognitively busy and thus fails to select the goal, or fails to notice the opportunity to do so, or just does not have the spare attentional capacity given the other things going on at the time—there are many possible slips "twixt cup and lip" when it comes to carrying out our intentions (Heckhausen, 1991).

Therefore, to the extent that an emotion regulation goal can be triggered automatically compared to consciously, it becomes a more reliable and consistent influence on us; it can also run effectively under busy conditions that would prevent the conscious goal process from operating (see Bargh & Thein, 1985); and it can take advantage of opportunities present in the environment that might otherwise have been missed because of conscious attention being directed elsewhere at the moment, or because there is not enough time right then to decide and prepare the correct response through conscious means.

One immediate potential benefit of research into nonconscious emotion regulation, then, would be the application of the findings to the treatment of life problems that heretofore have resisted conscious regulation attempts. For example, in the field of addiction counseling and treatment, the major difficulty is the overcoming of compelling direct environmental cues that trigger the craving and the behavioral routines long associated with satisfying it. Treatments that have traditionally focused on *conscious* means of behavior change do not apparently work very well (Sayette, 2004). Perhaps it is time to meet fire with fire in the case of treating such addictions. That is, it may be that a nonconscious emotion regulatory goal could succeed where conscious regulation attempts routinely fail.

This might sound too good to be true, but evidence already exists for this very process in the case of controlling unwanted stereotype influences on judgments of others. Moskowitz et al. (1999) showed that those participants who were committed to the goal of egalitarianism—of treating people from minority groups fairly—had developed an automatic, nonconscious goal of egalitarian treatment of others. More than that, the researchers were able to show that this goal was capable of *inhibiting* automatically activated stereotypes *before* they could influence the person's judgments. Remarkably, in these egalitarian participants, the group stereotypes did become activated automatically upon presentation of group-relevant stimuli, but were immediately *deactivated* by the nonconscious goal—all within less than a second. The strongest of the unwanted influences of the stimulus environment, then, including emotional experiences, might be best met with counteracting nonconscious regulatory goals—fighting fire with fire, as it were—instead of the conscious regulatory strategies that, in many cases at least, have not proven up to the job.

In sum, then, the study of nonconscious emotion regulation is a promising new direction for research and has the potential for exciting new insights regarding the role of emotions in our lives, as well as expanding our knowledge of nonconscious self-regulatory mechanisms. The significant advances that were made in other domains when the research spotlight turned to the automatic components of the phenomenon—stereotyping and prejudice, the attitude–behavior relation, interpersonal interaction, and goal pursuit, among others—stand as a promissory note to emotion researchers today.

ACKNOWLEDGMENTS

Preparation of this chapter was supported in part by Grant No. R01-MH60767 from the National Institute of Mental Health to John A. Bargh, and by a National Science Foundation predoctoral fellowship to Lawrence E. Williams. We thank Margaret Clark, Ezequiel Morsella, Noah Shamosh, and members of the ACME Lab for feedback on a previous version of this chapter.

NOTES

1. That participants engage in a mental process spontaneously, without being told to do so, as in the Jackson et al. (2003) study (see also Handley, Lassiter, Nickell, & Herchenroeder, 2004), is suggestive and consistent with the emotion regulation process being automatic but is not conclusive by itself (see below; also the excellent discussion of this issue by Uleman, 1989). People do many things in an experimental session without being explicitly instructed to do them, in part because of their assumptions about what the experiment is about and what is expected of them (e.g., demand effects).

2. Relevant to this point is the research program by Heckhausen, Gollwitzer, and colleagues on implemental versus deliberative mind-sets: this research has shown that it is a general feature of actional or "implemental" mind-sets (relative to "deliberative" or predecisional mind-sets), once the choice of action has been made, to deflect external impulses or suggestions for responses (e.g., priming effects), providing a kind of "tunnel vision" that keeps the person on track in pursuit of the desired goal (see Gollwitzer, 1999; Gollwitzer & Bayer, 1999).

REFERENCES

Aarts, H., & Dijksterhuis, A. (2003). The silence of the library: Environment, situational norm, and social behavior. *Journal of Personality and Social Psychology, 84,* 18–28.

Aspinwall, L. G., & Taylor, S. E. (1993). Effects of social comparison detection, threat, and self-esteem on affect, self-evaluation and expected success. *Journal of Personality and Social Psychology, 64,* 708–722.

Bandura, A. (1977). Self-efficacy: Toward a unifying theory of behavior change. *Psychological Review, 84,* 191–205.

Bargh, J. A. (1989). Conditional automaticity: Varieties of automatic influence in social perception and cognition. In J. S. Uleman & J. A. Bargh (Eds.), *Unintended thought* (pp. 3–51). New York: Guilford Press.

Bargh, J. A. (1990). Auto-motives: Preconscious determinants of social interaction. In E. T. Higgins & R. M. Sorrentino (Eds.), *Handbook of motivation and cognition* (Vol. 2, pp. 93–130). New York: Guilford Press.

Bargh, J. A. (1994). The Four Horsemen of automaticity: Awareness, efficiency, intention, and control in social cognition. In R. S. Wyer, Jr. & T. K. Srull (Eds.), *Handbook of social cognition* (2nd ed., pp. 1–40). Hillsdale, NJ: Erlbaum.

Bargh, J. A. (1996). Automaticity in social psychology. In E. T. Higgins & A. W. Kruglanski (Eds.), *Social psychology: Handbook of basic principles* (pp. 169–183). New York: Guilford Press.

Bargh, J. A. (1999). The cognitive monster: The case against controllability of automatic stereotype effects. In S. Chaiken & Y. Trope (Eds.), *Dual process theories in social psychology* (pp. 361–382). New York: Guilford Press.

Bargh, J. A. (2005). Bypassing the will: Towards demystifying the nonconscious control of social behavior. In R. Hassin, J. Uleman, & J. Bargh (Eds.), *The new unconscious* (pp. 37–58). New York: Oxford University Press.

Bargh, J. A. (Ed.). (2006). *Social psychology and the unconscious: The automaticity of higher mental processes.* Philadelphia: Psychology Press.

Bargh, J. A., & Chartrand, T. L. (1999). The unbearable automaticity of being. *American Psychologist, 54,* 462–479.

Bargh, J. A., & Chartrand, T. L. (2000). A practical guide to priming and automaticity research. In H. Reis & C. Judd (Eds.), *Handbook of research methods in social psychology* (pp. 253–285). New York: Cambridge University Press.

Bargh, J. A., & Gollwitzer, P. M. (1994). Environmental control over goal-directed action. *Nebraska Symposium on Motivation, 41,* 71–124.

Bargh, J. A., Gollwitzer, P. M., Lee-Chai, A. Y., Barndollar, K., & Troetschel, R. (2001). The automated will: Nonconscious activation and pursuit of behavioral goals. *Journal of Personality and Social Psychology, 81,* 1014–1027.

Bargh, J. A., & Thein, R. D. (1985). Individual construct accessibility, person memory, and the recall-judgment link: The case of information overload. *Journal of Personality and Social Psychology, 49,* 1129–1146.

Barker, R. G., & Wright, H. F. (1955). *Midwest and its children: The psychological ecology of an American town.* New York: Harper & Row.

Barkley, R. A. (2004). Attention-deficit/hyperactivity disorder and self-regulation: Taking an evolutionary perspective on executive functioning. In R. F. Baumeister & K. D. Vohs (Eds.), *Handbook of self-regulation* (pp. 301–323). New York: Guilford Press.

Calkins, S. D. (2004). Early attachment processes and the development of emotional self-regulation. In R. F. Baumeister & K. D. Vohs (Eds.), *Handbook of self-regulation* (pp. 324–339). New York: Guilford Press.

Calkins, S. D., & Hill, A. (2007). Caregiver influences on emerging emotion regulation: Biological and environmental transactions in early development. In J. J. Gross (Ed.), *Handbook of emotion regulation* (pp. 229–248). New York: Guilford Press.

Carver, C. S. (2004). Self-regulation of action and affect. In R. F. Baumeister & K. D. Vohs (Eds.), *Handbook of self-regulation* (pp. 13–39). New York: Guilford Press.

Carver, C. S., & Scheier, M. F. (1981). *Attention and self-regulation: A control-theory approach to human behavior.* New York: Springer.

Chartrand, T. L., & Bargh, J. A. (1996). Automatic activation of social information processing goals: Nonconscious priming reproduces effects of explicit conscious instructions. *Journal of Personality and Social Psychology, 71,* 464–478.

Chartrand, T. L., & Bargh, J. A. (1999). The chameleon effect: The perception–behavior link and social interaction. *Journal of Personality and Social Psychology, 76,* 893–910.

Chartrand, T. L., & Bargh, J. A. (2002). Nonconscious motivations: Their activation, operation, and consequences. In A. Tesser, D. A. Stapel, & J. V. Wood (Eds.), *Self and motivation: Emerging psychological perspectives* (pp. 13–41). Washington, DC: American Psychological Association.

Chen, M., & Bargh, J. A. (1999). Consequences of automatic evaluation: Immediate behavioral predispositions to approach or avoid the stimulus. *Personality and Social Psychology Bulletin, 25,* 215–224.

Custers, R., & Aarts, H. (2005). Positive affect as implicit motivator: On the nonconscious operation of behavioral goals. *Journal of Personality and Social Psychology, 89,* 129–142.

Damasio, A. R. (1996). The somatic marker hypothesis and the possible functions of the prefrontal cortex. *Philosophical Transactions of the Royal Society of London, B, 351,* 1413–1420.

Darwin, C. (1872). *The expression of the emotions in man and animals.* London: John Murray.

Davidson, R. J., & Irwin, W. (1999). The functional neuroanatomy of emotion and affective style. *Trends in Cognitive Science, 3,* 11–21.

Decety, J., & Sommerville, J. A. (2003). Shared representations between self and other: A social cognitive neuroscience view. *Trends in Cognitive Sciences, 7,* 527–533.

Devine, P. G. (1989). Stereotypes and prejudice: Their automatic and controlled components. *Journal of Personality and Social Psychology, 56,* 5–18.

Dijksterhuis, A., & Bargh, J. A. (2001). The perception–behavior expressway: Automatic effects of social perception on social behavior. In M. P. Zanna (Ed.), *Advances in experimental social psychology* (Vol. 33, pp. 1–40). San Diego: Academic Press.

Duckworth, K. L., Bargh, J. A., Garcia, M., & Chaiken, S. (2002). The automatic evaluation of novel stimuli. *Psychological Science, 13,* 513–519.

Erber, R., Wegner, D. M., & Therriault, N. (1996). On being cool and collected: Mood regulation in anticipation of social interaction. *Journal of Personality and Social Psychology, 70,* 757–766.

Fazio, R. H., Sanbonmatsu, D. M., Powell, M. C., & Kardes, F. R. (1986). On the automatic activation of attitudes. *Journal of Personality and Social Psychology, 50,* 229–238.

Ferguson, M. J., Bargh, J. A., & Nayak, D. A. (2005). After-affects: How automatic evaluations influence the interpretation of subsequent, unrelated stimuli. *Journal of Experimental Social Psychology, 41,* 182–191.

Fiske, S. T. (1989). Examining the role of intent: Toward understanding its role in stereotyping and prejudice. In J. S. Uleman & J. A. Bargh (Eds.), *Unintended thought* (pp. 253–283). New York: Guilford Press.

Fitzsimons, G. M., & Bargh, J. A. (2004). Automatic self-regulation. In R. F. Baumeister & K. D. Vohs (Eds.), *Handbook of self-regulation* (pp. 151–170). New York: Guilford Press.

Fitzsimons, G. M., & Bargh, J. A. (2003). Thinking of you: Nonconscious pursuit of interpersonal goals associated with relationship partners. *Journal of Personality and Social Psychology, 84,* 148–164.

Forgas, J. P., & Ciarrochi, J. V. (2002). On managing moods: Evidence for the role of homeostatic cognitive strategies in affect regulation. *Personality and Social Psychology Bulletin, 28,* 336–345.

Frith, C. D., & Wolpert, D. M. (Eds.). (2004). *The neuroscience of social interaction: Decoding, imitating, and influencing the actions of others.* New York: Oxford University Press.

Gallese, V., Fadiga, L., Fogassi, L., & Rizzolatti, G. (1996). Action recognition in the premotor cortex. *Brain, 119,* 593–609.

Gilbert, D. T., & Hixon, J. G. (1991). The trouble of thinking: Activation and application of stereotypic beliefs. *Journal of Personality and Social Psychology, 60,* 509–517.

Gollwitzer, P. M. (1999). Implementation intentions: Strong effects of simple plans. *American Psychologist, 54,* 493–503.

Gollwitzer, P. M., & Bayer, U. (1999). Deliberative versus implemental mindsets in the control of action. In S. Chaiken & Y. Trope (Eds.), *Dual process theories in social psychology* (pp. 403–422). New York: Guilford Press.

Gray, J. (2004). Integration of emotion and cognitive control. *Current Directions in Psychological Science, 13,* 46–48.

Gray, J. R., Schaefer, A., Braver, T. S., & Most, S. B. (2005). Affect and the resolution of cognitive control dilemmas. In L. F. Barrett, P. M. Niedenthal, & P. Winkielman (Eds.), *Emotion and consciousness* (pp. 67–94). New York: Guilford Press.

Gross, J. J. (1999). Emotion regulation: Past, present, future. *Cognition and Emotion, 13,* 551–573.

Haidt, J. (2001). The emotional dog and its rational tail: A social intuitionist approach to moral judgment. *Psychological Review, 108,* 814–834

Handley, I. M., Lassiter, G. D., Nickell, E. F., & Herchenroeder, L. M. (2004). Affect and automatic mood maintenance. *Journal of Experimental Social Psychology, 40,* 106–112.

Hebb, D. O. (1949). *Organization of behavior.* New York: Wiley.

Heckhausen, H. (1991). *Motivation and action.* New York: Springer.

Higgins, E. T. (1987). Self-discrepancy: A theory relating self and affect. *Psychological Review, 94,* 319–340.

Jackson, D. C., Mueller, C. J., Dolski, L., Dalton, K. M., Nitschke, J. B., Urry, H. L., et al. (2003). Now you feel it, now you don't: Frontal brain electrical asymmetry and individual differences in emotion regulation. *Psychological Science, 14,* 612–617.

Jostmann, N. B., Koole, S. L., van der Wulp, N. Y., & Fockenberg, D. A. (2005). Subliminal affect regulation: The moderating role of action vs. state orientation. *European Psychologist, 10,* 209–217.

Koole, S. L., & Jostmann, N. B. (2004). Getting a grip on your feelings: Effects of action orientation and external demands on intuitive affect regulation. *Journal of Personality and Social Psychology, 87,* 974–990.

Kruglanski, A. W. (1996). Goals as knowledge structures. In E. T. Higgins & A. W. Kruglanski (Eds.), *Social psychology: Handbook of basic principles* (pp. 493–520). New York: Guilford Press.

Lakin, J., & Chartrand, T. L. (2003). Using nonconscious behavioral mimicry to create affiliation and rapport. *Psychological Science, 14,* 334–339.

Larsen, R. J., & Prizmic, Z. (2005). Affect regulation. In L. F. Barrett, P. M. Niedenthal, & P. Winkielman (Eds.), *Emotion and consciousness* (pp. 40–61). New York: Guilford Press.

LeDoux, J. E. (1996). *The emotional brain.* New York: Simon & Schuster.

Lerner, J. S., Small, D. A., & Loewenstein, G. (2004). Heart strings and purse strings: Carry-over effects of emotions on economic transactions. *Psychological Science, 15,* 337–341.

Loewenstein, G. (2007). Affective regulation and affective forecasting. In J. J. Gross (Ed.), Handbook of emotion regulation (pp. 180-203). New York: Guilford Press.

Loewenstein, G., & Lerner, J. S. (2002). The role of affect in decision making. In R. Davidson, K. Scherer, & H. Goldsmith (Eds.), *Handbook of affective science* (pp. 619–642). New York: Oxford University Press.

MacCoon, D. G., Wallace, J. F., & Newman, J. P. (2005). Self-regulation: Context-appropriate balanced attention. In L. F. Barrett, P. M. Niedenthal, & P. Winkielman (Eds.), *Emotion and consciousness* (pp. 422–444). New York: Guilford Press.

Mauss, I. B., Evers, C., Wilhelm, F. H., & Gross, J. J. (2006). How to bite your tongue without blowing your top: Implicit evaluation of emotion regulation predicts affective responding to anger provocation. *Personality and Social Psychology Bulletin, 32,* 389–402.

McClure, S. M., Botvinick, M. M., Yeung, N., Greene, J. D., & Cohen, J. D. Conflict monitoring in cognition-emotion competition. In J. J. Gross (Ed.), *Handbook of emotion regulation* (pp. 204-226). New York: Guilford Press.

Merriam-Webster, Inc. (2002). *Webster's collegiate dictionary* (10th ed., p. 983). Springfield, MA: Author.

Mischel, W., & Ayduk, O. (2004). Willpower in a cognitive–affective processing system: The dynamics of delay of gratification. In R. F. Baumeister & K. D. Vohs (Eds.), *Handbook of self-regulation* (pp. 151–170). New York: Guilford Press.

Moors, A., & deHouwer, J. (2006). What is automaticity? An analysis of its component features and their interrelations. In J. A. Bargh (Ed.), *Social psychology and the unconscious: The automaticity of higher mental processes.* Philadelphia: Psychology Press.

Morsella, E. (2005). The functions of phenomenal states: Supramodular interaction theory. *Psychological Review, 112,* 1000–1021.

Moskowitz, G. B., Gollwitzer, P. M., Wasel, W., & Schaal, B. (1999). Preconscious control of stereotype activation through chronic egalitarianism. *Journal of Personality and Social Psychology, 77,* 167–184.

Mowrer, O. H. (1960). *Learning theory and behavior.* New York: Wiley.

Ochsner, K. N., Bunge, S. A., Gross, J. J., & Gabrieli, J. D. E. (2002). Rethinking feelings: An fMRI study of the cognitive regulation of emotion. *Journal of Cognitive Neuroscience, 14,* 1215–1229.

Ochsner, K. N., & Gross, J. J. (2004). Thinking makes it so: A social cognitive neuroscience approach to emotion regulation. In R. F. Baumeister & K. D. Vohs (Eds.), *Handbook of self-regulation* (pp. 229–255). New York: Guilford Press.

Ochsner, K. N., & Gross, J. J. (2007). The neural architecture of emotion regulation. In J. J. Gross (Ed.), *Handbook of emotion regulation* (pp. 87–109). New York: Guilford Press.

Oettingen, G., Grant, H., Smith, P. K., Skinner, M., & Gollwitzer, P. M. (in press). Nonconscious goal pursuit: Acting in an explanatory vacuum. *Journal of Experimental Social Psychology.*

Posner, M. I., & Rothbart, M. K. (1998). Attention, self-regulation, and consciousness. *Philosophical Transactions of the Royal Society of London, B, 353,* 1915–1927.

Rothbart, M. K., & Sheese, B. E. (2007). Temperament and emotion regulation. In J. J. Gross (Ed.), *Handbook of emotion regulation* (pp. 331–350). New York: Guilford Press.

Sassenberg, K., & Moskowitz, G. B. (2004). Don't stereotype, think different! Overcoming automatic stereotype activation by mindset priming. *Journal of Experimental Social Psychology, 41,* 506–514.

Sayette, M. A. (2004). Self-regulatory failure and addiction. In R. F. Baumeister & K. D. Vohs (Eds.), *Handbook of self-regulation* (pp. 447–465). New York: Guilford Press.

Simon, H. A. (1967). Motivational and emotional controls of cognition. *Psychological Review, 74,* 29–39.

Spencer, S. J., Fein, S., Wolfe, C. T., Fong, C., & Dunn, M. A. (1998). Automatic activation of stereotypes: The role of self-image threat. *Personality and Social Psychology Bulletin, 24,* 1139–1152.

Tetlock, P. (2002). Social functionalist frameworks for judgments and choice: Intuitive politicians, theologians, and prosecutors. *Psychological Review, 109,* 451–471.

Uleman, J. S. (1989). A framework for thinking intentionally about unintended thoughts. In J. S. Uleman & J. A. Bargh (Eds.), *Unintended thought.* New York: Guilford Press.

Wegner, D. M., & Bargh, J. A. (1998). Control and automaticity in social life. In D. Gilbert, S. Fiske, & G. Lindzey (Eds.), *Handbook of social psychology* (4/e). Boston: McGraw-Hill.

Wilson, T. D., & Brekke, N. (1994). Mental contamination and mental correction: Unwanted influences on judgments and evaluations. *Psychological Bulletin, 116,* 117–142.

Winkielman, P., Berridge, K. C., & Wilbarger, J. L. (2005). Emotion, behavior, and conscious experience: Once more without feeling. In L. F. Barrett, P. M. Niedenthal, & P. Winkielman (Eds.), *Emotion and consciousness.* New York: Guilford Press.

Zemack-Rugar, Y., Bettman, J. R., & Fitzsimons, G. J. (2005). *Effects of specific, nonconscious emotions on self-control behavior.* Manuscript submitted for publication, Duke University.

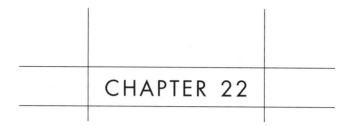

CHAPTER 22

Adult Attachment Strategies and the Regulation of Emotion

PHILLIP R. SHAVER
MARIO MIKULINCER

In the past 20 years, attachment theory (Bowlby, 1969/1982, 1973, 1980) has become one of the most influential conceptual frameworks for understanding emotion regulation. Although Bowlby did not devote much attention to abstract theorizing about emotion itself (he included only a single brief chapter about it in Volume 1 of *Attachment and Loss*), his writings were motivated by clinical and ethological observations of humans and other primates who were experiencing, expressing, and regulating emotions such as affection, anxiety, anger, grief, and despair. He was especially interested in the anxiety-buffering function of close relationships and the capacity for dysfunctional relationships to generate negative emotions and, in the extreme, to precipitate debilitating forms of psychopathology. Bowlby (1973, 1980) characterized the stable individual differences in emotion regulation that emerge from prolonged reliance on particular "attachment figures," people who provide either adequate or inadequate protection, safety, support, and guidance concerning emotions and emotion regulation.

With the accumulation of empirical knowledge about what Bowlby called the attachment behavioral system, individual differences in attachment orientations, and emotion regulation in infancy and adulthood, Bowlby's ideas (as elaborated and tested initially by Ainsworth, Blehar, Waters, & Wall, 1978) have been extended, tested, and organized into a theoretical model (e.g., Fraley & Shaver, 2000; Mikulincer & Shaver, 2003; Shaver & Mikulincer, 2002). The model clarifies the emotion-regulatory function of the attachment system and explains many of the emotional correlates and consequences of individual differences in attachment-system functioning. In this chapter, we elaborate on these individual differences and provide a detailed review of empirical

446

studies that have examined attachment-related variations in coping with stress, managing attachment-related threats, and regulating or defending against particular emotional states.

ATTACHMENT THEORY: BASIC CONCEPTS

Bowlby (1969/1982) claimed that human beings are born with an innate psychobiological system (the *attachment behavioral system*) that motivates them to seek proximity to significant others (*attachment figures*) in times of need. This system accomplishes basic regulatory functions (protection from threats and alleviation of distress) in human beings of all ages, but it is most directly observable during infancy and early childhood (Bowlby, 1988). Bowlby (1973) also described important individual differences in attachment-system functioning depending on the availability, responsiveness, and supportiveness of attachment figures. Interactions with attachment figures who are available and responsive in times of need facilitate the optimal functioning of the attachment system and promote a *sense of attachment security*. This pervasive sense of security is based on implicit beliefs that the world is generally safe, that attachment figures are helpful when called upon, and that it is possible to explore the environment curiously and engage effectively and enjoyably with other people. This sense of security is rooted in positive mental representations of self and others, which Bowlby called internal working models.

Unfortunately, there are darker alternatives to this condition, which develop when attachment figures are not reliably available and supportive, fail to provide adequate relief from distress, and cause a child who is dependent on them to form negative working models of self and others and to develop defensive *secondary attachment strategies*. (Direct security seeking is viewed as the *primary strategy*.) Secondary attachment strategies take two major forms: *hyperactivation* and *deactivation* of the attachment system (e.g., Cassidy & Kobak, 1988).

Hyperactivation (which Bowlby, 1969/1982, called protest) is characterized by intense efforts to attain proximity to attachment figures and insistent attempts to induce a relationship partner, viewed as insufficiently available or responsive, to provide more satisfying and reassuring care and support. Hyperactivating strategies include clinging, controlling, and coercive behaviors; cognitive and behavioral efforts to establish physical contact and a sense of merger or "oneness"; and overdependence on relationship partners for protection (Shaver & Mikulincer, 2002). People who rely on hyperactivating strategies compulsively seek proximity and protection, and they are chronically hypersensitive to signs of possible rejection or abandonment. In contrast, deactivation involves inhibition of proximity-seeking inclinations and actions, suppression or discounting of threats that might activate the attachment system, and determination to handle stresses alone (a defensive stance that Bowlby, 1969/1982, called compulsive self-reliance). People who rely on these strategies tend to maximize autonomy and distance from relationship partners, experience discomfort with closeness and intimacy, and strive for personal strength and control of relationship partners.

When studying individual differences in the functioning of the attachment system in adolescence and adulthood, attachment researchers have focused on a person's *attachment style*—the chronic pattern of relational expectations, emotions, and behaviors that results from internalization of a particular history of attachment experiences (Fraley & Shaver, 2000). Beginning with Ainsworth et al.'s (1978) studies of infant–

caregiver attachment, continuing through Hazan and Shaver's (1987) conceptualization of romantic love as an attachment process, and followed up in many recent studies by social and personality psychologists (reviewed by Mikulincer & Shaver, 2003), researchers have found that individual differences in attachment style can be measured along two orthogonal dimensions, attachment-related *avoidance* and *anxiety* (Brennan, Clark, & Shaver, 1998). A person's position on the avoidance dimension indicates the extent to which he or she distrusts others' goodwill and relies on deactivating strategies for coping with attachment insecurities. A person's position on the anxiety dimension indicates the degree to which he or she worries that relationship partners will be unavailable in times of need and relies on hyperactivating strategies for dealing with these worries. People who score low on both dimensions enjoy a dispositional sense of felt security, are likely to have had a security-supporting attachment history, and are said to be secure or to have a secure attachment style.

ATTACHMENT STRATEGIES AND EMOTION REGULATION

Theoretical Background

According to attachment theory (Cassidy & Kobak, 1988; Main, 1990; Shaver & Mikulincer, 2002), attachment orientations or styles include a variety of cognitive, affective, and behavioral maneuvers that can alter, obstruct, or suppress the generation, activation, and expression of emotions. These strategies guide the process of emotion regulation and shape a person's appraisals, feelings, and action tendencies.

In analyzing the regulatory processes associated with different attachment strategies, we rely on an updated version of Shaver, Schwartz, Kirson, and O'Connor's (1987) model of the emotion process (see Figure 22.1). This model is based on both theoretical considerations (e.g., Frijda, 1986; Lazarus, 1991) and ordinary people's accounts of their emotional experiences (e.g., Shaver et al., 1987; Smith & Ellsworth, 1987) and has been used to conceptualize both emotions and emotional development (e.g., Fischer, Shaver, & Carnochan, 1990). In the model, emotions, considered to be organized sets of thought and action tendencies supported by specific physiological processes, are generated by the appraisal of external or internal events in relation to a person's goals and

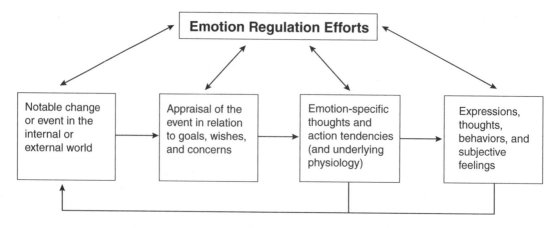

FIGURE 22.1. Flowchart model of the emotion process (based on Shaver et al., 1987).

concerns. The resulting emotions are experienced and expressed through changes in the cognitive accessibility of various mental contents and in action tendencies, behaviors, and subjective feelings (Oatley & Jenkins, 1996). Both the generation and the expression of emotions are affected by regulatory efforts, which can alter, obstruct, or suppress appraisals, concerns, action tendencies, and subjective feelings.

According to Shaver et al. (1987) and Oatley and Jenkins (1996), emotion generation depends on a perceived change in the environment, especially an unexpected, surprising, or personally relevant change. These changes are automatically, and often unconsciously, appraised in relation to a person's needs, goals, wishes, and concerns. If the perceived changes are favorable to goal attainment, the resulting emotions are hedonically positive. If the changes are unfavorable, the resulting emotions are hedonically negative. The particular emotions that emerge depend on the specific pattern of concerns and appraisals that get activated (e.g., Lazarus, 1991; Shaver et al., 1987). When a specific appraisal pattern occurs, a corresponding kind of emotion, including its evolutionarily functional action tendencies and physiological substrates (e.g., changes in respiration, blood pressure, neurochemistry, and muscle tension), follows automatically. These consequences can be manifested in thoughts, feelings, or actions; expressed both verbally and nonverbally; and measured in numerous ways.

Shaver et al. (1987) claimed, based partly on existing research and partly on their research participants' narratives, that regulatory efforts can alter the entire emotion process. If there is no reason to postpone, dampen, redirect, or deny the emerging emotion, the action tendencies are automatically expressed in congruent thoughts, feelings, and behaviors. However, when there are other goals in play (e.g., social norms, personal standards, and self-protective defenses) that make experience, enactment, and expression of an emotion undesirable, regulatory efforts are called into service to alter, obstruct, or suppress the emotion and bring about a more desirable emotional state or at least the outward appearance of a more desirable state.

In this model, regulatory efforts can be directed toward various parts of the emotion process. The most direct regulatory maneuvers are problem-solving efforts aimed at ending or changing the events that elicited the emotion. Regulatory maneuvers can also be directed at the appraisals that link external events to emotional reactions. Reappraisal can contribute to problem solving by calming a person and allowing him or her to deploy problem-solving resources more effectively, or even render problem solving unnecessary if the problem is deemed unsolvable or the person is unwilling or unable to engage in the necessary problem-solving steps (Lazarus & Folkman, 1984). In any case, these two coping reactions, problem solving and reappraisal, can eliminate many undesirable emotions and make it unnecessary to take further regulatory steps (Gross, 1999; Gross & Thompson, this volume). However, when problem solving or reappraisal is insufficient to eliminate aversive emotions, regulation efforts may be directed at the emotional state itself, including its physiological underpinnings. Alternatively, regulatory efforts can dissociate the emotion from its appearance in thoughts, feelings, and behaviors. In other words, the emotion's access to conscious awareness may be blocked and its overt expression suppressed.

Attachment Security and the Constructive Regulation of Emotions

According to Shaver and Mikulincer (2002), a sense of attachment security facilitates security-based strategies of emotion regulation, which are aimed at alleviating distress, maintaining comfortable, supportive intimate relationships, and increasing personal adjustment through constructive, flexible, and reality-attuned coping efforts. Moreover, they sustain what Shaver and Mikulincer (2002), following Fredrickson (2001), called a broaden-and-build cycle of attachment security, which expands a person's resources for maintaining equanimity and mental health in times of stress, broadens the person's perspectives and capacities, and facilitates incorporation of mental representations of security-enhancing attachment figures into the self. This broaden-and-build process allows securely attached people to maintain an authentic sense of personal efficacy, resilience, and optimism even in situations in which attachment figures are absent or social support is unavailable (Mikulincer & Shaver, 2004).

During emotion regulation, a sense of attachment security sustains problem-solving efforts and reappraisal attempts. When confronted with external or internal changes or events that would typically elicit undesirable emotions, securely attached individuals can generate instrumental problem-solving strategies (e.g., analyzing situations, planning effective strategies, and inhibiting interfering thoughts or actions) and mobilize available sources of social support to assist problem solving (e.g., by providing material aid, information, or advice) or sustain motivation and problem-solving efforts by soothing, supporting, and affirming the threatened or troubled individual.

Secure people's constructive approach to problem solving results from their interactions with attachment figures who are (or were) sensitive and responsive to expressed bids for proximity, protection, and support. (See Calkins & Hill, and Thompson & Meyer, this volume.) During supportive interactions with attachment figures, secure people learn (or learned, in the past) that their own actions are often sufficient to reduce distress and remove obstacles, and that seeking support from others is an effective means to enhance problem solving. Two other aspects of interactions with security-enhancing attachment figures facilitate problem solving. One common prerequisite for problem solving is recognizing that one's initial course of action is ineffective. Experiencing, or having experienced, attachment figures as loving and supportive allows secure people to revise erroneous beliefs without excessive fear of criticism, humiliation, or rejection. Problem solving also often requires the opening up of existing knowledge structures, incorporation of new information, and flexible adjustment of knowledge structures to current reality demands. Secure people's self-confidence allows them to open their cognitive structures to new information and flexibly adjust their plans for dealing realistically with environmental imperatives (Mikulincer, 1997). Moreover, believing implicitly that support will generally be available if needed, secure people can creatively explore a problematic or challenging situation while tolerating ambiguity and uncertainty.

Secure people can also reappraise situations, construe events in relatively benign terms, symbolically transform threats into challenges, hold on to an optimistic sense of self-efficacy, and attribute undesirable events to controllable, temporary, or context-dependent causes. This stance toward appraisals is sustained by deeply ingrained positive beliefs (or working models) about self and world (Mikulincer & Shaver, 2003). While interacting with available and supportive attachment figures, secure individuals have learned that distress is manageable and external obstacles surmountable. Moreover, they know they can effectively exert control over many threatening events. Their optimistic, hopeful mental representations promote self-soothing reappraisals of aversive events, assist in problem solving, and sustain effective emotion regulation.

Having managed emotion-eliciting events or reappraised them in relatively benign terms, secure individuals often do not need to alter or suppress other components of the emotion process. They make what Lazarus (1991) called a short-circuit of threat, sidestepping the interfering and dysfunctional aspects of emotions while retaining their functional, adaptive qualities. As a result, secure people can generally remain open to their emotions, express and communicate their feelings openly and accurately to others, and experience them fully in their own thoughts and feelings. Such people do not generally have to deny, exaggerate, or distort their emotional experiences.

Secure people can attend to their own distress without fear of being overwhelmed or losing control. For individuals whose attachment figures have been available and responsive, expression of negative emotions has usually led to distress-alleviating interventions by a caregiver. The person with good attachment figures learns that distress can be expressed honestly without the relationship being at risk, and this fosters an increasingly balanced way of experiencing and expressing emotions—with a sensible goal in mind and without undue hostility, vengeance, or anxiety about loss of control or loss of the relationship. According to Cassidy (1994), "the experience of security is based not on the denial of negative affect but on the ability to tolerate negative affects temporarily in order to achieve mastery over threatening or frustrating situations" (p. 233). In other words, for relatively secure individuals, "emotion regulation" does not require avoidance or denial of emotions.

Another aspect of secure people's experience of emotions is self-reflective capacity—the ability to notice, think about, and understand mental states (Fonagy, Steele, Steele, Moran, & Higgit, 1991)—which facilitates recognition of the functional aspects of emotions and the integration of emotional experience into one's sense of self. According to Fonagy et al. (1991), interactions with available and supportive attachment figures provide secure individuals with the capacity to understand and articulate their emotional experiences. Fonagy et al. (1991) described the security-enhancing caregiver of an infant as able "to reflect on the infant's mental experience and re-present it to the infant translated into the language of actions the infant can understand. The baby is, thus, provided with the illusion that the process of reflection of psychological processes was performed within its own mental boundaries. This is the necessary background to the evolution of a firmly established reflective self" (p. 207). This process, although it may sound mysterious when described by a psychoanalyst, can and has been empirically documented in studies using the Adult Attachment Interview (AAI; George, Kaplan, & Main, 1985; see review by Hesse, 1999) and Fonagy, Target, Steele, and Steele's (1998) measure of "mentalization" or "reflective functioning."

Avoidant Attachment and the Inhibition of Emotional Experience

According to attachment theory, avoidant (deactivating) strategies are motivated by the desire to suppress pain and distress caused by frustration of bids for proximity to and support from cool, distant, or rejecting attachment figures (Cassidy & Kobak, 1988). As mentioned earlier, the way to attain this goal is to squelch frustrating bids for proximity and inhibit painful activation of the attachment system. As a result of practicing this strategy, avoidant individuals learn to downplay threats and stop monitoring the whereabouts and availability of attachment figures, because focusing on threats or worrying about attachment figures reactivates the attachment system (Kobak, Cole, Ferenz-Gillies, Fleming, & Gamble, 1993). Instead, avoidant individuals tend to emphasize their self-reliance and self-efficacy while disparaging or dismissing other people's needs for intimacy or social support (Bowlby, 1988).

When regulating their emotions, avoidant people attempt to block or inhibit any emotional state that is incongruent with the goal of keeping their attachment system deactivated (Mikulincer & Shaver, 2003). These inhibitory efforts are directed mainly at fear, anxiety, anger, sadness, shame, guilt, and distress, because these emotions are associated with threats and feelings of vulnerability. In addition, anger often implies emotional involvement or investment in a relationship, and such involvement is incongruent with avoidant people's preference for independence and self-reliance (Cassidy, 1994). Moreover, fear, anxiety, sadness, shame, and guilt can be viewed as signs of personal weakness or vulnerability, all of which contradict the avoidant person's desired sense of personal strength and self-reliance.

Avoidant individuals also attempt to block or inhibit emotional reactions to potential or actual threats to attachment-figure availability (rejection, betrayal, separation, loss), because such threats are direct triggers of attachment-system activation. Like secure people, avoidant ones attempt to downregulate threat-related emotions. However, whereas secure people's regulatory attempts usually promote communication, compromise, and relationship maintenance, avoidant people's efforts are aimed mainly at keeping the attachment system deactivated, regardless of the deleterious effect this can have on a relationship.

The avoidant approach to emotion regulation can interfere with problem solving and reappraisal. To succeed at problem solving or reappraisal, people often have to admit that their beliefs were mistaken or their behaviors misguided, and they have to open their knowledge structures to new information. Avoidant individuals are reluctant to acknowledge that they were wrong, because being wrong calls their sense of competence and superiority into question. They may be unable to accept new information if it generates uncertainty or confusion and implies a need for help. Even engaging in flexible problem solving can generate threats related to possible failure or admission that some problems are unsolvable or beyond one's control, either absolutely or when tackled alone (Mikulincer, 1998a).

Deactivating strategies cause people to avoid noticing their own emotional reactions. Avoidant individuals often deny or suppress emotion-related thoughts and memories, divert attention from emotion-related material, suppress emotion-related action tendencies, or inhibit or mask verbal and nonverbal expressions of emotion (Kobak et al., 1993; Mikulincer & Shaver, 2003). By averting the conscious experience and expression of unpleasant emotions, avoidant individuals make it less likely that emotional experiences will be integrated into their cognitive structures and that they will use them effectively in information processing or social action. During many frustrating and painful interactions with rejecting attachment figures, they have learned that acknowledging and displaying distress leads to rejection or punishment (Cassidy, 1994).

Bowlby (1980) described avoidant inhibition and denial of emotional experiences in terms of "defensive exclusion" and "segregated mental systems." This was his way of retaining some of previous psychoanalysts' insights regarding psychological defenses. (See also Westen & Blagov, this volume.) When avoidant people encounter threats, either personal or relational, that activate their attachment system, they try to block related appraisals, concerns, feelings, memories, and action tendencies from consciousness. Over time, this kind of defensive exclusion distorts perceptions and memories, as can be seen in many experiments (e.g., Fraley, Garner, & Shaver, 2000) and in the AAI (George et al., 1985; Hesse, 1999). Even when threat- or attachment-related material is encoded, it tends to be processed at a shallow level because this results in fewer unpleasant associations with other thoughts and memories (Mikulincer & Shaver, 2003).

Attachment Anxiety and the Intensification of Undesirable Emotions

Unlike secure and avoidant people, who tend to view negative emotions as goal-incongruent states that should either be managed effectively or suppressed, anxiously attached individuals tend to perceive these emotions as congruent with attachment goals, and they therefore tend to sustain or even exaggerate them. Attachment-anxious people are guided by an unfulfilled wish to cause attachment figures to pay more attention and provide more reliable protection (Cassidy & Kobak, 1988; Mikulincer & Shaver, 2003). As explained previously, one way to attain this goal is to keep the attachment system chronically activated (i.e., in a state of hyperactivation) and intensify bids for attention until a satisfying sense of attachment security is attained. Chronically attachment-anxious individuals tend to exaggerate the presence and seriousness of threats and remain vigilant regarding possible attachment-figure unavailability (Kobak et al., 1993). They also tend to overemphasize their sense of helplessness and vulnerability, because signs of weakness and neediness can sometimes elicit other people's attention and care (Cassidy & Berlin, 1994).

Hyperactivation of negative emotions can render problem solving irrelevant. In fact, problem solving may thwart an anxious person's desire to perpetuate problematic situations and continue expressing neediness and dissatisfaction. Moreover, problem solving works against the anxious person's self-construal as helpless and incompetent; too much competence might result in loss of attention and support from attachment figures.

How is anxious hyperactivation sustained? One method is to exaggerate the appraisal process, perceptually heightening the threatening aspects of even fairly benign events, hold on to pessimistic beliefs about one's ability to manage distress, and attribute threat-related events to uncontrollable causes and global personal inadequacies (Mikulincer & Florian, 1998). This self-defeating appraisal process is sustained by negative beliefs about both self and world (Collins & Read, 1994; Shaver & Clark, 1994). Although these beliefs are initially developed in the context of emotionally negative interactions with unavailable or unreliable attachment figures, they are sustained by cognitive biases that overgeneralize past attachment injuries and inappropriately apply memories of injuries to new situations (Mikulincer & Shaver, 2003).

Another regulatory technique that heightens the experience and expression of threat-related emotions is shifting attention toward internal indicators of distress (Cassidy & Kobak, 1988; Shaver & Mikulincer, 2002). This maneuver involves hypervigilant attention to the physiological components of emotional states, heightened recall of threat-related experiences, and rumination on real and potential threats (Main & Solomon, 1986; Mikulincer & Shaver, 2003). Another hyperactivating strategy is to intensify negative emotions by favoring an approach, counterphobic orientation toward threatening situations or making self-defeating decisions and taking ineffective courses of action that are likely to end in failure. All these strategies create a self-amplifying cycle of distress, which is maintained cognitively by ruminative thoughts and feelings even after a threat objectively disappears.

Just as avoidant individuals can block or segregate memories of negative experiences, anxious people can mentally link such experiences tightly together, so that one negative thought or memory triggers a flood of others (Shaver & Mikulincer, 2002). Speaking in terms of associative memory networks, one cognitive node with a negative emotional tag can automatically spread its activation to other negatively tinged cognitive nodes, causing all of them to become highly available in working memory. This pattern of cognitive activation gives prominence to emotional implications of information and favors the organization of cognitions in terms of simple, undifferentiated affective features, such as the extent to which the information is threatening or implies rejection. Attachment-anxious people therefore suffer from a chaotic mental architecture pervaded by negative emotion (Main, Kaplan, & Cassidy, 1985). Main (1990) described this "state of mind with respect to attachment" as involving high levels of confusion, ambivalence, and incoherence, all of which have been amply documented in studies using the AAI (Hesse, 1999).

Interestingly, although hyperactivating and deactivating strategies lead to opposite patterns of emotional expression (intensification vs. suppression), both result in dysfunctional emotional experience. Whereas avoidant people miss the adaptive aspects of emotional experiences by blocking mental access to emotions, anxious people fail to take advantage of adaptive possibilities because their attention is riveted on threatening and disruptive aspects of emotional experience instead of its potentially functional aspects. As a result, they may perceive themselves as helpless to control the self-amplifying, ruminative flow of painful thoughts and feelings.

One might wonder why anxious people would remain immune to social feedback indicating that hyperactivation of distress is self-defeating and unlikely to lead to security. One answer is that hyperactivation of the attachment system sometimes succeeds in getting a relationship partners' attention, thereby temporarily heightening the anxious person's senses of relief and security. This kind of partial reinforcement schedule is thought to explain the link between inconsistent parenting and the creation of anxious attachment in early childhood (Cassidy & Berlin, 1994). In addition, once established, schematic processing—either persisting in seeing what one expects to see or influencing events so that they confirm one's expectations—can be self-sustaining even if it produces emotional pain and distress. It can be deceptively reassuring to know that one's worst fears are realized, thereby confirming one's predictions.

Empirical Evidence for Attachment-Related Differences in Emotion Regulation

There is now a large body of evidence supporting the analysis we have just provided in abstract theoretical terms. The findings consistently and coherently support the hypothesized links between attachment security and constructive patterns of emotion regulation, attachment avoidance and emotional inhibition, and attachment anxiety and distress intensification.

Coping with Stressful Events

Stressful events are major triggers of negative emotions and they often give rise to regulatory efforts. If attachment-related mental and behavioral strategies are involved in emotion regulation, they should be evident in the way people appraise and cope with stressful events.

Attachment strategies clearly influence the appraisal of stressful events (e.g., Alexander, Feeney, Hohaus, & Noller, 2001; Berant, Mikulincer, & Florian, 2001; Birnbaum, Orr, Mikulincer, & Florian, 1997; Mikulincer & Florian, 1998), with attachment anxiety being associated with distress-intensifying appraisals (appraising threats as extreme and coping resources as deficient). For avoidant individuals the findings are less consistent. Most studies have found that avoidant people report a pattern of appraisal similar to that shown by their secure counterparts. However, some studies have found that attachment avoidance, like attachment anxiety, is associated with a more pessimistic, distress-intensifying pattern of appraisal when people confront undeniable and uncontrollable traumatic events (e.g., Berant et al., 2001; Mikulincer & Florian, 1998). Intense and prolonged stress seems to shatter avoidant people's characteristic defenses and causes them to look like anxiously attached people. (This fits with the theoretical idea that both of these attachment patterns originated as ways of coping with intense feelings of insecurity in relation to attachment figures.)

With regard to coping strategies, several studies have supported our theoretical analysis of attachment-style differences in coping with both attachment-related and attachment-unrelated stressful situations (e.g., Berant et al., 2001; Birnbaum et al., 1997; Lussier, Sabourin, & Turgeon, 1997; Mikulincer & Florian, 1998; Mikulincer, Florian, & Weller, 1993; Schmidt, Nachtigall, Wuetrich, & Strauss, 2002). Whereas securely attached people tend to score relatively high on measures of support seeking and problem-focused coping, anxiously attached people rely on emotion-focused coping, and avoidant people rely on distancing coping. Also compatible with our analysis, avoidant attachment is associated with using repression as a defense (Mikulincer & Orbach, 1995; Vetere & Myers, 2002) and with behavioral blunting—using distraction to avoid confronting stressors (Feeney, 1995). In a recent study, for example, Turan, Osar, Turan, Ilkova, and Damci (2003) found that insulin-dependent diabetics scoring higher on attachment avoidance reported higher reliance on cognitive distancing and passive resignation as coping strategies, which in turn were associated with poor adherence to medical treatment.

Relations between attachment style and coping strategies were addressed in a 6-year longitudinal study of a large sample of people ranging in age from late adolescence to late adulthood (Zhang & Labouvie-Vief, 2004). The researchers found that, although adult attachment style was relatively stable over a 6-year period, there was also some fluidity associated with variations in coping strategies and mental health. Specifically, an increase in attachment security over the 6-year study period covaried with increases in problem-focused coping and perceived well-being as well as with decreases in distancing/avoidance coping and depressive symptoms. These findings fit with the characterization of felt security as a resilience resource that helps a person maintain emotional equanimity without extensive use of defenses (Mikulincer & Shaver, 2003).

Interestingly, three studies have revealed a significant association between avoidant attachment and emotion-focused coping. This seemingly uncharacteristic coping response for avoidant individuals may help to identify the contextual boundaries of deactivating strategies. In two studies (Lussier et al., 1997; Shapiro & Levendosky, 1999), heightened emotion-focused coping was observed in reaction to conflicts with close relationship partners. In the third study, Berant et al. (2001) found that avoidant mothers of newborns tended to rely on distancing coping if their infant was born healthy or with only a mild congenital heart defect (CHD), but they seemed to use emotion-focused coping if they gave birth to a child with a life-endangering CHD. It seems, therefore, that avoidant defenses, which are often sufficient for dealing with minor stressors, can fail when people encounter severe and persistent stressors. This conclusion is consistent with Bowlby's (1980) idea that avoidant people's segregated mental systems cannot be held outside consciousness indefinitely and that traumatic events can resurrect or reactivate distress that had previously been segregated and sealed off from consciousness.

Management of Attachment-Related Threats

Attachment strategies are also manifest in the ways people deal with attachment-related threats. In a pair of studies, Fraley and Shaver (1997) examined attachment-style differences in suppression of separation-related thoughts. Participants wrote continuously about whatever thoughts and feelings they were experiencing while being asked to suppress thoughts about a romantic partner leaving them for someone else. In the first study, the ability to suppress these thoughts was assessed by the number of times separation-related thoughts appeared in participants' stream-of-consciousness writing following the suppression period. In the second study, this ability was assessed by the level of physiological arousal (skin conductance) during the suppression task—the lower the arousal, the greater the presumed ability to suppress the thoughts.

The findings corresponded with attachment-related strategies for processing separation-related thoughts. Attachment anxiety was associated with poorer ability to suppress separation-related thoughts, as indicated by more frequent thoughts of loss following the suppression task and higher skin conductance during the task. In contrast, attachment avoidance was associated with greater ability to suppress separation-related thoughts, as indicated by less frequent thoughts of loss following the suppression task and lower skin conductance during the task. A recent functional magnetic resonance imaging (fMRI) study (Gillath, Bunge, Shaver, Wendelken, & Mikulincer, 2005) shows that these attachment-style differences are also evident in patterns of brain activation and deactivation when people are thinking about breakups and losses and when attempting to suppress such thoughts. (See also Ochsner & Gross, this volume.)

In a recent pair of studies, Mikulincer, Dolev, and Shaver (2004) replicated and extended Fraley and Shaver's (1997) findings while assessing, in a Stroop color-naming task, the cognitive accessibility of previously suppressed thoughts about a painful separation. Findings indicated that avoidant individuals were able to suppress thoughts related to the breakup; for them, such thoughts were relatively inaccessible, and their own positive self-traits became (presumably for defensive reasons) more accessible. However, their ability to maintain this defensive stance was disrupted when a cognitive load—remembering a 7-digit number—was added to the experimental task. Under high cognitive load, avoidant individuals exhibited ready access to thoughts of separation and negative self-traits. That is, the suppressed material resurfaced in experience and behavior when a high cognitive demand was imposed. We suspect that a similar resurfacing occurs when a high emotional demand is encountered.

Fraley et al. (2000) probed the regulatory mechanisms underlying avoidant individuals' deactivation of attachment-related threats. They asked whether deactivating strategies operate in a *preemptive* manner (e.g., by deploying attention away from attachment-related threats or encoding them in only a very shallow fashion) or a *postemptive*)manner (by repressing material that had been encoded). Participants listened to an interview about attachment-related threats and were asked to recall details from the interview either immediately afterward or at various delays ranging from half an hour to 21 days. An analysis of forgetting curves plotted over time revealed that avoidant individuals initially encoded less information about the interview than did less avoidant persons, and the two groups forgot the information at about the same rate. Thus, it seems that avoidant deactivating strategies at least sometimes act in a preemptive manner, by blocking threatening material from awareness and memory from the start.

Experiencing and Managing Death Anxiety

Adult attachment studies have also examined how attachment strategies affect the experience and management of specific emotional states. A number of studies conducted in Mikulincer's laboratory have focused, for example, on attachment-style differences in the strength of death anxiety (Florian & Mikulincer, 1998; Mikulincer, Florian, & Tolmacz, 1990), unconscious or preconscious indications of this fear (responses to projective Thematic Apperception Test [TAT] cards; Mikulincer et al., 1990), and the accessibility of death-related thoughts (the number of death-related words a person produces in a word-completion task; Mikulincer & Florian, 2000; Mikulincer, Florian, Birnbaum, & Malishkevich, 2002). Attachment-anxious individuals were found to intensify death concerns and keep death-related thoughts active in working memory. That is, attachment anxiety was associated with heightened fear of death at both conscious and unconscious levels, and with heightened accessibility of death-related thoughts even when no death reminder was present. Avoidant individuals' suppression of death concerns was inferred from a dissociation between their conscious claims and unconscious dynamics: Avoidance was related to low levels of self-reported death anxiety but also to heightened death-related content in responses to a projective TAT measure.

A related line of research examined attachment-style differences in the way people manage the anxiety evoked by death reminders. In a study by Mikulincer and Florian (2000), secure people reacted to mortality salience with heightened thoughts of symbolic immortality—a transformational, constructive strategy that, while not solving the unsolvable problem of death, leads a person to invest in his or her children's care and to engage in creative, growth-oriented activities whose products will live on after the person dies. Secure people have also been found to react to mortality salience with a heightened desire for intimacy (Mikulincer & Florian, 2000) and a heightened willingness to engage in social interaction (Taubman Ben-Ari, Findler, & Mikulincer, 2002). In contrast, people with an anxious or avoidant attachment style reacted to death reminders with more severe judgments and punishments of moral transgressors (Mikulincer & Florian, 2000). In other words, insecure people relied on what Greenberg, Pyszczynski, and Solomon (1997) call "culturally derived defenses"—adherence to a cultural world view and defensive enhancement of self-esteem. For anxious individuals, adhering to a shared cultural world view may be a way to gain greater love and acceptance from members of their group. For avoidant persons, the major issues are self-reliance and control, which benefit from the defensive enhancement of self-esteem (Hart, Shaver, & Goldenberg, 2005).

Experiencing and Managing Anger

Adult attachment research has also examined the experience and management of anger. In three studies, Mikulincer (1998b) found that securely attached people held optimistic expectations of their partner's responses during anger episodes and reacted with anger toward a partner only when there were clear contextual cues about the partner's hostile intent. Moreover, secure people's recollections of anger-eliciting episodes reflected functional attempts to rectify a relationship problem (what Bowlby, 1973, called the "anger of hope"). Secure people were constructively focused on repairing their relationship with the instigator of anger, engaging in adaptive problem solving, and expressing anger outward in a controlled and nonhostile way. Anxious people's anger experiences were quite different and were characterized by negative expectations concerning their partner's responses during anger episodes, reacting with angry and hostile feelings toward the partner even when there were no clear cues about the partner's hostile intentions, being prone to intense anger, experiencing uncontrollable feelings of anger, and ruminating excessively on these feelings.

Avoidant people's deactivating strategies resulted in what Mikulincer (1998b) called "dissociated anger." Although avoidant individuals did not report intense anger, they exhibited heightened hostility and physiological arousal. They also attributed hostility to their partner even when there were clear contextual cues concerning the partner's nonhostile intent, and they used distancing strategies for coping with anger rather than using anger constructively to repair or improve the relationship.

Insecure people's reports of anger proneness and hostility have been documented in other studies as well (e.g., Kobak & Sceery, 1988; Muris, Meesters, Morren, & Moorman, 2004; Troisi & D'Argenio, 2004). For example, Kobak and Sceery (1988) found that insecure attachment, as assessed by the AAI, was associated with greater hostility toward friends (which was easily noticed by the friends). Using self-report attachment scales, Woike, Osier, and Candela (1996) found that attachment anxiety was associated with writing more violent and hostile stories in response to projective TAT cards. Attachment anxiety has also been associated with relationship violence (e.g., Bartholomew & Allison, 2006).

Observational studies of anger in actual social interactions also provide evidence concerning the dysfunctional nature of insecure people's anger. Two studies examined anger reactions during conflicts in which partners were asked to identify an unresolved problem in their relationship and discuss and try to resolve it (Kobak et al., 1993; Simpson, Rholes, & Phillips, 1996). Whereas Kobak et al. (1993) assessed attachment patterns with the AAI and focused on interactions between teens and their mothers, Simpson et al. (1996) used a self-report attachment scale and focused on interactions between romantic partners. Despite these differences in assessment methods and types of relationships, both studies revealed that attachment insecurity, especially attachment anxiety, disrupts emotional equilibrium during interpersonal conflicts and elicits anger toward one's relationship partner. In the Kobak et al. (1993) study, insecure teens displayed more dysfunctional anger and less cooperative and problem-solving dialogue with their mothers. In Simpson et al.'s (1996) study, attachment anxiety was associated with displays and reports of anger and hostility during the conversation.

Other studies examined anger reactions while participants performed a frustrating, difficult cognitive task alone or with the help of a friend (Zimmermann, Maier, Winter, & Grossmann, 2001). Findings revealed that securely attached adolescents (as assessed by the AAI) displayed functional anger during the cognitive task; that is, their self-reported anger was associated with better task performance. In contrast, insecure adolescents displayed dysfunctional anger, including more disruptive behavior toward their friend (e.g., rejecting the friend's suggestions) and poorer task performance. In other words, insecure people's anger seemed to disrupt both their social interactions and their ability to solve problems.

Rholes, Simpson, and Orina (1999) examined overt manifestations of anger among support seekers and support providers in an anxiety-provoking situation. Women were told they would engage in an anxiety-provoking activity and were asked to wait with their dating partner for the activity to begin. During this 5-minute stressful waiting period, the reactions of the support seekers (women) and support providers (men) were unobtrusively videotaped. Each couple was then told that the woman would not have to endure the stressful activity after all, and each couple was unobtrusively videotaped during a 5-minute "recovery" period. The videotapes documented the dysfunctional nature of insecure participants' anger during both "stress" and "recovery" periods. In the stress period, women's avoidance was associated with more intense anger toward their partner, and this was particularly common when the woman was especially distressed and received relatively little support from her partner. In addition, men's avoidance was associated with more intense anger, and this was particularly common if their partner was more distressed. In the recovery period, women's attachment anxiety was associated with more intense anger toward their partners, and this was particularly true if they were more upset during the stress period or had sought more support from a partner.

These findings imply that avoidant men's lack of confidence in their ability to care for and support a distressed partner might have elicited greater anger toward her. Moreover, avoidant women's lack of confidence in their partner's support might have caused them to become more disappointed and angry while seeking support. Anxious women's lack of confidence in their partner's support seemed to elicit anger only after the threat had been lifted and support was no longer needed. Thus, anxious' women strong need for support and reassurance might counteract or lead to suppression of their angry feelings during support seeking. However, these feelings resurface once "support seeking" ends, which illustrates the way hyperactivating strategies tend to perpetuate distress-related feelings. (Interestingly, this is the same kind of behavior exhibited by anxious infants after they reunite with their mother following a laboratory separation period, as first documented by Ainsworth et al., 1978.)

The Experience of Jealousy

Adult attachment studies have also examined associations between attachment strategies and romantic jealousy. In general, more secure people tend to report mild emotional reactions to jealousy-eliciting events, fewer interfering thoughts and worries in response to these events, and greater use of constructive coping strategies, such as openly discussing feelings and concerns with the partner and attempting to put the relationship back on a better course (Guerrero, 1998; Leak, Gardner, & Parsons, 1998; Sharpsteen & Kirkpatrick, 1997).

Attachment-anxious people tend to experience jealousy in intense and dysfunctional ways, allowing it to ignite other negative emotions, overwhelm their thought processes, and erode relationship quality. Specifically, anxious people experience fear, guilt, shame, sadness, and anger during jealousy-eliciting events; report high levels of suspicion and worries during these events; and cope with them by expressing hostility toward the partner and engaging in more surveillance (mate-guarding) behaviors (Guerrero, 1998; Sharpsteen & Kirkpatrick, 1997).

Avoidant individuals, like their secure counterparts, do not react to jealousy-eliciting episodes with strong negative emotions or disrupted cognition. However, they are the least likely to engage in coping efforts aimed at restoring relationship quality (Guerrero, 1998). Instead, they prefer to avoid discussing the problem and overlook the jealousy-eliciting event. This pattern of responses is an example of deactivating strategies and is likely to contribute to relationship cooling and dissolution.

Cognitive Access and the Architecture of Emotional Experiences

Several studies have examined attachment-style differences in people's access to emotion-relevant information and the organization of this information in associative memory networks. In an experimental study of emotional memories, Mikulincer and Orbach (1995) asked participants to recall early experiences of anger, sadness, anxiety, or happiness, and memory retrieval time was used as a measure of cognitive accessibility. Participants also rated the intensity of focal and associated emotions in each recalled event. Avoidant people exhibited the poorest access (longest recall latencies) to sad and anxious memories, anxious people had the quickest access to such memories, and secure people fell in between. In the emotion-rating task, avoidant individuals rated focal emotions (e.g., sadness when retrieving a sad memory) and nonfocal emotions (e.g., anger when retrieving a sad memory) as less intense than secure individuals, whereas anxious individuals reported experiencing very intense focal *and* nonfocal emotions when asked to remember examples of anxiety, sadness, and anger. In other words, anxious people exhibited their usual rapid and extensive spread of activation among negative memories, whereas avoidant people had trouble accessing negative memories and seemed to report fairly shallow memories when they reported any at all.

Avoidant people's poor access to emotions is also evident in studies examining the coherence between conscious self-reports of emotional experience and less conscious, more automatic expressions of these experiences. (We assume that higher concordance between these measures indicates better mental access to emotional experiences). For example, Dozier and Kobak (1992) examined access to emotions during the AAI and found that avoidant people expressed few negative feelings during the interview but showed high levels of physiological arousal (heightened electrodermal activity) while speaking about their relationships with parents. Spangler and Zimmerman (1999) examined attachment-style differences (based on the AAI) in reactions to emotional film scenes and found that avoidant people, as compared with secure ones, evinced a greater discrepancy between their ratings of the emotional quality of the scenes and their mimicry responses to these scenes (measured with electromyography of the smile and frown muscles). Specifically, the frown muscles of avoidant people, which are usually interpreted as indicating negative emotions, were consistently activated at a low level regardless of the emotional quality of the scene. Zimmerman et al. (2001) extended these findings to the experience of anger and sadness during a problem-solving task. In that study, avoidant people (identified with the AAI) were characterized by a greater discrepancy (than seen in secure people) between self-reports and facial expressions of anger and sadness.

In examining the decoding of emotional stimuli, Niedenthal, Brauer, Robin, and Innes-Ker (2002) asked people to watch computerized videos in which a face that initially displayed a particular emotional expression gradually changed to a different expression, and to stop the display at the point at which the initial expression disappeared from the face. Fearfully avoidant individuals (those scoring high on both avoidance and anxiety) thought they saw the offset of happy and angry facial expressions earlier than did secure individuals, suggesting a tendency to minimize the encoding of emotion-relevant information and rapidly distance from it. In contrast, anxiously attached individuals saw the offset of these expressions later than secure individuals, suggesting a tendency to maintain the encoding of emotional stimuli for a longer time. Interestingly, the addition of a distress-eliciting condition led fearfully avoidant people to react like anxious ones, suggesting that distress arousal might have interfered with their ability to distance themselves from emotional stimuli.

Summary

Research findings reported to date provide a rich picture of attachment-related differences in emotion regulation. Secure and avoidant people attempt to manage and downregulate threat-related emotions. However, whereas security-based strategies act mainly on the emotion-generation end of the emotion process, using what Gross (1999) called antecedent-focused emotion regulation, and on increasing the likelihood that emotions will have constructive, functional effects, avoidant strategies act mainly on the emotion experience and expression end of the process and therefore tend to block mental access to emotions, a process Gross (1999) called response-focused emotion regulation. In a third approach to emotion regulation, anxious individuals, using hyperactivating strategies, actually intensify and perpetuate negative emotions by acting on all components of the emotion process.

CONCLUSIONS

In summarizing recent research on adult attachment patterns and their implications for emotion regulation, we have shown that attachment security is associated with appraisals and regulation efforts that are compatible with a balanced, open mind, generally low levels of stress and distress, and constructive approaches to relationship maintenance. The two major dimensions of insecure attachment are associated with organized strategies for dealing with painful experiences in previous attachment relationships.

Avoidance and attachment-system deactivation are reactions to important relationships in which attachment figures, often beginning with one or both parents, reacted negatively to expressions of need, vulnerability, and negative emotions. To cope with that powerfully painful relationship influence, avoidant people have learned to downplay threats (i.e., try not to appraise events as threatening), suppress or deny feelings of vulnerability and negative emotions, and view themselves as superior, autonomous, and properly unemotional. This does not keep them from reacting to relationship partners with frustration, hostility, and denigration or from boosting their own self-esteem in the face of mortality threats and relationship losses by focusing disproportionately on their own strengths and other people's weaknesses.

Attachment anxiety and attachment-system hyperactivation are reactions to important relationships in which attachment figures, often beginning with one or both parents, reacted inconsistently to a person's expressions of need, vulnerability, and negative emotions, sometimes rewarding them but at other times frustrating or ignoring them. This caregiver regimen causes a person to believe that constant vigilance, worry, and expressions of need, vulnerability, and retaliatory anger pay off, because they sometimes do capture a relationship partner's attention. Unfortunately, they can also alienate a person from initially favorable and loving relationship partners and produce exactly what the anxious person does not want: rejection and abandonment. Thus, what began as a response to a partial reinforcement schedule of attention and support, and what became a pattern of noisy negativity, seems to the anxious person to confirm his or her expectations and worst fears.

These different patterns of emotion and defense have been documented in a remarkable variety of studies using experimental, interview, and observational techniques. They are now being illuminated further by neuroscientific studies. They provide strong specific support for Bowlby and Ainsworth's attachment theory and its extension into the realm of adult relationships (Mikulincer & Shaver, 2003), as well as more general support for the once-discredited psychodynamic approach to personality (Shaver & Mikulincer, 2005). Research based on attachment theory also suggests therapeutic methods for dysfunctional emotion regulation. Further development and assessment of these methods will contribute to improved lives and relationships.

REFERENCES

Ainsworth, M. D. S., Blehar, M. C., Waters, E., & Wall, S. (1978). *Patterns of attachment: Assessed in the strange situation and at home.* Hillsdale, NJ: Erlbaum.

Alexander, R., Feeney, J. A., Hohaus, L., & Noller, P. (2001). Attachment style and coping resources as predictors of coping strategies in the transition to parenthood. *Personal Relationships, 8,* 137–152.

Bartholomew, K., & Allison, C. (2006). An attachment perspective on abusive dynamics in intimate relationships. In M. Mikulincer & G. S. Goodman (Eds.), *Dynamics of romantic love: Attachment, caregiving, and sex* (pp. 102–127). New York: Guilford Press.

Berant, E., Mikulincer, M., & Florian, V. (2001). The association of mothers' attachment style and their psychological reactions to the diagnosis of infant's congenital heart disease. *Journal of Social and Clinical Psychology, 20,* 208–232.

Birnbaum, G. E., Orr, I., Mikulincer, M., & Florian, V. (1997). When marriage breaks up: Does attachment style contribute to coping and mental health? *Journal of Social and Personal Relationships, 14,* 643–654.

Bowlby, J. (1982). *Attachment and loss: Vol. 1. Attachment* (2nd ed.). New York: Basic Books. (Original work published 1969)

Bowlby, J. (1973). *Attachment and loss: Vol. 2. Separation: Anxiety and anger.* New York: Basic Books.

Bowlby, J. (1980). *Attachment and loss: Vol. 3. Sadness and depression.* New York: Basic Books.

Bowlby, J. (1988). *A secure base: Clinical applications of attachment theory.* London: Routledge.

Brennan, K. A., Clark, C. L., & Shaver, P. R. (1998). Self-report measurement of adult attachment: An integrative overview. In J. A. Simpson & W. S. Rholes (Eds.), *Attachment theory and close relationships* (pp. 46–76). New York: Guilford Press.

Cassidy, J. (1994). Emotion regulation: Influence of attachment relationships. In N. A. Fox & J. J. Campos (Eds.), The development of emotion regulation: Biological and behavioral considerations. *Monographs of the Society for Research in Child Development, 59,* 228–249.

Cassidy, J., & Berlin, L. J. (1994). The insecure/ambivalent pattern of attachment: Theory and research. *Child Development, 65,* 971–981.

Cassidy, J., & Kobak, R. R. (1988). Avoidance and its relationship with other defensive processes. In J. Belsky & T. Nezworski (Eds.), *Clinical implications of attachment* (pp. 300–323). Hillsdale, NJ: Erlbaum.

Calkins, S. D., & Hill, A. (2007). Caregiver influences on emerging emotion regulation: Biological and environmental transactions in early development. In J. J. Gross (Ed.), *Handbook of emotion regulation* (pp. 229–248). New York: Guilford Press.

Collins, N. L., & Read, S. J. (1994). Cognitive representations of attachment: The structure and function of working models. In K. Bartholomew & D. Perlman (Eds.), *Attachment processes in adulthood* (pp. 53–92). London: Jessica Kingsley.

Dozier, M., & Kobak, R. R. (1992). Psychophysiology in attachment interviews: Converging evidence for deactivating strategies. *Child Development, 63,* 1473–1480.

Feeney, J. A. (1995). Adult attachment and emotional control. *Personal Relationships, 2,* 143–159.

Fischer, K. W., Shaver, P. R., & Carnochan, P. (1990). How emotions develop and how they organize development. *Cognition and Emotion, 4,* 81–127.

Florian, V., & Mikulincer, M. (1998). Symbolic immortality and the management of the terror of death: The moderating role of attachment style. *Journal of Personality and Social Psychology, 74,* 725–734.

Fonagy, P., Steele, M., Steele, H., Moran, G. S., & Higgit, M. (1991). The capacity for understanding mental states: The reflective self in parent and child and its significance for security of attachment. *Infant Mental Health Journal, 12,* 201–218.

Fonagy, P., Target, M., Steele, H., & Steele, M. (1998). *Reflective-functioning manual for application to adult attachment interviews.* London: University College London.

Fraley, R. C., Garner, J. P., & Shaver, P. R. (2000). Adult attachment and the defensive regulation of attention and memory: Examining the role of preemptive and postemptive defensive processes. *Journal of Personality and Social Psychology, 79,* 816–826.

Fraley, R. C., & Shaver, P. R. (1997). Adult attachment and the suppression of unwanted thoughts. *Journal of Personality and Social Psychology, 73,* 1080–1091.

Fraley, R. C., & Shaver, P. R. (2000). Adult romantic attachment: Theoretical developments, emerging controversies, and unanswered questions. *Review of General Psychology, 4,* 132–154.

Fredrickson, B. L. (2001). The role of positive emotions in positive psychology: The broaden-and-build theory of positive emotions. *American Psychologist, 56,* 218–226.

Frijda, N. H. (1986). *The emotions.* New York: Cambridge University Press.

George, C., Kaplan, N., & Main, M. (1985). *The Adult Attachment Interview.* Unpublished manuscript, Department of Psychology, University of California, Berkeley.

Gillath, O., Bunge, S. A., Shaver, P. R., Wendelken, C., & Mikulincer, M. (2005). Attachment-style differences in the ability to suppress negative thoughts: Exploring the neural correlates. *NeuroImage, 28,* 835–847.

Greenberg, J., Pyszczynski, T., & Solomon, S. (1997). Terror management theory of self-esteem and cultural worldviews: Empirical assessments and conceptual refinements. In P. M. Zanna (Ed.), *Advances in Experimental Social Psychology* (Vol. 29, pp. 61–141). San Diego: Academic Press.

Gross, J. J. (1999). Emotion and emotion regulation. In O. P. John & L. A. Pervin (Eds.), *Handbook of personality: Theory and research* (2nd ed., pp. 525–552). New York: Guilford Press.

Gross, J. J., & Thompson, R. A. (2007). Emotion regulation: Conceptual foundations. In J. J. Gross (Ed.), *Handbook of emotion regulation* (pp. 3–24). New York: Guilford Press.

Guerrero, L. K. (1998). Attachment-style differences in the experience and expression of romantic jealousy. *Personal Relationships, 5,* 273–291.

Hart, J. J., Shaver, P. R., & Goldenberg, J. L. (2005). Attachment, self-esteem, worldviews, and terror management: Evidence for a tripartite security system. *Journal of Personality and Social Psychology, 88,* 999–1013.

Hazan, C., & Shaver, P. R. (1987). Romantic love conceptualized as an attachment process. *Journal of Personality and Social Psychology, 52,* 511–524.

Hesse, E. (1999). The Adult Attachment Interview: Historical and current perspectives. In J. Cassidy & P. R. Shaver (Eds.), *Handbook of attachment: Theory, research, and clinical applications* (pp. 395–433). New York: Guilford Press.

Kobak, R. R., Cole, H. E., Ferenz-Gillies, R., Fleming, W. S., & Gamble, W. (1993). Attachment and emotion regulation during mother–teen problem solving: A control theory analysis. *Child Development, 64,* 231–245.

Kobak, R. R., & Sceery, A. (1988). Attachment in late adolescence: Working models, affect regulation, and representations of self and others. *Child Development, 59,* 135–146.

Lazarus, R. S. (1991). *Emotion and adaptation.* New York: Oxford University Press.

Lazarus, R. S., & Folkman, S. (1984). *Stress, appraisal, and coping.* New York: Springer.

Leak, G. K., Gardner, L. E., & Parsons, C. J. (1998) Jealousy and romantic attachment: A replication and extension. *Representative Research in Social Psychology, 22,* 21–27.

Lussier, Y., Sabourin, S., & Turgeon, C. (1997). Coping strategies as moderators of the relationship between attachment and marital adjustment. *Journal of Social and Personal Relationships, 14,* 777–791.

Main, M. (1990). Cross-cultural studies of attachment organization: Recent studies, changing methodologies, and the concept of conditional strategies. *Human Development, 33,* 48–61.

Main, M., Kaplan, N., & Cassidy, J. (1985). Security in infancy, childhood, and adulthood: A move to the level of representation. *Monographs of the Society for Research in Child Development, 50,* 66–104.

Main, M., & Solomon, J. (1986). Discovery of an insecure-disorganized/disoriented attachment pattern. In M. W. Yogman, W. Michael, & T. B. Brazelton (Eds.), *Affective development in infancy* (pp. 95–124). Westport, CT: Ablex.

Mikulincer, M. (1997). Adult attachment style and information processing: Individual differences in curiosity and cognitive closure. *Journal of Personality and Social Psychology, 72,* 1217–1230.

Mikulincer, M. (1998a). Adult attachment style and affect regulation: Strategic variations in self-appraisals. *Journal of Personality and Social Psychology, 75,* 420–435.

Mikulincer, M. (1998b). Adult attachment style and individual differences in functional versus dysfunctional experiences of anger. *Journal of Personality and Social Psychology, 74,* 513–524.

Mikulincer, M., Dolev, T., & Shaver, P. R. (2004). Attachment-related strategies during thought-suppression: Ironic rebounds and vulnerable self-representations. *Journal of Personality and Social Psychology, 87,* 940–956.

Mikulincer, M., & Florian, V. (1998). The relationship between adult attachment styles and emotional and cognitive reactions to stressful events. In J. A. Simpson & W. S. Rholes (Eds.), *Attachment theory and close relationships* (pp. 143–165). New York: Guilford Press.

Mikulincer, M., & Florian, V. (2000). Exploring individual differences in reactions to mortality salience: Does attachment style regulate terror management mechanisms? *Journal of Personality and Social Psychology, 79,* 260–273.

Mikulincer, M., Florian, V., Birnbaum, G., & Malishkevich, S. (2002). The death-anxiety buffering function of close relationships: Exploring the effects of separation reminders on death-thought accessibility. *Personality and Social Psychology Bulletin, 28,* 287–299.

Mikulincer, M., Florian, V., & Tolmacz, R. (1990). Attachment styles and fear of personal death: A case study of affect regulation. *Journal of Personality and Social Psychology, 58,* 273–280.

Mikulincer, M., Florian, V., & Weller, A. (1993). Attachment styles, coping strategies, and posttraumatic psychological distress: The impact of the Gulf War in Israel. *Journal of Personality and Social Psychology, 64,* 817–826.

Mikulincer, M., & Orbach, I. (1995). Attachment styles and repressive defensiveness: The accessibility and architecture of affective memories. *Journal of Personality and Social Psychology, 68,* 917–925.

Mikulincer, M., & Shaver, P. R. (2003). The attachment behavioral system in adulthood: Activation, psychodynamics, and interpersonal processes. In M. P. Zanna (Ed.), *Advances in experimental social psychology* (Vol. 35, pp. 53–152). New York: Academic Press.

Mikulincer, M., & Shaver, P. R. (2004). Security-based self-representations in adulthood: Contents and processes. In W. S. Rholes & J. A. Simpson (Eds.), *Adult attachment: Theory, research, and clinical implications* (pp. 159–195). New York: Guilford Press.

Muris, P., Meesters, C., Morren, M., & Moorman, L. (2004). Anger and hostility in adolescents: Relationships with self-reported attachment style and perceived parental rearing styles. *Journal of Psychosomatic Research, 57,* 257–264.

Niedenthal, P. M., Brauer, M., Robin, L., & Innes-Ker, A. H. (2002). Adult attachment and the perception of facial expression of emotion. *Journal of Personality and Social Psychology, 82,* 419–433.

Oatley, K., & Jenkins, J. M. (1996). *Understanding emotions.* Cambridge, MA: Blackwell.

Ochsner, K. N., & Gross, J. J. (2007). The neural architecture of emotion regulation. In J. J. Gross (Ed.), *Handbook of emotion regulation* (pp. 87–109). New York: Guilford Press.

Rholes, W. S., Simpson, J. A., & Orina, M. M. (1999). Attachment and anger in an anxiety-provoking situation. *Journal of Personality and Social Psychology, 76,* 940–957.

Schmidt, S., Nachtigall, C., Wuethrich, M. O., & Strauss, B. (2002). Attachment and coping with chronic disease. *Journal of Psychosomatic Research, 53,* 763–773.

Shapiro, D. L., & Levendosky, A. A. (1999). Adolescent survivors of childhood sexual abuse: The mediating role of attachment style and coping in psychological and interpersonal functioning. *Child Abuse and Neglect, 23,* 1175–1191.

Sharpsteen, D. J., & Kirkpatrick, L. A. (1997). Romantic jealousy and adult romantic attachment. *Journal of Personality and Social Psychology, 72,* 627–640.

Shaver, P. R., & Clark, C. L. (1994). The psychodynamics of adult romantic attachment. In J. M. Masling & R. F. Bornstein (Eds.), *Empirical perspectives on object relations theory* (Vol. 5, pp. 105–156). Washington, DC: American Psychological Association.

Shaver, P. R., & Mikulincer, M. (2002). Attachment-related psychodynamics. *Attachment and Human Development, 4,* 133–161.

Shaver, P. R., & Mikulincer, M. (2005). Attachment theory and research: Resurrection of the psychodynamic approach to personality. *Journal of Research in Personality, 39,* 22–45.

Shaver, P. R., Schwartz, J., Kirson, D., & O'Connor, C. (1987). Emotion knowledge: Further exploration of a prototype approach. *Journal of Personality and Social Psychology, 52,* 1061–1086.

Simpson, J. A., Rholes, W. S., & Phillips, D. (1996). Conflict in close relationships: An attachment perspective. *Journal of Personality and Social Psychology, 71,* 899–914.

Smith, C. A., & Ellsworth, P. C. (1987). Patterns of appraisal and emotion related to taking an exam. *Journal of Personality and Social Psychology, 52*, 475–488.

Spangler, G., & Zimmermann, P. (1999). Attachment representation and emotion regulation in adolescents: A psychobiological perspective on internal working models. *Attachment and Human Development, 1*, 270–290.

Taubman Ben-Ari, O., Findler, L., & Mikulincer, M. (2002). The effects of mortality salience on relationship strivings and beliefs: The moderating role of attachment style. *British Journal of Social Psychology, 41*, 419–441.

Thompson, R. A., & Meyer, S. (2007). Socialization of emotion regulation in the family. In J. J. Gross (Ed.), *Handbook of emotion regulation* (pp. 249–268). New York: Guilford Press.

Troisi, A., & D'Argenio, A. (2004). The relationship between anger and depression in a clinical sample of young men: The role of insecure attachment. *Journal of Affective Disorders, 79*, 269–272.

Turan, B., Osar, Z., Turan, J. M., Ilkova, H., & Damci, T. (2003). Dismissing attachment and outcome in diabetes: The mediating role of coping. *Journal of Social and Clinical Psychology, 22*, 607–626.

Vetere, A., & Myers, L. B. (2002). Repressive coping style and adult romantic attachment style: Is there a relationship? *Personality and Individual Differences, 32*, 799–807.

Westen, D., & Blagov, P. S. (2007). A clinical–empirical model of emotion regulation: From defense and motivated reasoning to emotional constraint satisfaction. In J. J. Gross (Ed.), *Handbook of emotion regulation* (pp. 373–392). New York: Guilford Press.

Woike, B. A., Osier, T. J., & Candela, K. (1996). Attachment style and violent imagery in thematic stories about relationships. *Personality and Social Psychology Bulletin, 22*, 1030–1034.

Zhang, F., & Labouvie-Vief, G. (2004). Stability and fluctuation in adult attachment style over a 6-year period. *Attachment and Human Development, 6*, 419–437.

Zimmermann, P., Maier, M. A., Winter, M., & Grossmann, K. E. (2001). Attachment and adolescents' emotion regulation during a joint problem-solving task with a friend. *International Journal of Behavioral Development, 25*, 331–343.

CHAPTER 23

Interpersonal Emotion Regulation

BERNARD RIMÉ

> Every painful experience tears up. But what makes it unbearable is that the
> one who suffers it feels set apart from the world. Shared, it ceases at least to
> be an exile.
>
> —DE BEAUVOIR (1972, p. 169)

In contemporary research, emotions are predominantly defined as arising when an individual attends to a situation and sees it as relevant to his or her goals (see Gross & Thompson, this volume). Most often, however, the classic homeostatic perspective proposed by physiologist Walter Cannon (1915/1929) still prevails in the way emotions are conceived. Accordingly, they are primarily seen as short-lived processes whose function is to eliminate the eliciting situation, thus bringing the individual back to a state of equilibrium. Emotion generation is described as involving a sequence of processes—situation, attention, cognitive change or appraisal, response—and an emotion would end with the final step of the sequence. Even if recursive processes occurring within the sequence can complicate the picture (see Gross & Thompson, this volume), nothing seems to happen beyond the situation–response sequence. Hereafter, it will be insisted that emotions very generally do not end with this sequence. Studies conducted in the last decades revealed that emotional episodes are virtually always followed by longer-term cognitive and social effects. In particular, individual emotional experiences elicit important social behaviors by which the actor informs his or her social partners of what happened and shares with them related thoughts and feelings.

Emotion regulation is a process through which an emotion can be dampened, intensified, or simply maintained (Gross & Thompson, this volume). According to Gross (1998), the potential targets of emotion regulation consist of each element in the emotional sequence: situation selection and modification, attentional deployment, cognitive change, response modulation. Yet, when emotions are seen as involving important manifestations taking place beyond the emotional sequence, a somewhat broader definition of emotion regulation is needed. Emotional memories remain active for some time after every emotional sequence and they thus have an impact on the individual well beyond this sequence. These aftermaths motivate important regulation attempts, most of which involve communication and social interaction. This is consistent with the view according to which the emotion regulation definition encompasses "changes in the emotion itself *or in other psychological processes, such as memory or social interaction*" (Cole, Martin, & Dennis, 2004, p. 320, emphasis added). In the perspective of this chapter, the normal fate of an emotional memory is to reach a dormant stage at which it stops having an impact on the current experience. In this context, *emotional recovery* defines the degree to which an individual is freed from the current impact of a given emotional memory. At complete recovery of an emotional episode, there is no more urge to think or to talk about it.

Whereas psychologists who investigate adults generally considered emotion regulation as a process occurring essentially within the person, child psychologists have established the fundamental interpersonal nature of emotion regulation among children. The gap between these two points of view could easily be filled by viewing the evolution from childhood to adult age as involving the growing ability to self-regulate emotion. Though this is definitely right in part, we should nevertheless be cautious with our cultural propensity to consider mature psychological processes essentially from an individualistic perspective. Considering how deep caregivers are involved in the regulation of a child's emotional life, can we expect adults' emotions to be entirely regulated by their self alone?

In this chapter, we first consider the evidence documenting interpersonal dimensions of emotion regulation. We then focus on the functions fulfilled by social behaviors with regard to the regulation of the emotion. Strong beliefs exist according to which the mere verbalization of an emotional experience induces emotional recovery. What do empirical data tell us about this? This chapter attempts to specify what people get and what they do not get from engaging in social expressive behaviors after an emotion.

THE SOCIAL SHARING OF EMOTIONS: OVERVIEW

Janoff-Bulman (1992) noted that people who went through a traumatic experience later evidence a seemingly insatiable need to tell others about it as if they felt coerced into talking. Although scarce, empirical data coming from studies about traumatic circumstances and severe life events confirmed the pervasiveness of this phenomenon. A need to talk was mentioned by 88% of rescuers operating in a North Sea oil platform disaster (Ersland, Weisaeth, & Sund, 1989), by 88% of people who had recently lost a relative (Schoenberg, Carr, Peretz, Kutscher, & Cherico, 1975), and by 86% of patients with a recent diagnosis of cancer (Mitchell & Glickman, 1977). Yet, data revealed that the need to talk after an emotion is in no manner limited to trauma or major negative life events. It develops after everyday positive and negative emotional events as well. This is what we found by investigating "the social sharing of emotion."

The social sharing of emotion entails a description, in a socially shared language, of an emotional episode to some addressee by the person who experienced it (Rimé, 1989; Rimé, Mesquita, Philippot, & Boca, 1991a). It usually develops in the period immediately following the episode, in discourse in which the protagonist tells one or several other persons about the emotion-eliciting circumstances and related thoughts and feelings. After an emotion, people undertake sharing in 80–95% of the cases (Rimé et al., 1991a; Rimé, Noël, & Philippot, 1991b; for reviews, see Rimé, 2005; Rimé, Philippot, Mesquita, & Boca, 1992; Rimé, Finkenauer, Luminet, Zech, & Philippot, 1998). This propensity is not dependent on education. It was evidenced at comparable levels whether people held a university degree or had an elementary school education. It was also observed with comparable importance in places as diverse as Asian, North American, and European countries (Mesquita, 1993; Rimé, Yogo, & Pennebaker, 1996; Singh-Manoux, 1998; Singh-Manoux & Finkenauer, 2001; Yogo & Onoe, 1998). The type of primary emotion felt in the episode is no more critical with regard to sharing. Episodes that involved fear, or anger, or sadness were shared as often as episodes of happiness or of love. However, emotional episodes involving shame and guilt were shared at a somewhat lesser degree (Finkenauer & Rimé, 1998). Laboratory studies confirmed that exposure to an emotion-eliciting condition provokes sharing (Luminet, Bouts, Delie, Manstead, & Rimé, 2000). Generally initiated very early after the emotion, sharing is typically a repetitive phenomenon in which more intense emotions are shared more repetitively and for a longer period (Rimé, 2005; Rimé et al., 1998). Emotional episodes are typically shared often or very often, and with a variety of target persons. Follow-up data showed that for a given emotional episode, emotion sharing decreases over the days or weeks subsequently (Rimé et al., 1998). Thus, progressive extinction is the normal fate of sharing. The length of the extinction period depends on the intensity of the emotion. However, sharing sometimes persists which indicates a failure to recover from the episode (Rimé et al., 1998).

THE PARADOX OF SOCIAL SHARING

Clearly, whether positive or negative, people share their emotional experiences equally with others. However, when doing so, they reexperience mental images of the event as well as related feelings and bodily sensations (Rimé et al., 1991b). For positive episodes, sharing them should reactivate positive emotional feelings and memories. It thus makes sense that people are motivated to socially share positive episodes further and further. Langston (1994) indeed demonstrated that the sharing of positive emotional episodes involves a process of "capitalization" in which positive events are seen not as problems to be surmounted or coped with but as opportunities on which to seize or "capitalize." Capitalization refers to the process of beneficially interpreting positive events (cf. Bryant, 1989, who used the term "savoring"). Capitalizing on a positive event can be achieved in at least three different ways: (1) by making it more memorable to the self (by marking the event's occurrence in some expressive fashion such as jumping, bragging, celebrating, etc.), (2) by seeking social contacts and letting others know about the event, and (3) by maximizing the event's significance (e.g., by increasing one's perceived control of the event). In two different studies (Langston, 1994), expressive displays such as communicating the positive events to others were indeed associated with an enhancement of positive affect far beyond the benefits due to the valence of the positive events themselves. Addressing openly the social sharing of positive emotions, Gable, Reis, Impett, and Asher (2004) confirmed these findings. In addition, they found that close relationships in which one's partner typically responds enthusiastically to capitalization were associated with higher relationship well-being (e.g., intimacy and daily marital satisfaction). Thus, sharing positive emotions not only increases positive affect at the intrapersonal level but it also enhances social bonds.

By contrast, in the case of negative episodes, the sharing process reactivates nega-tive emotional feelings, and memories and should thus be experienced as markedly aversive. A logical prediction is thus that more negative experiences should elicit less sharing. Yet, correlations between intensity of negative emotion and extent of sharing are systematically in the opposite direction (for a thorough review, see Rimé et al., 1998). Moreover, the sharing of negative emotional experiences is generally not found aversive. In one of our studies, participants first described in a detailed manner a past emotional experience of joy, sadness, fear, or anger, according to a random assignment. They then rated how far describing this experience was pleasant or painful (Rimé et al., 1991b). Not surprisingly, those who described an experience of joy rated it as more pleasant than those who described a negative episode. More surprising was that report-ing an episode of fear, sadness, or anger was rated by only a minority as painful. When participants in this study were asked whether they would be willing to undertake shar-ing another emotional memory of the same kind as the first one, virtually all of them agreed whatever the valence of the emotion involved. There is thus a paradox here. Even when it reactivates aversive experiences, sharing is a behavior in which people engage quite willingly.

If people are so eager to engage in a social process in which they may experience aversive affects, they ought to be driven by some powerful incentive. What could be the reward? Common sense offers a ready-made answer. It is generally assumed that verbal-izing an emotional memory can transform it and reduce a significant part of its emo-tional load. Zech (2000) found that 89% of respondents in a large sample of laypersons (n = 1024) endorsed the view that talking about an emotional experience is relieving. If data could confirm this view in demonstrating that verbalizing an emotion actually brings "emotional recovery," then the paradox would clear up. People would tolerate the reexperience involved in social sharing because of the final benefit it provides them. We thus examined this question in a respectable number of studies (Rimé et al., 1998; Zech & Rimé, 2005).

IS EMOTION SHARING A SOURCE OF EMOTIONAL RECOVERY?

In various studies, we investigated whether the extent of naturally developed sharing of an emotional experience would predict the degree of emotional recovery for this expe-rience (for a review, see Rimé et al., 1998). These studies always involved the assessment of three critical variables: (1) the initial intensity of the emotion elicited by the episode, (2) the extent of social sharing that was developed after, and (3) the intensity of the emotion elicited when the memory of the episode was reactivated later. The difference between (1) and (3) served to index emotional recovery. In line with common assump-tions, we predicted a positive correlation between the extent of social sharing and the degree of emotional recovery. To our surprise, the collected data never supported this prediction. Very generally, our correlative data were in line with the null hypothesis and perfectly inconsistent with the view that sharing an emotional experience would reduce the emotional load of this experience. For instance, we investigated characteristics of episodes which people had never shared (Finkenauer & Rimé, 1998). In two different studies, when shared and secret emotional episodes were compared for the intensity of the emotion they still elicited at recall, no significant difference was observed. No data supported the prediction that secret events would remain more intense than shared ones. To sum up, the correlative studies consistently suggested that *merely verbalizing* an emotional experience is irrelevant to emotional recovery.

Our correlative studies were paralleled by experimental investigations in which participants were assigned to various sharing conditions. We assessed how far these conditions affected emotional recovery (Zech, 2000; Zech & Rimé, 2005). In some experiments, students interviewed relatives about a recent negative emotional event. In others, participants extensively shared with an experimenter the most upsetting event of their life. Sharing conditions were created by instructing participants to emphasize either the factual aspects of the target emotional episode or its feeling aspects. Control conditions involved talking about a nonemotional topic. The emotional impact of the target episode was assessed before the sharing interview, immediately after, and again some days later. In one study, additional assessments were conducted 2 months later. Contrary to expectations, no effect of sharing condition was found on indices of emotional impact in any study. Thus, in regard to emotional recovery, the results of these experimental studies were as disappointing as those of the correlative ones.

The abundance of null findings finally led us to acknowledge that, despite stereotypes, socially sharing an emotion does not bring emotional recovery. Research on the social sharing of emotion was not alone in accumulating null findings. Comparable observations were made for psychological debriefings. Currently implemented immediately after traumatic events, debriefing procedures gather exposed individuals in small groups in which they have to describe to one another in a detailed manner what happened, express their thoughts concerning the event, and communicate "what was the worst thing in the situation." The technique thus clearly involves sharing emotions. Its purpose is to prevent posttraumatic stress disorders and thus to contribute to emotional recovery (e.g., Mitchell & Everly, 1995). However, recent meta-analytic reviews of controlled trials consistently concluded that debriefings have no efficacy in reducing symptoms of posttraumatic stress disorders or other trauma-related symptoms (Arendt & Elklit, 2001; Rose & Bisson, 1998; Van Emmerik, Kamphuis, Hulsbosch, & Emmelkamp, 2002). Adverse effects were even sometimes found. All in all, these observations strongly suggested that mere sharing cannot change emotional memories. Such a conclusion makes sense with regard to adaptation, as emotional memories carry important information for future situations. If their emotion-arousing capacities could be altered by mere talking, it would be deleterious to the fruits of our experience (Rimé, 1999).

The foregoing, conclusion were sometimes understood as contradicting the well-known findings from the "writing cure" (e.g., Pennebaker, 1997; for reviews, see Frattorili, in press; Lepore & Smyth, 2002). Examining effects of disclosing past traumas in written form, Pennebaker and his colleagues observed it to be associated with later health benefits as assessed by physician visits, reported symptoms, immunological functions, or other indices of health. These findings were commonly understood as supporting the view that simply "putting emotion into words" brings emotional recovery. However, in these studies, participants did not express themselves about a specific episode but, rather, about as many past emotional events as they wanted (e.g., Pennebaker & Beall, 1986). Thus, writing studies did not test whether putting a *specific* emotional episode into words leads to *recovery*, nor did they assess (through, e.g., intrusive thoughts about the event, searching for meaning in the event, intensity of emotional arousal when recalling the event, etc.) the residual impact that a specific episode still has (for a detailed discussion, see Pennebaker, Zech, & Rimé, 2001; Rimé, 1999). Also, observing health effects after expressive writing inductions does not allow us to infer that emotional recovery was the mediator variable. Processes through which expressive writing led to such effects are still under investigation (Frattaroli, 2006; Pennebaker, 2002).

BENEFITS FROM SHARING AN EMOTION

If experimental studies of the social sharing of emotion yielded null findings for emotional recovery, they simultaneously opened on interesting observations (Zech & Rimé, 2005). In questionnaires completed at follow-up, participants who had shared their emotions consistently rated their participation in the study as much more beneficial than participants in control conditions involving either sharing facts only or sharing nonemotional experiences. As compared to the latter, the former rated their session as more beneficial globally (e.g., it was useful), as more emotion relieving (e.g., it made them feel good), as more cognitively helpful (e.g., it helped them in putting order in themselves), and as more beneficial at an interpersonal level (e.g., they experienced comforting behaviors from the part of the recipient). Interestingly, the parallel between sharing and psychological debriefing holds here too. Indeed, victims of a trauma who took part in psychological debriefing frequently report that their participation was useful and beneficial.

A further paradox is thus met. On the one hand, sharing an emotion fails to alleviate the load of the shared emotional memory. On the other hand, participants who shared their emotions experienced a good number of benefits. At least, the latter findings were consistent with people's marked proclivity to share their emotions no matter how negative they were. However, it might be that participants who reported benefits inferred them from the widespread beliefs holding that sharing is beneficial. In some of our experiments, participants' beliefs in this regard were collected before the sharing situation (Zech & Rimé, 2005). We could thus check how far these beliefs predicted the benefits reported after sharing and we observed that a part of the variance of these benefits was indeed due to previous beliefs that participants held. But a substantial part of this variance was left unexplained by this factor.

It should thus be concluded that whereas talking about an emotional memory fails to have a significant effect on the emotional impact of this memory, people actually experience benefits from doing it. How can we make sense of this paradoxical conclusion? What exactly is gained from emotion sharing? To be in a better position to consider such questions, we explore successively three different subsets of questions. First, what exactly is involved in the impact of an emotional experience and what are the regulation needs that such an experience elicits? Second, what are people looking for when they engage in sharing? What are the motives they allege? After all, every layperson has a long past experience in sharing and should thus be aware of benefits one can get from sharing. Third, how do listeners react and respond to sharing? Answers to the latter question should inform us of what is actually offered to sharing persons in sharing situations.

IMPACT OF AN EMOTIONAL EXPERIENCE
AND REGULATION NEEDS

For laypersons, but also for many clinical and scientific psychologists, observations disconfirming that sharing brings emotional recovery are shocking. In current life indeed, when a negative emotional experience happened, it is ubiquitously recommended to "get it off one's chest." Distress situations in general elicit both simplistic approaches and simplistic interventions due to the fact that nonvictims dramatically underestimate a victim's situation (e.g., Coates, Wortman, & Abbey, 1979; Goffman, 1963; Wortman & Lehman, 1985). As the predominant concern of bystanders is generally a quick resolution of the crisis, simple solutions such as eliminating the cause or extricating the victim from the problematic situation prevail (Burleson, 1985; O'Keefe & Delia, 1987). Comforting interventions often consist of low-level imperatives focused on action, and recommendations such as "get it off your chest . . . !" are typical. In reality, negative emotional experiences have complex consequences because they affect the person on many different levels. Next, we list eight such levels (Rimé, 2005). For each of them, we also specify regulation needs to be met for overcoming it.

Eight Levels of Impact

With the loss or deprivation of a physical, material, social, or moral object, a negative emotion always encompasses some frustration of goals, so that a first level of the impact of the episode is *motivational* (Carver & Scheier, 1990; Mandler, 1984). For this impact to be overcome, the person has to abandon the frustrated goals and/or reorganize his or her hierarchy of motives. Under the form of fear, anger, sadness, shame, or the like (e.g., Frijda, 1986; Scherer, 1984), the *emotional* impact properly said constitutes a second level. It elicits strong social needs for appeasement, comforting, love, care, availability, proximity, and/or physical contact (e.g., Bowlby, 1969; Harlow, 1959), as well as concrete material help and assistance through action (e.g., Thoits, 1984). At a third level, a *cognitive* impact results from the fact that by disconfirming expectations, an emotional event challenges the person's representations of reality (e.g., Epstein, 1990, 1991; Horowitz, 1976, 1979). Overcoming this impact requires modification of schemas and integration of new information. A fourth level is found in the *symbolic* impact. Emotional events indeed have implications for important symbolic constructions such as views of oneself, views of others, and views of the world (e.g., Janoff-Bulman, 1992), sense of control, sense of invulnerability, sense of coherence (e.g., Taylor, 1983; Taylor & Brown, 1988), and the like. To overcome this impact, the person needs to develop the cognitive work and social communication proper to restore his or her symbolic system. Part of this restoration may also require positive experiences in effective action. At a fifth level, a negative experience has an impact on *action*. A goal frustration generates some degree of helplessness so that a temporary reduction of the person's capacity to act may result (e.g., Seligman, 1975). This capacity does not build up through cognitive work or interpersonal communication but in behavior and action. Restoration should thus develop in action too, and in severe cases, the contribution of external social support may be needed. At a sixth level, a *social* impact of the negative emotional experience takes the form of alienation. Because of the uncommon character of their experience, victims often develop feelings of estrangement and are treated by others as aliens or strangers (e.g., Wortman & Lehman, 1985). Therefore, powerful needs for social recognition and validation, for listening and understanding, for unconditional acceptance and for social integration are aroused. A seventh level regards the *self*. Key functions of the self encompass planning, prevision, control, organization of action, and reaching goals. Thus, a goal frustration threatens the self, causing a drop in self-esteem (e.g., Epstein, 1973). Support from others, reassurance, and expression of esteem will help to overcome these effects, together with new successful experiences in concrete action. Finally, an emotional experience has an impact on *memory*. The emotional memory which was set up in the episode is activated easily by numerous associative cues (e.g., Lang, 1979; Leventhal, 1984). If the appraisal of the reactivated memory is the same as the initial appraisal of the event, it will trigger the same emotions again and again. For overcoming this impact, cognitive reframing and reappraisal are required.

Central and Collateral Effects

The foregoing analysis shows that the impact of a negative emotional experience is complex and multifaceted. However, two broad classes of effects could be distinguished in this list.

A first class, obvious to everyone, is largely documented by scientific work and might be labeled central effects of an emotional experience. Such effects result from rapid and automatic meaning analyses of supervening events (e.g. Frijda, 1986, 2006; Scherer, 1984). For example, if meanings such as "goal blocked," "danger," "no control," and "no escape" are elicited, a variety of emergency reactions develop in the person's body, and this person simultaneously experiences fear. Central effects involve both a signaling and an executive function (Frijda, 1986, 2006; Oatley & Jenkins, 1996): The emotion-eliciting situation will become the center of attention and automatic action tendencies will temporarily control the behavior. The components of this experience are then stored in a complex memory network (Lang, 1979; Leventhal, 1984). Such materials can easily be activated and recalled via associative links in later situations.

Though they pervade the eight-level picture just sketched, effects of the second class are far from being obvious, and it even took scientists a long time to become aware of their existence (e.g., Bulman & Wortman, 1977; Epstein, 1973, 1990, 1991; Janoff-Bulman, 1992; Taylor, 1983; Taylor & Brown, 1988). We can label them "collateral consequences" of emotional experiences. They result from unattainment of goals, discomfirmation of expectations and schemas, shattering of symbolic constructions, and so forth. In emotional experiences, indeed, the meaning analysis goes beyond the specific emotion-eliciting situation. Situation-specific meanings such as "goal blocked," "danger," "no control," and "no escape" easily spread to broader meanings such as "the world is unsafe," "I am vulnerable and helpless," I am not in control," "I did poorly," and "life is unfair." Such meanings affect how the person views the world and how this person views him- or herself. In other words, they pervade the person's symbolic universe. In current life, the person behaves in a context of apparent order and meaning thanks to which he or she can face the world. Emotional events undermine this delicate architecture. They disconfirm expectations, models, and world views. Traumatic situations have been shown to be particularly deleterious in this regard (Epstein, 1973, 1990; Janoff-Bulman, 1992; Parkes, 1972). But any emotion has some impact on this symbolic architecture because emotion precisely develops at its fissures—or where things are unexpected and/or go out of control. By making fissures apparent, emotion makes us feel the weakness of the construction. This causes collateral emotional feelings under the form of anxiety, insecurity, helplessness, estrangement, alienation, loss of self-esteem, and so forth. *In other words, negative emotional experiences have a subtle and most often ignored consequence of temporary destabilization.*

Three Classes of Regulation Needs

The picture just sketched not only showed that the impact of a negative emotional experience is complex and multifaceted but also manifests that such experiences elicit a large variety of regulation needs. To obtain a simpler picture, these regulation needs can be categorized under three broad classes (see Table 23.1). A first one groups *socioaffective needs* such as basic comforting, concrete social support, social integration, and esteem support. They all result from the destabilizing effect of the emotional episode. Their fulfillment rests on the active contributions from the social environment.

TABLE 23.1. Three Classes of Regulation Needs after a Negative Emotional Experience

Socioaffective needs
- Appeasement, comforting, love, care, contact (level 2)
- Social support and backup in action (level 5)
- Understanding, recognition, social validation, social integration (level 6)
- Support, esteem, reassurance (level 7)

Cognitive needs
- Abandonment of goals, reorganization of motives (level 1)
- Modifying schemas and representations (level 3)
- Re-creation of meaning, restoration of the symbolic system (level 4)
- Reframing, new appraisal of the emotional event (level 8)

Action needs
- Concrete help and assistance (level 2)
- Re-creation of meaning, restoration of the symbolic system (level 4)
- Restoration of mastery and control through action (level 5)
- Successful experience through action (level 7)

A second class gathers *cognitive needs*, such as reorganization of motives, modification of schemas, re-creation of meaning and reframing, which open on a variety of cognitive tasks. Completing them allows the person to overcome perseveration of the episode impact (mental rumination, intrusive thoughts, intrusive imagery, preoccupation, etc.). Social contributions through comparison, suggestion, or incitation may play a critical role in this respect.

Finally, a third category comprising *action needs* reminds us of something which is often overlooked in the investigation of emotional expression and emotional recovery. Emotional experiences may damage facets of the person which were built up in experience and action, as is the case for example, for feelings of control, feelings of mastery, and self-esteem. As a consequence, emotional restoration requires the contribution of new experiences developed through concrete actions. By action needs, it is thus meant that actions undertaken by the person who experienced the emotion and/or members of this person's social network are most often requested for this person to achieve full emotional recovery. For instance, for a horse rider who fell from a horse, whatever their useful contribution to emotional recovery, no cognitive processing and no socioaffective interaction could substitute the action of riding a horse again. Only through such an action could the rider fully reconstruct his or her feelings of control, mastery, self-confidence, and so forth, which were damaged by the fall. Acting has self-constructing consequences that no word and no sympathy can replace.

The more the various regulation needs just listed are met, the more the impact of the eliciting emotional experience will be surmounted. Now, what is the contribution of emotion sharing in this regard? As emotion sharing consists of symbolic interactions, it can involve the planning of action but not action as such. Action such as riding the horse again will by definition develop outside the frame of interpersonal sharing situations. Thus, one of the three classes of regulation needs considered escapes sharing as such. How far can sharing meet the two remaining classes? Exploring motives that people allege for engaging in sharing and examining how listeners react and respond to sharing should be informative in this regard.

MOTIVES FOR SHARING EMOTIONS

What are the motives that people allege for engaging in sharing? Four sets of data are available in this regard. The first was obtained from a group of psychology students enrolled in an advanced class on emotion (Finkenauer & Rimé, 1996). After recalling a recent emotional experience they had shared, they were asked to list all the possible reasons why they had engaged in sharing. Next, working as a group, they had to eliminate their duplicates and group items with similar content into clusters. They thus reached a list of 69 motives which could be grouped under eight categories labeled as in Table 23.2. In a second study (Delfosse, Nils, Lasserre, & Rimé, 2004), a pool of 200 items were collected from non-psychology students who also referred to a recent emotional experience they had shared. Judges uninformed of previous findings then grouped these 200 items under the smallest possible number of classes. They obtained nine categories (Table 23.2) which were nicely consistent with the previous ones, as eight of them had a clear counterpart in the eight categories previously obtained. In a third study, Nils, Delfosse, and Rimé (2005) had some 100 male and female participants recruited in university libraries recalling a recent emotional episode they had shared. Each of them was then asked to mention five different reasons why they did so, which elicited 517 responses. Their responses were submitted to a systematic categorization technique ("heap-up" method, see Bardin, 1991) by judges blind to previous findings who thus obtained 11 classes of motives. Two of them involved tautological answers (e.g., "I shared because the event was strong"; "I shared because I have felt a need to talk") and are thus not considered here. The remaining nine classes of motives (Table 23.2) showed a very good fit with those from previous studies. They indeed matched six of the eight classes collected in the study by Finkenauer and Rimé (1996) and seven of the nine classes obtained by Delfosse et al. (2004). Finally, motives for sharing were also considered in a study examining the sharing of negative consumer experiences. To this aim, Wetzer, Zeelenberg, and Pieters (2005) developed a questionnaire relying on a literature review of theories about social sharing, word-of-mouth communication, and social interaction. Their review led them to adopt seven different motives as questionnaire dimensions. One of them, "revenge" (e.g., "I wanted the service provider to lose customers"), specific to the context of consumption situations, is not relevant here. Each of the other six classes (Table 23.2) had an exact correspondent in the categories of Delfosse et al. (2004). The consistency across studies is thus striking despite differences in approach.

The last column of Table 23.2 displays the 12 classes of motives for sharing emotions obtained when the four reviewed studies are considered together. What is their relevance to sharing situations and to emotion regulation? Some of the motives do not concern social partners in important respects. Rehearsing the episode or venting it does not necessitate an active contribution of the target person. Other motives such as entertaining or informing and warning the target do not aim at emotion regulation. By contrast, all remaining motives in the list manifest considerable demands addressed to social targets in view of emotion regulation. Social sharing partners are indeed expected to provide contributions as diverse as help and support, comfort and consolation, legitimization, clarification and meaning, and advice and solutions. And this long list of specific social solicitations is still augmented with less specific and more personally involving demands to the sharing partner, such as attention, bonding, and empathy.

Thus, motives alleged for socially sharing emotions reveal an overabundance of social demands with regard to emotion regulation. Obviously, these motives massively

TABLE 23.2. Classes of Motives for Socially Sharing an Emotion Evidenced in Four Studies

Finkenauer & Rimé (1996)	Delfosse, Nils, Lasserre, & Rimé (2004)	Nils, Delfosse, & Rimé (2005)	Wetzer, Zeelenberg, & Pieters (2005)	Summary of motives for sharing
Rehearsing; reexperiencing	Reminding; reexperiencing, remembering, rehearsing			Rehearsing
Venting; expressing, searching for relief, getting steam off	Catharsis: venting, finding relief, alleviating	Affective motives: venting, catharsis, search for relief	Venting: to get it off one's chest	Venting
Obtaining comfort: support, listening, sympathy, help	Social support: being listened to, receiving help/support	Social motives: seeking help and support	Support search: seeking comfort, moral support, or understanding	Help and support
		Socioaffective motives: being consoled, comforted		Comfort/consolation
		Social approval motives: being legitimized, approved, understood		Legitimization, validation
Finding understanding: explanation, meaning	Understanding: analyzing what happened, finding meaning/order	Cognitive motives: cognitive clarification, finding words, etc.	Advice search: obtaining information about the thoughts and feelings of others	Clarification and meaning
Obtaining advice: feedback, guidance	Knowing other person's view: receiving advice, finding solutions	Sociocognitive motives: receiving advice, suggestions, solutions		Advices and solutions
Being in touch: relating, escaping loneliness	Social bonding: escaping loneliness/ feeling of abandonment	Sociorelational motives: strengthening social links	Bonding: decreasing interpersonal distance and strengthening social bonds	Bonding, strengthening social links
	Empathy: touching/moving others, feeling oneself closer to others	Affecting the target: moving the listener		Arousing empathy
Receiving attention: impressing others	Gaining attention: distinguishing oneself, eliciting interest			Gaining attention
			Entertaining; "lubricating social interactions"	Entertaining
Informing others: warning	Informing others: bringing them one's experience	Informing one's close circle of one's experience or of one's condition	Warning: helping others by warning them about negative consequences of a particular action	Informing and/or warning

meet socioaffective regulation needs. They also meet some cognitive regulation needs such as finding clarification and meaning. Yet, major cognitive needs such as abandonment of goals, reorganization of motives, reconstruction of schemas, reframing, and reappraisal of the event are simply absent from social demands for regulation. This may in part result from the fact that participants simply might not be aware of such motives and thus might be unable to report them in investigations relying on self-reports. Yet, very likely, there is more. Theoretical views of goal-blocking situations and their consequences consistently stressed that initial responses to goal-blocking involves invigoration, repetitive behaviors, and concentration on the initial goal (e.g., Dembo, 1931; Klinger, 1975; Martin & Tesser, 1989). In other words, early after an emotion—which is precisely when most sharing takes place—people generally refuse to abandon their frustrated goals, they do not consider modifying their hierarchy of motives, they stick to their existing schemas, they do not want to change their representations, they stand by their initial appraisal of the emotional situation, they do not feel ready to reframe it or to change their perspective. There are thus motivational reasons why cognitive needs, which all require distancing from perspectives that prevailed at the time of the emotion, were not mentioned by respondents among motives for sharing emotions. Yet, as we demonstrate later, completion of these cognitive needs is particularly critical to emotional recovery.

SOCIAL EFFECTS OF THE SHARING OF EMOTION

What can we learn from the study of how recipients respond to emotion sharing? When they are brought together, three findings from this study reveal an interesting interpersonal dynamic which develops in sharing situations (Christophe & Rimé, 1997). First, when they rated the intensity of their primary emotions while listening, sharing listeners manifested a remarkable salience of the emotion of interest. Collected on 7-point scales, the average rating of interest exceeded the value of 6.00, suggesting that most recipients rated this particular scale at maximal level. This corroborates the fascination exerted by emotional materials on human beings (Rimé, Delfosse, & Corsini, 2005). As was stressed by Pennebaker and Harber (1993), there are of course limits to this fascination (see also Herbette & Rimé, 2004). Yet, listeners are generally much opened to emotional episodes. We are as eager to listen to emotional narratives as we are to watch a traffic accident, to look at a building in flames, or to attend emotional stories displayed on TV, newspapers, movies, novels, plays, dramas, operas, songs, images, and so on. A second finding confirmed that hearing an emotional story is emotion eliciting. A clear positive linear relation occurred between the emotional intensity of the episode heard and the intensity of the listeners' emotion. Third, responses displayed by sharing listeners varied dramatically as a function of intensity of the shared episode. For low-intensity episodes, listeners' responses mostly consisted of verbal manifestations. Such responses decreased linearly with the increasing intensity of the shared episode. Conversely, the higher the intensity of the episode heard, the more recipients displayed nonverbal behaviors such as touching, body contact, taking into the arms, or kissing. In sum, at increasing levels of emotional intensity, sharing interactions became decreasingly verbal and increasingly nonverbal.

The interpersonal dynamic which develops in the sharing of emotions can thus be sketched as follows. A person *A* who experienced an emotion feels the need to share this experience and shares it effectively with a person *B*. The latter manifests a strong interest for the narrative. This stimulates sharing and person *A* consequently expresses emotions more and more. The enhanced expression arouses emotions in person *B*. A reciprocal stimulation of emotion develops in this manner in the dyad which leads to enhanced empathy and to emotional communion. The empathetic feelings experienced by person *B* stimulate a willingness to help and support person *A*. If the emotional intensity of the episode shared is high, person *B* is likely to reduce his or her verbal communication and to switch to a nonverbal mode, with body contact or touching. Altogether, such a situation is proper to induce an increased liking of *B* for *A*. And *A*, who received from *B* attention, interest, empathy, support, and help, will similarly experience enhanced liking for this sharing target. In sum, the dynamic just sketched manifests that emotion sharing has the potential to bring the sender and the receiver closer to one another (Collins & Miller, 1994). As sharing addresses most often people who already count among intimates (Rimé et al., 1998), it is thus instrumental in maintaining, refreshing, and strengthening important social bonds. The practical significance of the process is considerable. In brief, it means that every time someone is faced with an emotion-eliciting situation, his or her closest social ties will be drawn tighter in the next minutes or hours. Enhanced social integration is thus a very likely consequence of the physiological and psychological turmoil resulting from an emotional situation.

Exposure to the narrative of an emotional experience can induce considerable emotional changes in the listener (Archer & Berg, 1978; Christophe, 1997; Christophe & Rimé, 1997; Lazarus, Opton, Monikos, & Rankin, 1965; Shortt & Pennebaker, 1992; Strack & Coyne, 1983). In confirmation of the general prediction that emotion elicits sharing, listeners of sharing were found to later share with others the heard narrative, in a "secondary sharing" (Christophe & Rimé, 1997; Curci & Bellelli, 2004). The extent of secondary sharing and the number of persons with whom it occurred varied as a function of the emotional intensity felt by the listener in the primary sharing. Also, listeners exposed to a highly emotional sharing manifested secondary sharing more extensively than those exposed to either a moderate or a low-intensity sharing. Thus, once an emotion is shared, there is a high probability that the target would share it too. Would the process extend further? A target of secondary sharing may also experience emotion when listening and thus may further share the episode heard in a "tertiary sharing." Emotions heard in a secondary sharing were indeed found to be shared again with one new listener for one-third of the participants and with several new listeners for another third of them (Christophe, 1997). In sum, sharing an emotion leads to the spreading of emotional information, thus revealing that emotional episodes propagate very easily across social networks. It can be calculated that when some intense emotional event affects someone in a community, 50 to 60 members of this community would be informed of it within the next hours by virtue of the propagation process. From intimates to intimates, most people in the community will know what happened to one of them. This propagation of emotional information has many implications. It means that emotion elicits intragroup communication. It means that members of a community keep track of the emotional experiences affecting their peers. It also means that in a group, the shared social knowledge about emotional events and emotional reactions is continuously updated as a function of new individual experiences. As emotions generally occur when events are unexpected or unpredicted and as such events generally require rapid and appropriate responding, the spreading of information about emotional situations and responses in a social group appears as a particularly efficient prevention tool with regard to future emotion-eliciting situations.

THE ACTUAL CONTRIBUTION OF SHARING
TO EMOTION REGULATION

We can now reconsider the paradoxes encountered in investigating sharing of emotion and examine how far observations reviewed in the latter three sections could help us in resolving them. These paradoxes can be summed up as follows. Sharing an emotion necessarily involves the reactivation of the emotional experience. In the case of negatively valenced episodes, sharing should thus be aversive. Yet, people are found to be extremely eager to engage in sharing whatever the valence of the experience. They generally assume that doing so would bring them emotional recovery with respect to the shared experience. However, assessing the evolution of the emotional impact of a shared experience failed to reveal significant recovery effects. Yet, participants who shared experiences reported abundant benefits of having done so. Do materials considered earlier shed light on these contrasting observations?

Examining the impact of an emotional experience manifested the variety of regulation needs involved. They consisted of, respectively, socioaffective needs, cognitive needs, and action needs. Motives that people allege for sharing are massively in line with regulation needs of the first category: they look for help and support, comfort and consolation, legitimization, attention, bonding, empathy, advice, and solutions. Listeners' responses in sharing nicely meet these expectations, as they involve attention, interest, empathy, support, nonverbal comforting, and help. Thus, sharing covers particularly well the socioaffective regulation needs elicited by emotional experiences. By contrast, cognitive needs are relatively overlooked by sharing. Major aspects of the cognitive regulation of the emotional experience—abandonment of goals, reorganization of motives, reframing, and new appraisal of the emotional event—are simply absent from motives to sharing. Does this mean that they are by definition excluded from sharing, as is the case for action needs? Certainly not. Abandonment of goals, modification of schemas, re-creation of meaning, reframing, or reappraisal of the event are all needs that could benefit from the contribution of interpersonal symbolic interactions. Yet, responses adopted by sharing listeners are making this possibility very unlikely. When shared emotions are intense, listeners' use of verbal mediators reduces and they switch to the nonverbal mode, thus leaving less opportunity for cognitive work and still more place to manifestations of the socioaffective kind. In addition, as stressed before, most of the social sharing of an emotion takes place early after this emotion, a stage at which people generally are obsessed with their frustrated goals. They do not consider modifying their hierarchy of motives, they stick to their existing schemas, they do not want to change their representations, they stand by their initial appraisal of the emotional situation, they do not feel ready to reframe it nor to change their perspective. To sum up, in regard to cognitive processing in naturally occurring sharing, there is no offer and there is no demand. Thus, if naturally developed sharing seems particularly well suited for the fulfillment of socioaffective needs resulting from the impact of an emotional episode, this is certainly not the case for cognitive needs.

Paradoxes may now be resolved. People develop sharing abundantly and quite willingly after an emotional experience because it brings them socioaffective contributions from their sharing partners, thus granting them completion of their socioaffective regulation needs. Rather than preventing the development of sharing, reactivation effects are actually playing a major instrumental role in the interpersonal dynamic that sharing instigates. Indeed, the more the sharing person would feel and express emotions, the more the sharing partner would respond along socioaffective lines, thus providing help and support, comfort and consolation, legitimization, attention, bonding, empathy, advices, and solutions. Because of the interpersonal dynamic it naturally favors, the sharing process is thus remarkably efficient to buffer destabilizing consequences of negative emotional episodes, which result from the disconfirmed expectations, models, and world views, and which manifest themselves in anxiety, insecurity, helplessness, estrangement, alienation, loss of self-esteem, and so forth. In other words, naturally developed sharing is perfectly suited for relieving what we described earlier as the *collateral consequences* of a negative emotional episode, and thus, for restoring the person's stability, at least temporarily. The immediate and strong completion of his or her socioaffective needs is in fact the source of the important benefits the sharing person reports after every social sharing situation. These perceived benefits will fuel laypersons' beliefs that sharing is helpful and relieving. Because people are indiscriminant about the multifaceted impact of their emotional experiences, they equate emotional relief and emotional recovery.

Indeed, the fact that the sharing of emotion was instrumental in buffering the collateral consequence of a negative emotional episode is irrelevant to the regulation of *central effects* of such an experience and, thus, leaves emotional recovery unachieved. Central effects of emotional experiences result from automatic meaning analyses and from the storage of components of the related experience in long-term memory. In the absence of cognitive work on this material, it will elicit the same set of emotional manifestations every time it is activated and recalled. Thus, relieving effects obtained from the socioaffective process involved in naturally developed sharing are expected to be temporary and to vanish rapidly once the sharing situation is over. Whereas the social sharing of emotion is a normal component of emotional responding in the early phase following an emotional episode, a perseveration of the need to share the same experience in the longer term is indicative of poor recovery and suggests deficits in the completion of related cognitive work.

Completion of cognitive work involving abandonment of goals and reorganization of motives, modification of schemas, re-creation of meaning, reframing, or reappraisal of the event is thus critical for achieving emotional recovery. Yet, we noted that people are not prone to develop such work in the immediate aftermath of an emotional experience. We also noted that naturally developed sharing is unlikely to bring it up. Practical recommendations in this regard are thus double. First, cognitive work should better not be undertaken early after an emotional experience. Early after a negative emotional experience, completion of socioaffective needs is primarily what the person needs. In this regard, any available human being with sense and sensibility may provide some useful contribution, though most often the person's circle of intimates is expected to play the preponderant role. Second, if the person's need to share fails to extinguish over time and if preoccupations with the episode do disturb current adaptation, cognitive work should take place. Sharing developed with professional psychologists or psychotherapists will then provide the person the appropriate guidance and support for completing the needed cognitive work.

CONCLUDING COMMENTS

As Schachter (1959) foresaw it in his classic studies around "emotion and affiliation" and "misery seeks company," a formidable and mostly ignored social process develops in the wake of emotions. Emotional experiences, whether positive or negative, elicit a social sharing process that is generally repetitive and directed toward a variety of targets. Such a process signals interpersonal regulatory attempts that people need to develop in the aftermath of an emotional experience. The question thus arises of what is at stake in these interpersonal regulatory efforts undertaken after an emotion.

In the case of a positive emotional episode, regulatory efforts are obviously not oriented toward the reduction or buffering of the experienced emotions. To the contrary, what is at stake in this case is to maintain, sustain, and prolong as much as possible the experienced positive affects. By doing so, people can enhance their self-esteem and self-confidence, and in this manner, they are able to improve their general well-being. Studies showed that communicating the positive events to others was indeed associated with an enhancement of positive affect far beyond the benefits due to the valence of the positive events themselves. In addition, the process of sharing positive emotions was shown to enhance social bonds. Thus, the interpersonal regulatory efforts developed after an emotion not only involve capitalization at the benefit of the person who experienced the emotion, but they also entail benefit sharing with members of this person's social network.

In the case of a negative emotional episode, regulatory efforts should reduce the negative affects aroused by the emotional memory. Their implicit purpose would thus be to bring this memory to the dormant stage, or to a stage at which it would no longer return to the person's mind. As a result, this person's attentional capacities would become fully available for current tasks. In this chapter, we considered that the regulation work resulting from a negative emotional experience is not an univocal task. Collateral or destabilizing effects of such an experience elicit socioaffective needs which naturally developed sharing is well suited to buffer. However, the central effects of the negative emotional experience may prolong its impact through activation of its long-term memory representation. Regulating central effects requires important cognitive work which is much less easily achieved and is nevertheless critical to emotional recovery. Moreover, it should be stressed that, as was the case for positive emotions, the social sharing of negative emotions has important consequences for the social network of the concerned person. We noted that sharing is instrumental in maintaining, refreshing, and strengthening important social bonds. We also noted that through a process of social propagation of emotion sharing, members of a community keep track of the emotional experiences affecting their peers. In addition, we remarked that due to the sharing process, in a group, the shared social knowledge about emotional events and emotional reactions is continuously updated as a function of new individual experiences.

In our Western culture, we predominantly conceive emotion as a process taking place deep inside the physiological and subjective universe of the person. It is thus stimulating to explore interpersonal and social aspects of emotion regulation. It does not spontaneously come to our mind that when someone experiences an emotion, people around this person play a critical role in the regulation of this experience. Yet, is it so surprising? Considering the conditions under which emotional life is shaped in child development, the answer is no.

To start with, newborns are only able to send emotional signals. For a long time, every adaptational responses to these signals come from the baby's social environment. A long-term contract known as *attachment* develops between the baby and members of this social milieu. Attachment represents a resource that the infant activates when under stress (Bowlby, 1969). Thus, in stressful situations, attachment figures provide children with the essence of every later socioaffective response: presence, appeasement, contact, comforting, support, and so forth. Under their socioaffective protection, the child develops abilities to construe the environment he or she explores, thus setting up cognitive tools for preventing further emotional stressors. Parents also talk to their child far before the latter is able to understand language. In emotional situations in particular, the child is talked to abundantly. In such talks, the emotion-eliciting situation and the child's feelings and responses to it are labeled, causes and effects are identified, remedies are mentioned, and regulatory advices are formulated. In this manner, the child's emotional consciousness emerges and develops in a framework entirely defined from the caregiver's perspective. Young children are already so well aware that adults aptly carry emotional meanings that already in their first year of life, they manifest social referencing (Baldwin & Moses, 1996; Feinman & Lewis, 1983; Klinnert, Emde, Butterfield, & Campos, 1986; Sorce, Emde, Campos, & Klinnert, 1985; Striano & Rochat, 2000). They explore an adult face when exposed to a puzzling situation and they refer to the facial signals for defining the situation as innocuous, dangerous, or pleasant, thus demonstrating how heavily they rely on adults for emotional meaning. In addition, because of adults' conversations or because of tales they are told, children are exposed daily to innumerable emotion narratives in which they learn what can happen and how they could or should react (Brunner, 1990). As soon as he or she can talk, a child is actively trained by adults in telling stories and reporting what happened in their absence (Fivush, 1994; Fivush, Haden, & Reese, 1999). Last but not least, all along their development, children are equipped by attachment figures and their substitutes with common sense and symbolic constructions through which they will be protected from the emotional impact of raw reality (Berger & Luckmann, 1967).

Thus, for every individual, both emotional meaning and meanings that buffer emotions originate from the social milieu. It may then not come as a surprise that when, later in life, individuals confront an emotional experience, their most systematic response is to address the social milieu.

REFERENCES

Archer, R. L., & Berg, J. H. (1978). Disclosure reciprocity and its limits: A reactance analysis. *Journal of Experimental Social Psychology, 14,* 527–540.
Arendt, M., & Elklit, A. (2001). Effectiveness of psychological debriefing. *Acta Psychiatrica Scandinavica, 104,* 423–437.
Baldwin, D. A., & Moses, L. J. (1996). The ontogeny of social information gathering. *Child Development, 67,* 1915–1939.
Bardin, L. (1991). *L'analyse de contenu* [Content analysis]. Paris: Presses Universitaires de France.
Berger, P. L., & Luckmann, T. (1967). *Social construction of reality.* Garden City, NY: Doubleday.
Bowlby, J. (1969). *Attachment and loss: Vol. 1. Attachment.* New York: Basic Books.
Bruner, J. (1990). *Acts of meaning.* Cambridge, MA: Harvard University Press.
Bryant, F. B. (1989). A four factor model of perceived control: Avoiding, coping, obtaining, and savoring. *Journal of Personality, 57,* 773–797.
Bulman, R., & Wortman, C. B. (1977). Attributions of blame and coping in the "real world": Severe accidents victims react to their lot. *Journal of Personality and Social Psychology, 35,* 351–363.
Burleson, B. R. (1985). The production of comforting messages: Social–cognitive foundations. *Journal of Language and Social Psychology, 4*(3–4), 253–212.
Cannon, W. B. (1929). *Bodily changes in pain, hunger, fear and rage.* New York: Appleton. (Original work published 1915)
Carver, C. S., & Scheier, M. F. (1990). Origins and functions of positive and negative affect: A control-process view. *Psychological Review, 97,* 19–35.
Christophe, V. (1997). *Le partage social des émotions du point de vue de l'auditeur* [Social sharing of emotion under the angle of the listener]. Unpublished doctoral dissertation, Université de Lille III, France.

Christophe, V., & Rimé, B. (1997). Exposure to the social sharing of emotion: Emotional impact, listener responses and the secondary social sharing. *European Journal of Social Psychology*, 27, 37–54.

Coates, D., Wortman, C. B., & Abbey, A. (1979). Reactions to victims. In I. H. Frieze, D. Bar-Tal, & J. S. Carrol (Eds.), *New approaches to social problems* (pp. 461–489). San Francisco: Jossey-Bass.

Cole, P., Martin, S., & Dennis, T. (2004). Emotion regulation as a scientific construct: Methodological challenges and directions for child development research. *Child Development*, 75, 317–333.

Collins, N. L., & Miller, L. C. (1994). Self-Disclosure and liking: A meta-analytic review. *Psychological Bulletin*, 116, 457–475.

Curci, A., & Bellelli, G. (2004). Cognitive and social consequences of exposure to emotional narratives: Two studies on secondary social sharing of emotions. *Cognition and Emotion*, 18, 881–900.

de Beauvoir, S. (1972). *Tout compte fait* (All things considered). Paris: Gallimard.

Delfosse, C., Nils, F., Lasserre, S., & Rimé, B. (2004). Les motifs allégués du partage social et de la rumination mentale des émotions: Comparaison des épisodes positifs et négatifs. *Cahiers Internationaux de Psychologie Sociale*, 64, 35–44.

Dembo, T. (1931). Der anger als dynamisches problem [Anger as a dynamic problem]. *Psychologische Forschung*, 15, 1–144.

Epstein, S. (1973). The self-concept revisited, or a theory of a theory. *American Psychologist*, 28, 404–416.

Epstein, S. (1990). Cognitive–experiential self-theory. In L. Pervin (Ed.), *Handbook of personality: Theory and research* (pp. 165–192). New York: Guilford Press.

Epstein, S. (1991). The self-concept, the traumatic neurosis, and the structure of personality. In D. Ozer, J. M. Healey, Jr., & A. J. Stewart (Eds.), *Perspectives on personality* (Vol. 3, Part A, pp. 63–98). London: Jessica Kingsley.

Ersland, S., Weisaeth, L., & Sund, A. (1989). The stress upon rescuers involved in an oil rig disaster. "Alexander Kielland" 1980. *Acta Psychiatrica Scandinavica*, 80, 38–49.

Feinman, S., & Lewis, M. (1983). Social referencing at ten months: A second-order effect on infants' responses to strangers. *Child Development*, 54, 878–887.

Finkenauer, C., & Rimé, B. (1998). Socially shared emotional experiences vs. emotional experiences kept secret: Differential characteristics and consequences. *Journal of Social and Clinical Psychology*, 17, 295–318.

Finkenauer, F., & Rimé, B. (1996). *Motives for sharing emotion*. Unpublished raw data.

Fivush, R. (1994), Constructing narrative, emotion, and self in parent–child conversations about past. In U. Neisser & R. Fivush (Eds.), *The remembering self: Construction and accuracy in the self-narrative* (pp. 136–156). New York: Cambridge University Press.

Fivush, R., Haden, C., & Reese, E. (1999). Remembering, recounting, and reminiscing: The development of autobiographical memory in social context. In D. C. Rubin (Ed.), *Remembering our past: Studies in autobiographical memory* (pp. 341–359). New York: Cambridge University Press.

Frattaroli, J. (2006). Experimental disclosure and its moderators: A meta-analysis. *Psychological Bulletin*, 132, 823–865.

Frijda, N. (1986). *The emotions*. Cambridge, UK: Cambridge University Press.

Frijda, N. (2006). *The laws of emotion*. Mahwah, NJ: Erlbaum.

Gable, S. L., Reis, H. T., Impett, E. A., & Asher, E. R. (2004). What do you do when things go right? The intrapersonal and interpersonal benefits of sharing positive events. *Journal of Personality and Social Psychology*, 87, 228–245.

Goffman, E. (1963). *Stigma: Notes on the management of spoiled identity*. Englewood Cliffs, NJ.: Prentice Hall.

Gross, J. J., & Thompson, R. A. (2007). Emotion regulation: Conceptual foundations. In J. J. Gross (Ed.), *Handbook of emotion regulation* (pp. 3–24). New York: Guilford Press.

Gross, J. J. (1998). The emerging field of emotion regulation: An integrative review. *Review of General Psychology*, 2, 271–299.

Harlow, H. F. (1959, June). Love in infant monkeys. *Scientific American*, 200, 68–74.

Herbette, G., & Rimé, B. (2004). Verbalization of emotion in chronic pain patients and their psychological adjustments. *Journal of Health Psychology*, 9, 661–676.

Horowitz, M. J. (1976). *Stress response syndromes*. New York: Aronson.

Horowitz, M. J. (1979). Psychological response to serious life events. In V. Hamilton & D. M. Warburton (Eds.), *Human stress and cognition: An information processing approach* (pp. 235–263). Chichester, UK: Wiley.

Janoff-Bulman, R. (1992). *Shattered assumptions. Towards a new psychology of trauma*. New York: Free Press.

Klinger, E. (1975). Consequences of commitment to and disengagement from incentives. *Psychological Review, 82*, 1–25.

Klinnert, M. D., Emde, R. N., Butterfield, P., & Campos, J. J. (1986). Social referencing: The infant's use of emotional signals from a friendly adult with mother present. *Developmental Psychology, 22*, 427–432.

Lang, P. J. (1979). A bio-informational theory of emotional imagery. *Psychophysiology, 16*, 495–512.

Langston, C. A. (1994). Capitalizing on and coping with daily-life events: Expressive responses to positive events. *Journal of Personality and Social Psychology, 67*, 1112–1125.

Lazarus, R. S., Opton, E. M., Monikos, M. S., & Rankin, N. O. (1965). The principle of short-circuiting of threat: Further evidence. *Journal of Personality, 47*, 909–917.

Lepore, J. L., & Smyth, J. M. (2002). *The writing cure. How expressive writing promotes health and emotional well-being*. Washington, DC: American Psychological Association.

Leventhal, H. (1984). A perceptual–motor theory of emotion. *Advances in Experimental Social Psychology, 17*, 117–182.

Luminet, O., Bouts, P., Delie, F., Manstead, A. S. R., & Rimé, B. (2000). Social sharing of emotion following exposure to a negatively valenced situation. *Cognition and Emotion, 14*, 661–688.

Mandler, G. (1984). *Mind and body: Psychology of emotion and stress*. New York: Norton.

Martin, L. L., & Tesser, A. (1989). Toward a motivational and structural theory of ruminative thought. In J. S. Uleman & J. A. Bargh (Eds.), *Unintended thought* (pp. 306–326). New York: Guilford Press.

Mesquita, B. (1993). *Cultural variations in emotion: A comparative study of Dutch, Surinamese and Turrkish people in the Netherlands*. Unpublished doctoral dissertation, University of Amsterdam, The Netherlands.

Mitchell, G. W., & Glickman, A. S. (1977). Cancer patients: Knowledge and attitude. *Cancer, 40*, 61–66.

Mitchell, J. T., & Everly, G. S. (1995). Critical incident stress debriefing (CISD) and the prevention of work-related traumatic stress among high risk occupational groups. In G. S. Everly & J. M. Lating (Eds.), *Psychotraumatology. Key papers and core concepts in post-traumatic stress* (pp. 267–280). New York: Plenum Press.

Nils, F., Delfosse, C., & Rimé, B. (2005). *Partage social des émotions : Raisons invoquées et médiateurs perçus* [Social sharing of emotions: Alleged reasons and perceived mediators]. Manuscript submitted for publication. University of Louvain at Louvain-la-Neuve, Belgium.

Oatley, K., & Jenkins, J. M. (1996). *Understanding emotions*. Cambridge, MA: Blackwell

O'Keefe, B., & Delia, J. (1987). Psychological and interactional dimensions of communicative development. In H. Giles & R. St. Clair (Eds.), *Recent advances in language, communication and social psychology* (pp. 41–85). London: Erlbaum.

Parkes, C. M. (1972). *Bereavement: Studies of grief in adult life*. London, UK: Tavistock

Pennebaker, J. W. (1997). Writing about emotional experiences as a therapeutic process. *Psychological Science, 8*, 162–166.

Pennebaker, J. W. (2002). Writing about past emotional events: From past to future. In J. L. Lepore & J. M. Smyth (Eds.), *The writing cure: How expressive writing promotes health and emotional well-being* (pp. 281–291). Washington, DC: American Psychological Association.

Pennebaker, J. W., & Beall, S. (1986). Confronting a traumatic event: Toward an understanding of inhibition and disease. *Journal of Abnormal Psychology, 95*, 274–281.

Pennebaker, J. W., & Harber, K. D. (1993). A social stage model of collective coping: The Loma Prieta Earthquake and Persian Gulf War. *Journal of Social Issues, 49*, 125–145.

Pennebaker, J. W., Zech, E., & Rimé, B. (2001). Disclosing and sharing emotion: Psychological, social and health consequences. In M. Stroebe, W. Stroebe, R. O. Hansson, & H. Schut (Eds.), *New handbook of bereavement: Consequences, coping, and care* (pp. 517–544). Washington, DC: American Psychological Association.

Rimé, B. (1989). Le partage social des émotions. In B. Rimé & K. Scherer (Eds.), *Les émotions* (pp. 271–303). Neuchâtel, Switzerland: Delachaux et Niestlé.

Rimé, B. (1999). Expressing emotion, physical health, and emotional relief: A cognitive social perspective. *Advances in Mind–Body Medicine, 15*, 175–179.

Rimé, B. (2005). *Le partage social des émotions* [The social sharing of emotions]. Paris: Presses Universitaires de France.

Rimé, B., Delfosse, C., & Corsini, S. (2005). Emotional fascination: Responses Elicited by Viewing Pictures of September 11 attack. *Cognition and Emotion, 19*, 923–932.

Rimé, B., Finkenauer, C., Luminet, O., Zech, E., & Philippot, P. (1998). Social sharing of emotion: New evidence and new questions. In W. Stroebe & M. Hewstone (Eds.), *European review of social psychology* (Vol. 9, pp. 145–189). Chichester, UK: Wiley.

Rimé, B., Mesquita, B., Philippot, P., & Boca, S. (1991a). Beyond the emotional event: Six studies on the social sharing of emotion. *Cognition and Emotion, 5,* 435–465.

Rimé, B., Noël, P., & Philippot, P. (1991b). Épisode émotionnel, réminiscences cognitives et réminiscences sociales. *Cahiers Internationaux de Psychologie Sociale, 11,* 93–104

Rimé, B., Philippot, P., Boca, S., & Mesquita, B. (1992). Long lasting cognitive and social consequences of emotion: Social sharing and rumination. In W. Stroebe & M. Hewstone (Eds.), *European Review of Social Psychology* (Vol. 3, pp. 225–258). Chichester, UK: Wiley.

Rimé, B., Yogo, M., & Pennebaker, J. W. (1996). *Social sharing of emotion across cultures.* Unpublished raw data.

Rose, S., & Bisson, J. (1998). Brief early psychological interventions following trauma: A systematic review of the literature. *Journal of Traumatic Stress, 11,* 697–710.

Schachter, S. (1959). *The psychology of affiliation.* Stanford, CA: Stanford University Press.

Scherer, K. R. (1984). Emotion as a multicomponent process: A model and some cross-cultural data. In P. Shaver (Ed.), *Review of personality and social psychology* (Vol. 5, pp. 37–63). Beverly Hills, CA: Sage.

Schoenberg, B. B., Carr, A. C., Peretz, D., Kutscher, A. H., & Cherico, D. J. (1975). Advice of the bereaved for the bereaved. In B. Schoenberg, I. Gerber, A. Wiener, A. H. Kutscher, D. Peretz, & A. C. Carr (Eds.), *Bereavement: Its psychological aspects* (pp. 362–367). New York: Columbia University Press.

Seligman, M. E. P. (1975). *Helplessness: On depression, development and health.* San Francisco, Freeman.

Shortt, J. W., & Pennebaker, J. W. (1992). Talking versus hearing about Holocaust experiences. *Basic and Applied Social Psychology, 13,* 165–179.

Singh-Manoux, A. (1998). *Les variations culturelles dans le partage social des émotions* [Cultural variations in social sharing of emotions]. Unpublished doctoral dissertation, Université de Paris X-Nanterre, France.

Singh-Manoux, A., & Finkenauer, C. (2001). Cultural Variations in social sharing of emotions: An intercultural perspective on a universal phenomenon. *Journal of Cross-Cultural Psychology, 32,* 647–661.

Sorce, J. F., Emde, R. N., Campos, J. J., & Klinnert, M. D. (1985). Maternal emotional signaling: Its effect on the visual cliff behavior of 1-year-olds. *Developmental Psychology, 21,* 195–200.

Strack, F., & Coyne, J. C. (1983). Shared and private reaction to depression. *Journal of Personality and Social Psychology, 44,* 798–806.

Striano, T., & Rochat, P. (2000). Developmental link between dyadic and triadic social competence in infancy. *British Journal of Developmental Psychology, 17,* 551–562.

Taylor, S. E. (1983). Adjustment to threatening events. A theory of cognitive adaptation. *American Psychologist, 38,* 1161–1173.

Taylor, S. E., & Brown, J. D. (1988). Illusion and well-being: A social psychological perspective on mental health. *Psychological Bulletin, 103,* 193–210.

Thoits, P. A. (1984). Coping, social support, and psychological outcomes. In P. Shaver (Ed.), *Review of personality and social psychology* (Vol. 5, pp. 219–238). Beverly Hills, CA: Sage.

Van Emmerik, A. A., Kamphuis, J. H., Hulsbosch, A. M., & Emmelkamp, P. M. (2002). Single session debriefing after psychological trauma: A meta-analysis. *Lancet, 360,* 766–771.

Wetzer, I. M., Zeelenberg, M., & Pieters, R. (2005). *Motivations for socially sharing emotions: Why being specific matters.* Manuscript submitted for publication. Department of Psychology, Tilburg University, The Netherlands.

Wortman, C. B., & Lehman, D R. (1985). Reactions to victims of life crises: Support attempts that fail. In I. G. Sarason & B. R. Sarason (Eds.), *Social support: Theory, research, and applications* (pp. 463–489). Dordrecht, The Netherlands: Martinus Nijhoof.

Yogo, M., & Onoe, K. (1998, August 4–8). *The social sharing of emotion among Japanese students.* Poster session presented at ISRE '98, the biannual conference of the International Society for Research on Emotion, held in Wuerzburg, Germany.

Zech, E. (2000). *The effects of the communication of emotional experiences.* Unpublished doctoral dissertation. Louvain-la-Neuve, Belgium: University of Louvain

Zech, E., & Rimé, B. (2005). Is it talking about an emotional experience helpful? Effects on emotional recovery and perceived benefits. *Clinical Psychology and Psychotherapy, 12,* 270–287.

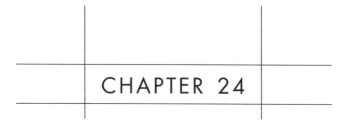

CHAPTER 24

The Cultural Regulation of Emotions

BATJA MESQUITA
DUSTIN ALBERT

Happiness is the norm in American culture (D'Andrade, 1984; Wierzbicka, 1994). Natural though this desire to be actively happy may seem to most American readers, the norm of happiness is in fact grounded in specific cultural meanings and practices (Tsai, Knutson, & Fung, 2006). High-activation happiness is valued because, in American contexts, it signals that one has successfully managed the central cultural tasks of standing out, fulfilling one's personal and material goals, and being unique (Hochschild, 1995). A constant smile and a friendly demeanor exhibits to other Americans a "good inner self" and psychological well-being (Markus & Kitayama, 1994; Wierzbicka, 1994).

The norm of happiness is far from universal. During her stay with the Ifaluk (on a Pacific atoll), the anthropologist Catherine Lutz was reprimanded for smiling at a girl who acted happy. The Ifaluk condemn this emotion, because it is thought to lead to a neglect of duties (Lutz, 1987) that are central to the social organization of Ifaluk life. The pursuit of high-activation happiness also seems discouraged in many East Asian cultures that live according to the Confucian tradition. According to this tradition, emotions should be cultivated as the means to harmonious human relationships. High-activation happiness does not fit this goal, as it may elicit jealousy in others (Edwards, 1996) or inappropriately emphasize autonomy (Heine, Lehman, Markus, & Kitayama, 1999).

These descriptions show that the norms for emotion, and thus the endpoints of emotion regulation, may differ greatly among cultures. Not only do American cultural models condone high-activation happiness, they also facilitate the experience of yielding to and enhancing this emotion and its expression. Cultures in which the expression of personal success and self-reliance is considered threatening to harmonious human relationships are likely to prevent or inhibit the experience and expression of this type of happiness.

The main goal of this chapter is to show that emotion regulation is always embedded in the meanings and practices that constitute the sociocultural world, which we describe as *cultural models of self and relating*. From the point of view of an individual-centered model of emotion regulation (Gross, 1998; Gross & Thompson, this volume), the importance of culture to emotion regulation is most clearly seen in the cultural constitution of emotion regulatory goals. Whereas emotion regulation may be universally motivated by the individual's need to establish and maintain adaptive relationships, and to feel and act consistent with the kind of self one wants to be (Thompson, 1991), cultural models play a crucial role in defining the specific goals for such relationships and selfhood (Markus & Kitayama, 1991). Furthermore, we argue that culture regulates emotion at the individual level by making emotional responses that are aligned with cultural models chronically accessible. In this way, culture increases the likelihood of an emotional response when it is consistent with the model and decreases its likelihood when it is inconsistent with the model.

A further objective of this chapter is to go beyond the conception of emotion regulation as an individual process and to discuss emotion regulation at a sociocultural level. We argue that cultural practices themselves—the actual social worlds in which the individual engages—contribute in important ways to emotion regulation. First, sociocultural regulation occurs by providing specific opportunities for emotion experiences and endowing those experiences with meaning. For example, American social life is characterized by practices that highlight individuals' general value and specific achievements, including the frequent exchange of compliments and encouragements as well as institutionalized award ceremonies. Engaging in these ubiquitous practices promotes the frequent experience of happiness and pride and infuses these emotions with specific cultural meanings associated with the conditions of their experience. Furthermore, culture provides the contexts for normative modes of emotional expression, from the ritual (e.g., birthday celebrations and funerals) to the mundane (e.g., conversations between girlfriends and after-work drinks with colleagues). Finally, sociocultural regulation takes the form of the reward and punishment contingencies—the positive or negative responses of other people—that saturate the social environment. In this chapter we discuss instances of the cultural regulation of emotion at both the individual and sociocultural level.

To provide a foundation for our discussion of the cultural regulation of emotion, we first define and describe cultural models of self and relating. Next, we discuss our assumptions about emotion and emotion regulatory processes, positioning our views with respect to contemporary models. We then discuss the cultural regulation of emotion at the level of situation selection, situation modification, attentional deployment, appraisal, and behavior. We conclude by highlighting the ways in which a focus on sociocultural processes contributes to the literature on emotion regulation.

CULTURAL MODELS OF SELF AND RELATING

Cultural models of self and relating are, at the same time, forms of knowledge and practices (Bruner, 1986, 1990; D'Andrade, 1984; D'Andrade & Strauss, 1992; Holland, Lachicotte, Skinner, & Cain, 1998; Holland & Quinn, 1987; Markus & Kitayama, 1991;

Markus, Mullally, & Kitayama, 1997; Shweder & Haidt, 2000). They are models of the social reality in that culture, as well as models of the normative. Cultural models importantly constitute a person's reality, because they focus attention, they guide perception, they lend meaning, and they imbue emotional value. Therefore, a cultural model is decisive for what one's world is like (Bruner, 1986), and reflects the cultural "answers" to existential questions, such as how to be a person and how to maintain relationships (D'Andrade, 1984; D'Andrade & Strauss, 1992; Holland & Quinn, 1987). In this section, we discuss North American and Japanese cultural models as examples.

According to middle-class American models of self and relating, the individual should be independent and free from others, as well as stand out among them (Kim & Markus, 1999; Rothbaum, Pott, Azuma, Miyake, & Weisz, 2000; Triandis, 1995). Consequently, it is very important that individuals think of themselves as possessing the positive characteristics that enable them to be autonomous and self-reliant; hence, there is an emphasis on self-esteem (Heine et al., 1999; Hochschild, 1995). Close relationships are not necessarily less valued than in cultures with interdependent models of self and relating (e.g., Japan), but the meaning and dynamics of relationships in American contexts strongly reflect independence concerns (Rothbaum et al., 2000). Relationships are evaluated for the extent to which they meet one's personal needs, and conflicts are viewed as inevitable due to the frequent expression and negotiation of those needs (Rothbaum et al., 2000). Furthermore, mutual approval—enhancing each other's self-esteem—is an important quality of friendship (Kitayama & Markus, 2000), and relationships in general are expected to contribute to one's pursuit of personal achievement and happiness (Rothbaum et al., 2000; Triandis, 1994).

In contrast, according to the prevalent model of self and relating in Japanese cultural contexts, individuals experience themselves as interdependent—that is, in relation to others, belonging to social groups, or significantly and reciprocally enmeshed in families, communities, or work groups (Kanagawa, Cross, & Markus, 2001; Kondo, 1990; Markus & Kitayama, 1991). The dominant goals of the self are to be like others and to enhance the fit between what one is doing and what is expected (Heine et al., 2001; Kim & Markus, 1999; Lebra, 1992, 1994; Oishi & Diener, 2003). Self-improvement is a persistently salient concern, as it is necessary for meeting relational expectations (Karasawa, 2001; Lewis, 1995b; Mesquita & Markus, 2004). To self-improve, individuals need to be aware of their shortcomings; hence, the focus on negative information about oneself (Kitayama, Matsumoto, Markus, & Norasakkunkit, 1997). Close relationships are based on the fulfillment of role-based obligations and the demonstration of loyalty to significant social ingroups (Rothbaum et al., 2000). The degree to which relationships meet one's personal needs is deemphasized, and conflict is avoided in favor of conciliatory behaviors meant to preserve relational harmony.

This contrast between American and Japanese cultures illustrates that people in different sociocultural contexts live different realities—or systems of practices and meanings—that we call cultural models of self and relating. Individuals' understandings, feelings, and acts never occur in a social vacuum but, rather, must be situated in these cultural models.

Heterogeneity in Models

It should be noted that a focus on cultural models of self and relating does not mean that people in a given context are homogeneous clones of one another (Markus et al., 1997). First, there is more than one cultural model in a given situation. Multiple models relating to a variety of possible identifications (e.g., gender, ethnicity, and occupation) exist and compete for an individual's attention and engagement.

Second, no two individuals in a culture will engage a given model in exactly the same way. An individual's particular representations of a model are specific to his or her learning history within that culture and level of engagement with specific cultural meanings and practices. What is critical is that even if individuals have not fully internalized the cultural models, those models are still reflected in the practices in which these individuals engage, the reward structures that are in place for them, and the expectations of others in their lives (Shweder, 1991, 1999). Thus, cultural models set the reality boundaries within which self, relationships, and goals are defined, formed, and promoted (Bruner, 1986).

Cultural Models Theory

Cultural models theory highlights that social and psychological processes are saturated with meaning, and in this way they are carriers of culture. Cultural models should thus not be conceived as predictors of psychological processes; rather, they are *manifest* in psychological (and other) processes, including emotions. It is precisely the systematic approach and conceptualization of meaning that can be counted as cultural models theory's greatest credit. A focus on meaning is relatively new to psychology.

It would be possible, within certain models, to make predictions about the specific psychological contents to be found. However, in this chapter the focus is on describing cultural differences in a systematic way and making them understandable through their fit with cultural models. The chapter is inductive, rather than hypothesis testing.

EMOTION AND EMOTION REGULATION

We conceive of emotions as multicomponential processes that materialize largely in accordance with their sociocultural contexts (Mesquita, 2003; Mesquita & Markus, 2004). Thus, we postulate that multiple facets of emotion, such as the antecedent situation, appraisal, and behavioral readiness and means, together constitute the emotion process (Frijda, 1986; Lang, 1988; Oatley, 1992; Oatley & Johnson-Laird, 1987; Scherer, 1984). Emotions, in this view, are not invariant, discrete events, but rather they are aggregates of the outputs from the different aspects of emotion (Barrett, in press-a, in press-b; Frijda, 1986; Mesquita, 2003; Russell, 2003).

At each point of the emotion, cultural models of self and relating afford emotional responses that fit with and promote the culturally normative and modal ways of being a person and having a relationship, whereas they reduce the likelihood of emotional responses that violate cultural models of self and relating (Mesquita, 2003). The process of emotion is thus considered flexible and adaptive to the specific contexts in which it takes place. As a consequence, the patterns of emotional outputs are thought to vary across instances of emotions, people, and, importantly, cultural contexts. This view of emotions is in contrast to theories that posit a biologically based repertoire of discrete emotional response programs (e.g., Ekman, 1992; Izard, 1994; Johnson-Laird & Oatley, 1992). In the latter view, one of a small set of emotions is thought to be elicited by a given environmental stimulus or appraisal and subsequently to unfold as a relatively invariant pattern of physiological response, subjective experience, and expressive behavior.

These two views of emotion also lead to different conceptualizations of emotion regulation. For instance, the conceptualization of emotions as discrete events with a set of invariant responses underlies current two-factor models of emotion regulation (e.g., Gross, 1998; Gross & Thompson, this volume). A discrete emotion is thought to be automatically triggered by some antecedent process and then regulated by a separate set of processes. In other words, this approach posits a "natural" emotion that is generated and would be observable as invariant if it were not obscured by the individual's regulatory efforts.

Our view of emotions leads us to a different conception of emotion regulation. Following Campos, Frankel, and Camras (2004), we postulate that the processes responsible for emotion generation and emotion regulation are ontologically indistinguishable. This is clearly illustrated by the common case of people regulating their emotions before they are even generated. For instance, people downregulate their negative emotions before they are elicited by selecting favorable environments and developing habitual, "preemptive" appraisal styles. In our view, all emotion experience is regulated.

Little is known about response selection in emotion. We assume that the level of accessibility and projected rewards of emotional responses will affect their selection, as these factors are responsible for response selection in other psychological domains. This is the case for emotion generation and emotion regulation alike. Our theory concurs with Gross's process model of emotion regulation (Gross, 1998; Gross & Thompson, this volume) that emotions are regulated at a number of key component levels, with the exception that we consider the components of regulation to be indistinguishable from components constituting the generative process. The conceptual language of emotion regulation fits both.

Much emotion regulatory work is performed automatically. However, we also consider conscious, effortful emotion regulation as a distinct component of the emotion process. With this inclusive definition of emotion regulation in mind, we discuss some evidence that emotion regulation is shaped by cultural models of self and relating.

CULTURAL MODELS CONSTITUTE EMOTION REGULATION

The cultural shaping of emotions is suggested by cultural differences in the prevalence and nature of particular emotions but can be established with more confidence when these differences are readily understood and accounted for by differences in cultural models of self and relating (Mesquita, 2003). Cultural models regulate emotions, first, by patterning the situations one encounters in the world, such that there is a relatively high frequency of situations affording emotions that are consistent with the cultural models, and a relatively low frequency of situations that would elicit emotions that are inconsistent with the model. Furthermore, cultural models are organizing principles of the actual emotions occurring because they promote the selection of model-consistent responses throughout the emotion process (e.g., situation selection and modification, attentional deployment, appraisal, and behavior), while inhibiting the selection of responses that are incompatible with the model (Mesquita, 2003).

Congruence with cultural models will increase the salience of a response (in terms of its desirability), and thus its probability of activation. Incongruent responses will be highly salient as well (in terms of their undesirability) and thus more likely to be avoided (Strack, Schwarz, Bless, & Kuebler, 1993). Cultural models therefore are apparent in the activation of responses for every facet of the emotion process through modulation of the desirability and undesirability salience of each potential response. We stress that cultural models shape the *probabilities* for response activation within a given context in a manner that tends to align an individual's experience and expression of emotion with those cultural models. This leaves open the possibility that at times responses emerge that are incongruent with the prevailing cultural model. This mechanism applies to emotion components that are typically associated with the emotion-generation process, as well as conscious, effortful emotion regulation.

We now review evidence for the manifestation of cultural models of self and relating at the level of situation selection and modification, attentional deployment, appraisal, and behavior.

Situation Selection

One major path of emotion regulation has been coined "situation selection," described as "approaching or avoiding certain people, places, or objects in order to regulate emotions" (Gross, 1998, p. 283). Given that cultural realities, including the relative prevalence of different types of situations are shaped in ways that reflect and perpetuate cultural models of self and relating, these realities always represent an *a priori* selection of situations. It is thus in the first place, through their embodiment in the worlds as encountered, that cultural models regulate emotions. Furthermore, cultural models are reflected in motivational focus (e.g., approach vs. avoidance) at the level of the individual, thus shaping individual selection of situations. We provide examples of situation regulation that have in common that they serve particular models of self and relating and at the same time affect the ensuing emotions.

Sociocultural Situation Selection

Culture-level situation selection can promote or inhibit the occurrence of certain emotions. As referred to before, many American situations serve to make individuals feel special and unique and promote happiness and feeling good about the independent self (D'Andrade, 1984). Contemporary American schools seem to be geared toward promoting the happiness of their students. "Show-and-tell" practices as early as preschool make the individual child feel important and special, and thus promote happiness, and so do the many smiley faces, stickers, and gift-box rewards for every achievement, however small. In his most recent book, psychologist Richard Nisbett (2003) describes how the school board in his hometown even "debated whether the chief goal of the schools should be to impart knowledge or inculcate self-esteem" (p. 55). Similarly, American advertisements emphasize the uniqueness of each individual, the right of choice and freedom (Kim & Markus, 1999). We speculated at the beginning of this chapter that engagement in those practices promotes and sustains happiness and that emotion is indeed frequent in American contexts (Diener & Suh, 1999; Diener & Tov, in press).

In contrast, Japanese models tend to construe individuals-in-relationship and emphasize the continuing obligation to accommodate others, fulfill one's roles, and perfect one's contributions in order to approach others' expectations or cultural ideals in general (Heine et al., 1999). Many of the practices that constitute Japanese models of self and relating may be thought to promote anticipatory fear or shame. An example is the Japanese practice of *hansei* (self-reflection or self-criticism). *Hansei* involves focusing on one's shortcomings and on possible improvements in the future. *Hansei* is institutionalized at elementary schools (Karasawa, 2001; Lewis, 1995a), where children at the end of each day are encouraged to search for their inadequacies and weaknesses so that they can look for ways to improve those in order to meet the group's standards. The constant awareness of one's shortcomings is conducive to the experience of emotions such as anticipated fear and shame. In support of this idea, shame has been described as an emotion prevalent in the Japanese context (Benedict, 1946; Doi, 1973; Heine et al., 1999), and it is more frequently reported by Japanese than by North Americans (Mesquita et al., 2006).

Cultural models of self and relating also shape the quality and dynamics of daily interactions between people, thus affording opportunities for model-consistent emotion experiences. A number of comparative studies have suggested that North American and East Asian social interactions differ substantially, creating the contexts for divergent emotions. As before, North American practices facilitate and promote a relatively high frequency of happiness and pride, whereas East Asian practices engender greater degrees of wariness and shame. For instance, in a comparison of situations in North American and Japanese contexts, Kitayama et al. (1997) found relatively more North American situations that afforded self-enhancement and relatively more Japanese situations that afforded self-criticism. Thus, comparative results suggest that in conversations, Japanese have more *reason* to feel ashamed and that Americans have more *reason* to feel happy.

Cultural differences in the regulation of emotion situations can be clearly seen in early childrearing practices as well. Several studies suggest that Japanese mothers structure their children's environment in a way that encourages relative stability and moderation of emotion, whereas American mothers provide for greater situational variability, thus increasing the probability that the child will experience a range of both positive and negative emotions (Rothbaum et al., 2000). Japanese mothers lull and comfort their infants more by soothing, relationship-focused vocalizations and by maintaining close proximity to their children. In doing so, it seems that Japanese mothers' behaviors create a safe and stable environment, thus decreasing the probability of the child experiencing strong negative emotions (Rothbaum et al., 2000). On the other hand, American mothers' speech appears to orient their children more toward objects in the environment, and American mothers allow their children more exploratory activity and use more distal proximity strategies (e.g., eye contact) than do Japanese mothers (Rothbaum et al., 2000). The opportunity for exploration may render the environment a place of more excitement and positive emotions but also one with greater potential for negative emotions.

In sum, culture regulates emotion situations by shaping the quality and dynamics of specific practices and patterns of social interaction in a manner that affords emotion experiences and expressions that are consistent with the prevalent cultural models of self and relating. This is well illustrated by the comparison between North American and East Asian cultures. Whereas the experience and expression of emotions— particularly positive ones—are important markers of the independent self in North American cultural models (Lutz, 1987), in East Asian models strong emotions are seen to distract from one's ability to fulfill role obligations and thus to preserve relational harmony, a primary cultural ideal (Suh, Diener, Oishi, & Triandis, 1998). Thus, emotion moderation in general, and the practice of emotions oriented to self-improvement in particular, is the ideal and actual pattern of emotions in these East Asian cultures (Kitayama & Markus, 2000), and East Asian environments appear maximally suited to produce this pattern. Developmental research provides a close look at how cultural models are embodied in the ways that parents structure children's physical and interpersonal environments, thus providing the parameters for children's emotion experience. Furthermore, the limited adult literature suggests that cultural meanings and practices shape human environments (occupational settings, mass entertainments, religious institutions, etc.) throughout the lifespan in ways that have important implications for emotion experience. More comparative research is needed to understand the ways in which the different structures of social environments differentially shape emotions.

Situation Selection at the Level of the Individual

There is some evidence that different cultural models not only structure the social environment in distinct ways but also affect the relative motivational focus of individuals on either avoiding negative or approaching positive situations (e.g., Elliott, Chirkov, Kim, & Sheldon, 2001; Lee, Aaker, & Gardner, 2000). Whereas the dominant focus in American contexts appears to be on the *accomplishment* of positive outcomes, East Asians and Russians have been found to be more concerned with *avoiding* failures to meet social expectations. Importantly, this internalization of cultural goals functions in parallel with the cultural structuring of environments to support models of self and relating.

The relative focus of a cultural model on either approach or avoidance may have implications for the patterns of emotion experienced by individuals engaging the model. Higgins, Shah, and Friedman (1997) found evidence that a prevention focus fosters relaxation or relief when the goals are achieved and anxiety when the goals are not reached. On the other hand, these authors found that a promotion focus affords feelings of happiness when the goals are achieved and feelings of sadness when the goals are not met.

In a cross-cultural vignette study on success and failure, Lee et al. (2000) found that the American group, consistent with what should be hypothesized on the basis of their cultural focus on promotion, reported a higher intensity of happiness/depressed emotions than relief/anxiety emotions. Conversely, a Chinese group, consistent with their focus on prevention, reported a higher intensity of relief/anxiety than happiness/depressed emotions. This is some first evidence that the differences in situation selection at the level of approach or avoidance are related to differences in the prevalent types of emotions.

In sum, cultural models of self and relating motivate the selection of situations, which itself can be seen as a form of emotion regulation. Situation selection can take place at the sociocultural or the individual level, but in both cases it renders certain emotions more and others less likely to occur.

Situation Modification and Attentional Deployment

Sociocultural forces may also be instrumental in what have been called *situation modification* and *attentional deployment* (Gross, 1998; Gross & Thompson, this volume). Social practices often are geared toward aligning situations with cultural models of self and relating. First, they do so by motivating individuals to modify their own situations and redeploy their own attention in ways that support the achievement of culturally sanctioned goals. Thus, at the individual level, we assume that the fine-tuning of situations and one's focus of attention within them function via the same basic mechanisms that operate for individual-level situation selection. For instance, it is reasonable to expect that the cultural differences in approach and avoidance motivation that were described earlier would extend beyond the selection of situations to their modification, and to the types of environmental cues to which one's attention is habitually drawn (or from which one's attention is habitually averted). More generally, we argue that cultural models of self and relating function as the maps by which individuals navigate the social world, and thus as an important reference point for individual situation selection and attentional deployment.

There is evidence suggesting that independent and interdependent cultural contexts may motivate individuals to deploy attention to relatively different types of social information when making emotion judgments. In a recent comparative study, Japanese and Americans were presented with cartoon stimuli depicting a central person who expressed anger, sadness, or happiness, surrounded by four other people whose facial expressions varied independently from the central person (Masuda, Ellsworth, Mesquita, Leu, & Veerdonk, 2005). Respondents were asked to rate the central person's emotions. Consistent with an independent model, Americans in this study judged the central person's emotions by expression alone, disregarding the emotions of the surrounding people. Consistent with an interdependent model, however, the Japanese *did* consider the emotions of the other people in the picture. Thus, when assessing the central person's emotions, Japanese were affected by the emotional expressions of others in the situation, not just by the expression of the central person. For example, Japanese gave higher anger ratings to an angry central person if the other people in the situation were angry as well, relative to situations in which the other people were not angry. Furthermore, an eye-tracking procedure confirmed that Japanese participants scanned the periphery of the images, which contained the other characters, to a greater degree than did the Americans. It seems plausible that in Japanese contexts, attention is directed toward all of the participants in a social situation, and that this practice supports interdependent goals.

In addition, other people in the environment support the alignment of one's emotion experience with cultural models by adjusting the situation and funneling attention for the individual. Caregiver–child interactions that center on emotions are an obvious example. Caregivers often either change the situation or shift the child's attention to make the child's emotions consistent with cultural models. As the cultural models differ, caretaker attempts to regulate emotion differ as well.

The different strategies by which caretakers may regulate a child's course of emotion is illustrated by a study comparing two groups of Nepali mothers, Tamang and Chhetri-Brahmin (Cole & Tamang, 1998). The mothers were asked what they would do if their 4- or 5-year-old child was angry at them. The majority of Tamang mothers, whose Buddhist models centered on social harmony by way of egalitarianism, compassion, and tolerance, reported that they would give the children food and cajole them in order to make them happy. This strategy could be described as both situation modification and attentional deployment. On the other hand, the majority of Chhetri-Brahmin mothers, whose Hindu cultural models taught them the value of spiritual purity, social order, and disciplined action, reported they would tell their child to behave, to study, and to go to school. The Chhetri-Brahmin mothers tended not to change the situation but, rather, tried to change their children's behavior, in part by telling them to concentrate on more important matters like school; their regulation strategy thus relied on attentional deployment and possibly behavioral suppression.

Much infant/child research has demonstrated the importance of caregiver efforts in regulating children's emotions (for a review, see Diamond & Aspinwall, 2003). As we have argued in this chapter, the goals that guide caregivers' regulation strategies are importantly informed by cultural models of self and relating, and this is nicely illustrated by the aforementioned Nepali example. However, emotion regulation by others does not cease in childhood or adolescence; even after children mature enough to internalize effective emotion regulation strategies of their own, significant social partners continue to contribute regulatory efforts across the lifespan. This can be observed through such adult interpersonal practices as the provision of comfort and support, the expression of empathy, the redirection of attention, or suggestions for cognitive reframing of emotionally salient information (Diamond & Aspinwall, 2003). Furthermore, the level of regulatory activity exhibited by others in one's environment is likely related to the prevalent cultural models of self and relating. For example, research with Turkish and Surinamese immigrants in the Netherlands showed a greater degree of "social sharing" of emotions by these interdependent groups, relative to independent Dutch participants (Mesquita, 2001). Interdependent groups solicited more problem-solving commitment related to emotion events from relational partners, and in turn, they perceived greater concern and commitment from those partners. In sum, an individual's social environment tends to be instrumental in changing one's emotional context, as well as refocusing one's attention in ways that make the emotion more consistent with cultural models of self and relating.

Appraisal Regulation

The way people appraise a situation importantly constitutes the emotional experience (Mesquita & Ellsworth, 2001). Appraisal always takes place in the context of cultural models of self and relating. That is, people make sense of emotional situations with reference to the cultural meanings and practices of being a (good) person and having (appropriate) relationships. Appraisal *is* meaning making, and meaning making is always cultural. Therefore, the emotional meaning of an event must be a cultural meaning. However, this does not mean that initial appraisals are always the most rewarding ones in a particular situation. If the initial interpretation of an event is not congruent with one's (culturally informed) goals, this may be a reason for subsequent reappraisal (Gross, 1998; Mesquita & Frijda, 1992). Rather than viewing initial appraisal and cognitive change as fundamentally distinct processes, we propose that both are subject to the same forces. Both take into account what the modal and normative ways of being a person in the world are. We discuss here the instantiation of cultural models in appraisals as well as the mechanisms for "correcting" appraisals that are "out of line" in a given situation.

One obvious way in which cultural models of self and relating constitute appraisals is by providing the schemas against which a given situation is appraised. Thus, when the world is felt to be a predictable place, the same event may be interpreted differently than when the world is considered unpredictable and fate is held as the determining force. In trying to explain the near absence of frustration and anger among Tahitians (relative to North Americans), the anthropologist Robert Levy points to "a shared common sense that individuals have very limited control over nature and over the behavior of others; [and] that . . . if one does not strive and force things, reality will inevitably take care of the individual" (Levy, 1978, p. 226). Thus, as Levy notes, a universe so defined is "*cognitively* less frustrating than those cultures which define realities in which almost anything is possible to individuals" (p. 226). The general expectation that the world is minimally rewarding, and that there is no way to force rewards, leads to a lower prevalence of anger.

The Tahitian perspective on life contrasts with middle-class American models that place an emphasis and value on control and predictability (Mesquita & Ellsworth, 2001). In middle-class American contexts, a view of the world as malleable prevails. Primary control tends to be a dominant response, reflecting the assumption that circumstances can be made to fit one's personal goals (Morling, Kitayama, & Miyamoto, 2002; Weisz, Rothbaum, & Blackburn, 1984). Paradoxically, when there is a sense of control, this may render events that are inconsistent with one's goals more frustrating (Frijda, 1986). Hence, there is a relative emphasis on agency in Western appraisals of antecedent situations (Smith & Ellsworth, 1985).

Cultural models thus provide the backdrop against which events are meaningful. A sense that the world is a predictable place—that is, a place in which agents make a difference (Markus & Kitayama, 2003)—not only makes any lack of agency more salient but also renders the experience more unpleasant. This is illustrated by a study by Roseman and colleagues in which Indian and American college students reported instances of anger, sadness, and fear and rated their experiences on several appraisal dimensions (Roseman, Dhawan, Rettek, & Naidu, 1995). Cultural models for Indian college students are less likely to make salient the possibility of successful control of one's circumstances than are cultural models for American students (Miller, Bersoff, & Harwood, 1990). Consistent with this understanding, Indian college students rated self-reported emotional events to be less "incongruent with their motives" than did their American counterparts. As expected, Indian students also reported lower overall intensities of both sadness and anger, and, moreover, these cultural differences in emotion intensity were fully mediated by the perception that the event was less discrepant with goals. Although the link between the cultural emphasis on controllability and the perception of goal relevance was not measured, we suggest that cultural representations of agency—the extent to which individual control is emphasized—affected the perception of a discrepancy between emotional events and personal goals, and in turn influenced the intensity of felt sadness and anger.

Cultural models of self and relating also specify the source of meaning for events. This is an aspect of appraisal not usually attended to by appraisal theories, but it may have very important implications for how people perceive and act on situations, and how likely they are to change their appraisals once they have formed. It appears that whereas independent cultural models emphasize the subjective meaning of events, interdependent cultural models tend to situate meaning making in the social situation more than in the individual.

One example of perceiving meaning as situation-based emerged from a study comparing emotion reports in different cultural contexts within the Netherlands. In this study, the interdependent Surinamese and Turkish immigrants considered their emotional experience more intersubjectively true—or "obvious"—than did the independent Dutch respondents (Mesquita, 2001). Turkish and Surinamese respondents assumed to a larger extent than Dutch respondents that another person in their position would have had similar feelings and thoughts about the situation and would have acted in a way similar to them as well. Thus, whereas the meaning of emotional events in the Dutch group was considered subjective and open to different appraisals ("I did not like that behavior"), emotional events in the interdependent groups were seen as providing information about the world and thus leaving less room for interindividual variation in appraisal ("one cannot take a relationship with that person seriously"). It seems likely that such "obviousness" reduces the susceptibility of an appraisal to cognitive change.

Furthermore, there are several studies showing that in more interdependent cultural models, the meaning of events can be tied to other people's feelings. In this case, too, the meanings are located outside the individual self. In a comparison of American and Japanese respondents from both university student and community samples, Mesquita et al. (2006) found that Japanese respondents reported more appraisals that reflected an awareness of the meaning of the situation for the other person in a relational dyad, as well as the meaning of the situation for a generalized other. This study consisted of standardized interviews that asked respondents to relate experiences that fit with certain stimulus situations, such as a situation of offense. Respondents reported a situation from their past, and their emotion narratives were recorded and later coded. The narratives suggested that, in the negative situations in particular, Japanese considered the meaning of the events for other people. For example, more than 40% of the Japanese, versus none of the Americans, explained an offense situation from the perspective of a third person or a generalized other, an appraisal that can be seen to reflect an outside-in perspective. In addition, in the offense situation, 56% of the Japanese compared to only 5% of the Americans tried to understand or sympathize with the offender. These outside-in appraisals, like sympathizing and taking the perspective of another person, also appeared to have behavioral consequences. For example 60% of the Japanese reported doing nothing in the offense situation.

We have argued that cultural models appear to differ with regard to their perspective on the source of situational meaning—the ideas about where meaning comes from. Interdependent cultural models emphasize the perspective of others. Paradoxically, this may have two diametrically opposed effects. On the one hand, an individual assuming that meanings are subject to social consensus may feel that his or her appraisal of the situation is obvious, and that appraisals are thus not subject to regulation. On the other hand, interdependent cultural models may suggest that the individual's perspective should be broadened to include the meaning of the situation to others. In the latter case, a difference in perspective between self and others is assumed. Taking the perspective of another person or a generalized other may open an individual's appraisal to regulation. Accordingly, evidence suggests that emotional experience is more influenced by one's immediate relational context in interdependent than independent cultures (Oishi, Diener, Scollon, & Biswas-Diener, 2004).

In sum, cultural models of self and relating are seen to function as both a schematic backdrop against which meaning is created and a set of practices that specify the source of emotional meaning in the person–environment interaction.

Cultural Regulation of Behavior

Cultural models appear to regulate action readiness (i.e., behavioral goals) and actual behavior as well. First, the models provide normative and descriptive representations of self and others as well as schemas and goals for relationships and thus afford certain goals of behavior. Furthermore, cultural models define the effective and desirable cultural practices for a given context and thus shape the particular behavioral means that are chosen to fulfill those aims.

Action Readiness

Cultural differences in reported action readiness have been shown to reflect the models of self and relating that are prevalent in a context. A study by Frijda, Markam, Sato, and Wiers (1995) provided evidence for the differential importance of general themes of action readiness for independent and interdependent cultural groups, and the consistency of these differences with the groups' respective models of self and relating. In this study, Dutch, Indonesian and Japanese participants were asked to recall instances of given emotions, and rate these emotions on 36 standardized action-readiness items. Separate factor analyses by culture suggested five universal action-readiness factors: moving away, moving toward, moving against, want help, and submission. However, the relative importance of themes of action readiness differed across cultures, and the cultural models of the three groups offer plausible explanations for these variations.

Moving away and *moving against* were more important for distinguishing between emotions in the Dutch group than they were for either of the other groups. The Dutch cultural model of seeking independence, if necessary through opposition (as a way of expressing oneself [Stephenson, 1989; Van Der Horst, 1996]), may explain the significance of these action-readiness modes for Dutch emotion experience. On the other hand, *moving toward* and *submission* explained more emotion variance in the Indonesian and Japanese groups than in the Dutch. This fits with our understanding of the models of these two Asian cultures, which appear to be centrally concerned with promoting goals of relational harmony (Markus et al., 1997), either by reducing social distance (moving toward) or by fitting in and making oneself acceptable to the other person (submission). Thus, the action-readiness responses (or behavioral goals) in each cultural context fit their respective models of self and relating.

Likewise, there is evidence that in comparable situations, or following comparable emotional experiences, behavioral goals may culturally vary in ways that can be understood from the prevalent models of self and relating. For example, there is indication that the behavioral goals of shame differ across cultures (Bagozzi, Verbeke, & Gavino, 2003; Mesquita & Karasawa, 2004). Whereas shame in independent Western contexts is associated with an appraisal that the event is incongruent with one's identity goals, and that it is caused by one's own stable characteristics (Tracy & Robins, 2004), shame in interdependent East Asian cultures appears related to the assessment that an event is incongruent with *relationship goals*—one's obligations to others, to one's parents, to the nation, etc.—and that it brings dishonor on the groups to which one belongs. The answers to East Asian shame are self-improvement and the public sharing of shame, both ways to reassert oneself as a member of one's social group. These behavioral goals are completely different from the common Western response, wanting to disappear, which may be understood as an appropriate response to ultimate, unchangeable failure (cf. Bagozzi et al., 2003). Thus, behavioral goals vary along with the appraisals of situations that are implicated by different cultural models of self and relating.

Behavioral Means

There is also evidence for cultural differences in the specific behavioral *means* that are used to realize behavioral goals. First, cultural models of self and relating may be understood to regulate behavioral means by setting the parameters of acceptable (or preferred) behavior. Ethnographic work suggests, for example, that culture-specific behaviors sometimes are chosen to serve emotional goals without being disruptive of prevalent cultural models (Mesquita & Frijda, 1992). This is illustrated by the Balinese reaction to frightening events—falling asleep—which can be understood as a culture-specific means of achieving the dominant behavioral goal of avoidance (Bateson & Mead, 1942). Falling asleep satisfies, at least subjectively, the goal of reducing one's exposure to threat while avoiding the emotional disruption that other fear responses are felt to cause. Therefore, falling asleep can be considered a culturally effective means to accomplish the goal of avoidance (or "moving away").

Cultural models may also specify the preferred contexts and practices for behavioral expression, as is the case for rituals. "Rituals consist of prescribed behavior modes that remove the need to expose one's individual feelings. Yet at the same time, they form opportunities to vent one's emotions in a socially acceptable way" (Mesquita & Frijda, 1992, p. 197). A good example of a ritual that appears to provide an institutionalized means for expressing emotional behaviors that would otherwise conflict with the prevailing cultural model was described for the Philippine Ilongots by the anthropologist Michelle Rosaldo. In this small community, ingroup harmony was essential for survival of the group. Ilongots, therefore, saw it as a communal responsibility to regulate emotions that could threaten the harmony of the group. Liget—an emotion denoting energy, passion, and anger simultaneously—was one of those threatening emotions (Rosaldo, 1980). A ritual of headhunting was in place, should feelings of liget arise. When one or more Ilongot men experienced the heavy feeling of liget, a group of them would go out to kill an outsider. After the beheading, the Ilongot men came home purged of violence, and the community celebrated the overcoming of liget by singing together. The ritual thus directed the behavioral intentions elicited by liget toward an outgroup target, channeling a potentially intraculturally disruptive behavior into one that reinforced the solidarity of the group. Rituals may be understood as prototypes for the mechanisms by which sociocultural practices afford opportunities to express (or act on) emotions in culturally supported ways.

In sum, cultural models not only specify the relational goals of emotions but also determine the meaning, and therefore the appropriateness and effectiveness, of certain behaviors in specific contexts. Finally, cultures may create specific contexts and means for emotional behavior, often in prescribed and culturally modeled ways.

CONCLUSION

There is substantial evidence for the cultural regulation of emotions, conceived here as the sum of cultural mechanisms that function to bring individual and group emotional experience in line with models of self and relating. Cultural models of self and relating are reflected in the creation and modification of events, the deployment of attention, the culturally provided meanings of the situation, the encouraged perspective on appraisal, and the behavioral goals and means for emotion. There is thus "redundancy" in the cultural regulation of emotions (Levy, 1978), such that cultural models shape emotions into congruence at many different loci as well as in many different ways. Thus, we suggest that although conscious, effortful regulation is one of the ways in which emotions are brought into alignment with cultural models of self and relating, it is not the only one. In fact, we would go further to propose that cultural regulation is most likely to target automatic response selection, given that voluntary processes require cognitive resources. Allowing ourselves an anthropomorphic perspective on culture for a sentence, one could say that effortful emotion regulation is "culture's" last resort for shaping emotions in a culturally normative fashion, only to be used when all other ways failed.

One of the main contributions of a cultural perspective to the literature on emotion regulation is to show that emotion regulation is not merely an intrapersonal process. Rather, emotions are importantly regulated by the ways in which our worlds are structured and our lives are organized. Thus, we have suggested that cultural regulation takes place both at the structural level of cultural practices and at the level of culturally primed psychological tendencies. We have illustrated how emotion is regulated at the level of cultural practices through the structuring of social situations and the dynamics of social interactions; close others' attempts to modify situations themselves, one's focus of attention within situations, or the meaning that is derived from them; and the opportunities afforded for emotional behavior. Cultural regulation at the level of individual psychological tendencies is also evident, exemplified by cultural differences in motivational orientations either to seek out or to avoid certain situations; the prevalent perspective applied to situations and the meanings that are salient within them; and the behavioral tendencies that are associated with given emotions. Cultural practices and psychological tendencies coconstitute emotional experiences and expressions that are aligned with prevailing cultural models of self and relating.

More important, a cultural focus on emotion regulation contributes to the literature a focus on the *content* of the endpoints of regulation. It is generally assumed that emotion regulation serves an individual's social adjustment. For example, Gross and colleagues noted that "we frequently experience strong emotions that need to be managed if we are to keep our appointments, careers, and friendships" (Gross, Richards, & John, in press, p. 2). Clearly, then, emotion regulation is motivated by the need to maintain relationships with others, to present ourselves properly, and perhaps—as we have suggested previously—to live up to our self-ideals and goals. However, knowing that emotion regulation serves relational goals does nothing to explicate the exact nature of the regulation. In this chapter, we have proposed that the expectations, definitions, goals, and practices for self and relationships are importantly contextualized by the sociocultural contexts in which we live—the cultural models of self and relating.

REFERENCES

Bagozzi, R. P., Verbeke, W., & Gavino, J. C. (2003). Culture moderates the self-regulation of shame and its effects on performance: The case of salespersons in the Netherlands and the Philippines. *Journal of Applied Psychology, 88*(2), 219–233.

Barrett, L. F. (in press-a). Are emotions natural kinds? *Perspectives on Psychological Science.*

Barrett, L. F. (in press-b). The experience of emotion: A social psychological model. *Personality and Social Psychology Bulletin.*

Bateson, G., & Mead, M. (1942). Balinese character. In *Special Publications: New York Academy of Sciences* (pp. 1–47). New York: New York Academy of Sciences.

Benedict, R. (1946). The chrysanthemum and the sword. Patterns of Japanese culture. Boston: Houghton Mifflin.

Bruner, J. (1986). *Actual minds, possible worlds.* New York: Plenum Press.

Bruner, J. (1990). *Acts of meaning.* Cambridge, MA: Harvard University Press.

Campos, J. J., Frankel, C. B., & Camras, L. (2004). On the nature of emotion regulation. *Child Development, 75*(2), 377–394.

Cole, P. M., & Tamang, B. L. (1998). Nepali children's ideas about emotional displays in hypothetical challenges. *Developmental Psychology, 34*, 640–646.

D'Andrade, R. G. (1984). Culture meaning systems. In R. A. Shweder & R. A. Levine (Eds.), *Culture theory: Essays on mind, self, and emotion* (pp. 88–119). Cambridge, UK: Cambridge University Press.

D'Andrade, R. G., & Strauss, C. (1992). *Human motives and cultural models.* Cambridge, UK: Cambridge University Press.

Diamond, L. M., & Aspinwall, L. G. (2003). Emotion regulation across the life span: An integrative perspective emphasizing self-regulation, positive affect, and dyadic processes. *Motivation and Emotion, 27*, 125–156.

Diener, E., & Suh, E. (1999). National differences in subjective well-being. In E. Diener & D. Kahneman (Eds.), *Well-being: The foundations of hedonic psychology* (pp. 434–450). New York: Russell Sage.

Diener, E., & Tov, W. (in press). Culture and subjective well-being. In S. Kitayama & D. Cohen (Eds.), *Handbook of cultural psychology*. New York: Guilford Press.

Doi, L. T. (1973). *The autonomy of dependence*. Tokyo, Japan: Kodansha.

Edwards, P. (1996). Honor, shame and humiliation in modern Japan. In O. Leaman (Ed.), *Friendship East and West philosophical perspectives* (pp. 34–155). London: Curzon.

Ekman, P. (1992). An argument for basic emotions. *Cognition and Emotion, 6*(3/4), 169–200.

Elliott, A., Chirkov, V., Kim, Y., & Sheldon, K. (2001). A cross-cultural analysis of avoidance (relative to approach) personal goals. *Psychological Science, 12*, 505–510.

Frijda, N. H. (1986). *The emotions*. Cambridge, UK: Cambridge University Press.

Frijda, N. H., Markam, S., Sato, K., & Wiers, R. (1995). Emotion and emotion words. In J. A. Russell, J. Fernández-Dols, A. S. R. Manstead, & J. C. Wellenkamp (Eds.), *Everyday conceptions of emotion: An introduction to the psychology, anthropology, and linguistics of emotion* (pp. 121–143). New York: Kluwer Academic/Plenum.

Gross, J. J. (1998). The emerging field of emotion regulation: an integrative review. *Review of General Psychology, 2*, 271–299.

Gross, J. J., Richards, J. M., & John, A. P. (in press). Emotion regulation in everyday life. In D. K. Snyder, J. A. Simpson, & J. N. Hughes (Eds.), *Emotion regulation in families: Pathways to dysfunction and health*. Washington DC: American Psychological Association.

Gross, J. J., & Thompson, R. A. (2007). Emotion regulation: Conceptual foundations. In J. J. Gross (Ed.), *Handbook of emotion regulation* (pp. 3–24). New York: Guilford Press.

Heine, S. J., Kitayama, S., Lehman, D. R., Takata, T., Ide, E., Leung, K., et al. (2001). Divergent consequences of success and failure in Japan and North America: An investigation of self-improving motivations and malleable selves. *Journal of Personality and Social Psychology, 81*(4), 599–615.

Heine, S. J., Lehman, D. R., Markus, H. R., & Kitayama, S. (1999). Is there a universal need for positive self-regard. *Psychological Review, 106*(4), 766–794.

Higgins, E., Shah, J., & Friedman, R. J. (1997). Emotional responses to goal attainment: Strength of regulatory focus as a moderator. *Journal of Personality and Social Psychology, 72*, 515–525.

Hochschild, J. L. (1995). What is the American dream? In J. L. Hochschild (Ed.), *Facing up to the American dream: Race, class and the soul of the nation* (pp. 15–38). Princeton: Princeton University Press.

Holland, D., Lachicotte, W., Jr., Skinner, D., & Cain, C. (1998). *Identity and agency in cultural worlds*. Cambridge, MA: Harvard University Press.

Holland, D., & Quinn, N. (1987). *Cultural models in language and thought*. Cambridge, UK: Cambridge University Press.

Izard, C. E. (1994). Innate and universal facial expressions: Evidence from developmental and cross-cultural research. *Psychological Bulletin, 115*, 288–299.

Johnson-Laird, P. N., & Oatley, K. (1992). Basic emotions, rationality and folk theory. *Cognition and Emotion, 6*(3/4), 201–223.

Kanagawa, C., Cross, S. E., & Markus, H. R. (2001). "Who am I?" The cultural psychology of the conceptual self. *Personality and Social Psychology Bulletin, 27*(1), 90–103.

Karasawa, M. (2001). Nihonnjinnni okeru jitano ninnshiki: Jikohihan baiasuto tasyakouyou baiasu [A Japanese mode of self-making: Self criticism and other enhancement]. *Japanese Journal of Psychology, 72*(4), 198–209.

Kim, H., & Markus, H. R. (1999). Deviance or uniqueness, harmony or conformity? A cultural analysis. *Journal of Personality and Social Psychology, 77*(4), 785–800.

Kitayama, S., & Markus, H. R. (2000). The pursuit of happiness and the realization of sympathy: Cultural patterns of self, social relations, and well-being. In E. Diener & E. Suh (Eds.), *Subjective well-being across cultures* (pp. 113–161). Cambridge, MA: MIT Press.

Kitayama, S., Matsumoto, D., Markus, H. R., & Norasakkunkit, V. (1997). Individual and collective processes in the construction of the self: Self-enhancement in the US and self-criticism in Japan. *Journal of Personality and Social Psychology, 72*(6), 1245–1267.

Kondo, D. (1990). *Crafting selves: Power, gender, and discourses of identity in a Japanese workplace*. Chicago: University of Chicago Press.

Lang, A. (1988). What are the data of emotion? In V. Hamilton, G. H. Bower, & N. H. Frijda (Eds.), *Cognitive perspectives on emotion and motivation* (Vol. 44, pp. 173–191). Dordrecht, The Netherlands: Kluwer.

Lebra, T. S. (1992). Self in Japanese culture. In N. E. Rosenberger (Ed.), *Japanese sense of self*. New York: Oxford University Press.

Lebra, T. S. (1994). Mother and child in Japanese socialization: A Japan–US comparison. In P. M. Greenfield & R. R. Cocking (Eds.), *Cross-cultural roots of minority child development* (pp. 259–274). Hillsdale: Erlbaum.

Lee, A. Y., Aaker, J. L., & Gardner, W. L. (2000). The pleasures and pains of distinct self-construals: The role of interdependence in regulatory focus. *Journal of Personality and Social Psychology, 78*(6), 1122–1134.

Levy, R. I. (1978). Tahitian gentleness and redundant controls. In A. Montagu (Ed.), *Learning non-aggression: The experience of non-literate societies* (pp. 222–235). New York: Oxford University Press.

Lewis, C. C. (1995a). *Educating hearts and minds*. New York: Cambridge Press.

Lewis, C. C. (1995b). The roots of discipline: Community and commitment. In C. C. Lewis (Ed.), *Educating hearts and minds* (pp. 101–123). New York: Cambridge University Press.

Lutz, C. (1987). Goals, events, and understanding in Ifaluk emotion theory. In N. Quinn & D. Holland (Eds.), *Cultural models in language and thought*. New York: Cambridge University Press.

Markus, H. R., & Kitayama, S. (1991). Culture and self: Implications for cognition, emotion, and motivation. *Psychological Review, 98*(2), 224–253.

Markus, H. R., & Kitayama, S. (1994). The cultural construction of self and emotion: Implications for social behavior. In S. Kitayama & H. R. Markus (Eds.), *Emotion and culture: Empirical studies of mutual influence* (pp. 89–130). Washington, DC: American Psychological Association.

Markus, H. R., & Kitayama, S. (2003). Models of agency: Sociocultural diversity in the construction of action. In J. J. Berman & V. Murphy-Berman (Eds.), *Cross-cultural differences in perspectives on the self* (Vol. 49, pp. 18–74). Lincoln: University of Nebraska Press.

Markus, H. R., Mullally, P. R., & Kitayama, S. (1997). Selfways: Diversity in modes of cultural participation. In U. Neisser & D. A. Jopling (Eds.), *The conceptual self in context: Culture, experience, self-understanding* (pp. 13–61). New York: Cambridge University Press.

Masuda, T., Ellsworth, P. C., Mesquita, B., Leu, J., & Veerdonk, E. (2005). *Putting the face in context: Cultural differences in the perception of emotions from facial behavior*. Unpublished manuscript, University of Michigan, Ann Arbor, MI.

Mesquita, B. (2001). Emotions in collectivist and individualist contexts. *Journal of Personality and Social Psychology, 80*(1), 68–74.

Mesquita, B. (2003). Emotions as dynamic cultural phenomena. In R. Davidson, H. Goldsmith & K. R. Scherer (Eds.), *The handbook of the affective sciences* (pp. 871–890). New York: Oxford University Press.

Mesquita, B., & Ellsworth, P. C. (2001). The role of culture in appraisal. In K. R. Scherer & A. Schorr (Eds.), *Appraisal processes in emotion: Theory, methods, research.* (pp. 233–248). New York: Oxford University Press.

Mesquita, B., & Frijda, N. H. (1992). Cultural variations in emotions: A review. *Psychological Bulletin, 112*(2), 179–204.

Mesquita, B., & Karasawa, M. (2004). Self-conscious emotions as dynamic cultural processes. *Psychological Inquiry, 15*, 161–166.

Mesquita, B., Karasawa, M., Haire, A., Izumi, S., Hayashi, A., Idzelis, M., et al. (2006). *What do I feel?: The role of cultural models in emotion representations*. Unpublished manuscript, Wake Forest University, Winston-Salem, NC.

Mesquita, B., & Markus, H. R. (2004). Culture and emotion: Models of agency as sources of cultural variation in emotion. In N. H. Frijda, A. S. R. Manstead, & A. H. Fischer (Eds.), *Feelings and emotions: The Amsterdam symposium* (pp. 341–358). Cambridge, MA: Cambridge University Press.

Miller, J. G., Bersoff, D. M., & Harwood, R. L. (1990). Perceptions of social responsibilities in India and the United States: Moral imperatives on personal decisions? *Journal of Personality and Social Psychology, 58*, 33–47.

Morling, B., Kitayama, S., & Miyamoto, Y. (2002). Cultural practices emphasize influence in the United States and adjustment in Japan. *Personality and Social Psychology Bulletin, 28*(3), 311–323.

Nisbett, R. E. (2003). *The geography of thought. How Asians and Westerners think differently . . . and why*. New York: Free Press.

Oatley, K. (1992). *Best laid schemes: The psychology of emotions*. New York: Cambridge University Press.

Oatley, K., & Johnson-Laird, P. N. (1987). Towards a cognitive theory of emotions. *Cognition and Emotion, 1*(1), 29–50.

Oishi, S., & Diener, E. (2003). Goals, culture, and subjective well-being. *Personality and Social Psychology Bulletin, 29*(8), 939–949.

Oishi, S., Diener, E., Scollon, C. N., & Biswas-Diener, R. (2004). Cross-situational consistency of affective experiences across cultures. *Journal of Personality and Social Psychology, 86*, 460–472.

Rosaldo, M. Z. (1980). *Knowledge and passion: Ilongot notions of self and social life.* New York: Cambridge University Press.

Roseman, I., Dhawan, N., Rettek, S., & Naidu, R. K. (1995). Cultural differences and cross-cultural similarities in appraisals and emotional responses. *Journal of Cross Cultural Psychology, 26*(1), 23–48.

Rothbaum, F., Pott, M., Azuma, H., Miyake, K., & Weisz, J. (2000). The development of close relationships in Japan and the United States: Paths of symbiotic harmony and generative tension. *Child Development, 71*(5), 1121–1142.

Russell, J. A. (2003). Core affect and the psychological construction of emotion. *Psychological Review, 110*(1), 145–172.

Scherer, K. R. (1984). Emotion as a multicomponent process: A model and some cross-cultural data. In P. R. Shaver (Ed.), *Review of personality and social psychology* (Vol. 5, pp. 37–63). Beverly Hills, CA: Sage.

Shweder, R. A. (1991). *Thinking through cultures.* Cambridge, MA: Harvard University Press.

Shweder, R. A. (1999). Why cultural psychology? *Ethos, 27*(1), 62–73.

Shweder, R. A., & Haidt, J. (2000). The cultural psychology of emotions: Ancient and new. In M. Lewis & J. M. Haviland-Jones (Eds.), *Handbook of emotions* (2nd ed., pp. 397–414). New York: Guilford Press.

Smith, C. A., & Ellsworth, P. C. (1985). Patterns of cognitive appraisal in emotion. *Journal of Personality and Social Psychology, 48*, 813–838.

Stephenson, P. H. (1989). Going to McDonalds in Leiden: Reflections on the concept of self and society in the Netherlands. *Ethos, 17*, 226–247.

Strack, F., Schwarz, N., Bless, H., & Kuebler, A. (1993). Awareness of the influence as a determinant of assimilation versus contrast. *European Journal of Social Psychology, 23*(1), 53–62.

Suh, E., Diener, E., Oishi, S., & Triandis, H. C. (1998). The shifting basis of life satisfaction judgments across cultures: Emotion vs norms. *Journal of Personality and Social Psychology, 74*, 482–493.

Thompson, R. A. (1991). Emotional regulation and emotional development. *Educational Psychology Review, 3*, 269–307.

Tracy, J. L., & Robins, R. W. (2004). Putting the self into self-conscious emotions: A theoretical model. *Psychological Inquiry, 15*, 103–125.

Triandis, H. C. (1994). *Culture and social behavior.* New York: McGraw-Hill.

Triandis, H. C. (1995). *Individualism and collectivism.* Boulder, CO: Westview Press.

Tsai, J. L., Knutson, B., & Fung, H. H. (2006). Cultural variation in affect valuation. *Journal of Personality and Social Psychology, 90*, 288–307.

Van Der Horst, H. (1996). *The low sky: Understanding the Dutch.* Den Haag, The Netherlands: Scriptum Books.

Weisz, J. R., Rothbaum, F. M., & Blackburn, T. C. (1984). Standing out and standing in: The psychology of control in America and Japan. *American Psychologist, 39*(9), 955–969.

Wierzbicka, A. (1994). Emotion, language, and cultural scripts. In S. Kitayama & H. R. Markus (Eds.), *Emotion and culture: Empirical studies of mutual influence* (pp. 133–196). Washington, DC: American Psychological Association.

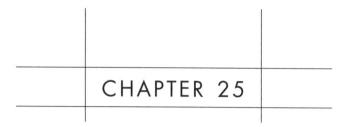

CHAPTER 25

Emotion Regulation and Religion

FRASER WATTS

In considering the role of religion in emotion regulation, it is important to note that both "emotion" and "religion" are terms whose meaning has changed considerably. The first section of the chapter considers changing concepts, first of religion and then of emotion. The central point is that the Christian tradition has a rich history of reflection on emotion that antedates "psychology," and which includes concepts that may have continuing value.

Subsequent sections deal with the contribution of different aspects of religion to emotion regulation, distinguishing particularly between religious belief and religious practice. The section on religious practice plays particular attention to the role of medi-tation in emotion regulation. In fact, there has been more concern about the regulation of specific emotions such as guilt anger than about emotion regulation in general and, to illustrate this, the second half of this chapter is devoted to more detailed discussion of these two emotions.

Academic literature on religion and emotion has not been a central aspect of the psychology of religion, though Corrigan, Crump, and Kloos (2000) have performed an invaluable service in collating a bibliography. Corrigan's own research on the interface of religion and emotion has been particularly important (Corrigan, 2002, 2004). Watts (1997) has discussed religion from the standpoint of emotion theory, and Emmons (2005) has recently provided a helpful overview of work on the interface of religion and emotion. Unfortunately, emotion regulation has not often been considered explicitly in the context of religion, though there are several relevant lines of theory and research on which it is possible to draw.

CHANGING CONCEPTS OF RELIGION AND EMOTION

"Religion" changed its meaning and significance considerably during the Enlightenment. For someone like Aquinas, religion was a relatively incidental matter, and meant something like "rule of life." However, the growing distinction between religious and secular areas of life has radically transformed what people mean by "religion." It is only now that there are many areas of life that exist outside the influence of religion that "religion" has come to refer to a rather specialized area of human functioning. Another key change is that Western Christianity (and perhaps more recently Western Buddhism) has become a collective cultural movement which people join or leave at will, often on the basis of an explicit decision. In contrast, to be a Hindu or a Jew is more a designation of cultural identity than it is a statement about what, in the West, we would now call religion. This chapter focuses predominantly on the Judeo-Christian tradition, which has been the main focus of study in the psychology of religion. Psychologists have studied Christianity more extensively than any other religion, and modern psychology has a richer dialogue with Christian theology than with any other tradition of religious thought. Nevertheless, reference is made to other religions where appropriate. For example, when considering the contribution of meditation to emotion regulation, Buddhism is considered as well as Christianity.

The concept of "emotion" came to prominence during the 19th century, as William Reddy (2001) and others have described. Of course, the term "emotion" had been used before, but it had not been the dominant way of conceptualizing what we now call emotion. The earlier terminology was explicitly embedded in moral and religious discourse in a way that contrasts markedly with how "emotion" was used by the end of the 19th century when it was introduced as an explicitly secular and scientific concept (Dixon, 2003). The earlier range of terms for what is now called emotion was in some ways much richer, and important conceptual distinctions were made between different terms. The simplification of terminology that took place when this rich vocabulary was replaced by a single undifferentiated category of emotion was in many ways regrettable, as there was much of value in the earlier distinctions.

The most important distinction was that between passions and affections, which were regarded as having different moral significance. Violent passions were a moral problem and required regulation. In contrast, the gentler and more cognitive "affections" were an important part of human moral functioning. Far from needing regulation, the affections contributed to the human capacity for self-regulation. If there is any validity to this distinction between passions and affections, it is highly relevant to the subject of emotion regulation. The terminology of "passions" and "affections" has probably been lost beyond retrieval, but some such distinction may need to be invented in other terms. For example, the distinction has been made between basic emotions that are not dependent on self-schemas and complex emotions that are, for example, Oatley (1992). That may have some overlap with the old distinction between passions and affections.

Revivalists such as Jonathan Edwards and Isaac Watts tried to steer a path between two extremes concerning emotion. On the one hand, like many others in the 18th century, they were concerned about how "ungoverned passions break all the bonds of human society and peace, and would change the tribes of mankind into brutal herds, or make the world a mere wilderness of savages" (Watts, 1746). On the other hand, they did not want a coldly intellectual approach to religion that neglected "homely sensations" such as hope, fear, love, and joy. The middle ground to which they aspired required a clear distinction between affections, which were an aid to religious understanding and devotion and more violent forms of emotion that were disruptive of it.

It is another important aspect of the earlier approach to what we would now call emotions that they were placed much more explicitly in a moral context. Emotions were a key aspect of what used to be called moral psychology. With the development of a more explicitly scientific approach to emotions in the latter part of the 19th century the sense of the moral context and significance of emotions was lost. However, there has recently been a revival of interest in the moral significance of emotions by philosophers such as Rom Harré (1983) and Justin Oakley (1992), and by psychologists such as Paul Rozin (Rozin, Lowery, Imada, & Haidt, 1999). There is now increasing recognition that assumptions about the moral order are an important part of the context within which emotions arise. For example, anger often arises when assumptions about proper behavior are breached. Emotions also play an important role in maintaining that moral order. For example, anger can help to maintain moral norms.

The earlier thinking about the emotions was less preoccupied than the present-day age with the distinction between positive and negative emotions. The central issue for people now is how to manage or overcome negative emotions and to achieve a state of positive emotional contentment (e.g., Baumeister, 2005). It is essentially a hedonistic approach to emotions that has as its central focus whether emotions are a source of pleasure or distress. That is foreign to the earlier moral and religious approach. At the risk of oversimplification, the question with which we are now concerned is how best to regulate the emotions and the contribution that religion can make to that goal. We are more concerned with the contribution that religion can make to emotion regulation and less concerned with the contribution of emotions to moral and religious life.

The key dichotomy within human experience for someone like Ignatius of Loyola, a Spanish mystic of the 16th century (1491–1556) was between consolations and desolations (Meissner, 1992). At first, this dichotomy might sound rather like the distinction between positive and negative experiences. However, Ignatius wanted to distinguish experiences that draw people closer to God (as consolations do) from experiences that separate them from him (as desolations do). The impact of the emotions on closeness to God was, for Ignatius, a much more central concern than whether or not the emotions were pleasurable. There is probably very little connection between the two criteria. So, for example, positive emotions would be no more likely to draw people closer to God than negative ones.

RELIGIOUS BELIEFS AND EMOTION REGULATION

Religion is a multifaceted phenomenon, and different aspects of religion make different contributions to emotion regulation. For example, Glock and Stark (1965) distinguished ritualistic, ideological, experiential, intellectual, and consequential aspects of religion. Several similar schemes have been proposed (Hood, Spilka, Hunsberger, & Gorsuch, 1996, Table 1.2). However, for the purpose of considering the implications of religion for emotion regulation, the most important distinction is probably that between religious belief and religious practice, and these are now considered in turn.

Religion provides an unusually comprehensive framework of meaning, which is central to its distinctive contribution to its emotion regulation. The religious framework can be used to make sense of a variety of events and circumstances that would normally be emotionally destabilizing. Reframing potentially stressful events is an important aspect of coping with emotional stress, and religion can play a key role in reframing.

A wide range of empirical studies have found that religion plays a significant role in helping people to cope with stress or to protect them against it. For example, McIntosh, Silver, and Wortman (1993) found that religious parents coped better with infant death and concluded that such better coping was mediated though social support, cognitive processes, and the ability to find meaning. As has been noted already, religion is multifaceted and can potentially contribute to how people cope with emotional stress in a great variety of ways. For example, the support of a religious community, the framework of meaning provided by religious beliefs, and the sense of the presence and support of God are all likely to play a part in emotion regulation, but in significantly different ways. Some aspects of religion will be more helpful in particular cases than others.

The percentage of people who use religious coping has been rather variable from study to study, as Pargament (1997) has pointed out. This variability is probably due to differences in the kind of people and stresses studied and the methodologies used by particular researchers. It seems that severe stress can push people to extremes in their view of religion as a way of coping. Some people who are not normally religious turn to religion under severe stress to help them cope. Other people, under severe stress, turn against religion though, as McIntosh et al. (1993) found in their study of coping with infant death, it is people whose religious beliefs were never strong who are most likely to abandon them under stress. Clearly, there are complex patterns here, and no simple relationship between religion and coping. However, the overall conclusions reached by Pargament from the research that he reviews are religion is used in coping more widely than is often supposed, and that it provides a relatively effective mode of coping.

Pargament makes an interesting and important distinction between whether stress leads people to preserve what is familiar in their religion or to transform it. Often there are elements of both, and it is not possible to maintain a sharp distinction between preservation and transformation modes of religious coping. So, for example, religious perseverance may be accompanied by a reframing of ideas about God, people, or events. Equally, conversion or deconversion under stress may also include elements of continuity with the person's religious past. So, Pargament's distinction between preservation and transformation is perhaps best taken as drawing attention to the way in which continuity and change are intertwined in religious coping, rather than as a distinction between two completely different forms of religious coping.

There has recently been developing interest in the impact of religious beliefs on attributions (e.g., Spilka, Hood, Hunsberger, & Gorsuch, 2003), which promises in turn to shed light on how religion may contribute to emotion regulation. Causal attributions play an important role in moderating the emotional impact of events. So, the religious practice of attributing events to God, in addition to the more usual internal or external attributions, seems likely to have considerable emotional significance. In general, broadening causal attributions to include attributions to God seems likely to moderate the more extreme emotional reactions to events that might otherwise occur. For example, successes and failures will have less emotional impact if they are attributed to God, as well as internally. Attributions to God seem to function as an unusual kind of attribution that does not fall neatly in either the internal or external category (Watts, Nye, & Savage, 2002).

Further advances to our understanding of how religious beliefs contribute to emotional transformation will depend on a more specific theory of religious cognition. Watts (2004; Watts et al., 2002) is developing such a theory, using the general combative architecture of interacting cognitive subsystems (ICS; Teasdale & Barnard, 1993), which has proved applicable to a wide range of phenomena in cognitive psychology. ICS makes a distinction between two meanings systems which constitute the central engine of cognition. One is "propositional," which encodes cognition in nonemotional form, and in a way that is readily capable of articulation. The other is a more intuitive cognitive subsystem, the "implicational" system, which encodes meanings in a denser, more schematic way, that requires transformation into a different cognitive code before articulation is possible.

ICS is one of a number of multilevel cognitive theories of emotion (Williams, Watts, Macleod, & Matthews, 1997). An early example was Howard Leventhal's perceptual–motor theory, which distinguished between perceptual–motor, schematic, and conceptual levels (Leventhal, 1984). The schematic level is in some ways like implicational cognition, and the conceptual level is in some ways like prepositional cognition. However, ICS is a more rigorous theory in which assumptions are made more explicit; it has also been applied more widely and is based on a wider range of empirical data.

Religious beliefs could be encoded either at the propositional or the implicational level. However, there are aspects of religious belief that suggest that it is characteristically implicational. Implicational cognition is schematic in that it generalizes across different instances; that is also true of religious cognition. For example, the death and resurrection schema in Christian thinking arises out of beliefs about Jesus but also applies to painful experiences being followed by renewal in the life of the believer. In addition, implicational cognition has more direct links with affect than propositional, and religious belief has been recognized in the classic Christian tradition as a "knowledge of the heart," rather than a dryly intellectual matter.

Though there appear to be close empirical links between religious belief, emotional transformation, and practical coping, Paul Lauritzen (1992) has argued that there is a network of common assumptions that has made it difficult to recognize these links. His starting point is the observation that theory and practice often seem strangely disconnected in moral and philosophical theology, despite the relevance of religious beliefs to the practical lives of believers. He argues that this disconnection between theory and practice arises from seeing morality too much as a matter of duty and obligation, which in turn leads to leaving emotion out of consideration. He urges the value of moral theories that emphasize virtue and character, rather than duty and obligation, and argues that they can more readily find a place for emotion in connecting theory and practice.

Lauritzen (1992) also argues for the role of a deep and rich self-understanding in linking religious belief with practical life and suggests that narrative modes of self-understanding may be particularly helpful. Theories that emphasize rich and socially embedded ways of conceptualizing the self can more easily accommodate the role of emotion, though this in turn depends on reconceptualising emotions and seeing them "not as irrational, biologically primitive forces, but as meaningful experiences embedded in social practices" (p. 108). Religion affects both social schemas and self-schemas, and both in turn influence emotions.

The cognitive approach to emotion has become increasingly prominent and has been important in making clear the link between religious beliefs and emotions. If emotions are assumed to be largely independent of cognition, it is hard to see how religious beliefs could influence emotion; a more cognitive approach to emotion makes it easier to see how religious beliefs are relevant to emotional life. Robert C. Roberts (1982) explains:

[B]ecause emotions are construals, and construals always require some "terms," and the "terms" of the Christian emotions are provided by the Christian story, there is a necessary connection between the Christian emotions and the Christian story. So people who don't want to think of the spiritual life in terms of emotions and feelings because they believe that emotions are "subjective" and cut off from "doctrine" and thinking can lay their fears to rest. Emotions are no less tied to concepts than arguments and beliefs are. (p. 21)

Though cognition and emotion have often been seen as separate, in recent decades there has been a significant movement in both psychology and philosophy toward recognizing the close relationship that exists between them. For example, John Bowker (2005) has argued that our view of aesthetics, morality, and religion should all be based on the assumption that cognition and emotion are intertwined. It is not necessary to consider how we can move from one to the other (or derive one from the other) as they are never separate in the first place. In a similar vein, Mark Wynn (2005) has argued for the value of a cognitive approach to emotion in overcoming the disjunction between the supposedly objective intellectual content of religious beliefs and the emotional form of religious practice.

RELIGIOUS PRACTICE AND EMOTION REGULATION

We now turn to examining how religious practices contribute to emotion regulation. Some religious practices, such as prayer, draw very explicitly on religious beliefs. Indeed, prayer can be seen at the human level as an exercise in the religious reframing of events (e.g., Watts, 2001). Some reframing in prayer involves past events. For example, confession involves the identification of events to which guilt is an appropriate reaction, and thanksgiving involves the identification of events for which gratitude is an appropriate reaction. On the other hand, intercessory prayer provides an opportunity for identifying and reframing hopes and anxieties about the future. The empirical study of the contribution of prayer to emotion regulation is still at a very early stage. However, it seems likely to be an important arena of religious emotion regulation.

Religious practices often have significant effects on people's states of arousal, as Eugene d'Aquili and Andrew Newberg (1999), among others, have pointed out. Some religious practices, such as rhythmic dancing or chanting, tend to increase arousal levels, whereas other religious practices, notably meditation, tend to reduce them. Because arousal affects emotion, these two groups of religious practices will regulate emotion in very different ways. High-arousal practices may help to induce an ecstatic state, whereas the value of low-arousal practices may reside more in their capacity to regulate negative emotions.

Meditation is probably the religious practice with most interesting implications for emotion regulation and is worth considering in some detail. Though meditation has always been an important strand of Christian religious practice, it is even more central to Buddhism, and both faith traditions are considered in this section. Meditation illustrates in an interesting way a shift in the relationship between religious and emotional objectives. Meditation has traditionally been undertaken primarily for religious reasons. However, people have become increasingly aware that the practice of meditation has significant implications for emotional regulation. The result is that meditation is now undertaken by many people as much for its contribution to emotion regulation as for religious reasons.

When people are meditating, various techniques are employed to liberate them from distracting thoughts and feelings. It is impossible to move toward any deep state of meditation when practitioners are currently in the grip of strong emotions such as anger, guilt, or anxiety. Contemporary psychological research highlights the linkage between regulation of thoughts and regulation of emotions. Many emotional states seem to be maintained by emotional thoughts. It has been shown, for example, that depression is maintained by negative thoughts. A vicious circle can arise in which a depressed mood gives rise to negative thoughts, and negative thoughts in turn increase depressed mood (Teasdale & Barnard, 1993). Controlling distracting thoughts through the practice of meditation would tend also to lead to an abatement of strong emotional states. A virtuous cycle may then be established in which a calm, meditational state is facilitated by an absence of negative thoughts, and in turn helps to keep negative thoughts at bay. Much advice on the control of negative thoughts can be found in traditional literature on spiritual practices. An interesting Christian example is the 17th-century Christian text, *Holy Wisdom*, by Augustine Baker (d. 1641) (Baker, 1657/1964) that is unusually rich in practical advice. For example, he advises people to simply "neglect" distracting intrusive thoughts rather than struggle to exclude them from their minds.

Concerns might be expressed, from the perspective of modern psychology, about the regulation of emotion in the context of meditation. It might be argued that it involves an unhealthy "bottling up" of emotion, which would be better acknowledged and expressed. However, there are several reasons why this argument is not convincing. Concern over the nonexpression of emotion is often linked to an acceptance of a hydraulic model of emotion in which failure to express emotion is seen as analogous to the damming of a flow of water, causing pressure and tension. However, though this hydraulic model of emotion is implicit in much Freudian and post-Freudian thinking, it has received little scientific support and certainly cannot be accepted uncritically. These issues are explored more fully elsewhere in this book (e.g., Thompson & Meyer, this volume).

Emotion regulation in the context of meditation involves restraint about the *expression* of emotion, and indeed about giving way to strong emotions in ways that may not be externally observable, in emotional ruminations, for example. However, the emotional restraint characteristic of meditation does not imply any lack of *awareness* of emotions. This is a distinction that has often been overlooked in counseling psychology, and it is worth remembering that Freud's primary concern was about the repression of emotions to the point where they were excluded from consciousness rather than about the suppression of emotional expression.

It has often been claimed that meditation, rather than blunting emotional awareness, leads to enhanced awareness of emotions. For example, Rudolf Steiner (1962), speaking of those undergoing training in spiritual practices, remarks:

> The pupil shall by all means rejoice over what is joyful and sorrow over what is sorrowful. It is the outward expression of joy and sorrow, of pleasure and pain that he must learn to control. If he honestly tries to attain this, he will soon discover that he does not grow less, but actually more sensitive to everything in his environment that can cause emotions of joy or pain. (pp. 247–248)

It is also worth recalling here the distinction between passions and affections made in the moral psychology of the Enlightenment. Meditation is probably facilitated by the regulation of the passions (i.e., strong emotions that dominate their entire consciousness). However, the practice of meditation in no way requires the control of gentler affections. Indeed, a key aspect of the distinction between passions and affections has always been that passions impair human understanding whereas, at least in Christian spiritual practice, affections are often seen as enhancing it.

Even though I have argued that meditation only requires an absence of very strong emotions, rather than complete emotional detachment, it is probably the case that many people pursue meditation in a way that maximizes emotional detachment. The degree of emphasis on emotional detachment no doubt depends to some extent on the religious tradition; for example, there may be an even stronger tendency to seek emotional detachment in Buddhist than in Christian meditation. There are indications from empirical research on Christian meditation practiced by Carmelite nuns that emotional detachment is not actually helpful in meditation. Mallory developed a questionnaire that made a distinction between nuns who had a positive approach to the contemplative life that emphasized the love of God and those who had a negative view that emphasized the rejection of all desires. Analysis showed that advances in contemplative prayer, as reflected in criteria derived from the writings of St John of the Cross, were quite closely correlated with a positive emphasis on God's love, whereas they showed no correlation with an emphasis on renunciation of desire (Mallory, 1977).

There has recently been much psychological interest in mindfulness, in which people learn to focus attention selectively on the present. There is evidence that people who have trained to achieve mindfulness are better attuned to their emotions, have a greater capacity for self-regulation, and have a higher sense of well-being (Brown & Ryan, 2003). Mindfulness has been used in conjunction with cognitive therapy of depression and appears to enhance its effectiveness (Segal, Williams, & Teasdale, 2002).

Mindfulness can be formulated in terms of ICS, to which reference has already been made (Teasdale & Barnard, 1993). This model of cognition assumes that multiple cognitive operations are normally proceeding simultaneously. In contrast, Teasdale and his colleagues propose that in mindfulness this "multitasking" is suspended and the peripheral subsystems are largely closed down, so that the implicational subsystem can operate in a way that is unimpeded by a cross-talk with other subsystems (Teasdale, Segal, & Williams, 1995). In terms of ICS, mindfulness appears to be a state in which implicational cognition is favored over propositional cognition.

One significant aspect of this theory of mindfulness is that implicational cognition (unlike propositional cognition) has a direct link to body states that represent an affective form of cognition. According to this view, the kind of cognition that comes to prominence in mindfulness, far from being one in which emotion has no role, is one that is characteristically emotional. However, the emotions involved are those that the moral psychologists of the Enlightenment would have called affections, rather than passions. An analogy can be drawn between the affective, intuitive religious meanings toward which mindfulness leads and the affective cognition used by psychotherapists in the form of countertransference. Therapists are trained to pay attention to their emotional reactions to patients, though such reactions are usually a matter of gentle and subtle emotions rather than strong passions. Careful attention by therapists to their feelings about a client may elucidate things about the client that would otherwise be difficult to access. In a similar way, meditation may lead to an emotionally engaged form of intuition.

RELIGIOUS PERSPECTIVES ON GUILT

Religion provides a broad framework for considering particular emotions. Though the reduction of negative emotions is often an appropriate objective, a religious perspective will also want to consider when and how negative emotions can be transformed to serve a constructive purpose. The substantial research literature on methods of emotion regulation has focused very largely on reducing negative emotions. Such reduction is often simply assumed to be a worthwhile objective, but from a religious perspective, that assumption is questionable. As we have already seen, from a Christian point of view, it is more important whether experiences affect people's relationship to God than whether they are pleasurable or not.

Guilt provides an interesting illustration of this point. It is tempting to assume that guilt is an unpleasant emotion with psychologically harmful effects, and that any methods of emotion regulation that would reduce it or eliminate it are desirable. However, from a Christian point of view, there is clearly potential value in guilt. It has a role in making people aware that their patterns of conduct are morally inappropriate and in motivating people to modify their behavior.

At first glance, there may seem to be something of a clash here between the perspectives of religion and contemporary psychology about guilt, with psychology emphasizing the deleterious effects of guilt and religion emphasizing its potential value. However, reconciliation can be achieved by distinguishing between different kinds of guilt. Some guilt, as Freud recognized, is neurotic and excessive, both in the range of situations in which it occurs and because the magnitude of the guilt reaction is disproportionate to the conduct that triggered it. That is the kind of guilt that psychological approaches to emotion regulation have been most concerned to reduce, and a religious perspective would accept such guilt reduction as a worthwhile objective.

In contrast, as Freud would have recognized, there can also be guilt that is realistic in the sense that it is a proper response to inappropriate or maladaptive conduct. Psychology tends to emphasize the dangers of excessive guilt, whereas religion tends to emphasize the function of realistic guilt. However, neither need have a quarrel with the other; they are focusing essentially on different kinds of guilt, and once a distinction is made between them, the apparent conflict falls away. The constructive role of guilt can be seen as an example of the more general function of emotions. Indeed, Keith Oatley (1992) has argued that it is the key function of emotions to occur at key junctures in goals and plans and to lead to the adoption of more appropriate goals and plans. Psychological research supports the view that guilt promotes prosocial behavior and the maintenance of good interpersonal relationships (Baumeister, Stillwell, & Heatherton, 1994).

It is part of the value of introducing a religious perspective to emotion regulation that it emphasizes distinctions between emotional reactions that are superficially similar but differ in important ways. Having made this distinction in connection with guilt, it is not difficult to see that there are parallel distinctions to be made about a range of other emotions. Many negative emotions can have a constructive role, and it may be more important for people to respond to emotions appropriately than to try to regulate them out of existence. For example, depression may occur in situations in which people are experiencing a chronic and pervasive lack of satisfaction and personal fulfillment, with important psychological needs unmet. In that situation, it may be important to restructure life in a way that redresses that problem rather than merely attempt to rectify the depression.

A key feature of the Christian approach to guilt is that it tries to assure people that they are forgiven (Watts et al., 2002). Religious teaching on guilt sometimes draws attention to problematic conduct, but it does so in the context of also emphasizing that there is a solution to the guilt to which it leads. The Christian practice of sacramental confession to a priest emphasizes both guilt and forgiveness, but which of the two is experienced more strongly by a particular person probably depends on his or her background mental and emotional state. Just as people are inclined to remember selectively mood-congruent material (Williams et al., 1997), so too whether people who go to sacramental confession focus mainly on guilt or forgiveness probably depends on whether their background psychological state is predominantly positive or negative.

It has been suggested that we are currently living in a culture that is less guilt-focused than used to be the case (Baumeister & Exline, 1999). Our culture may be more a narcissistic one that gives rise to feelings of shame rather than guilt (Watts, 2001). The essence of the distinction, as usually made by psychologists, is that guilt is a reaction to observable behavior whereas shame arises from a more pervasive sense of what kind of people we are. Current religious practices probably address the regulation of guilt more effectively than they do shame, an imbalance that needs to be redressed. There may have been too much emphasis in the Christian tradition on individual sacramental confession as an approach to the emotion regulation of guilt. Grainger has recently emphasized how broader aspects of Christian liturgy can also contribute to the religious alleviation of excessive guilt feelings (Grainger, 2004).

RELIGIOUS PERSPECTIVES ON ANGER

In the final section of this chapter I consider the regulation of anger in detail from a religious perspective. Anger has probably been considered more extensively from a religious point of view than any other emotion (e.g., Campbell, 1986). Christians, like many others in society, have often found it hard to know what to think about anger and what to do about it in practice. However, there are a number of points at which a religious framework makes a distinctive contribution to issues about anger. The discussion of anger proceeds in four sections. First, I place the Christian approach to anger in the broader context of world faith traditions; then I consider the implications of assumptions about divine anger for human anger. Next I examine the close relationship between anger and moral assumptions, and finally I discuss the ways in which religion contributes to anger regulation.

Anger and World Religions

Though this section continues to focus mainly on Christianity, it is worth noting initially that the world's faith traditions are quite diverse in their approach to anger. Stratton (1923), in a helpful comparative survey, identifies three main approaches. According to his scheme, Judaism, Islam, and Zoroastrism are "irate and martial religions" that take a positive view of anger; Taoism, Vishnuism, Buddhism and Jainism are "un-angry religions" that see no useful place for anger; whereas Christianity and Confucianism are "the religions of anger-supported love" that see a selective role for anger in the service of positive objectives. Of course, such a broad classification ignores the diversity that can be found within different religions, though it is a useful first approximation.

There is a rich Buddhist literature on anger (Nhââat, 2001) that generally sees anger as something entirely negative and to be overcome. In the West, Stoicism, though more a philosophy than a faith tradition, took a similar view. Schimmel (1997) draws interesting similarities between the Judeo-Christian and stoic approach to the regulation of anger. Though Stratton is probably correct in suggesting that Christianity takes a more moderate view of anger most faith traditions, avoiding the extremes of both "martial" and "un-angry" religions, a rich variety of views can be found within the Christian tradition.

It is consistent with Stratton's framework that different views of anger can be found in the Hebrew Bible and the Christian New Testament. Texts that emphasize God's anger are to be found almost entirely in the Hebrew Bible (Baloian, 1992). However, the idea that the Judaic approach endorses anger, whereas the Christian approach harnesses anger in the context of love, can be overdone. It is not possible to maintain that Jesus, as presented in the Gospels, is free of anger, or that the New Testament presents an anger-free religion. Some of the words attributed to Jesus in the Gospels read like the words of an angry man. Nevertheless, there seems to be some reticence in the Gospels about explicitly attributing anger to Jesus. When people in the Synagogue accuse him of healing on the Sabbath Day, he looked round at them with anger (Mark 3.5). Also, when the disciples sought to interfere with people bringing children to Jesus, Jesus was indignant (Mark 10. 14). Interestingly, these explicit references to the anger of Jesus are found only in Mark's gospel. Though the other synoptic Gospels tell the same stories, they leave the anger of Jesus implicit. This may reflect a gathering unease, even within the 1st century, about the implications of the anger of Jesus.

Such explicitly pastoral advice about anger as can be found in the New Testament epistles clearly encourages circumspection about anger without requiring that it be completely eliminated. For example, St. Paul's "let not the sun go down on your anger" (Ephesians 4. 26) and St. James" "be slow to anger" (James 1. 19) both imply a careful management of anger, within the implicit assumption that it will sometimes arise. In general, it seems that Stratton is correct in discerning, in the New Testament, a position on anger that lies between, say, Judaism and Buddhism.

Divine and Human Anger

The anger of God has often caused discomfort to theologians, and this concern goes back to Lactantius" *Dies Ira Dei*, written in the 4th century. However, his assumptions about the embeddedness of anger in social hierarchies no longer carry conviction. According to Lactantius, God's anger is justifiable because of his position of authority; similarly human anger can be justifiable for those in authority. So, he suggests that human anger is justifiable when people in authority are moved, by anger, to correct the misdeeds of those in their charge. Closely linked to this approach to anger based on social hierarchy is the notion that anger is justified when people are in the right. As Stearns (Stearns & Stearns, 1986) comments, the premodern view assumed "that anger is justifiable when one is on the right side, and that God, always on the right side, may be angry . . . " (p. 48). This can be taken to legitimize the anger of the zealous servants of God. However, there is a sense in which no human being can presume to be as much in the right as God and therefore to have the same entitlement to anger.

By the 18th century, attitudes were changing in a way that rendered God a more explicit model for human conduct than had been the case previously. One aspect of this was that God was seen as having a "personality" in a way that had not previously been considered (Webb, 1934). Among diary materials, those of Dudley Ryder (1715–1716) illustrate the new thinking (Stearns & Stearns, 1986). His discussion of anger is explicitly based on the likeness of God to a good man. It was no longer possible to assume that anger was acceptable for God but not for humans; the anger of God was becoming a more relevant model for humans.

This development has made all the more important another approach to the problem of anger, one foreshadowed by Lactantius, namely, the distinction between different kinds of anger. Lactantius" distinction is between "just" and "unjust" anger; though these different forms of anger might also be labeled "constructive" and "vengeful" anger. This distinction was relatively novel with Lactantius, but it has fathered many subsequent distinctions, such as Fromm's (1977) between malignant and benign aggression. The fine details of Lactantius" distinction are probably no longer of practical importance. However, there is still much to be said for the line of argument that identifies the anger of God as being of one kind rather than another (e.g., constructive rather than vengeful) and concludes from this that one kind of anger, but not the other, is acceptable for human beings.

The anger of God continues to be a problem for Christian theologians, and Campbell distinguishes three main contemporary responses to this problem (Campbell, 1986). One is to simply disregard references to the anger of God as inconsistent with the predominant Biblical view. A second approach is to make a sharp distinction between divine and human anger, and to see God's anger as reflecting his holiness. The third, and most recent, approach is to see God's anger as arising from his passionate involvement with creation.

Moral Aspects of Anger

Anger, at least in contemporary North America and Europe, seems to be a more benign and constructive phenomenon than is often supposed, and many religions would want to emphasize its potential value. One of the most thorough surveys of anger available (Averill, 1982) indicates that most anger is directed toward family and friends rather than enemies or strangers. Further, it is relatively rare for anger to issue in violence or aggression. Indeed, most expressions of anger are constructive in intention.

Much current public concern about anger seems to arise from a misunderstanding about the nature of anger and the failure to distinguish it from rage. Darwin played a crucial role in propagating the view that anger and indignation "differ from rage only in degree" (Tavris, 1982), though it is arguable that there is a qualitative distinction to be made between them. In the older terminology rage is clearly a "passion," whereas anger can be more an "affection." Darwin's wish to abolish the distinction between rage and anger reflects the attempt in the latter part of the 19th century to abandon the religiously based distinction between passions and affections.

Whether or not we become angry depends critically on our assumptions about whether certain conduct is morally acceptable or not. We only become angry when our standards of conduct are breached. Rage, in contrast, is not a moral emotion in that sense; neither is annoyance. As Averill's survey showed, people can make a clear distinction between anger and annoyance. Though there is a tendency for anger to be more intense than annoyance, the critical distinction is that we become angry only when we regard ourselves as being justified in our reactions, whereas this is not a requirement for annoyance. In a similar vein, Ortony, Clore, and Collins (1988) in their careful taxonomy of emotions have argued that anger requires not just an unpleasant event but a blameworthy one. In this, they argue that anger is the opposite of gratitude. An important feature of the attribution of blame is whether or not those who thwart us are judged to have acted deliberately. The assumption of intentionality seems to be a necessary prerequisite of anger.

Anger exposes a person's moral assumptions and attributions of blame, and these constitute a central focus for modern cognitive therapy for anger. These moralistic assumptions and attributions would also be a central focus for a religious approach to anger. Where anger reaches problematic and pathological proportions, this is frequently found to be the outcropping of idiosyncratic and intolerant moral values. For example, an excessively angry person cannot allow that someone who has angered them may have defensible standards of conduct, albeit ones that are different in detail from their own. There is also frequently an excessive tendency in angry people to assume that people's annoying acts are committed deliberately.

The relationship between anger and morality is probably a reciprocal one. Anger is a reflection of a person's moral sensibilities, and a person with no morality might be incapable of an emotional reaction that could strictly be labeled "anger." However, anger may also contribute to our moral sensibilities, as Rudolph Steiner (1983) argued in an intriguingly entitled lecture, "The Mission of Anger." According to his view, we first "judge" an event implicitly by reacting with anger. This helps us to learn to make more conscious any deliberate evaluations. Thus, says Steiner (1983), "In certain respects, anger is an educator. It arises in us as an inner experience before we are mature enough to form an enlightened judgement of right and wrong" (p. 26). The claim is that anger is a reflection of moral sensibilities that are implicit rather than explicit, and that it can contribute to the development of those sensibilities.

The role of anger in the development of some of the prominent moral leaders of the 20th century is something that could be argued in detail for people such as Mahatma Ghandi and Martin Luther King. We live in a world in which there is much to be angry about, and a link between anger and moral values can be fruitful. "Liberation" theology has recently made fruitful contact with anger and in South America in particular has provided some of the rationale for resistance to oppressive political regimes.

In general, emotions become problematic when they persist beyond the episode that originally evoked them and have no moral basis. They then become not an authentic emotional response but a self-maintaining mood that feeds on itself, often by constant rehearsal of stereotyped thoughts about the unacceptability of other people's conduct. Such self-talk is a key focus of the cognitive therapy of anger and can form a useful part of pastoral counseling. Christian use of forgiveness similarly strikes at processes which maintain anger artificially, so that people are released from anger that is so prolonged that "the sun goes down on it" (Ephesians 4. 26).

Religion and Anger Regulation

These are various ways in which religion can make a contribution to the regulation of anger. Lauritzen (1992) sets out three distinct ways in which Christian beliefs can influence anger, and a somewhat similar analysis could no doubt be developed for other faith traditions.

The first kind of transformation arises from Lauritzen's basic analysis of anger as playing a key role in maintaining retributive justice. In this first kind of religious transformation, this basic function of anger is maintained, but religious values affect what people become angry about. For example, they may be less likely to become angry about personal pleasures being frustrated and more likely to become angry about immoral conduct. The social function of anger is unchanged, but a religious perspective affects which things trigger anger.

In Lauritzen's second kind of religious influence on anger, a clear distinction is made between that which is appropriate to humanity and that which belongs properly to God. The framework of Christian belief can be seen as switching the responsibility for judgment and justice to God, thus making it unnecessary for human anger to still serve the purpose of maintaining retributive justice. Anger may still be deemed to be warranted in the same circumstances and may still serve the function of maintaining retributive justice, but it is God's anger that is appropriate to this function, rather than human anger.

The third way in which anger is affected by religion is that anger is transcended entirely. The believer becomes so caught up in the religious story about God's work of salvation that anger and resentment no longer arise and are no longer seen as appropriate. A broader perspective of God's work of salvation becomes so dominant that maintaining retributive justice by anger seems irrelevant. Religious life involves such a radical transformation of how human situations and priorities are perceived that anger becomes irrelevant.

Anger also creates opportunities for the practice of forgiveness, which creates an alternative way of formulating the impact of anger on religion. One of the central contributions of Christian teaching to the management of anger is the possibility of release from anger by the forgiveness of others, and it is a field in which religious ideas have migrated into psychology and given rise to a rich research literature (Worthington, 2005). There are two interestingly different approaches in the therapeutic psychology of forgiveness, each with its own distinctive theological resonance (Watts, 2004).

The work of Enright (e.g., Enright & North, 1998) has emphasized the value of the detached reframing of whatever has provoked anger, and to need forgiveness. There are some antecedents of this approach in the sermons of Bishop Butler (1970) in the 18th century, whose approach would now be seen in terms of the psychology of attributions. Rather than assuming that an injury has been done deliberately, he argues that we should be more inclined to attribute the actions of others to "inadvertence and mistake," and to recognizie our own contribution as well as that of the other person. From this perspective, it can also be helpful, in withdrawing from the attributions that are giving rise to anger, to regard judgment as belonging to God, rather than to human beings. Such reframing facilitates detachment from a perception of a particular situation that is giving rise to anger.

An alternative approach to forgiveness, particularly highlighted in the work of Worthington (1998), puts the emphasis on empathy with the person who needs to be forgiven, and Watts (2004) has suggested that this approach to forgiveness has resonance with Christian thinking about incarnation. Humanity stood in need of forgiveness by God, and the Christian assumption is that God responded to that human need by identifying himself empathically with humanity. Worthington's approach emphasizes that replacing anger with forgiveness depends on empathy. Both divine and human forgiveness can thus be seen as proceeding by an empathic identification with the transgressor.

Though the management of anger may sometimes be an appropriate objective of pastoral care, too much pastoral advice on anger has accepted rather uncritically the assumption that anger is best managed out of existence. There is a place for this approach, but it does not amount to an adequate religious appreciation of the potential value of anger. I have tried to outline the assumptions on which a more positive religious view of anger can be built.

FUTURE DIRECTIONS

In most chapters in this handbook, discussion about future research directions is a matter of building on an already developing research program. However, in the case of religion, there is so far relatively little systematic research. However, the most promising line of empirical research so far is concerned with the role of religion in coping, and such research is the best lead to build on in future work.

It is clear that religious coping strategies are often quite widely employed. What is less clear is how significant a difference they make to the effectiveness of coping. They might make a really important contribution, and in this chapter I have indicated some of the reasons why they might do so. However, on the other hand, it might just be that religious people tend to couch their coping strategies in religious terms, but that doing so does not make any decisive difference. That is not an easy matter to investigate and can probably only be studied naturalistically rather than through experimental manipulation. However, it is an important issue to address.

If religion does play a useful role in coping, there is a further question about *how* it does so, and the two principal hypotheses are social and cognitive. Religion may provide people with a valuable network of social support. Indeed, if religious people live up to the teaching about altruistic love that is to be found in most faith traditions, the social support of their religious community might be particularly helpful. The other principal hypothesis is that religion helps through providing a cognitive framework, and that is the approach that has been more thoroughly explored in this chapter. However, we are so far largely at the level of trying to understand how religion *might* affect cognitive aspects of coping, and there is scope for much more research on how it actually does so. It is then an important matter how far the beneficial effects of religion are mediated though an improved capacity to regulate emotional states, as David Pizarro and Peter Salovey (2002) have suggested. The social and cognitive features of religious organizations may, at their best, make them "emotionally intelligent."

An important consideration to take into account in future research is the diversity of religious people. Indeed, in other areas of the psychology of religion, a comparison of religious and nonreligious people has often not been particularly fruitful, largely because religious people differ so much among themselves. It has often been more fruitful to compare different kinds of religious people with one another. For example, Allport's distinction between intrinsic and extrinsic religious people has been crucial in studying how religion relates to mental health and social prejudice (see Spilka et al., 2003). It would not be surprising if the same was true of emotion regulation, and a key prerequisite for future research is to identify which aspects of religious diversity are particularly relevant in this area.

Finally, it seems that research on religion and emotion regulation will be more fruitful if it is addressing relatively specific questions. Certainly, religious people cannot simply be grouped together as though they were all the same. As we have seen in connection with anger, religious traditions take quite divergent approaches, and even within a particular religious tradition there can be important differences. To get meaningful results, it will be important to study homogeneous religious populations. Also, it may be more fruitful to study the regulation of particular emotions, rather than emotion regulation generally. For example, the issues that arise in connection with anger and guilt are significantly different, and the contribution of religion to the regulation of other emotions such as depression and anxiety would be different again. The principal recommendation for further research in this area is thus to examine specific questions that are as specific and well defined as possible.

REFERENCES

Averill, J. R. (1982). *Anger and aggression: An essay on emotion*. New York: Springer-Verlag.

Baker, A. (1964). *Holy wisdom*. Wheathampstead, UK: Anthony Clarke Books. (Original work published 1657)

Baloian, B. E. (1992). *Anger in the Old Testament*. New York: P. Lang.

Baumeister, R. F. (2005). *The cultural animal: Human nature, meaning, and social life*. Oxford, UK: Oxford University Press.

Baumeister, R. F., & Exline, J. J. (1999). Virtue, personality and social relations: Self-control as the moral muscle. *Journal of Personality, 67*(6), 1165–1194.

Baumeister, R. F., Stillwell, A. M., & Heatherton, T. F. (1994). Guilt: An interpersonal approach. *Psychological Bulletin, 115*(2), 243–267.

Bowker, J. W. (2005). *The sacred neuron: Extraordinary new discoveries linking science and religion*. London: I. B. Tauris.

Brown, K. W., & Ryan, R. M. (2003). The benefits of being present: Mindfulness and its role in psychological well-being. *Journal of Personality and Social Psychology, 84*(4), 822–848.

Butler, J. (1970). Upon forgiveness of injuries. In T. A. Roberts (Ed.), *Butler's fifteen sermons* (pp. 80–89). London: SPCK.

Campbell, A. V. (1986). *The gospel of anger*. London: SPCK.

Corrigan, J. (2002). *Business of the heart: Religion and emotion in the nineteenth century*. Berkeley: University of California Press.

Corrigan, J. (2004). *Religion and emotion: Approaches and interpretations*. Oxford, UK: Oxford University Press.

Corrigan, J., Crump, E., & Kloos, J. M. (2000). *Emotion and religion: A critical assessment and annotated bibliography*. Westport, CT: Greenwood Press.

D'Aquili, E. G., & Newberg, A. B. (1999). *The mystical mind: Probing the biology of religious experience*. Minneapolis, MN: Fortress Press.

Dixon, T. (2003). *From passions to emotions: The creation of a secular psychological category*. Cambridge, UK: Cambridge University Press.

Emmons, R. (2005). Emotion and religion. In R. F. Paloutzian & C. L. Park (Eds.), *Handbook of psychology of religion and spirituality* (pp. 235–252). New York: Guilford Press.

Enright, R. D., & North, J. (1998). *Exploring forgiveness*. Madison: University of Wisconsin Press.

Fromm, E. (1977). *The anatomy of human destructiveness*. Harmondsworth, UK: Penguin.

Glock, C. Y., & Stark, R. (1965). *Religion and society in tension*. Chicago: Rand McNally.

Grainger, R. (2004). Forgiveness and liturgy. In F. N. Watts & L. Gulliford (Eds.), *Forgiveness in context: Theology and psychology in creative dialogue*. London: T & T Clark.

Harré, R. (1983). *Personal being: a theory for individual psychology*. London: Blackwell.

Hood, R. W., Spilka, B., Hunsberger, B., & Gorsuch, R. (1996). *The psychology of religion: An empirical approach* (2nd ed.). New York: Guilford Press.

Lauritzen, P. (1992). *Religious belief and emotional transformation: A light in the heart*. London: Associated University Presses.

Leventhal, H. (1984). A perceptual motor theory of emotion. In L. Berkowitz (Ed.), *Advances in experimental social psychology* (Vol. 17, pp. 117–182). New York: Academic Press.

Mallory, M. M. (1977). *Christian mysticism: Transcending techniques*. Assen: van Gorcum.

McIntosh, D. N., Silver, R. C., & Wortman, C. B. (1993). Religion's role in adjustment to a negative life event: Coping with the loss of a child. *Journal of Personality and Social Psychology, 65*(4), 812–821.

Meissner, W. W. (1992). *Ignatius of Loyola: The psychology of a saint*. New Haven: Yale University Press.

Nhâãat, H. (2001). *Anger: Buddhist wisdom for cooling the flames*. London: Rider.

Oakley, J. (1992). *Morality and the emotions*. London: Routledge.
Oatley, K. (1992). *Best laid schemes: The psychology of emotions*. Cambridge, UK: Cambridge University Press.
Ortony, A., Clore, G. L., & Collins, A. (1988). *The cognitive structure of emotions*. Cambridge, UK: Cambridge University Press.
Pargament, K. I. (1997). *The psychology of religion and coping: Theory, research, practice*. New York: Guilford Press.
Pizarro, D., & Salovey, P. (2002). Religious systems as "emotionally intelligent" organizations. *Psychological Inquiry, 13*(3), 220–222.
Reddy, W. M. (2001). *The navigation of feeling: A framework for the history of emotions*. Cambridge, England: Cambridge University Press.
Roberts, R. C. (1982). *Spirituality and human emotion*. Grand Rapids, MI: Eerdmans.
Rozin, P., Lowery, L., Imada, S., & Haidt, J. (1999). The CAD triad hypothesis: A mapping between three moral emotions (contempt, anger, disgust) and three moral codes (community, autonomy, divinity). *Journal of Personality and Social Psychology, 76*(4), 574–586.
Schimmel, S. (1997). *The seven deadly sins: Jewish, Christian, and classical reflections on human psychology*. Oxford, UK: Oxford University Press.
Segal, Z. V., Williams, J. M. G., & Teasdale, J. D. (2002). *Mindfulness-based cognitive therapy for depression: A new approach to preventing relapse*. New York: Guilford Press.
Spilka, B., Hood, R. W., Hunsberger, B., & Gorsuch, R. (2003). *The psychology of religion: An empirical approach* (3rd ed.). New York: Guilford Press.
Stearns, C. Z., & Stearns, P. N. (1986). *Anger: The struggle for emotional control in America's history*. Chicago: University of Chicago Press.
Steiner, R. (1962). *Occult science* (F. Adams & M. Adams, Trans.). London: Rudolf Steiner Press.
Steiner, R. (1983). *Metamorphoses of the soul: Paths of experience: 18 public lectures 1909–10* (C. Davy & C. von Arnim, Trans., 2nd ed.). London: Rudolf Steiner Press.
Stratton, G. M. (1923). *Anger: Its religious and moral significance*. London: Allen & Unwin.
Tavris, C. (1982). *Anger, the misunderstood emotion*. New York: Simon & Schuster.
Teasdale, J. D., & Barnard, P. J. (1993). *Affect, cognition and change*. Hillsdale, NJ: Erlbaum.
Teasdale, J. D., Segal, Z. V., & Williams, J. M. G. (1995). How does cognitive therapy prevent depressive relapse and why should attentional control (mindfulness) training help? *Behaviour Research and Therapy, 33*, 25–39.
Thompson, R. A., & Meyer, S. (2007). Socialization of emotion regulation in the family. In J. J. Gros (Ed.), *Handbook of emotion regulation* (pp. 249–268). New York: Guilford Press.
Watts, F. N. (1997). Psychological and religious perspectives on emotion. *Zygon, 32*(2), 243–260.
Watts, F. N. (2001). Shame, sin and guilt. In A. I. McFadyen & M. Sarot (Eds.), *Forgiveness and truth* (pp. 53–70). Edinburgh, Scotland: T & T Clark.
Watts, F. N. (2004). Christian theology. In F. N. Watts & L. Gulliford (Eds.), *Forgiveness in context: Theology and psychology in creative dialogue*. London: T & T Clark.
Watts, F. N., Nye, R., & Savage, S. B. (2002). *Psychology for Christian ministry*. London: Routledge.
Watts, I. (1746). *The Doctrine of the passions explained and improved: Or, a brief and comprehensive scheme of the natural affections of mankind*. Coventry: Luckman. (Original work published 1729)
Webb, C. C. J. (1934). *God and personality*. London: Allen & Unwin.
Williams, J. M. G., Watts, F. N., Macleod, C., & Matthews, A. (1997). *Cognitive psychology and emotional disorders* (2nd ed.). Chichester, UK: Wiley.
Worthington, E. L. (1998). *Dimensions of forgiveness: Psychological research and theological perpsectives*. Philadelphia: Templeton Foundation Press.
Worthington, E. L. (2005). *Handbook of forgiveness*. New York: Routledge.
Wynn, M. (2005). *Emotional experience and religious understanding: Integrating perception, conception and feeling*. Cambridge, UK: University Press.

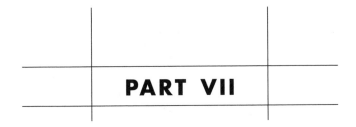

PART VII

CLINICAL APPLICATIONS

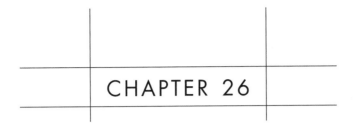

CHAPTER 26

Emotion Regulation and Externalizing Disorders in Children and Adolescents

BENJAMIN C. MULLIN
STEPHEN P. HINSHAW

Within the past two decades, the field of child development has experienced a surge of research attention on the regulation of emotion. This burgeoning literature has helped to expose the centrality of emotional processes to various aspects of healthy development (see Eisenberg, Hofer, & Vaughn, this volume) and to elucidate the interrelationships between cognitive, social, and emotional aspects of childhood (Cole, Martin, & Dennis, 2004). As this book attests, the range of scientists interested in emotion regulation is rapidly growing, yielding a better understanding of the multilevel factors that may influence our experience and expression of emotions.

Recently, investigators have begun to apply knowledge of emotion regulation to the study of psychopathology in children and adolescents. The applicability of emotion regulation research to clinical phenomena is potentially far-reaching, given the prominence of emotional disturbance in many forms of pathology. In fact, even a cursory examination of current diagnostic manuals in psychiatry reveals that emotion-related problems are central to the descriptions as well as diagnostic criteria for many if not most forms of psychopathology (American Psychiatric Association, 2000). Not only will clinical investigators and clinicians benefit from what is learned in emotion regulation research, but this research effort may be aided by a developmental psychopathology perspective in which normal and abnormal emotion regulation trajectories can be studied side by side, with the potential for mutual elucidation (Cicchetti & Cohen, 2006). That is, understanding clinical conditions in which emotion dysregulation is salient should aid in informing the field about general processes of emotion regulation.

In this chapter we examine the relationship between emotion regulation and externalizing disorders, the most common form of childhood psychopathology (Kazdin, 1995). The externalizing label is applied to numerous forms of problem behavior, ranging from hyperactivity/impulsivity and social problems to antisocial behavior and aggression. Although externalizing disorders have traditionally been conceptualized as problems of behavior and cognition rather than affect (see Quay & Hogan, 1999), these conditions are inextricably tied in with emotional processes. In fact, their very depictions include disorganized, explosive, and defiant patterns of affect and behavior, which interfere with learning, social maturation, and the rights of others (American Psychiatric Association, 2000). Thus, on the face of it, emotion and emotion regulation would appear to be centrally involved in such conditions.

Beyond face validity per se, a small but developing body of research indicates that deficits in emotion regulation may coincide with the disinhibitory problems of attention-deficit/hyperactivity disorder (ADHD) and may represent a key mechanism in the emergence of particular forms of antisocial behavior (Barkley, 1997; Olson, Sameroff, Kerr, Lopez, & Wellman, 2005; Silk, Steinberg, & Morris, 2003). A central goal for research in this area is to link normally developing processes of emotion regulation to the timing and manifestations of clinical disorders of the externalizing spectrum. Given the multiple definitions of emotion regulation in current use and given the incomplete knowledge base about the unfolding of emotion regulation strategies and processes across childhood and adolescence (Cole et al., 2004), this remains an elusive goal at present. As we emphasize throughout this chapter, it is crucial to consider specific forms of the relevant behavior patterns when examining emotional and emotion regulatory processes, as it increasingly appears that deficits in emotion regulation are relevant to some but not all forms of externalizing behavior. Because global portrayals of externalizing behavior as indicative of emotion dysregulation may obscure rather than clarify important associations, we emphasize specificity of linkages to the extent allowed by the current literature. Finally, despite considerable speculation as to the importance of emotion dysregulation for externalizing psychopathology, research in this area is of relatively recent origin, with a range of definitions and research paradigms utilized to tap emotion regulation and dysregulation. Hence, a review of basic models and research methods is in order.

MODELS OF EMOTION REGULATION AND RELATIONS WITH PSYCHOPATHOLOGY

Emotion Regulation: Definitions and Differentiations

To appreciate the developmental roots of emotion regulation, we first turn to the important area of temperament. The influential model of Rothbart defines temperament as individual differences in reactivity and self-regulation with respect to emotion, attention, and motor activity (Rothbart & Bates, 1998). This and other models of temperament posit that such response tendencies become evident extremely early in development, revealing strongly psychobiological underpinnings (at the same time, these tendencies persist throughout the lifespan and become inextricably intertwined with experience). Reactivity, in the context of emotion, refers to individual, perhaps dispositional, differences in basic emotional responsiveness to eliciting stimuli. Negative reactivity, for example, would reflect a temperamental proneness to irritability, anger, or fear in response to environmental triggers. Regulation, in contrast, would refer to an individual's ability to modulate that reactivity through a variety of cognitive and behavioral processes. Importantly, these regulatory processes show tremendous development throughout the periods of toddlerhood, early childhood, and preadolescence.

One component of Rothbart's model, effortful control, is particularly germane to our discussion of emotion regulation (for elaboration, see Eisenberg et al., this volume; and Rothbart & Sheese, this volume). *Effortful control* represents "the ability to inhibit a dominant response in order to perform a subdominant response" (Posner & Rothbart, 2000). Consequently, effortful control is often employed to dampen emotional reactivity (Eisenberg & Spinrad, 2004). This control is achieved through the voluntary management of attentional resources, including the capacities to focus or shift attention between stimuli and to inhibit behavioral responses. In an anger-arousing situation, this process could mean shifting attention away from the source of anger (e.g., another child who has stolen one's toy) and inhibiting the dominant behavioral response (e.g., physical retaliation). Inhibiting a behavioral response is itself proposed as a core means by which all of us regulate our emotional states (Eisenberg et al., 2000). That is, refraining from a physical response to frustration may prevent emotional escalation and instead have a soothing effect.

Additional forms of emotion regulation are likely to occur through involuntary, or *reactive* forms of control (Eisenberg & Spinrad, 2004). These automatic responses to emotional stimuli may include the reorienting of attention or distraction, which can occur without conscious awareness and serve to modulate one's emotional experience and aid in the inhibition of an emotion-related behavioral response. For additional work on the complex construct of inhibition, we recommend the masterful review of Nigg (2000), which posits a number of separable forms of inhibitory processes.

Gross and Thompson (this volume) conceptualize emotion regulation as a series of processes that can be both automatic and voluntary (as well as conscious and unconscious), which may occur either before or after the activation of an emotion and which serve to amplify, maintain, or diminish its intensity. Clearly, this definition of emotion regulation embodies many of the aforementioned ideas from temperament theory. The relationship between temperament and emotion may be best expressed through a metaphor from Saarni, Campos, Camras, and Witherington (2006, p. 273): "temperament is rather like a season of the year, whereas emotions are the mercurial weather conditions that shift from day to day, demanding adjustment and accommodation on a frequent basis" (p. xx). Thus, temperament does not dictate the nature of each emotional experience but instead has a general influence on a child's ability to regulate a range of emotions. A child high in negative temperamental reactivity may well be capable of instances of positive reactivity (e.g., exuberance) but will generally respond in an angry or fearful fashion to evocative stimuli. For a more complete discussion of the complex relationship between temperament, emotions, and emotion regulation, please see Rothbart and Sheese (this volume).

Clinical research employing these concepts has typically focused on the relationship between the *dys*regulation of emotion and symptomatology associated with various disorders. Cole, Michel, and Teti (1994a) separated dysregulation into two forms—*overregulated* and *underregulated*—arguing that most forms of psychopathology result from either underregulating or overregulating the intensity or expression of particular emotions. This dichotomy (or, more likely, continuum) could potentially map onto more descriptive classifications of behavior disorders of childhood and adolescence. The most fundamental of these contains, at one anchor, *internalizing* problems (including sadness and other indicators of depression, anxiety, social withdrawal, and somatic concerns), and at the other, *externalizing* problems (involving the focus of the current chapter, namely, disinhibited, aggressive, and antisocial behavior). Although it seems reasonable to place at least some forms of externalizing behavior at the "under-regulated" end of the continuum, it is less clear whether internalizing problems truly reflect an overregulation of positively valenced emotions or an underregulation of negative emotions such as fear.

As Cole et al. (1994a) admit, this model may be oversimplifying a complex set of processes, and the concept of emotion regulation has evolved to allow more careful applications to the processes underlying psychopathology. Indeed, it is important to be mindful of the difference between an emotion and its regulation (Cole et al., 1994a; Gross & Thompson, this volume). The mere presence of sadness or anger does not in itself indicate overregulation or underregulation; these emotions have important survival value and allow us to appraise situations and act accordingly. We certainly would not want them to be regulated into nonexistence. However, as our understanding of the mechanisms behind internalizing and externalizing problems increases, it seems likely that children extreme on these behavioral dimensions will show patterns of under-regulating certain emotions while overregulating others. For example, children with severe anxiety may lack the ability to effectively diminish the intensity of experienced fear while simultaneously constricting their experience of positive, approach-valenced emotions. Similarly, children in the externalizing spectrum may not underregulate all of their emotions. Yet, as we argue in the subsequent sections, children prone to reactive forms of aggression struggle to regulate their experience of emotions such as anger.

Externalizing Psychopathology: Dimensional and Categorical Perspectives

What precisely do we mean by psychopathology in the "externalizing" spectrum? When investigators in the middle of the last century began to apply factor-analytic methods to understand the nature of child behavior problems, analyzing quantitative ratings of a range of symptoms, two large factors consistently emerged: (1) problems of the internalizing spectrum and (2) externalizing problems, including impulsive and hyperactive behaviors as well as anger, defiance, aggression, and antisocial actions. A large number of factor-analytic investigations have replicated this essential distinction (e.g., Achenbach, 1991). It is noteworthy that problems related to impulse control, attentional focus, and motoric overactivity fall somewhere in between the two poles of internalizing and externalizing in broadband factor-analytic work; they typically yield dimensions of behavior that are separable from either internalizing or externalizing dimensions in finer-grained data analyses. Thus, as emphasized below, explanatory power typically increases when one separates aggression and antisocial behavior on the one hand from inattention, impulsivity, and hyperactivity on the other.

Two key points are immediately salient. First, even though internalizing and externalizing factors have usually been found to constitute orthogonal dimensions, actual samples of youth (particularly those with clinical-range problems) typically display positive associations between these two domains, which can be of substantial magnitude (Achenbach, 1991). Thus, it is a mistake to think that youngsters with externalizing problems are necessarily free of depression or anxiety—an important complication for investigations of emotion regulation (or other relevant processes) in relation to externalizing behavior patterns and a major complexity for those designing interventions. Second, each of these broad dimensions includes a number of partially independent subdimensions. Thus, the internalizing domain can be separated into depression versus anxiety versus preoccupation with bodily pains (among others). Pertinent to this chapter, the externalizing domain comprises several important subtypes.

1. As just noted, patterns of inattention, impulsivity, and hyperactivity are statistically associated with aggression and antisocial behavior in most samples, but they diverge from these latter behaviors in important ways (Hinshaw, 1987; Waschbusch, 2002). That is, they have different patterns of risk and causal factors, with inattention/impulsivity/hyperactivity linked more to genetic and psychobiological causal influences and aggressive behavior more specifically associated with aberrant parenting and other psychosocial risks. Furthermore, they have partially distinct long-term developmental trajectories (for a review, see Hinshaw, 1999). Placing these domains together into one, large externalizing category may mask differences of clinical and conceptual importance.

2. Further differentiation is also salient. For instance, *inattention* is differentiable from *hyperactivity* and *impulsivity* (Hinshaw, 2001; Milich, Balentine, & Lynam, 2001). Inattentive behavior patterns predict academic underachievement and social isolation, whereas hyperactivity and impulsivity are more closely linked with peer rejection and with externalizing features related to aggression.

3. Crucially, the domain of aggression and antisocial behavior is not homogeneous. As summarized in Hinshaw and Lee (2003), several subareas are quite important to distinguish.

First, *overt aggression* (fights, verbal assaults, physical confrontations) is separable from both *covert* manifestations of antisocial behavior (such as theft, destruction of property, lying, and cheating) and so-called *indirect aggression*—behavior patterns that involve harming the reputation of another through talking behind his or her back or destroying reputations. This latter construct is synonymous with (but not identical to) *relational aggression,* prevalent in girls and involving malicious gossip and other means of aligning with certain peers to exclude or damage the reputation of another.

Second, within the domain of overt aggression, *verbal* versus *physical* forms are separable, displaying differing developmental trajectories and correlates. Another important distinction is made between planful, proactive aggression (which overlaps with the construct of instrumental aggression)—involving calculated means of obtaining resources important to the self—and hostile, reactive, or retaliatory aggression, which by definition features a more explosive and angry presentation, linked with frustration and threat. As we highlight subsequently, emotion regulation processes are differentially linked with this important subdivision.

So far, we have been discussing psychopathology viewed continuously, as constituting dimensions of behavior. Another tradition in psychopathology is that of categorical entities or clinical diagnoses. The debate over whether psychopathology is best characterized in terms of underlying dimensions versus distinct taxa or categories is a long and contentious one. In their incisive review, Pickles and Angold (2003) aptly point out that such perspectives are complementary rather than diametrically opposed: Depending on one's framework, psychopathology exhibits both categorical and dimensional features, much in the same way that light simultaneously exhibits both continuous (wave) and discrete (photon-related) properties.

In the categorical tradition, clinicians and investigators concerned with externalizing psychopathology have focused on the clinical disorders of ADHD as well as the disruptive behavior disorders of oppositional defiant disorder (ODD) and conduct disorder (CD). Each of these has a constituent list of symptoms, associated features, typical age of onset, and developmental course; diagnoses are assigned on the basis of developmentally extreme, pervasive, and persistent symptom patterns that yield substantial impairment (American Psychiatric Association, 2000).

Specifically, ADHD includes the two symptom domains of inattention/disorganization and hyperactivity/impulsivity. Age of onset is typically before 7 years of age. Children displaying the former pattern are diagnosed with the Inattentive subtype; they typically do not show much evidence of aggression or antisocial behavior. Children with the latter pattern constitute the Hyperactive/Impulsive type, and those with high levels of both symptom profiles (constituting the majority who are referred for assessment and treatment) are diagnosed with the Combined type. The latter two are prone to evidence noncompliant and aggressive behavior patterns (American Psychiatric Association, 2000; see also Barkley, 2003). Across all three types, the prevalence of ADHD is believed to be between 5% and 8% of the child and adolescent population, with a male:female ratio of approximately 3:1 in community samples and higher among clinic-referred youth.

Although ADHD is viewed by some social critics as a modern-day diagnosis for mildly bothersome children or a means of pathologizing normal-range behavior patterns, when the diagnosis is carefully made, children and adolescents with ADHD show substantial impairments, including marked risk for school failure and discordant family interactions, a greatly increased risk for rejection by their peers, lowered levels of independence, and surprisingly high rates of accidental injury (Barkley, 2003; Hinshaw, 2002b; Hinshaw, Sami, Treuting, Carte, & Zupan, 2002). The impairments associated with ADHD are highly likely to persist into adolescence and adulthood. Thus, ADHD is a condition mandating clinical attention; research into its underlying mechanisms is proceeding at a rapid pace.

Moving to the disruptive behavior disorders, ODD refers to a persistent pattern of rule-breaking, irritable, hostile, and noncompliant behaviors, serving as a precursor to serious antisocial behavior in perhaps a third of all cases. Emotional dyscontrol is implicit in such symptoms. CD, on the other hand, connotes a more severe category of youth who violate the rights of others or show serious rule breaking. The CD diagnosis includes a combination of overtly aggressive behaviors (e.g., fighting and assault) and covert antisocial activities (e.g., lying and cheating). Moreover, unlike ODD, the diagnostic criteria for CD do not include affective disturbance per se, although as we discuss later, affective problems may be relevant for certain individuals within this category.

An important subdivision exists for CD with respect to age of onset. That is, children who begin to display serious antisocial activities before the age of 10 years are quite likely to reveal a constellation of risk factors that include early neuropsychological difficulties, hostile and inconsistent parenting (with a strong likelihood of early patterns of insecure attachment), an extremely high male:female ratio, and a propensity for comorbidity with ADHD that begins early in development (see Moffitt, 1993). This relatively small subgroup (perhaps 2–3% of the population) is highly likely to show persistent patterns of aggression and antisocial behavior across the lifespan (Moffitt & Caspi, 2001). Indeed, a number of investigators have estimated that this subgroup may be responsible for nearly half of the criminal activity in a given society (Hinshaw & Lee, 2003). On the other hand, patterns of adolescent-onset CD are far more normative, more evenly spread between the sexes, and prone to desist following adolescence (although more lasting problems may be evident in some cases). Thus, the age of onset of serious aggression and antisocial behavior appears to mark an important diagnostic distinction.

In our next sections, we consider the relevance of emotion and emotion regulation first for ADHD and then for conduct problems/aggression

EMOTION REGULATION AND ADHD

In his influential unifying theory of ADHD, Barkley (1997) proposed that primary deficits in behavioral inhibition would result in downstream problems with several executive functions. In brief, behavioral inhibition occurs when a child withholds a dominant response; this inhibition then allows the coming online of important executive functions such as working memory, internalization of speech (which includes problem solving and self-questioning), and—of central importance for this chapter—the regulation of affect and arousal. Theoretically, deficits in inhibitory control would interfere with motor control, resulting in the symptom of hyperactivity. They would also prevent the display of measured emotional responding and self-regulation. Thus, Barkley's clear contention is that a fundamental deficit in inhibitory control would yield disruptions to regulatory executive processes in children with ADHD. Such youth would consequently be expected to exhibit emotional reactivity, to be relatively unable to anticipate emotionally charged events (because of reduced capacity for forethought), to have problems in evaluating the impact of their actions on others in emotionally charged situations, and to have a propensity for showing low capacity to regulate their emotional states in the service of achieving a goal.

How are such inhibitory deficits to be understood in the context of effortful control (see Posner & Rothbart, 2000)? Such constructs certainly overlap, but Barkley's conception of inhibitory deficits as related to ADHD is narrower than that of most views of effortful control. The latter include not only the suppression of a prepotent response but also the voluntary allocation and shifting of attention to relevant stimuli. One of the needs of emerging and overlapping fields of research—specifically emotion regulation and developmental psychopathology—is to align definitions and paradigms so that different research efforts can build on one another.

Given the centrality of inhibitory deficits in ADHD, the prediction from Barkley's model is that poor emotion regulation should be ubiquitous in individuals with this disorder (excepting the Inattentive type, which, Barkley contends, does not exhibit the fundamental deficit in inhibition). Yet evidence is mixed, as we discuss next. One key problem is that much of the research on this topic has not accounted for the frequent association of ADHD with aggression and antisocial behavior; in categorical terms, it has not accounted for the comorbidity of ADHD with ODD or CD. As a result, emotion regulatory deficits attributed to ADHD may actually pertain to underlying patterns of aggression. Unless this diagnostic association is accounted for, results are difficult to interpret.

Consistent with Barkley's conceptualization, irritability, hostility, and emotional lability and inflexibility have all been observed as part of the clinical picture for ADHD (Barkley, 1990, 1997; Cole, Zahn-Waxler, & Smith, 1994b; Landau & Milich, 1988). However, experimental research has not yielded support for any particular pattern of ADHD-related emotional deficits. Some studies have documented higher negative and positive emotional reactivity in children with ADHD than in comparison children (Maedgen & Carlson, 2000). Evidence for impaired emotional inhibition has also been found (Walcott & Landau, 2004). Another investigation failed to find higher levels of emotional reactivity yet did show that boys with ADHD were generally less empathic than their healthy peers—a provocative result given the importance of empathic responding for interpersonal relationships (Braaten & Rosen, 2000) and the linkages of certain temperamental and emotion regulatory patterns with the development of empathy (Rothbart & Sheese, this volume). Other studies have identified impaired emotion recognition in youth with ADHD, which is attributed to a failure to properly attend to emotional cues (Cadesky, Mota, & Schachar, 2000). In addition, levels of ADHD symptomatology have been negatively correlated with accurate identification of emotions in oneself and in others (Norvilitis, Casey, Brooklier, & Bonello, 2000). Overall, a range of emotion-related problems and deficits has been attributed to ADHD, yet each investigation within the small set of relevant studies has tended to utilize idiosyncratic methods and measures, leading to a lack of consistency across findings (see Cole et al., 2004, for a critique of this general state of affairs within research on emotion regulation).

Furthermore, with the exception of Cadesky et al. (2000), the aforementioned reports did not control for the presence of aggression or conduct problems or create subgroups to reflect the presence of these symptoms in their ADHD samples. A key investigation from our own laboratory argues that it is the presence of associated aggression that carries with it the presence of emotion regulation problems (Melnick & Hinshaw, 2000). In this report, we examined boys with ADHD with and without comorbid aggression, as well as nondiagnosed comparison boys, placing them in an experimental task in which frustration was elicited. Specifically, when interacting with his parents, each boy was given an engaging model to build, from which two key pieces had been excluded by the investigative team without prior knowledge of the family. Every boy and family in the sample noticed the missing pieces, yet great variability in subsequent responses occurred. We were particularly interested in emotional reactivity and emotion regulation.

Observational measures, coded from videotapes of the interchanges, revealed that the highly aggressive subgroup of boys with ADHD showed both higher emotional reactivity and lowered quality of emotion regulation strategies than did either the ADHD subgroup low on aggression or the comparison sample. Indeed, the latter two groups did not differ significantly on either emotional dimension. Because the ADHD subgroups were equated on levels of hyperactivity/impulsivity, we argued for a within-population distinction between children with ADHD with and without aggression (Hinshaw, 1987; Jensen, Martin, & Cantwell, 1997). That is, we claimed that high levels of emotional reactivity and problems in emotion regulation may not characterize all youth with ADHD but pertain only to the subgroup exhibiting concurrent aggression. From this admittedly oversimplified model, ADHD is characterized by problems in attention and impulse control and is linked to deficits in executive functions (e.g., planning, set maintenance, and set shifting) as well as clear problems in academic achievement, but it is not necessarily characterized by significant emotion dysregulation unless externalizing behavior patterns (particularly aggression) accompany the ADHD symptoms.

Clearly, such work requires replication. Furthermore, the observational coding of the emotion patterns, which constitute a strength of the investigation in one respect, is not ideal for inferring such internal emotion regulation strategies as cognitive reappraisal. That is, emotion comprises partially distinct aspects of facial displays, internal experiences, observable behaviors, and physiological response patterns; measuring only one or two of these channels will yield an incomplete picture of emotion or emotion regulation. In addition, micro-observational paradigms are required to distinguish reactivity from regulation (although some models view this distinction as potentially artificial; see Gross & Thompson, this volume). Still, the noteworthy finding was that observable reactivity (which tended to be explosive in the ADHD–aggressive subgroup) and observable dysregulation (which was characterized by a failure to use soothing, coping, or distraction strategies in this group) were specific to the subgroup with comorbid ADHD and aggression.

Overall, Barkley's theoretical model of ADHD—which posits a fundamental deficit of inhibitory control leading to problems with the display of key executive functions, including regulation of affect—has placed emotion regulation as a major facet of this disorder. Symptom lists and clinical lore also attest to the ubiquity of emotional lability, explosiveness, and difficulties in "coming down" from excitable states as part and parcel of ADHD. Yet existing research has suffered from several core difficulties: (1) a lack of attention to paradigms that can differentiate emotional reactivity from emotion regulation; (2) a failure to engage in cross-modal measurement of either form of emotion; and (3) a lack of appreciation of the *specificity* of any emotion regulation deficits to ADHD per se as opposed to conditions that are frequently comorbid with this disorder, particularly the disruptive disorders of ODD or CD. The findings of Melnick and Hinshaw (2000), however, do not entirely oppose Barkley's theory, as it may be that deficits in behavioral inhibition, when of sufficient severity, are responsible for both the emotion regulation problems and the associated aggression. Nonetheless, generalization of such findings to other paradigms tapping emotion regulation, to girls with this condition, and to other comorbid conditions is essential for uncovering specificity of linkages between clinical disorders and emotion regulatory deficits (see Hinshaw, 2003; for a review). Crucial in this regard will be investigations of high-risk toddlers and preschoolers, who can be followed prospectively through developmental periods crucial to the establishment of emotion regulation and effortful control strategies.

EMOTION REGULATION AND CONDUCT PROBLEMS/AGGRESSION

Evidence continues to mount linking poor emotion regulation, and particularly negative emotional reactivity, to conduct problems in children and adolescents. Children with high levels of negative reactivity tend to display strong and consistently aversive emotional reactions to environmental events, ranging from anger and irritability to fear (Frick & Morris, 2004). Such emotions have been linked to conduct problems and aggression both cross-sectionally (Eisenberg et al., 2001; Hubbard et al., 2002; Olson et al., 2005; Shields & Cicchetti, 1998; Silk et al., 2003) and prospectively (Bates, 1991; Caspi, 2000; Eisenberg et al., 1997). Not surprisingly, negative emotional reactivity seems to play the largest role in antisocial behaviors that themselves comprise highly aroused responses to environmental stimuli (Frick & Morris, 2004).

As noted earlier, investigators have made an important distinction between aggressive acts that occur as emotionally charged, defensive reactions to perceived threat, labeled *reactive aggression*, and those that constitute unprovoked, premeditated behaviors typically meant to achieve personal gain, labeled *proactive aggression* (Price & Dodge, 1989). Not surprisingly, high negative reactivity and poor emotion regulation are associated with reactive but not proactive aggression (Hubbard et al., 2002; Shields & Cicchetti, 1998). In particular, children who consistently exhibit reactive aggressive behaviors tend to display particular sociocognitive biases that may be linked closely with poor emotion regulation. These involve diminished capacity to attend to social cues, leading to misinterpretation and incorrect processing of social information (Crick & Dodge, 1996; Dodge & Coie, 1987). At the same time, such sociocognitive deficits tend to predict emotion dysregulation, highlighting the circular and transactional nature of emotion–cognition linkages.

Emotional arousal may also limit a child's ability to correctly evaluate potential responses to social information. Consequently, in their social interactions, reactive-aggressive children have been shown to attend selectively to signs of hostility, to take ambiguous information from social interactions and attribute hostile intentions from their peers, and to retrieve aggressive responses to perceived threat rapidly and indiscriminately (Asarnow & Callan, 1985; Crick & Dodge, 1996). Escalating displays of negative reactivity in these children are believed to contribute to their high levels of peer rejection and peer victimization, which are then likely to reinforce their hostile sociocognitive biases (Dodge, Lochman, Harnish, Bates, & Pettit, 1997). Once again, transactional patterns linking sociocognitive biases, emotion processing, and peer response characterize the developmental patterns of youth with reactive aggression.

In addition to hostile sociocognitive biases, it may simply be more difficult for a child prone to intense negative reactions to inhibit aggressive responses. In a heightened state of anger, a child is more likely to lash out at another child impulsively without considering the consequences (Hubbard et al., 2002). In fact, reactive–aggressive children exhibit more heightened physiological signs of emotional arousal than their proactive–aggressive and nonaggressive peers, suggesting that they may be "hotheaded" and physically primed for aggressive responses (Hubbard et al., 2002). It is unclear whether this arousal reflects a chronic overabundance of negative affect or a vulnerability to emotional provocation; both problems suggest the intermingling of high reactivity and low regulation. Although it might appear that reactivity would constitute the more salient dimension with respect to aggressive behavior, the intertwined nature of reactivity and regulation places a premium on paradigms that can yield more specific information on each process.

Relating to a core theme from the previous section, very little of the research on emotion dysregulation in youth prone to reactive aggression has considered comorbidity. That is, it may well be that the impulsivity characteristic of reactive–aggressive children and adolescents is most likely to occur in those who display combinations of aggression and ADHD. Once again, we caution investigators to be as specific as possible in their designations of diagnostic subgroups or associated dimensions of pathology, to prevent claims about emotion regulation–psychopathology linkages that are confounded.

Youth tending toward proactive aggression display a different sociocognitive pattern, with a proclivity for estimating considerable personal gains from aggressive behavior but failing to show the cue-reading and hostile-attribution biases characteristic of reactive–aggressive children and adolescents (for a review, see Coie & Dodge, 1998). It is therefore tempting to conclude that the sociocognitive and emotional faculties of aggressive children can be reliably distinguished based on the type of aggressive acts they tend to commit. Yet many youth referred for treatment display a combination of reactive and proactive aggression, precluding simplistic, dichotomous models.

With that caveat in mind, it appears that poor emotion regulation plays a lesser role in the commission of covert antisocial behaviors, such as stealing and lying, which are not typically characterized by heightened negative affect (Frick, O'Brien, Wootton,

& McBurnett, 1994). It may actually be the case that both proactive aggression and covert forms of antisocial behavior are characterized by *under*arousal and a lack of emotional reactivity (Lahey, Hart, Pliszka, Applegate, & McBurnett, 1993). In other words, despite the frequent overlap of multiple forms of antisocial behavior in the same individual, the dimensions encompassing planful, instrumental, and covert forms of this type of behavior may signal a more cold-blooded and less emotionally reactive style. Furthermore, in their research on antisocial children, Frick and colleagues (Barry et al., 2000; Frick, Barry, & Bodin, 2000) identified a subset of youth demonstrating callous–unemotional traits (e.g., lack of empathy, absence of guilt, and shallow emotional range), which are thought to represent precursors of the core features of classical adult psychopathy (Cleckley, 1976). Antisocial children who exhibit such a lack of emotionality tend to display more severe conduct problems than those antisocial children low on callous–unemotional traits, (Caputo, Frick, & Brodsky, 1999; Lynam, 1998; Wootton, Frick, Shelton, & Silverthorn, 1997). Research has mushroomed in the last few years on this subgroup of children and adolescents, who may be at marked risk for severe antisocial behavior later in life (see, e.g., special issue of *Journal of Abnormal Child Psychology*; Salekin & Frick, 2005).

Although this prepsychopathic, hypoemotional group of antisocial youth seem distinct from the overly reactive group described earlier, their pathways to aggressive behavior may not be entirely dissimilar. Indeed, callous–unemotional children are not only prone to covert, highly planned antisocial behaviors but are also likely engage in overt, spontaneous aggressive acts as well. In fact, disinhibition is a central feature of this psychopathic profile in children (Frick et al., 2000), just as it is a defining feature of reactive forms of aggression and just as impulsive behavior is a hallmark of adult psychopathy. Specifically, the disinhibition exhibited by children with callous–unemotional traits is characterized by low levels of fear in threatening situations and poor responsiveness to punishment cues (Frick et al., 2000; Kagan & Snidman, 1991).

Behavioral disinhibition may interact with callous–unemotional traits in a number of ways. For example, low levels of fear may result in unresponsiveness to parental discipline, ambivalence about parental or peer disapproval, and low levels of anxiety in response to one's own misbehavior (Frick et al., 2000). These factors conceivably combine to produce a child who is unafraid of being disciplined, unmotivated to behave appropriately, and unable to feel remorse for his or her misbehavior. This pattern differs from the reactive–aggressive children described earlier, who may behave aggressively in a more defensive manner due to heightened emotional reactions (e.g., anger or fear). Thus, it is possible that (1) problems with emotion regulation are characteristic of only certain types of reactive, highly aroused aggressive acts, but that (2) disinhibition represents a risk factor for reactive aggressive acts as well as those that are propelled by need for sensation seeking and a lack of particular emotions (i.e., empathy and remorse).

Although reactive–aggressive and callous–unemotional behavior patterns show disparate developmental trajectories, sociocognitive biases, and patterns of emotional dysfunction, investigations into their neurobiological bases reveal considerable overlap, at least in this early stage of research. For example, theoretical accounts of reactive aggression and psychopathy both implicate hypoactivity of the orbitofrontal cortex and amygdala (Blair, 2003; Davidson et al., 2000). The amygdala is involved in aversive conditioning (LeDoux, 1998) and may be implicated in registering and regulating expressed anger (Davidson, Putnam, & Larson, 2000). Abnormalities in this structure (or its functionality) could potentially explain both the underreactivity of psychopathic individuals, due to a lack of fear in situations with the potential for punishment, and the dysregulated anger expressions of individuals prone to reactive aggression. Although it is difficult to derive substantive conclusions about the neuroaffective processes underlying aggressive behavior from these studies, rapid improvements in imaging techniques should ultimately provide a more nuanced understanding of these two classes of externalizing behaviors.

Overall, research on linkages between emotional processes and conduct problems/ aggression is proliferating. A host of sociocognitive information-processing deficits and biases appear to characterize youth with reactive–aggressive tendencies; these are linked in transactional fashion with problems in emotion recognition and emotion regulation. Comorbidity of such children with ADHD is often, however, underexplored. Children and adolescents characterized by proactive aggression display a distinct profile of sociocognitive processes; emotion dysregulation may not pertain as readily to such youth or to the class of antisocial behavior known as covert. On the other hand, still another conceptualization of aggressive and antisocial activities, termed "callous–unemotional" and thought to be a precursor of later psychopathic tendencies, is believed to be characterized by emotional underreactivity, prompting poor response to punishment cues, and interacting with sensation-seeking tendencies to propel a pernicious course of antisocial behavior. Neurobiological studies with adults have identified anatomical and functional abnormalities in individuals prone to violent behavior but have yet to conclusively distinguish between reactively aggressive and callous–unemotional individuals. Given the exciting work occurring in this area at present, a review of the linkages between emotion regulation and conduct problems/aggression a decade from now should yield a more complete and comprehensible set of findings.

FUTURE DIRECTIONS

Space limitations preclude more than a headline review of future directions for this important area of investigation. Still, each of these points should provide for important research contributions in the coming years.

1. The emergence of risk for serious forms of externalizing behavior during infancy and toddlerhood, along with the emergence of effortful control and emotion regulation during these same developmental periods, means that prospective investigations must begin early in development. Indeed, as Tremblay (2000) has emphasized, longitudinal investigations into aggression have largely been hampered by a failure to capture the first years of life, when the origins of chronic aggression may first be evident. He argues that investigators hoping to study these complex developmental phenomena must be willing to recruit pregnant women to ensure that data collection begins in infancy, if not prenatally. This type of longitudinal design would allow documentation of the earliest displays of emotionality and regulation and enable the examination of myriad environmental factors (e.g., prenatal, perinatal, social, familial and peer-related) that may influence emotional and behavioral trajectories.

2. Relatedly, it will be vitally important to assess the complex physiological and genetic contributions to emotion regulation and externalizing psychopathology. A large and growing body of work has served to illuminate the neurological bases of aggression and other externalizing behaviors (Blair, 2004; Raine, 2002; Raine et al., 2005). Similarly, the rapidly growing field of affective neuroscience is increasingly able to provide

descriptions of the neural circuitry underlying emotion and emotion regulation (Ochsner et al., 2004; Ochsner & Gross, this volume; Davidson, Fox, & Kalin, this volume). Very little work, unfortunately, has bridged the gap between these literatures to investigate the role of basic physiological emotion processes in externalizing behaviors.

A 2000 paper by Davidson et al. did, however, make connections between research on individual differences in the physiology of emotion regulation and investigations documenting neuroanatomical and neurochemical abnormalities in individuals prone to impulsive aggression. The authors proposed that this particular type of aggressive behavior can be traced to improper function of a number of areas critically involved in the regulation of negative affect, including the orbital frontal cortex, amygdala, and the anterior cingulate cortex. Given the likelihood of substantial genetic influence on neurodevelopment, future investigations in this area will require genetically informative designs, employing multigenerational studies with twin and adoption methods. These paradigms will help distinguish the contributions of environment, genes, and the interaction between the two in the formation of both aggression, emotion regulation, and their shared neural substrates. Such investigations would benefit from the use of not only behavioral indicators but also emotion and emotion regulation paradigms.

3. The concepts of *multifinality* and *equifinality* will serve as important guides for understanding the range of developmental pathways involving emotion dysregulation. As defined by Cicchetti and Rogosch (1996), multifinality refers to the possibility of multiple developmental trajectories arising from the same original risk factor. For example, disparate outcomes characterize youth who begin life with either extremely inhibited or extremely disinhibited temperamental styles, revealing that developmental trajectories incorporate the cumulative effects of early, biologically loaded states (e.g., temperamental tendencies) with a range of environmental triggers and contexts. Similarly, early problems with emotion regulation may serve as antecedents to both internalizing and externalizing outcomes in later life, depending on a host of interactive factors and contexts.

Conversely, equifinality refers to the divergent pathways that may come to produce the same developmental outcome. For example, poor emotion regulation, poverty, violent neighborhoods, and physical abuse all represent childhood risk factors for adolescent aggression; these could work individually or jointly to yield externalizing behavior patterns. Equifinality signals that a given endstate may be the result of differing developmental processes.

In developmentally oriented investigations related to emotional processes, it will be crucial to examine the potential for both processes to be operating. In other words, (1) high emotional reactivity and poor emotion regulation may produce both internalizing and externalizing outcomes in the presence of divergent environmental triggers and contexts; and (2) divergent risk factors, including various difficulties with emotion and emotion regulation, may converge to produce aggressive behavior. Approaches that span the entire lifespan will be welcome in this endeavor (e.g., Williams, Ponesse, Schachar, Logan, & Tannock, 1999).

4. To the greatest extent possible, it will be useful for investigators to employ laboratory tasks or other paradigms that can effectively separate reactivity from regulation (see the authoritative conceptual review of Cole et al., 2004). Distinctions between these concepts are not always entirely clear; behavioral rating scales, in particular, are unlikely to provide much specificity, given the rather global nature of their constituent items as well as tendencies for adult informants to have difficulties in specifying distinct emotional or behavioral processes. Clarity may be enhanced by making greater use of

physiological measures of emotion, including indices of autonomic and neuroendo-crine reactivity and coding schemes of interactive sequences of behavior that can reliably and validly tap subcomponents of emotional processing. Still, the thoughtful conceptual model of Gross and Thompson (this volume) provides caution that emotion and its regulation may not be as distinct as sometimes claimed.

    5. Future investigations should address the role of environment and socialization in the genesis of emotion regulation. Emotion regulation strategies are thought to take root soon after birth, when infants learn to maintain affective homeostasis through the consistent responsivity of their caregivers (Tronick, 1989). Throughout childhood and adolescence, emotion regulation is likely to improve with cognitive and neurological development, but at the same time caregiver and peer environments undoubtedly influence the use of particular regulatory strategies (for a recent empirical investigation, see Chaplin, Cole, & Zahn-Waxler, 2005). It will be important to uncover the transactional processes that exist between dysregulated children and their parents or peers (see Campbell, 2002). For example, emotionally dysregulated children are likely to have charged negative responses to frustrating situations (e.g., being disciplined), which in turn may evoke a heightened negative response from parents, leading to further dysregulation from the child. It is a mistake to think that socialization experiences flow linearly to the development of emotion regulation, or vice versa; reciprocal and transactional processes are undoubtedly the rule.

    In our own study (Melnick & Hinshaw, 2000), we found evidence to support such interlocked processes, with maternal negativity during the frustration task (i.e., negative tone, disapproval, or exasperation toward the child) predicting poor overall regulation by the child. Understanding the temporal relations between such constructs is important: For instance, do child tendencies elicit negative parenting, does faulty socialization predict emotion dysregulation, or both? Better comprehension of such dyadic exchanges could produce clinical benefits, where treatments might be designed to help parents and their children learn to mutually defuse emotional confrontations.

    Finally, we highlight that many constituent processes are likely to reveal at least moderate heritability. In other words, temperamental dimensions, impulse control strategies, externalizing behavior patterns per se, and—one would assume—emotion regulatory processes all reveal genetic underpinnings, meaning that caregiver–child linkages may reflect genetic mediation as much as psychosocial transmission. Again, genetically informative designs are needed to understand the separations and linkages.

    6. As our understanding of the specificity of relationships between emotion regulation and externalizing behaviors improves, it will be imperative to design treatments that foster emotion regulation skills in disordered or at-risk children (i.e., those with aggressive-spectrum externalizing problems). A particularly appealing aspect of such intervention work is that it represents one of the few instances in human research in which experimental control can occur, given the random assignment of children (or families) to various intervention conditions. Far more use needs to be made of research design and data-analytic strategies that can allow for examination of key moderator variables and mediator processes, providing answers to such questions as (1) for whom particular interventions work most effectively and (2) what processes are most relevant for producing clinically meaningful change. Hinshaw (2002a) and Kraemer, Wilson, Fairburn, and Agras (2002) provide elaboration of the potential utility of moderation and mediation to be examined in the context of experimental work on treatment and prevention.

7. Because of the higher prevalence of serious externalizing problems among boys than girls, most of the extant literature in this area has been conducted with male samples. Thus, it is not clear whether links between poor emotion regulation and externalizing behavior (particularly reactive aggression) apply similarly to girls. Research has documented significantly lower rates of overt aggression in girls, but higher rates of relational aggression (referring, again, to means of indirectly retaliating against a peer by gossip, spreading rumors, or other means of social influence; see Hinshaw & Lee, 2003). It is unknown whether this form of aggressive behavior is associated with emotional arousal. Indeed, it is quite possible that poor emotion regulation in girls manifests in different ways than in boys, such as in depressive symptomatology (for a review, see Zahn-Waxler, 2001).

We are poorly informed, as well, to the applicability of current findings to children from diverse cultural backgrounds. A quick perusal of current literature on emotion dysregulation in children reveals the use of predominantly Caucasian, middle-class samples. Large, culturally diverse, gender-balanced samples would permit comparison of multiple emotion regulation trajectories and relationships to pathological outcomes. Raver (2004) presents an eloquent and sophisticated plea for the use of method equivalence and model equivalence tests to understand the applicability of emotion regulation strategies to diverse populations.

CONCLUSION

It is an exciting time to be working in the area of developmental psychopathology, given the convergence of information and paradigms from areas as diverse as molecular genetics and gene–environment interactions, neuroscience, socialization research, life-span approaches, and affective science to the thorny yet fascinating issues related to the development of significant behavioral and emotional disturbances in childhood and adolescence. We agree with Cole et al. (2004) that a concerted effort to deal with key measurement issues (including separation of emotion from its regulation, attention to temporal effects and contextual factors, and convergent methods and operations) is sorely needed, particularly in the application of emotion regulation strategies to psychopathology. At the same time, careful attention to such principles as continuous versus categorical models of psychopathology, specificity of emotion and emotion regulation linkages to discrete forms of externalizing behavior, and developmentally sensitive research designs are crucial to success in these endeavors. Conceptual linkages with temperament, effortful control, and contextual factors that influence the display of externalizing behavior are clearly needed in relevant research. Externalizing problems and conditions are costly to individuals, families, communities, and society at large; the promise of approaches that bring to bear the considerable power of emotion regulatory paradigms could yield unprecedented means of gaining conceptual and clinical understanding with regard to this domain of behavior.

ACKNOWLEDGMENTS

Work on this chapter was supported by National Institute of Mental Health Grant Nos. 45064 and 12009.

REFERENCES

Achenbach, T. M. (1991). *Manual for the Child Behavior Checklist 4/18 Profile 1991.* Burlington, VT: University Associates in Psychiatry.

American Psychiatric Association. (2000). *Diagnostic and statistical manual of mental disorders–Text revision* (4th ed.). Washington, DC: American Psychiatric Association.

Asarnow, J. R., & Callan, J. W. (1985). Boys with peer adjustment problems: Social cognitive processes. *Journal of Consulting and Clinical Psychology, 53*(1), 80–87.

Barkley, R. A. (1990). *Attention deficit hyperactivity disorder: A handbook for diagnosis and treatment.* New York: Guilford Press.

Barkley, R. A. (1997). Behavioral inhibition, sustained attention, and executive functions: Constructing a unifying theory of ADHD. *Psychological Bulletin, 121*(1), 65–94.

Barkley, R. A. (2003). Attention-deficit/hyperactivity disorder. In E. J. Mash & R. A. Barkley (Eds.), *Child psychopathology* (2nd ed., pp. 75–143). New York: Guilford Press.

Barry, C. T., Frick, P. J., DeShazo, T. M., McCoy, M. G., Ellis, M., & Loney, B. (2000). The importance of callous–unemotional traits for extending the concept of psychopathy to children. *Journal of Abnormal Psychology, 109,* 335–340.

Bates, J. E. (1991). Origins of externalizing behavior problems at eight years of age. In D. J. Pepler & K. H. Rubin (Eds.), *The development and treatment of childhood aggression* (pp. 167–193). Hillsdale, NJ: Erlbaum.

Blair, R. J. R. (2003). Neurological basis of psychopathy. *British Journal of Psychiatry, 182,* 5–7.

Blair, R. J. R. (2004). The roles of orbital frontal cortex in the modulation of antisocial behavior. *Brain and Cognition, 55,* 198–208.

Braaten, E. B., & Rosen, L. A. (2000). Self-regulation of affect in attention deficit-hyperactivity disorder (ADHD) and non-ADHD boys: Differences in empathic responding. *Journal of Consulting and Clinical Psychology, 68*(2), 313–321.

Cadesky, E. B., Mota, V. L., & Schachar, R. J. (2000). Beyond words: How do problem children with ADHD and/or conduct problems process nonverbal information about affect? *Journal of the American Academy of Child and Adolescent Psychiatry, 39,* 1160–1167.

Campbell, S. B. (2002). *Behavior problems in preschool children* (2nd ed.). New York: Guilford Press.

Caputo, A. A., Frick, P. J., & Brodsky, S. L. (1999). Family violence and juvenile sex offending: Potential mediating roles of psychopathic traits and negative attitudes toward women. *Criminal Justice and Behavior, 26,* 338–356.

Caspi, A. (2000). The child is the father of man: Personality continuities from childhood to adulthood. *Journal of Personality and Social Psychology, 78*(1), 158–172.

Chaplin, T. M., Cole, P. M., & Zahn-Waxler, C. (2005). Parental socialization of emotion expression; Gender differences and relations to child adjustment. *Emotion, 5,* 80–88.

Cicchetti, D., & Cohen, D. (2006). *Developmental psychopathology* (2nd ed.). New York: Wiley.

Cicchetti, D., & Rogosch, F. A. (1996). Equifinality and multifinality in developmental psychopathology. *Development and Psychopathology, 8*(4), 597–600.

Cleckley, H. (1976). *The mask of sanity* (5th ed.). St. Louis, MO: Mosby.

Coie, J. D., & Dodge, K. (1998). Aggression and antisocial behavior. In N. Eisenberg (Ed.), *Handbook of child psychology: Social, emotional and personality development* (5th ed., Vol. 3, pp. 779–862). New York: Wiley.

Cole, D. A., Michel, M. K., & Teti, L. O. (1994a). The development of emotion regulation and dysregulation: A clinical perspective. *Monographs for the Society for Research in Child Development, 59*(240), 73–100.

Cole, D. A., Zahn-Waxler, C., & Smith, D. (1994b). Expressive control during a disappointment: Variations related to preschoolers' behavior problems. *Developmental Psychology, 30,* 203–209.

Cole, P. M., Martin, S. E., & Dennis, T. A. (2004). Emotion regulation as a scientific construct: Methodological challenged and directions for future research. *Child Development, 75*(2), 317–333.

Crick, N. R., & Dodge, K. A. (1996). Social information-processing mechanisms in reactive and proactive aggression. *Child Development, 67,* 993–1002.

Davidson, R. J., Fox, A., & Kalin, N. H. (2007). Neural bases of emotion regulation in nonhuman primates and humans. In J. J. Gross (Ed.), *Handbook of emotion regulation* (pp. 47–68). New York: Guilford Press.

Davidson, R. J., Putnam, K. M., & Larson, C. L. (2000). Dysfunction in the neural circuitry of emotion regulation—A possible prelude to violence. *Science, 289*, 591–594.

Dodge, K. A., & Coie, J. D. (1987). Social-information processing factors in reactive and proactive aggression in children's peer groups. *Journal of Personality and Social Psychology, 52*, 1146–1158.

Dodge, K. A., Lochman, J. E., Harnish, J., Bates, J., & Pettit, G. S. (1997). Reactive and proactive aggression in school children and psychiatrically impaired chronically assaultive youth. *Journal of Abnormal Psychology, 106*, 37–51.

Eisenberg, N., Cumberland, A., Spinrad, T. L., Fabes, R. A., Shepard, S. A., Reiser, M., et al. (2001). The relations of regulation and emotionality to children's externalizing and internalizing problem behavior. *Child Development, 72*(4), 1112–1134.

Eisenberg, N., Fabes, R. A., Shepard, S. A., Murphy, B. C., Guthrie, I. K., Jones, S., et al. (1997). Contemporaneous and longitudinal prediction of children's social functioning from regulation and emotionality. *Child Development, 68*, 642–664.

Eisenberg, N., Guthrie, I. K., Fabes, R. A., Shepard, S. A., Losoya, S. H., Murphy, B. C., et al. (2000). Prediction of elementary school children's externalizing problem behaviors from attentional and behavioral regulation and negative emotionality. *Child Development, 71*(5), 1367–1382.

Eisenberg, N., Hofer, C., & Vaughan, J. (2007). Effortful control and its socioemotional consequences. In J. J. Gross (Ed.), *Handbook of emotion regulation* (pp. 287–306). New York: Guilford Press.

Eisenberg, N., & Spinrad, T. L. (2004). Emotion-related regulation: Sharpening the definition. *Child Development, 75*(2), 334–339.

Frick, P. J., Barry, C. T., & Bodin, S. D. (2000). Applying the concept of psychopathy to children: Implication for the assessment of antisocial youth. In C. B. Gacono (Ed.), *The clinical and forensic assessment of psychopathy* (pp. 3–25). Mahwah, NJ: Erlbaum.

Frick, P. J., & Morris, A. S. (2004). Temperament and developmental pathways to conduct problems. *Journal of Clinical Child and Adolescent Psychology, 33*(1), 54–68.

Frick, P. J., O'Brien, B. S., Wootton, J. M., & McBurnett, K. (1994). Psychopathy and conduct problems in children. *Journal of Abnormal Psychology, 103*, 700–707.

Gross, J. J., & Thompson, R. A. (2007). Emotion regulation: Conceptual foundations. In J. J. Gross (Ed.), *Handbook of emotion regulation* (pp. 3–24). New York: Guilford Press.

Hinshaw, S. P. (1987). On the distinction between attentional deficits/hyperactivity and conduct problems/aggression in child psychopathology. *Psychological Bulletin, 101*(3), 443–463.

Hinshaw, S. P. (1999). Psychosocial intervention for childhood ADHD: Etiologic and developmental themes, comorbidity, and integration with pharmacotherapy. In D. Cicchetti & S. L. Toth (Eds.), *Developmental approaches to prevention and intervention* (Vol. 9, pp. 221–269). Rochester, NY: University of Rochester Press.

Hinshaw, S. P. (2001). Is the inattentive type of ADHD a separate disorder? *Clinical Psychology: Science and Practice, 8*(4), 498–501.

Hinshaw, S. P. (2002a). Intervention research, theoretical mechanisms, and causal processes related to externalizing behavior patterns. *Development and Psychopathology, 14*, 789–818.

Hinshaw, S. P. (2002b). Is ADHD an impairing condition in childhood and adolescence? In P. S. Jensen & J. R. Cooper (Eds.), *Attention-deficit hyperactivity disorder: State of the science, best practices* (pp. 5-1–5-21). Kingston, NJ: Civic Research Institute.

Hinshaw, S. P. (2003). Impulsivity, emotion regulation, and developmental psychopathology: Specificity versus generality of linkages. *Annals New York Academy of Sciences, 1008*, 149–159.

Hinshaw, S. P., & Lee, S. (2003). Oppositional defiant and conduct disorders. In E. J. Mash & R. A. Barkley (Eds.), *Child psychopathology* (2nd ed.). New York: Guilford Press.

Hinshaw, S. P., Sami, N., Treuting, J. J., Carte, E. T., & Zupan, B. A. (2002). Preadolescent girls with attention-deficit/hyperactivity disorder: II. Neuropsychological performance in relation to subtypes and individual classification. *Journal of Consulting and Clinical Psychology, 70*(5), 1099–1111.

Hubbard, J. A., Smithmyer, C. M., Ramsden, S. R., Parker, E. H., Flanagan, K. D., Dearing, K. F., et al. (2002). Observational, physiological, and self-report measures of children's anger: Relations to reactive versus proactive aggression. *Child Development, 73*(4), 1101–1118.

Jensen, P. S., Martin, D., & Cantwell, D. P. (1997). Comorbidity in ADHD: Implications for research, practice, and DSM-V. *Journal of the American Academy of Child and Adolescent Psychiatry, 36*, 1065–1079.

Kagan, J., & Snidman, N. (1991). Temperamental factors in human development. *American Psychologist, 46*, 856–862.

Kazdin, A. E. (1995). *Conduct disorders in childhood and adolescence* (2nd ed.). Thousand Oaks, CA: Sage.

Kraemer, H. C., Wilson, G. T., Fairburn, C. G., & Agras, W. S. (2002). Mediators and moderators of treatment effects in randomized clinical trials. *Archives of General Psychiatry, 59*, 877–884.

Lahey, B. B., Hart, E. L., Pliszka, S., Applegate, B., & McBurnett, K. (1993). Neurophysiological correlates of conduct disorder: A rationale and a review of research. *Journal of Clinical Child Psychology, 22*, 141–153.

Landau, S., & Milich, R. (1988). Social communication patterns of attention-deficit-disordered boys. *Journal of Abnormal Psychology, 16*, 69–81.

LeDoux, J. (1998). *The emotional brain.* New York: Weidenfeld & Nicolson.

Lynam, D. (1998). Early identification of the feldgling psychopath: Locating the psychopathic child in the current nomenclature. *Journal of Abnormal Psychology, 107*, 566–575.

Maedgen, J. W., & Carlson, C. L. (2000). Social functioning and emotional regulation in the attention deficit hyperactivity disorder subtypes. *Journal of Clinical Child Psychology, 29*, 30–42.

Melnick, S., & Hinshaw, S. P. (2000). Emotion regulation and parenting in AD/HD and comparison boys: Linkages with social behaviors and peer preference. *Journal of Abnormal Child Psychology, 28*(1), 73–86.

Milich, R., Balentine, A. C., & Lynam, D. (2001). ADHD combined type and ADHD predominantly inattentive type are distinct and unrelated disorders. *Clinical Psychology: Science and Practice, 8*(4), 463–488.

Moffitt, T. E. (1993). Adolesence-limited and life-course-persistent antisocial behavior: A developmental taxonomy. *Psychological Review, 100*(4), 674–701.

Moffitt, T. E., & Caspi, A. (2001). Childhood predictors differentiate life-course persistent and adolescence-limited antisocial pathways among males and females. *Development and Psychopathology, 13*, 355–375.

Nigg, J. T. (2000). On inhibition/disinhibition in developmental psychopathology: Views from cognitive and personality psychology and a working inhibition taxonomy. *Psychological Bulletin, 126*(2), 220–246.

Norvilitis, J. M., Casey, R. J., Brooklier, K. M., & Bonello, P. J. (2000). Emotion appraisal in children with attention-deficit/hyperactivity disorder and their parents. *Journal of Attention Disorders, 4*(1), 15–26.

Ochsner, K. N., & Gross, J. J. (2007). The neural architecture of emotion regulation. In J. J. Gross (Ed.), *Handbook of emotion regulation* (pp. 87–109). New York: Guilford Press.

Ochsner, K. N., Ray, R. R., Cooper, J. C., Robertson, E. R., Chopra, C., Gabrieli, J. D. E., et al. (2004). For better or worse: Neural systems supporting the cognitive down- and up-regulation of negative emotion. *NeuroImage, 23*, 483–499.

Olson, S. L., Sameroff, A. J., Kerr, D. C., Lopez, N. L., & Wellman, H. M. (2005). Developmental foundations of externalizing problems in young children: The role of effortful control. *Development and Psychopathology, 17*, 25–45.

Pickles, A., & Angold, A. (2003). Natural categories of fundamental dimensions: On carving nature at the joints and the rearticulation of psychopathology. *Development and Psychopathology, 15*(3), 529–551.

Posner, M. I., & Rothbart, M. K. (2000). Developing mechanisms of self-regulation. *Development and Psychopathology, 12*, 427–441.

Price, J. M., & Dodge, K. A. (1989). Reactive and proactive aggression in childhood: Relations to peer status and social context. *Journal of Abnormal Child Psychology, 17*, 455–471.

Quay, H. C., & Hogan, A. E. (1999). *Handbook of disruptive behavior disorders* (Vol. 13). Dordrecht, Netherlands: Kluwer Academic.

Raine, A. (2002). Biosocial studies of antisocial and violent behavior in children and adolescents: A review. *Journal of Abnormal Child Psychology, 30*(4), 311–326.

Raine, A., Moffitt, T. E., Caspi, A., Loeber, R., Stouthamer-Loeber, M., & Lynam, D. (2005). Neurocognitive impairments in bos on the life-course persistent antisocial path. *Journal of Abnormal Psychology, 114*(1), 38–49.

Raver, C. C. (2004). Placing emotional self-regulation in sociocultural and socioeconomic contexts. *Child Development, 75*(2), 346–353.

Rothbart, M. K., & Bates, J. E. (1998). Temperament. In W. Damon (Ed.), *Handbook of child psychology: Vol. 3. Social, emotional, and personality development* (pp. 105–176). New York: Wiley.

Rothbart, M. K., & Sheese, B. E. (2007). Temperament and emotion regulation. In J. J. Gross (Ed.), *Handbook of emotion regulation* (pp. 331–350). New York: Guilford Press.

Saarni, C., Campos, J. J., Camras, L., & Witherington, D. (2006). Emotional development: action, communication, and understanding. In N. Eisenberg (Ed.), *Social, emotional and personality development* (Vol. 3). New York: Wiley.

Salekin, R. T., Frick, P. J. (2005). Psychopathy in children and adolescents: The need for a developmental perspective. *Journal of Abnormal Child Psychology, 33*(4), 403–409.

Shields, A., & Cicchetti, D. (1998). Reactive aggression among maltreated children: The contributions of attention and emotion dysregulation. *Journal of Clinical Child Psychology, 27*(4), 381–395.

Silk, J. S., Steinberg, L., & Morris, A. S. (2003). Adolescents' emotion regulation in daily life: Links to depressive symptoms and problem behavior. *Child Development, 74*(6), 1869–1880.

Tremblay, R. E. (2000). The development of aggressive behaviour during childhood: What have we learned in the past century? *International Journal of Behavioural Development, 24*(2), 129–141.

Tronick, E. Z. (1989). Emotions and emotional communication in infants. *American Psychologist, 44*, 112–119.

Walcott, C. M., & Landau, S. (2004). The relation between disinhibition and emotion regulation in boys with attention deficit hyperactivity disorder. *Journal of Clinical Child and Adolescent Psychology, 33*(4), 772–782.

Waschbusch, D. A. (2002). A meta-analytic examination of comorbid hyperactive-impulsive-attention problems and conduct problems. *Psychological Bulletin, 128*(1), 118–150.

Williams, B. R., Ponesse, J. S., Schachar, R. J., Logan, G. D., & Tannock, R. (1999). Development of inhibitory control across the life span. *Developmental Psychology, 35*, 205–213.

Wootton, J. M., Frick, P. J., Shelton, K. K., & Silverthorn, P. (1997). Ineffective parenting and childhood conduct problems: The moderating role of callous–unemotional traits. *Journal of Consulting and Clinical Psychology, 65*(2), 301–308.

Zahn-Waxler, C. (2001). The development of empathy, guilt, and internalization of distress: Implications for gender differences in internalizing and externalizing problems. In R. J. Davidson (Ed.), *Anxiety, depression, and emotion: Wisconsin symposium on emotion* (Vol. 1, pp. 222–265). New York: Oxford University Press.

CHAPTER 27

Incorporating Emotion Regulation into Conceptualizations and Treatments of Anxiety and Mood Disorders

LAURA CAMPBELL-SILLS
DAVID H. BARLOW

The last several decades have witnessed remarkable advances in psychosocial conceptualizations and treatments of anxiety and mood disorders. Many of these advances are grounded in cognitive and behavioral theory. As a result, maladaptive thinking and behavioral patterns have been recognized as important features of emotional disorders and as useful targets of treatment (Barlow, 2001; Beck, Rush, Shaw, & Emery, 1979). Empirical investigations of cognitive-behavioral treatments have supported the notion that altering negative beliefs and counterproductive behaviors can lead to clinically significant and durable change in anxiety and mood symptoms (Chambless et al., 1996).

Despite the positive contributions made by cognitive-behavioral theorists, significant room for improvement remains in the treatment of emotional disorders (Nathan & Gorman, 2002). Moreover, cognitive-behavioral accounts of anxiety and depression are incomplete in important ways. One shortcoming of cognitive-behavioral models is their tendency to reduce emotion to its associated thoughts and behaviors. The emphasis on cognition and behavior may have overshadowed recognition of fundamental disturbances in the way that individuals with these disorders experience and respond to their emotions. Indeed, recent work suggests that individuals with anxiety and mood disorders display a range of difficulties in dealing with emotions, including impaired understanding of emotions, more negative reactions to emotional experience, and greater difficulty repairing negative emotions than controls (Mennin, Heimberg, Turk, & Fresco, 2005; Turk, Heimberg, Luterek, Mennin, & Fresco, 2005).

Basic research on emotion regulation offers an exciting new perspective from which we can consider anxiety and mood disorders. In particular, this research provides opportunities to "fill in the blanks" left by dominant cognitive-behavioral theories. In this chapter, we suggest that individual differences in emotion regulation may relate to vulnerability and resilience to anxiety and mood disorders. We also provide numerous examples of how many clinical features of anxiety and mood disorders may be construed as maladaptive attempts to regulate unwanted emotions. Finally, we review a novel treatment approach for anxiety and mood difficulties that is informed by basic research on emotion regulation.

Before we turn to our main topics, it will be useful to clarify the definitions of terms used throughout this chapter. Our definitions of "emotion" and "emotion regulation" closely parallel those articulated by Gross and Thompson (this volume). We consider emotions to be multimodal phenomena that involve changes in subjective experience, physiology, and action tendencies. Emotions occur in response to internal or external stimuli that are meaningful to the organism's survival, well-being, or other goals. In certain situations, the subjective experience, physiological changes, or behavioral tendencies that are associated with an emotion increase the chances of successfully attaining a goal (e.g., activation of the sympathetic nervous system and the impulse to flee help achieve the goal of survival in a life-threatening situation).

When using the term "emotion regulation," we refer to cognitive and behavioral processes that influence the occurrence, intensity, duration, and expression of emotion. These processes may support upregulation or downregulation of positive or negative emotions. However, because anxiety and mood disorders are largely characterized by excessive negative emotion, we focus on downregulation of negative emotion. This choice does not imply that other forms of emotion regulation are not relevant to emotional disorders; for instance, individuals with depression may have deficient abilities to upregulate positive emotion.

We concur with Gross and Thompson's (this volume) assessment that mechanisms of emotion regulation can be placed on a continuum of automatic and effortless to conscious and effortful. Some emotion regulation processes—such as the activation of the parasympathetic nervous system to restore homeostasis following sympathetic arousal—are innate and automatic. Other regulatory strategies are likely acquired through classical conditioning, instrumental learning, or social learning (Masters, 1991). These strategies may require conscious modulation or may become relatively automatic as a result of repetition. All forms of emotion regulation (i.e., automatic, conscious, innate, and learned) may be integral to the psychopathology of anxiety and mood disorders.

One additional distinction is useful when considering the role of emotion regulation in psychopathology: the difference between modulation of acute versus more enduring states. Again following Gross and Thompson (this volume), we use the terms "emotion" to indicate acute states that occur in response to specific stimuli, "mood" to reflect enduring states that are relatively independent of specific triggers, and "affect" as an umbrella term that encompasses emotion and mood. We hypothesize that individuals with anxiety and mood disorders make counterproductive attempts to regulate acute affective episodes that lead to the exacerbation and persistence of unwanted emotion (ineffective emotion regulation). Moreover, we hypothesize that individuals with these disorders select maladaptive strategies for the long-term management of affect that contribute to the persistence of negative mood (ineffective mood regulation).

By "ineffective" we mean that an emotion or mood regulation strategy is either (1) unsuccessful in reducing the unwanted affect or (2) associated with long-term costs that outweigh the benefit of short-term reduction of affect. In contrast, we consider effective regulation to entail responses to affective states that allow for a minimization of subjective and physiological distress in conjunction with continued ability to pursue short-

and long-term goals that are important to the individual. Effective regulation probably involves a combination of selecting "good" strategies and being able to apply such strategies flexibly depending on contextual demands (e.g., Bonanno, Papa, LaLande, Westphal, & Coifman, 2004).

THE RELEVANCE OF INDIVIDUAL DIFFERENCES IN EMOTION REGULATION TO ANXIETY AND MOOD DISORDERS

Numerous empirical investigations have shown that different regulation strategies impact the subjective, physiological, and behavioral components of emotion in distinct ways. Two strategies that have been studied in detail are suppression and reappraisal. Suppression has been defined somewhat differently across studies but typically refers to efforts to hide what one is feeling (i.e., expressive suppression). At times, suppression also has referred to efforts to inhibit the emotional experience itself (i.e., trying not to *feel* certain emotions). In contrast, reappraisal entails thinking about an emotional stimulus or situation in a way that decreases emotional intensity. For example, while viewing a picture that depicts people crying at a funeral, a person might think that the deceased person is free from pain and in a good place.

Gross and colleagues have documented that individuals instructed to use suppression while viewing emotion-provoking films are successful in decreasing expressive behavior (Gross, 1998; Gross & Levenson, 1997). Suppression also decreases the subjective experience of positive emotion but has no effect on the subjective experience of negative emotion. Moreover, suppression is consistently associated with increased sympathetic arousal. Given that *decreased* arousal is a goal of efforts to regulate many negative emotions (e.g., anxiety and anger), suppression appears to have limited value as a negative emotion regulation strategy. Participants instructed to use reappraisal also are successful in decreasing expressive behavior; however, reappraisal reduces subjective negative emotion without increasing sympathetic arousal (Gross, 1998; Gross & Levenson, 1997). Therefore, reappraisal seems to be a relatively adaptive emotion regulation strategy that yields reductions in overt and subjective negative emotion without increasing physiological arousal.

Individual differences also exist in the availability and implementation of emotion regulation strategies. Due to temperamental differences or learning histories, individuals may acquire different propensities to use suppression, reappraisal, and other strategies. A study by Gross and John (2003) elucidated the impact of these differences on individuals' lives. This study showed that habitual use of reappraisal to manage emotions was associated with higher levels of positive affect overall and lower levels of negative affect overall. Reappraisal also correlated positively with interpersonal functioning and well-being. In contrast, habitual use of suppression was related to lower levels of positive affect overall and higher levels of negative affect overall. Moreover, suppression correlated negatively with interpersonal functioning and well-being. Although most individuals probably alternate between reappraisal and suppression depending on the situation, this investigation suggests that individuals who use reappraisal to manage emotions are relatively well adjusted, while individuals who rely on suppression are functioning more poorly. However, because the study was cross-sectional in nature, it is not possible to ascertain causal relationships between emotion regulation strategies, dispositional mood, interpersonal functioning, and well-being.

Gross and John's (2003) findings raise the intriguing possibility that maladaptive emotion regulation may contribute to anxiety and mood disorders. If people who habitually suppress their emotions experience increased negative emotion, decreased positive emotion, social problems, and decreased quality of life, might they also be more vulnerable to anxiety and mood disorders (especially when stress arises)? Moreover, if individuals who habitually reappraise emotions experience decreased negative emotion, increased positive emotion, better social functioning, and increased quality of life, might they also be resilient to stress and emotional disorders?

Several recent studies of clinical samples provide evidence that overreliance on suppression may contribute to anxiety disorders. When compared to control participants on self-report questionnaires, individuals with panic disorder endorsed more habitual "smothering" of anger, sadness, and anxiety (Baker, Holloway, Thomas, Thomas, & Owens, 2004). A recent study from our lab also showed that individuals with anxiety and mood disorders spontaneously used suppression more than controls when viewing an anxiety-provoking film (Campbell-Sills, Barlow, Brown, & Hofmann, in press). Finally, individuals with panic disorder reported that the suppression instructions they heard as part of an experiment were very similar to the strategies they used to manage anxiety in their daily lives (Levitt, Brown, Orsillo, & Barlow, 2004). Suppression may be particularly ineffective for these patients, given that individuals with anxiety disorders are often distressed by sympathetic arousal (Reiss, Peterson, Gursky, & McNally, 1986). In accordance with this hypothesis, we observed that use of suppression in a clinical sample correlated with increased negative affect and heart rate in response to an emotional film, poorer recovery from changes in negative affect, and decreased self-efficacy for managing future emotions (Campbell-Sills et al., in press; Campbell-Sills, Barlow, Brown, & Hofmann, in press).

Whether maladaptive emotion regulation is part of the causal chain leading to the manifestation of anxiety and mood disorders is currently unknown. However, recent evidence suggests that ineffective emotion regulation is part of the phenomenology of these disorders. More prospective research is needed in which emotion regulation is characterized for individuals who are then followed over time. Characterization of emotion regulation style should include not just use of single strategies but the ability to flexibly alter one's strategy based on contextual factors. This type of research design would allow investigation of the predictive value of emotion regulation styles in determining responses to stressors and incidence of anxiety and mood disorders.

EMOTION REGULATION AND CLINICAL FEATURES OF ANXIETY AND MOOD DISORDERS

In the previous section, we focused on suppression and reappraisal to illustrate how empirical studies of emotion regulation can inform our thinking about vulnerability and resilience to anxiety and mood disorders. In the current section, we argue that many clinical features of anxiety and mood disorders can be conceptualized as maladaptive attempts to regulate unwanted emotions. In making this argument, we incorporate a wider range of emotion regulation strategies into our discussion. We have chosen to organize this discussion of problematic emotion regulation strategies according to Gross's process model of emotion regulation (Gross & Thompson, this volume). According to this model, emotion regulation can occur at a variety of points along the temporal course of emotion generation. We assert that many of the most prominent and debilitating features of anxiety and mood disorders can be construed as problematic use of situation selection, situation modification, attentional deployment, cognitive change, and response modulation to regulate emotions. Although most of the strategies we discuss can be adaptive in certain situations, patients with emotional disorders often display an overreliance on them that maintains symptoms and disrupts functioning.

Maladaptive Situation Selection: Situational Avoidance and Social Withdrawal

All individuals regulate some of their emotions by choosing to enter certain situations and to avoid others during the course of their daily lives. For example, a person could decline a party invitation in order to prevent feelings of embarrassment that she has come to associate with social situations. Or a person could skip the Empire State Building on his tour of New York in order to avoid experiencing fear that he associates with high places.

In the case of several anxiety disorders, the use of situation selection to regulate emotion and mood becomes problematic because persistent avoidance of safe situations maintains pathological fear, negatively affects psychosocial functioning, and diminishes quality of life. The tendency to avoid situations manifests most obviously in panic disorder and the phobic disorders, when the affected individual avoids specific situations (e.g., enclosed spaces and public speaking) in order to decrease the likelihood of experiencing fear. Avoidance is a fear-regulation strategy that can be technically "effective" in the short term because it almost guarantees that the patient will not have to endure acute episodes of fear. However, avoidance also prevents habituation, or the natural abatement of fear that typically occurs when individuals confront feared situations repeatedly and stay in them for long periods of time. Furthermore, avoidance prevents people from learning that the worst-case scenario does not typically occur (e.g., ridicule does not usually happen in social situations).

Individuals with panic disorder with agoraphobia, social phobia, and specific phobia often find that their lives become limited due to situational avoidance. Their social, academic, occupational, and leisure pursuits can be severely restricted, leading to a marked decrease in quality of life. Other negative emotions may result such as frustration, sadness, and shame. Reliance on situation selection to manage feelings of fear is therefore counterproductive for many patients with anxiety disorders. Although the acute feelings of fear that would arise in certain situations are prevented, individuals often experience a net *increase* of negative emotion due to the distress and impairment associated with situational avoidance.

Avoidance also plays a role in mood disorders, where it most frequently takes the form of social withdrawal. Withdrawal from activities and social relationships may be a by-product of the anhedonia (i.e., decrease in the ability to experience pleasure) that frequently accompanies depressive episodes. Some have speculated that the decrease in activity that accompanies depression stems from adaptive functions such as conservation of resources in the face of loss (Beck, 1972) or elicitation of empathic responses from others during difficult times (Barnett, King, & Howard, 1979). It is possible that social withdrawal also is a method for regulating sadness. Individuals suffering from depression may predict that their sad feelings will worsen as a result of social activities, either because they will not "perform" well or because they will experience rejection that will worsen their self-esteem. Social withdrawal may be intended to regulate acute emotion (e.g., canceling a date in response to immediate feelings of sadness) or an enduring mood (e.g., continually staying home because one believes that socializing will provoke feelings of inadequacy and worsen overall mood).

Although social withdrawal may initially protect patients from negative social experiences, it leads to a dramatic reduction in positive experiences as individuals become further removed from their usual activities and relationships. This lack of positive experiences is hypothesized to worsen mood and decrease social support, ultimately leading to poorer health and well-being. Social withdrawal therefore constitutes a maladaptive affect regulation strategy and is often a main focus of psychosocial treatments for depression.

Maladaptive Situation Modification: Safety Signals

If complete avoidance of a situation is not possible or desirable, patients often turn to situation modification tactics to regulate negative emotions. Situation modification involves making changes to a situation that alter its emotional impact. An excellent example of situation modification is the use of safety signals. Safety signals are objects individuals use to reduce distress in feared situations. They are common across the anxiety disorders but are most widely recognized in panic disorder and phobic disorders. Examples of safety signals include anxiety medication, foods or beverages that are believed to alleviate or prevent anxiety symptoms, or cell phones that can be used if a need for help arises (Barlow, 1988).

Safety signals temporarily reduce fear and afford a sense of protection in feared situations, and therefore they can be construed as tools for emotion regulation. At first glance, use of safety signals may even seem like an effective form of emotional control—after all, these objects allow persons with excessive anxiety to enter feared situations and endure them with less distress. However, use of safety signals is counterproductive in the long term because security becomes associated with the "talisman" rather than the feared situation itself. In other words, the person never learns that the situation *itself* is safe, because safety and success are attributed to the presence of the safety aid.

To illustrate, suppose that a patient with panic disorder always takes her alprazolam bottle with her when she rides the subway. She rides the subway many times over the course of a year, which should promote habituation of the fear response to this situation. However, the patient has (consciously or unconsciously) attributed her safety in this situation to the availability of her medication, even though she has never taken a pill on the subway. One day she forgets her alprazolam at home and realizes this as she is riding through a subway tunnel. Once she is aware that the safety signal is not present, her mind and body respond as though the situation is dangerous and she has a panic attack. This experience reinforces her belief that the subway is not safe unless her alprazolam is readily available.

In this example, reliance on a safety signal prevented habituation of fear of riding the subway, even though the patient had repeatedly exposed herself to that situation. Reliance on the safety signal can therefore be conceptualized as a factor that maintains the patient's panic disorder. More generally, we suggest that use of safety signals is an example of a maladaptive situation modification that contributes to the persistence of anxiety disorders.

Maladaptive Attentional Deployment: Thought Suppression, Distraction, Worry, and Rumination

Many problematic emotion regulation strategies used by individuals with anxiety and mood disorders involve shifting attention either toward or away from the source of the negative emotion. Thought suppression involves efforts to control cognitive products such as verbal-linguistic thoughts and mental images. To make thoughts "go away," a person deliberately shifts his or her attention from the offending content onto some other target that is deemed acceptable (e.g., a "good" thought or a compensatory behavior). Thought suppression is most commonly associated with obsessive–compulsive disorder (OCD; Tolin, Abramowitz, Przeworski, & Foa, 2002); however, individuals with other anxiety and mood disorders also use this strategy to control unwanted thoughts (Beevers, Wenzlaff, Hayes, & Scott, 1999; Ehlers, Mayou, & Bryant, 2003). Most empirical studies have emphasized the paradoxical *increase* in unwanted thoughts that occurs subsequent to thought suppression (Wegner, Schneider, Carter, & White, 1987; Trinder & Salkovskis, 1994), leading to a general consensus that suppressing thoughts is counterproductive.

Individuals with anxiety and mood disorders do not attempt to suppress thoughts indiscriminately; rather, the thoughts they inhibit are negative in valence and elicit uncomfortable emotions such as anxiety, disgust, or sadness. Consistent with the general role of emotions as motivators of behavior, we argue that it is the subjective emotional experience attached to cognitions that motivates thought suppression. Therefore, thought suppression may be construed as a method of emotion regulation. More specifically, it can be considered a type of attentional deployment because it involves redirecting attention from a distressing thought to a more desirable target.

Cases of predominantly obsessional OCD offer the clearest illustration of how thought suppression may be conceptualized as emotion regulation gone awry. For individuals with clinical obsessions, certain thoughts induce an intense subjective experience involving anxiety, disgust, shame, and other negative emotions. Consider an individual who experiences repetitive, intrusive thoughts of harming a loved one (e.g., images of stabbing that person with a kitchen knife and the thought "I wish you were dead"). These thoughts produce intense anxiety and shame, and the desire to reduce these feelings leads the individual with OCD to shift her attention from the upsetting thoughts to compensatory thoughts (e.g., "I love you") and behaviors (e.g., folding her arms tightly across her chest to prevent herself from reaching for a knife).

Thought suppression may provide momentary relief from the anxiety and shame; however, research suggests that it also may produce a "rebound effect" in which more unwanted thoughts occur (Salkovskis & Campbell, 1994; Wegner et al., 1987). Rather than decrease feelings of anxiety and shame, a net increase of these emotions occurs. Moreover, thought suppression may prevent habituation to intrusive thoughts (Wegner & Zanakos, 1994) and increase the likelihood of OCD symptoms (Rassin, Murris, Schmidt, & Merckelbach, 2000), making it a problematic form of emotion regulation.

Distraction is another attentional strategy for emotion regulation that is frequently used by individuals with anxiety and mood disorders. Distraction involves reducing attention to internal or external emotional stimuli by focusing on less affectively charged thoughts or activities. For example, a patient with generalized anxiety disorder (GAD) who worries about the safety of loved ones may watch television when loved ones go out at night. Being immersed in a television program is a way to distract herself from unpleasant thoughts about loved ones getting into accidents and the feelings of anxiety that accompany these thoughts. On the other hand, a person who is afraid of flying may spend a flight playing video games to "drown out" the sights and sounds related to air travel, thereby reducing attention to stimuli that elicit fear.

Much like safety signals, distraction appears to be a beneficial emotion regulation strategy at first glance. Indeed, distraction may be adaptive when used in moderation in appropriate situations (e.g., having a cavity filled at the dentist). However, continual reliance on distraction may maintain symptoms of anxiety and mood disorders. In particular, when individuals are engaged in distraction, they are unable to effectively challenge anxious thinking or to take action to solve problems. Individuals with GAD often experience a worrisome thought ("I'm probably not going to get this report done on time") and immediately try to distract themselves, only to have another worrisome thought arise ("He will probably be mad when I tell him I can't be home for dinner tonight"). Patients report that they "hop" from worry to worry without ever resolving any of their concerns or problems. Part of treatment involves getting patients to stop and focus on their worrisome thoughts one by one, so that they can rationally evaluate them and outline actions for solving their problems. These strategies tend to be much more effective for managing feelings of anxiety in the long term as compared to distraction.

Gross and Thompson (this volume) have categorized worry and rumination as a form of attentional deployment called *concentration*, in that both of these cognitive processes involve focusing one's attention on the emotional aspects of a situation. Worry is a form of cognition that is verbal, future-focused, and imbued with a negative emotional tone. It is most prominently associated with GAD but may be present in any other anxiety or mood disorder. Mood disorders are often characterized by another form of persistent negative cognition called rumination. Rumination strongly resembles worry but usually involves dwelling on past and present negative circumstances rather than future events. It has been defined as, "thoughts and behaviors that focus the individual's attention on the negative mood, the causes and consequences of the negative mood, and self-evaluations related to the mood" (Rusting & Nolen-Hoeksema, 1998, p. 790). Worry and rumination are highly overlapping mental phenomena, as suggested by their high correlation and equally strong relationships to anxiety and depression (Fresco, Frankel, Mennin, Turk, & Heimberg, 2002).

The hypothesis that worry and rumination are attempts to regulate negative emotions is counterintuitive. Both forms of cognition seem to invite *more* negative emotion through their focus on negative events. However, research shows that many people (including those with anxiety and mood disorders) have positive beliefs about worry and rumination and view them as methods for reducing short- and long-term emotional discomfort. For example, individuals commonly believe that worrying helps them to prepare for upcoming situations, thereby helping them to avoid future discomfort (Wells, 1995; Wells & Carter, 2001). In addition, individuals with GAD (unlike nonpathological worriers) report that they use worry as a way to avoid thinking about other, more painful topics (Borkovec & Roemer, 1995). Depressed individuals perceive various benefits of rumination, including increasing self-awareness and understanding of one's depression, moving toward solving life problems, and preventing the occurrence of future mistakes (Papageorgiou & Wells, 2001; Watkins & Baracaia, 2001).

Borkovec and colleagues have advanced and gathered empirical support for the hypothesis that worry serves as a method for avoiding intense emotion and physiological arousal (Borkovec, 1994). Verbal–linguistic worry is relatively disconnected from autonomic arousal compared to mental imagery, which elicits a strong cardiovascular response (Vrana, Cuthbert, & Lang, 1986). Worrying also has been shown to reduce physiological arousal in response to laboratory stressors such as imagined public speaking (Borkovec & Hu, 1990). Thus, worrying may be a method for coping with a potential threat that prevents the somatic arousal typically associated with feared outcomes. The consequence of reduced arousal is hypothesized to negatively reinforce the process of worry (Borkovec, 1994).

The negative consequences of worrying usually outweigh any possible benefit derived from dampening the physiological arousal that would otherwise occur in response to emotional stimuli. For example, although worry is sometimes viewed as a vehicle for problem solving, it appears to lengthen decision-making times without achieving a more effective resolution of problems (Metzger, Miller, Cohen, Sofka, & Borkovec, 1990). Worry also is associated with low parasympathetic tone (Lyonfields, Borkovec, & Thayer, 1995) and may interfere with habituation to emotional material (Butler, Wells, & Dewick, 1995). Furthermore, when worry becomes persistent and uncontrollable, it often is accompanied by the symptoms of GAD (e.g., muscle tension and sleep disturbance).

Similarly, despite its perceived benefits, rumination has been shown to intensify and prolong depressed and angry moods in laboratory studies (Nolen-Hoeksema & Morrow, 1993; Rusting & Nolen-Hoeksema, 1998). Ruminative response style also predicts duration of depressive symptoms, severity of depressive symptoms, and less favorable response to treatment (Nolen-Hoeksema, Morrow, & Fredrickson, 1993; Schmaling, Dimidjian, Katon, & Sullivan, 2002). In a longitudinal study, rumination was found to mediate the relationships of other risk factors for depression (e.g., self-criticism) in the prediction of future major depressive episodes (Spasojevic & Alloy, 2001).

Individuals who worry and ruminate obviously do not deliberately seek the negative outcomes described previously. Rather, operant processes such as negative reinforcement or beliefs that worry and rumination have some value in long-term mood regulation most likely sustain these counterproductive cognitive patterns. Worry and rumination therefore may be subtle attentional forms of affect regulation that have unintended effects of exacerbating distress in the long term.

Maladaptive Cognitive Change: Rationalization

Individuals also alter the meanings they assign to emotion-provoking stimuli in order to regulate emotions. The research reviewed earlier suggests that many efforts to reappraise such stimuli are effective in reducing negative emotion (e.g., Gross, 1998). We support reappraisal as an effective emotion regulation strategy and have included it as a major component of the treatment of emotional disorders that we describe herein. In guiding patients in their efforts to use reappraisal, we help them to develop *realistic and evidence-based* reinterpretations of emotion-provoking situations. Patients find this more useful than "telling themselves" something about an emotional situation that is supposed to make them feel better. Simply thinking in a "Pollyanna" manner or rationalizing one's problems can actually be unhelpful forms of cognitive emotion regulation.

To understand why rationalization is an ineffective method for managing negative emotions, consider a student who is worried about his performance on a chemistry test. After the test, he may desperately try to provide reasons why a bad grade would not matter in order to avoid feeling anxious ("Who cares about chemistry?" "I probably won't even want to go to medical school anyway"). In this case, the person is unwilling to experience anxiety and so uses rationalization for the sole purpose of avoiding that feeling. However, the reinterpretation of the situation is invalid (e.g., the student in this example really does care about his grades and aspires to be a doctor) and therefore will reduce anxiety in a very superficial and temporary way. Rationalization differs from our use of reappraisal in treatment, which involves thinking through the likelihood of negative events and one's ability to cope in a *realistic* manner. Where the "rationalizer" might say, "This test doesn't matter anyway because I hate chemistry," the "reappraiser" might say, "I'll be disappointed if I get a bad grade on this test, but I can study harder next time and make up for it." Rationalization ultimately rings false and may hinder the individual from taking action that will help solve the problem at hand—therefore it is ineffective at resolving negative emotions and moods.

Maladaptive Response Modulation: Substance Use

Gross and Thompson (this volume) define response modulation as attempts to alter the subjective, physiological, or behavioral manifestations of emotion as directly as possible. We already have discussed the possibility that individuals with emotional disorders overuse suppression to regulate emotions. Suppression is a form of response modulation that does not appear to be particularly effective for managing negative emotions and may have undesirable consequences (e.g., increased sympathetic activation). Another problematic form of response modulation used by individuals with emotional disorders is substance use. Individuals with anxiety disorders frequently take medications that have a direct impact on physiological manifestations of emotion (e.g., benzodiazepines) and also report using alcohol and nonprescribed drugs to manage feelings of anxiety and sadness (Sbrana et al., 2005). Emotional disorders have high rates of comorbidity with substance use disorders (Kessler, Chiu, Demler, & Walters, 2005), which appears partly due to patients' efforts to "self-medicate" (Swendsen et al., 2000).

Reliance on alcohol and nonprescribed drugs to regulate negative emotions has clear costs including the legal, social, health, and occupational problems that accompany substance abuse and dependence. These costs quickly outweigh any benefit gained from short-term reduction of negative emotions. While prescribed medications are a helpful component of many treatment plans, cases also arise in which prescribed medication use is problematic. For instance, many patients with panic disorder become reliant on benzodiazepines to control the physiological arousal associated with anxiety. These patients may become unwilling to enter certain situations without taking a dose of medication. This behavior prevents the patient from experiencing habituation of fear and reinforces the fear of physiological arousal that contributes to panic disorder (Barlow, 1988). Therefore, some use of prescribed medication can be construed as a problematic form of response modulation that characterizes emotional disorders.

EMOTION REGULATION AND TREATMENT OF ANXIETY AND MOOD DISORDERS

Based in part on the emotion regulation theory and research reviewed earlier, we have developed a treatment protocol that targets three fundamental components of the major emotional disorders. We refer to this protocol as a unified treatment to convey its applicability to the full range of anxiety and unipolar mood disorders. The treatment has shown promising results in pilot studies and will soon be tested in a randomized clinical trial. A preliminary outline of the treatment appeared in Barlow, Allen, and Choate (2004) but is now considerably updated. Here we describe the conceptualization and tactics of this protocol as administered to individuals with anxiety and mood disorders. The short-term goal of treatment is modification of maladaptive cognitive and behavioral patterns (including maladaptive emotion regulation strategies), while the long-term goals are reduced incidence and intensity of disordered emotions and improved psychosocial functioning.

Following a standard educational phase common to most psychotherapeutic approaches, the three main components of the unified treatment are (1) *altering cognitive appraisals* through training in a cognitive emotion regulation strategy that is grounded in basic emotion research and traditional cognitive therapy techniques; (2) *facilitating action tendencies not associated with the "disordered" emotion* in order to create new behavioral habits that promote better functioning and eventual resolution of symptoms; and (3) *preventing emotional avoidance* or reducing patients' maladaptive attempts to regulate their emotions by avoiding uncomfortable thoughts, sensations, and situations.

Treatment involves provoking emotion through presentation of situational, internal, and somatic cues. In early treatment sessions, patients complete standard emotion inductions such as listening to music or viewing pictures that induce emotions such as anxiety, sadness, happiness, and disgust. Later in treatment, implementation of the protocol differs from patient to patient in the situational cues and exercises used. It should be noted that unlike traditional behavior therapies for anxiety disorders, "exposure" to the emotional cues is not conceptualized as the mechanism of action. Rather, successfully provoking emotions provides the necessary context for implementation of the three treatment strategies, which are described in detail in the sections that follow.

Cognitive Reappraisal

Cognitive change has been identified as one of the major categories of emotion regulation strategies, and reappraisal in particular has been shown to be a relatively effective means of achieving emotional control (Gross, 1998; Gross & John, 2003). These findings come as little surprise to clinical psychologists familiar with cognitive therapy. Since the 1970s, and under the enormous influence of Aaron T. Beck (Beck, 1972; Beck et al., 1979), clinicians have focused on the judgments that individuals make regarding events and their abilities to cope with these events. Beck first outlined the well-known "cognitive triad" of negative beliefs about the self, the world, and the future in his descriptions of thinking patterns characteristic of depression. Subsequently, the role of negative thinking was included in conceptualizations of anxiety disorders (Beck & Emery, 1985; Clark, 1986; Goldstein & Chambless, 1978).

Cognitive therapy has traditionally focused on evaluating the rationality of negative appraisals and substituting more realistic or evidence-based appraisals. This may seem like an attempt to suppress negative thoughts, and indeed it can be used in this way as Hayes and colleagues have pointed out (e.g., Hayes, Strosahl, & Wilson, 1999). Whereas we construe thought suppression as a generally unhelpful strategy, altering distorted appraisals of threat and negativity is an important goal of treatment. The emotion regulation literature reviewed previously provides clear evidence that reappraisal of stimuli before full activation of emotion has a salutary effect on the later manifestation of negative emotion (e.g., Gross, 1998). In a clinical setting, it also has been shown that patients with specific phobias who were instructed to reappraise their core threats experienced greater symptom reduction than those receiving exposure exercises without reappraisal (Kamphuis & Telch, 2000; Sloan & Telch, 2002). We therefore endorse use of cognitive reappraisal for emotion regulation, particularly in advance of emotion-provoking situations or before emotions have reached a peak level of intensity.

In our protocol, we emphasize two misappraisals that appear central to anxious and depressive thinking: (1) overestimating the probability of negative events happening, and (2) overestimating the consequences of that negative event if it did happen (e.g., Barlow & Craske, 2000). Patients are taught to recognize these appraisals and to use cognitive restructuring techniques to reappraise situations in an adaptive manner. For example, an individual with social phobia might identify numerous fearful cognitions she experiences prior to going to a party (e.g., "Nobody will talk to me"; "I'll blush and stammer if anyone does start a conversation, and it will be horrible"). Once her initial appraisal of the party is made explicit, she can determine whether her cognitions are distorted, and if so, she can reappraise the situation more realistically. In this case, the patient might recognize that she is overgeneralizing based on rare experiences of being left alone at parties and also magnifying the importance of anxiety symptoms such as blushing. This type of cognitive analysis leads to a more realistic and adaptive appraisal of the party situation (e.g., "I almost always find someone to talk to— I'm sure I will at this party too," "Even if I blush or stammer, I can still maintain a conversation and even enjoy myself"). Cognitive restructuring skills like the ones briefly illustrated in this example are practiced in advance of emotion-inducing situations, with the aim of altering the cognitive conditions under which the individual encounters emotion-provoking stimuli. This phase of treatment can provide symptom relief and facilitate application of the other treatment components in that it prepares patients to confront emotion-provoking stimuli.

Modifying Emotional Action Tendencies

As Izard pointed out in 1971, "the most efficient and generalized principles and techniques for emotion control [are] focused on the neuromuscular component of emotion striate muscle action and can initiate, amplify, attenuate, or inhibit an emotion" (p. 415). In other words, "the individual learns to act his way into a new way of feeling" (p. 410). As Barlow (1988) previously suggested, it is possible that the crucial function of exposure in the treatment of phobic disorders is to prevent action tendencies associated with fear and anxiety and to facilitate different action tendencies. Attention to action tendencies associated with various emotions constitutes a critical component of the unified treatment for emotional disorders.

While action *tendencies* may be construed as part of the actual emotional response (e.g., the impulse to flee is integral to the emotion of fear), they are typically not deterministic and therefore emotion-driven action can be considered a separate (and modifiable) event. As noted by Gross and Thompson (this volume), the ability to override emotion-driven action tendencies has important personal and social consequences. In the case of anxiety and mood disorders, this capacity is compromised and emotions govern behavior to an excessive degree. Individuals with these disorders are largely engaged in what we call emotion-driven behaviors (EDBs).

We conceptualize EDBs as behaviors that naturally emanate from certain emotional states and are adaptive in circumscribed situations. For instance, the act of running away when we become frightened is an EDB meant to protect us from whatever is frightening us. It is a behavior driven by the emotion to allow us to escape from life-threatening situations. Similarly, if something makes us angry, our action tendency may involve shouting at whoever caused the offense. Such behavior may be effective in allowing us to defend our rights against an attack. Facial expressions constitute another example of EDBs that are associated with particular emotions. Fearful, worried, and sad expressions are "behaviors" that are driven by their corresponding emotions and are adaptive in situations in which rapid communication with others is important.

An important aspect of human emotions is that because we have the ability to think about the future or the past, our thoughts can elicit emotional experiences in the absence of a situational trigger. If a person responds to the emotions elicited by thoughts about a future or past event, we can still construe the behavior as an EDB. For example, if someone with GAD becomes very worried about the safety of his family and frantically begins calling family members to see if they are safe, this is an EDB (because the behavior is driven by the emotion of anxiety). Similarly, a person with OCD may repeatedly wash her hands (another EDB) in response to thoughts of contamination and associated feelings of anxiety or disgust.

Although some EDBs (e.g., fleeing) are adaptive in a limited range of circumstances, the EDBs that characterize anxiety and mood disorders often prove counterproductive and create increasingly unfavorable conditions for the individual. These EDBs occur in response to *disordered* emotions that are excessive and/or inappropriate to the situational context. As such, these behaviors do not serve any of the positive functions of emotion (e.g., self-protection). At best, they function to regulate negative emotion in the short-term; however, as we discussed in the previous section there is usually a net increase of negative emotion in the long term when these strategies are used. Examples of EDBs associated with anxiety and mood disorders that produce such undesirable effects are escape from feared situations, social withdrawal, and compulsive rituals. Attempting to modify these EDBs is the second phase of treatment in the unified protocol.

In treatment, we present the idea that EDBs reinforce disordered emotion and ultimately maintain emotional disorders. At times patients with anxiety and mood disorders have difficulty recognizing their own EDBs because they have come to avoid most situations that would produce emotions intense enough to elicit them. Our unified treatment protocol assists patients in recognizing EDBs that occur in response both to emotion-provoking situations and to internal triggers such as cognitions, physical sensations, and emotions. Emotion-induction exercises are particularly helpful in this regard. Once patients are able to identify their characteristic EDBs, we support their efforts to refrain from these habitual response patterns. Patients identify and practice behavioral responses to situations, thoughts, emotions, and physical sensations that are incompatible with their usual EDBs.

The EDBs targeted in treatment range from obvious to subtle. An example of an obvious EDB might involve a patient with panic disorder quickly exiting a theater once he notices signs of anxiety. Because being in a theater is not a dangerous situation, the response of fleeing is unnecessary and counterproductive to the patient's goal of enjoying his leisure time. In treatment, the patient would be encouraged to override the EDB and remain in the theater. Moreover, he would be instructed to move to the center of a crowded aisle because this behavior would be even more contrary to his EDB. This alternative action conveys that the situation is safe and that there is no need to escape. We hypothesize that enacting such alternative behavior will ultimately decrease the emergence of the disordered emotion in that situation.

Another example of an obvious EDB is inactivity related to depression. An individual might wake up in a sad mood and be inclined to stay in bed all morning. Staying in bed is a behavior driven by the emotion of sadness—a feeling-state that generally causes humans to withdraw and conserve resources. Unless the patient is coping with an immediate loss, however, conserving resources is unlikely to be necessary or helpful (Beck, 1972). In treatment, a patient would be taught to view this behavior as an EDB and instructed to override it by engaging in some type of activity. Alternative actions could include taking a shower, going out for a brisk walk, or scheduling breakfast with a friend. These alternative behaviors are hypothesized to have a positive impact on the patient's emotional state and energy level. Indeed, treatments that focus solely on increasing activity levels have demonstrated efficacy for reducing depressive symptoms (Jacobson, Martell, & Dimidjian, 2001).

An example of a subtler EDB that is targeted in treatment is procrastination, which is especially prominent in GAD and mood disorders. A person may begin writing a term paper but repeatedly stop because writing the paper elicits anxious and depressive thoughts and emotions. Stopping writing is an example of an EDB because it is temporarily escaping a situation that elicits emotional discomfort. Although this "shutdown" from work provides some relief in the short term, the person usually feels worse later on because she still has the same concerns about the paper but also has additional pressure to write it quickly and feels badly about herself for putting it off. In treatment, we would increase awareness of procrastination as a maladaptive EDB and encourage alternative behavior such as deliberately starting anxiety-provoking tasks earlier than necessary.

Preventing Emotional Avoidance

Emotional avoidance is conceptualized as any strategy used to dampen the intensity of emotion during exposure to emotion-provoking stimuli. While we use the term "emotional avoidance" in treatment, these strategies are essentially methods of emotion regulation. Emotional-avoidance strategies are not always problematic; however, in the case of anxiety and mood disorders they are often used in a way that maintains psychopathology. In a general sense, continual use of emotional-avoidance strategies may prevent individuals from benefiting from the positive functions of emotion. Emotions provide us with important information about our internal and external environments, and it may be necessary for individuals to identify and understand their emotions before they decide if and how to regulate them. Beyond this general cost of sustained emotional avoidance, individuals can become reliant on avoidant tactics that reinforce disordered emotion, such as safety signals, thought suppression, and distraction.

Reduction of emotional avoidance is often considered in conjunction with modification of EDBs. As noted previously, modifying EDBs entails deliberately engaging in behavior that is incompatible with the original emotional action tendency. If a patient engages in some incompatible behavior during the course of treatment but is still not experiencing a significant level of emotion, he may be using some emotional-avoidance strategies. (This is mainly true at the beginning of treatment; of course, with sustained modification of EDBs the disordered emotion may not arise).

We address both behavioral and cognitive avoidance strategies in the unified protocol. In addition to targeting overt avoidance of feared situations, we also attempt to modify "subtle behavioral avoidance," which is essentially the use of situation modification to regulate unwanted emotions. In some cases, patients use subtle behavioral avoidance to reduce physiological arousal associated with strong emotion. For example, people with panic disorder may try to avoid perspiring by stripping away clothes or turning the thermostat down to prevent physical sensations that may trigger panic. People also use subtle behavioral avoidance to avoid subjective discomfort, such as a student planning her lunch at the cafeteria very early or late to avoid the embarrassment she feels when she runs into people she knows. As we discussed earlier, use of safety signals is another common form of subtle behavioral avoidance.

Cognitive avoidance strategies are also targeted in treatment but are difficult to identify because patients may not even be aware that they are using them. In many cases, cognitive avoidance strategies involve the use of attentional deployment to regulate negative emotions. Some common examples of cognitive avoidance strategies are distraction (e.g., reading a book, listening to music, and watching television) and "tuning out" (e.g., the person "pretends" he or she is not in the situation or does not fully engage in the experience of being in the situation).

In the unified treatment protocol, emotional avoidance is discouraged because it is a "band-aid" approach rather than a long-term solution to excessive anxiety and/or depression. Moreover, as we discussed in the previous section, emotional-avoidance behaviors can play a role in maintaining emotional disorders. During treatment, patients are taught to recognize their own emotional avoidance strategies through emotion-induction exercises. For example, a patient with social phobia who is asked to speak in front of a group might learn that she averts her gaze from audience members as a way to subtly control anxiety. Once patients have identified their usual emotional-avoidance tactics, they are instructed to refrain from them when they confront emotion-provoking situations. Behaviors that are encouraged in place of emotional avoidance vary by patient but often include doing the opposite of a usual behavioral pattern (e.g., the patient with panic disorder could wear many layers of clothes to increase sensations of warmth and perspiration or the patient with social phobia could go to lunch when the cafeteria is at its busiest). Instructing individuals to notice and focus on their subjective and somatic experience during emotion inductions also helps to counteract cognitive avoidance techniques of distraction and tuning out.

We hypothesize that instructing patients to confront emotion-provoking situations without their usual EDBs and emotional-avoidance tactics sets the stage for new learning to occur. Patients learn on conscious and unconscious levels that their negative predictions are unfounded and that they are strong enough to cope with situations and emotions effectively. In regulating their emotions, patients are taught to emphasize antecedent reappraisal of emotion-provoking situations in combination with tolerance of emotion once it has been activated. The behavioral changes they make eventually lead to fewer occurrences of disordered emotion and improved psychosocial functioning.

SUMMARY AND CONCLUSIONS

Basic research on emotion regulation can inform our conceptualizations and treatments of anxiety and mood disorders. A number of studies have already revealed the differential effects of emotion regulation strategies on dispositional mood, interpersonal functioning, and overall well-being. We have proposed that counterproductive efforts to regulate emotions are integral to the phenomenology and maintenance of anxiety and mood disorders. Many core features of these disorders (e.g., worry and behavioral avoidance) can be understood as maladaptive attempts to regulate uncomfortable or unwanted emotions. The unified treatment protocol outlined in our final section is one vision of how restructuring patients' emotion regulation habits may lead to alleviation of symptoms and improved functioning for individuals suffering from anxiety and mood disorders. Future research will examine the subjective, physiological, behavioral, and neural correlates of emotion regulation in individuals with anxiety and mood disorders, as well as test the efficacy of emotion regulation-focused treatment protocols.

REFERENCES

Baker, R., Holloway, J., Thomas, P. W., Thomas, S., & Owens, M. (2004). Emotional processing and panic. *Behaviour Research and Therapy, 42,* 1271–1287.

Barlow, D. H. (1988). *Anxiety and its disorders: The nature and treatment of anxiety and panic* (1st ed.). New York: Guilford Press.

Barlow, D. H. (2001). *Clinical handbook of psychological disorders: A step-by-step treatment manual.* New York: Guilford Press.

Barlow, D. H., Allen, L. B., & Choate, M. L. (2004). Towards a unified treatment for emotional disorders. *Behavior Therapy, 35,* 205–230.

Barlow, D. H., & Craske, M. G. (2000). *Mastery of your anxiety and panic (MAP3): Client workbook for anxiety and panic* (3rd ed.). San Antonio, TX: Psychological Corporation.

Barnett, M. A., King, L. M., & Howard, J. A. (1979). Inducing affect about self or other: Effects on generosity of children. *Developmental Psychology, 15,* 164–167.

Beck, A. T. (1972). *Depression: Causes and treatment.* Philadelphia: University of Pennsylvania Press.

Beck, A. T., & Emery, G., with Greenberg, R. L. (1985). *Anxiety disorders and phobias: A cognitive perspective.* New York: Basic Books.

Beck, A. T., Rush, A. J., Shaw, B. F., & Emery, G. (1979). *Cognitive therapy of depression.* New York: Guilford Press.

Beevers, C. G., Wenzlaff, R. M., Hayes, A. M., & Scott, W. D. (1999). Depression and the ironic effects of thought suppression: Therapeutic strategies for improving mental control. *Clinical Psychology: Science and Practice, 6,* 133–148.

Bonanno, G. A., Papa, A., LaLande, K., Westphal, M., & Coifman, K. (2004). The importance of being flexible: The ability to both enhance and suppress emotional expression predicts long-term adjustment. *Psychological Science, 15,* 482–487.

Borkovec, T. D. (1994). The nature, functions, and origins of worry. In G. C. L. Davey & F. Tallis (Eds.), *Worrying: Perspectives in theory, assessment, and treatment* (pp. 5–34). New York: Wiley.

Borkovec, T. D., & Hu, S. (1990). The effect of worry on cardiovascular response to phobic imagery. *Behaviour Research and Therapy, 28,* 69–73.

Borkovec, T. D., & Roemer, L. (1995). Perceived functions of worry among generalized anxiety disorder patients: Distraction from more emotionally distressing topics? *Behaviour Therapy and Experimental Psychiatry, 26,* 25–30.

Butler, G., Wells, A., & Dewick, H. (1995). Differential effects of worry and imagery after exposure to a stressful stimulus: A pilot study. *Behavioural and Cognitive Psychotherapy, 23,* 45–56.

Campbell-Sills, L., Barlow, D. H., Brown, T. A., & Hofmann, S. G. (2006). Effects of suppression and acceptance on emotional responses of individuals with anxiety and mood disorders. *Behaviour Research and Therapy, 44,* 1251–1263.

Campbell-Sills, L., Barlow, D. H., Brown, T. A., & Hofmann, S. G. (in press). Acceptability and suppression of negative emotion in anxiety and mood disorders. *Emotion.*

Chambless, D. L., Sanderson, W. C., Shoham, V., Johnson, S. B., Pope, K. S., Crits-Christoph, P., et al. (1996). An update on empirically validated therapies. *The Clinical Psychologist, 49,* 5–18.

Clark, D M. (1986). A cognitive approach to panic disorder. *Behaviour Research and Therapy, 24,* 461–470.

Ehlers, A., Mayou, R. A., & Bryant, B. (2003). Cognitive predictors of posttraumatic stress disorder in children: Results of a prospective longitudinal study. *Behaviour Research and Therapy, 41,* 1–10.

Frankl, V. E. (1960). Parodoxical intention: A logotherapeutic technique. *American Journal of Psychotherapy, 14,* 520–535.

Fresco, D. M., Frankel, A. N., Mennin, D. S., Turk, C. L., & Heimberg, R. G. (2002). Distinct and overlapping features of rumination and worry: The relationship of cognitive production to negative affective states. *Cognitive Therapy and Research, 26,* 179–188.

Goldstein, A. J., & Chambless, D. L. (1978). A reanalysis of agoraphobia. *Behavior Therapy, 9,* 47–59.

Gross, J. J. (1998). Antecedent- and response-focused emotion regulation: Divergent consequences for experience, expression, and physiology. *Journal of Personality and Social Psychology, 74,* 224–237.

Gross, J. J., & John, O. P. (2003). Individual differences in two emotion regulation processes: Implications for affect, relationships, and well-being. *Journal of Personality and Social Psychology, 85,* 348–362.

Gross, J. J., & Levenson, R. W. (1997). Hiding feelings: The acute effects of inhibiting negative and positive emotion. *Journal of Abnormal Psychology, 106,* 95–103.

Gross, J. J., & Thompson, R. A. (2007). Emotion regulation: Conceptual foundations. In J. J. Gross (Ed.), *Handbook of emotion regulation* (pp. 3–24). New York: Guilford Press.

Hayes, S. C., Strosahl, K. D., & Wilson, K. G. (1999). *Acceptance and commitment therapy: An experiential approach to behavior change.* New York: Guilford Press.

Izard, C. E. (Ed.). (1971). *The face of emotion.* New York: Appleton-Century-Crofts.

Jacobson, N. S., Martell, C. R, & Dimidjian, S. (2001). Behavioral activation treatment for depression: Returning to contextual roots. *Clinical Psychology: Science and Practice, 8,* 255–270.

Kamphuis, J. H., & Telch, M. J. (2000). Effects of distraction and guided threat reappraisal on fear reduction during exposure based treatments for specific fears. *Behaviour Research and Therapy, 38,* 1163–1181.

Kessler, R. C., Chiu, W. T., Demler, O., & Walters, E. E. (2005). Prevalence, severity, and comorbidity of 12-month DSM-IV disorders in the National Comorbidity Survey Replication. *Archives of General Psychiatry, 62,* 617–627.

Levitt, J. T., Brown, T. A., Orsillo, S. M., & Barlow, D. H. (2004). The effects of acceptance versus suppression of emotion on subjective and psychophysiological response to carbon dioxide challenge in patients with panic disorder. *Behavior Therapy, 35,* 747–766.

Lyonfields, J. D., Borkovec, T. D., & Thayer, J. F. (1995). Vagal tone in generalized anxiety disorder and the effects of aversive imagery and worrisome thinking. *Behavior Therapy, 26,* 457–466.

Masters, J. C. (1991). Strategies and mechanisms for the personal and social control of emotion. In J. Garber & K. A. Dodge (Eds.), *The development of emotion regulation and dysregulation* (pp. 182–207). Cambridge, UK: Cambridge University Press.

Mennin, D. S., Heimberg, R. G., Turk, C. L., & Fresco, D. M. (2005). Preliminary evidence for an emotion dysregulation model of generalized anxiety disorder. *Behaviour Research and Therapy, 43,* 1281–1310.

Metzger, R. L., Miller, M. L., Cohen, M., Sofka, M., & Borkovec, T. D. (1990). Worry changes decision-making: The effects of negative thoughts on cognitive processing. *Journal of Clinical Psychology, 46,* 78–88.

Nathan, P. E., & Gorman, J. M. (2002). *A guide to treatments that work* (2nd ed.). New York: Oxford University Press.

Nolen-Hoeksema, S., & Morrow, J. (1993). Effects of rumination and distraction on naturally occurring depressed mood. *Cognition and Emotion, 7,* 561–570.

Nolen-Hoeksema, S., Morrow, J., & Fredrickson, B. L. (1993). Response styles and duration of depressed moods. *Journal of Abnormal Psychology, 102,* 20–28.

Papageorgiou, C., & Wells, A. (2001). Metacognitive beliefs about rumination in recurrent major depression. *Cognitive and Behavioral Practice, 8,* 160–164.

Rassin, E., Murris, P., Schmidt, H., & Merckelbach, H. (2000). Relationships between thought-action fusion, thought suppression, and obsessive–compulsive symptoms: A structural equation modeling approach. *Behaviour Research and Therapy, 38,* 889–897.

Reiss, S., Peterson, R. A., Gursky, D. M., & McNally, R. J. (1986). Anxiety sensitivity, anxiety frequency, and the prediction of fearfulness. *Behaviour Research and Therapy, 24,* 1–8.

Rusting, C. L., & Nolen-Hoeksema, S. (1998). Regulating responses to anger: Effects of rumination and distraction on angry mood. *Journal of Personality and Social Psychology, 74,* 790–803.

Salkovskis, P. M., & Campbell, P. (1994). Thought suppression in naturally occurring negative intrusive thoughts. *Behaviour Research and Therapy, 32,* 1–8.

Sbrana, A., Bizzarri, J. V., Rucci, P., Gonnelli, C., Doria, M. R., Spagnoli, S., et al. (2005). The spectrum of substance use in mood and anxiety disorders. *Comprehensive Psychiatry, 46,* 6–13.

Schmaling, K. B., Dimidjian, S., Katon, W., & Sullivan, M. (2002). Response styles among patients with minor depression and dysthymia in primary care. *Journal of Abnormal Psychology, 111,* 350–356.

Sloan, T., & Telch, M. J. (2002). The effects of safety-seeking behavior and guided threat reappraisal on fear reduction during exposure: An experimental investigation. *Behaviour Research and Therapy, 40,* 235–251.

Spasojevic, J., & Alloy, L. B. (2001). Rumination as a common mechanism relating depressive risk factors to depression. *Emotion, 1,* 25–37.

Swendsen, J. D., Tennen, H., Carney, M. A., Affleck, G., Willard, A., & Hromi, A. (2000). Mood and alcohol consumption: An experience sampling test of the self-medication hypothesis. *Journal of Abnormal Psychology, 109,* 198–204.

Tolin, D. F., Abramowitz, J. S., Przeworski, A., & Foa, E. B. (2002). Thought suppression in obsessive–compulsive disorder. *Behaviour Research and Therapy, 40,* 1255–1274.

Trinder, H., & Salkovskis, P. M. (1994). Personally relevant intrusions outside the laboratory: Long-term suppression increases intrusion. *Behaviour Research and Therapy, 32,* 833–842.

Turk, C. L., Heimberg, R. G., Luterek, J. A., Mennin, D. S., & Fresco, D. M. (2005). Emotion dysregulation in generalized anxiety disorder: A comparison with social anxiety disorder. *Cognitive Therapy and Research, 29,* 89–106.

Vrana, S. R., Cuthbert, B. N., & Lang, P. J. (1986). Fear imagery and text processing. *Psychophysiology, 23,* 247–253.

Watkins, E., & Baracaia, S. (2001). Why do people ruminate in dysphoric moods? *Personality and Individual Differences, 30,* 723–734.

Wegner, D. M., Schneider, D. J., Carter, S. R., & White, T. L. (1987). Paradoxical effects of thought suppression. *Journal of Personality and Social Psychology, 52,* 5–13.

Wegner, D. M., & Zanakos, S. (1994). Chronic thought suppression. *Journal of Personality, 62,* 615–640.

Wells, A. (1995). Meta-cognitions and worry: A cognitive model of generalized anxiety disorder. *Behavioural and Cognitive Psychotherapy, 23,* 301–320.

Wells, A., & Carter, K. (2001). Further tests of a cognitive model of generalized anxiety disorder: Metacognitions and worry in generalized anxiety disorder, and panic disorder, social phobias, depression, and non patients. *Behavior Therapy, 32,* 85–102.

CHAPTER 28

Alcohol and Affect Regulation

KENNETH J. SHER
EMILY R. GREKIN

> Wine removes the cares pressing upon the minds of sorrowing mortals who,
> when filled with this juice of the grape, no longer need sleep and no longer
> remember their daily miseries. There is no other like cure for all their troubles.
> —EURIPIDES, *Bacchae* (~450 B.C.)

Historians and anthropologists have documented the prominent role of alcohol in the daily life of humans across diverse societies from the beginning of recorded history (Poznanski, 1959; Roueché, 1960). Indeed, there appears to be considerable evidence that many Neolithic cultures were well acquainted with alcohol and, writing in 1960, Berton Roueché noted that "all but three of the numerous Stone Age cultures that have survived into modern times have demonstrated an indigenous familiarity with alcohol" (p. 6). Thus, when we begin to examine the role of alcohol consumption in human behavior, we should appreciate that we are looking at a phenomenon that has been a significant part of human experience for thousands of years. In this chapter we provide an overview of research addressing two interrelated questions:

1. What are the effects of alcohol on emotion and other affective states?
2. To what extent and under what conditions do people use alcohol to regulate emotions and affect?

Toward these goals, we first consider the short- and long-term affective consequences of alcohol consumption, as well as those variables that moderate and mediate the alcohol/affect relation. We then consider relations between affective states and drinking drawing on general population surveys, comorbidity studies, experimental studies of emotion manipulation and drinking, studies of daily drinking and affect, and research on emotion and alcoholic relapse.

A GENERAL PERSPECTIVE
ON THE PSYCHOPHARMACOLOGY OF ALCOHOL

Before describing the relation between alcohol consumption and various affective states, we briefly discuss some general issues regarding the pharmacology of alcohol. Specifically, we wish to highlight the fact that the term "alcohol consumption" indexes a host of variables and that, when considering the effects of alcohol consumption, a number of parameters should be considered in order to specify the types of effects that might be expected from a given dose of ethanol.

Like all drugs, the effects of alcohol tend to be dose dependent. Typically, a "dose" is defined as the amount of alcohol administered (e.g., grams of pure ethanol per kilogram body weight) or the resulting blood alcohol concentration (BAC). Moreover, the effect of alcohol on the ascending limb of the BAC curve (i.e., when BAC is rising) often differs from the effect observed when BAC is falling, even at comparable BACs. Holdstock and de Wit (1998) reviewed existing studies examining the effect of BAC limb and dose on a variety of measures. They concluded that "at high doses, and during the descending limb of the alcohol dose-response curve, ethanol typically produces sedative-like effects. However, at low doses, and during the ascending limb, ethanol often has stimulant-like effects" (Holdstock & de Wit, 1998, p. 1903). In other words, limb effects appear to be dose dependent with the descending limb associated with sedation at higher doses. Presumably, most drinkers drink for immediate (i.e., rising limb) effects which are most proximal to consumption (and associated with greater reward). Punishing, sedative effects, however, are likely to be experienced by heavier drinkers, but these are somewhat delayed. These biphasic effects set up an inherent paradox for the drinker who uses alcohol as a response modulation strategy; although alcohol can bring about short-term emotion regulation it can also have a "rebound" effect—ultimately amplifying initial negative emotions.

Beyond the pharmacological effects of alcohol, beliefs about the consequences of alcohol consumption can be an important determinant of its affective and behavioral consequences. Marlatt, Demming, and Reid (1973) were the first researchers to demonstrate that expectancy (i.e., believing one has or has not consumed alcohol) can have powerful effects on behavior. They did this by experimentally crossing expected and actual beverage content so that the pharmacological effects of alcohol, the belief that one has consumed alcohol, and their interaction could be independently estimated (i.e., a balanced placebo design). Since then, numerous studies have demonstrated the role of expectancies on both internal affective states and observable behavior. Although, overall, the effect of expectancy on mood is small, expectancy does appear to increase the incidence of illicit social behaviors, supporting the hypothesis that expectancy provides an attributional excuse to engage in desired but socially prohibited acts (see Hull & Bond, 1986, for a review). These findings suggest that nonpharmacological aspects of drinking can serve an emotion regulation function to the extent they affect appraisal or other cognitive emotion regulation strategies.

Social context also plays a role in determining the affective consequences of drinking. In general, group drinking contexts promote self-reported euphoria and other positive emotions while solitary drinking promotes sedation and dysphoria (Doty & de Wit, 1995; Pliner & Cappell, 1974; Sher, 1985; Warren & Raynes, 1972). These findings suggest that the effectiveness of alcohol consumption as an emotion regulation strategy may depend on social context, with solitary drinking (itself, an indicator of a problematic drinking) a less effective emotional regulation strategy than social drinking.

Another important consideration in the alcohol/affect relationship is the frequent coadministration of other drugs (especially nicotine but also marijuana, cocaine, caffeine, and others) (see Sher, Wood, Richardson, & Jackson, 2005). Unfortunately, relatively few laboratory-based studies in humans coadminister alcohol with other psychoactive drugs. Notably, while some alcohol/drug interactions (e.g., interactions with nicotine) appear to result in reduced levels of intoxication, others (e.g., interactions with marijuana) appear to increase intoxication (or at least impairment). In the case of cocaine, simultaneous use produces a novel metabolic by-product (cocaethylene) that appears to have psychoactive properties of its own. Given that existing literature suggests that the use of multiple substances is common and that there are important alcoholx other drug interactions (Sher et al., 2005), understanding the real-world role of alcohol in regulating emotions and other affective states may require a more extensive consideration of other drugs that are concurrently used with alcohol.

It should be emphasized that there is great individual variation in susceptibility to intoxication due to both metabolic and pharmacodynamic factors (Ramchandani, Bosron, & Li, 2001a; Ramchandani, Kwo, & Li, 2001b). Many individual-difference variables have been studied as moderators of alcohol response, including genetic variation (indexed by family history and, more recently, by allelic variation in several candidate genes), personality traits (especially those associated with disinhibition, aggression, and negative emotionality), alcohol outcome expectancies, and cognitive functioning (especially those related to executive functioning) (see recent review by Sher & Wood, 2005). For present purposes, it is reasonable to assume that there are likely to be large individual differences in alcohol effects on a range of affective states as a function of dispositional variables. Further, it is likely that these differences are partially heritable and may relate to the predisposition to use alcohol as an emotion regulation strategy. That is, the degree to which alcohol is effective in altering emotional states is an important individual difference that likely influences whether someone uses alcohol as a response-modulation strategy.

THE EFFECT OF ALCOHOL ON AFFECTIVE STATES

Despite the prominent role of alcohol in the history of humankind, formal study of the psychological effects of alcohol is a relatively recent phenomenon. The scientific footing for the study of alcohol as an emotion regulation strategy was established by Masserman and Yum (1946) who conducted experiments on alcohol and "experimental neuroses" in cats. These studies demonstrated that fear and avoidance behavior could be reduced by the administration of alcohol. A decade later, Conger (1956) proposed a "drive-reduction" theory of alcohol. This theory (which would later be renamed the tension-reduction hypothesis [TRH]) posited that alcohol reduced "drives" (i.e., emotional–physiological states) associated with avoidance. Conger's theory, strongly entrenched in Hullian learning concepts, was specific to approach–avoidance situations and has held up to empirical scrutiny reasonably well . In contrast, studies which have defined "tension" more broadly (e.g., general life stress as opposed to approach–avoidance conflict), have not always found an alcohol/tension-reduction relationship (e.g., Greeley & Oei, 1999; Sher, 1987; Stritzke, Lang, & Patrick, 1996). Throughout most of the second half of the 20th century, the TRH and related concepts such as the "self-medication" hypothesis (e.g., Khantzian, 1990) were the dominant explanations for drinking behavior and figured predominantly not only in the alcohol literature but in more general behavioral explanations of drinking and alcoholism from both behavioral (e.g., Bandura, 1969) and psychodynamic (e.g., Khantzian, 1990) perspectives.

EFFECTS OF ALCOHOL ON EMOTIONAL STATES: DIRECT AND INDIRECT EFFECTS

The pharmacological agent, ethyl alcohol, has numerous effects on body systems, but for present purposes we restrict our discussion to brain systems that affect emotion and cognition. From a learning perspective, we can classify alcohol effects into three broad classes: (1) positive reinforcing effects (e.g., euphoric and arousing), (2) negative reinforcing effects (e.g., anxiolytic and antidepressant), and (3) punishing effects (e.g., depressant). For purposes of discussion, it is also useful to consider two broad classes of actions: (1) direct effects of alcohol on brain mechanisms controlling emotions (and on peripheral organs providing proprioceptive feedback on arousal) and (2) indirect effects of alcohol on emotions mediated via brain mechanisms regulating cognition (e.g., attention, memory, and appraisal). Although these two perspectives are not incompatible with each other, they tend to invoke different explanatory mechanisms and levels of analysis. Specifically, direct alcohol effects tend to invoke neurochemical explanations while indirect alcohol effects invoke higher-level cognitive theories.

Effects of Alcohol on Emotions: Direct Effects on Central Brain Mechanisms Underlying Various Affective States

It is sometimes said that alcohol is a "dirty drug" because it has effects on multiple, distinct neuropharmacological systems. Positively reinforcing effects of alcohol, such as euphoria and increased arousal, are thought to be largely associated with enhanced monoaminergic (e.g., dopamine and norepinephrine) and opioid peptide activity (National Institute on Alcohol Abuse and Alcoholism [NIAAA], 1997). For example, dopamine has been both directly and indirectly (i.e., neuromodulation of other neurotransmitters) implicated in the motor stimulation and euphoric effects of alcohol (Weiss & Koob, 1991). These dopamine-mediated effects have been found in both self-administration and injection studies and can be traced to ethanol-sensitive neurons in the "shell" of the nucleus accumbens (Di Chiara, 1997). The subjective experience of arousal in response to alcohol consumption has been linked to norepinephrine. Specifically, alcohol has a biphasic effect on norepinephrine; low doses of alcohol increase norepinephrine levels and alertness while high doses decrease norephinephrine levels and alertness (Fromme & D'Amico, 1999). Norepinephrine is concentrated in the locus coeruleus and may underlie the stimulant effects of low alcohol doses on the ascending limb of the blood alcohol curve (Fromme & D'Amico, 1999). Opioid peptides are also thought to partially mediate alcohol's positively reinforcing effects (Kranzler & Anton, 1994; Nevo & Hamon, 1995). Opioids have analgesic and reward properties that can lead to craving and that appear to be blocked by receptor antagonists such as naltrexone (Froehlich, 1997). While opioid neurons are found in a variety of different brain regions, those in the hypothalamus and pituitary gland may be particularly sensitive to alcohol administration (Fromme & D'Amico, 1999).

Alcohol's anxiolytic, sedative, and motor-impairing effects are thought to be mediated by alcohol's effects on the gamma-aminobutyric acid ($GABA_A$) receptor. Notably, drugs that facilitate GABA-ergic activity via their actions on subunits of the $GABA_A$

complex (e.g., benzodiazepines, alcohol, and other sedative drugs) have been shown to increase sedative and motor impairment effects in animals and to decrease passive avoidance (i.e., reduce conditioned inhibition or conflict) (Fromme & D'Amico, 1999). Moreover, drugs that act as "inverse agonists" and antagonists at the $GABA_A$ receptor have demonstrated the ability to counteract anxiolytic and impairing psychomotor effects of alcohol (Wood, Vinson, & Sher, 2001). $GABA_A$ receptors are spread throughout the brain and therefore affect multiple types of behaviors (sedation, motor impairment, anxiolysis, etc.) but $GABA_A$-mediated anxiolytic effects appear to be most associated with the distribution of the a-2 subunit in the hippocampus and cortical regions (Mohler, Fritschy, & Rudolph, 2002).

Although most rewarding effects of alcohol are thought to be centrally mediated, it is possible that some effects are mediated peripherally. For example, alcohol has been shown to have beta-blocking activity and, consequently, could reduce peripheral arousal (e.g., heart palpitation and tremor) in stressful situations, especially where physiological arousal itself creates an escalating cycle of arousal/anxiety (e.g., performance anxiety; see Sher, 1987, for a discussion of this issue). It should also be noted that one of alcohol's most punishing acute subjective effects (e.g., flushing) appears to be due to intermediary by-products of ethanol metabolism, (specifically, acetaldehyde, a toxic metabolite of alcohol), and it appears that many of the effects of acetaldehyde are manifested in the periphery.

Effects of Alcohol on Emotions: Indirect Effects Mediated via Effects on Cognitive Brain Mechanisms

A number of current theories suggest that alcohol's effects on emotion are mediated by cognition. We briefly describe three of these theories, namely Steele and Josephs's (1990) attention-allocation (or "alcohol myopia") theory, Hull's (1981) "self-awareness" theory, and Sayette's (1993a) "appraisal-disruption" theory. Common to all these theories is the recognition that the emotional effects of alcohol are highly variable, not only *between* individuals but also across time and situations *within* individuals, and that contextual effects are critical in understanding this variability. These cognitive theories place primary emphasis on the proposition that alcohol-related disruption of information processing lies at the heart of alcohol's effects on emotion.

Steele and Josephs's (1990) "alcohol myopia" theory proposes that alcohol's effects on emotion are mediated by attentional processes. Specifically, alcohol is posited to result in a narrowing of the scope of attention, limiting the ability to attend to multiple cues. Under these circumstances, only those situational cues that are most immediate and salient are likely to be attended to. As we have recently discussed (Sher & Wood, 2005; Sher et al., 2005), this hypothesis has received support across multiple domains and provides a coherent explanation as to how alcohol can lead to either an animated, euphoric, celebratory experience or to a depressive, "crying in one's beer" experience. For example, Steele and Josephs (1990) have shown that alcohol consumption followed by distracting pleasant or neutral stimuli can attenuate stress responses, but when no distraction is present, alcohol consumption either no longer reduces anxiety or produces anxiogenic effects.

Sayette's (1993a) appraisal-disruption theory proposes that alcohol disrupts the appraisal of a situation as benign or stressful by "constraining the spread of activation of information previously stored in nodes in a memory network" (Sayette, 1999, p. 260). That is, alcohol serves to diminish the elaboration and integration of new information that typically takes place when one is confronted with a stressor. According to Sayette, this perspective predicts that stress-reducing effects should be strongest when a stressor is experienced following (rather than prior to) intoxication because disruption of appraisal is more likely. In contrast, if alcohol is consumed following a stressor, little effect should be found. Although there have only been four studies directly comparing the temporal ordering of alcohol consumption and stressor exposure, this prediction is supported by existing research (Sayette, 1993a, 1999; Sayette, Martin, Perrott, Wertz, & Hufford, 2001).

Hull's (1987) "self-awareness" theory posits that alcohol interferes with cognitive processes necessary for maintaining a self-aware state. That is, under conditions of intoxication, individuals are less able to encode the self-relevance of various threats. According to this theory, alcohol should have greatest stress-reducing effects on stressors that are self-relevant (e.g., personal failure) and in individuals who are highly self-aware. Hull (1987) reviews support for this perspective which includes data demonstrating that (1) alcohol reduces self-awareness (e.g., as indicated by lower levels of self-referential speech, poorer recall of self-relevant words) and (2) alcoholics high in dispositional self-awareness are particularly likely to relapse when they experience stressors that are self-relevant.

Based on these cognitive theories, recent research has attempted to identify mediators of the alcohol/emotion relationship. For example, Curtin, Patrick, Lang, Cacioppo, and Birbaumer (2001, p. 527) related attentional processing (using the P3 component of the event-related potential) to conditions where threat cues were presented in isolation versus divided attention (visual–motor task plus threat cues) and fear was assessed using fear-potentiated startle and response latency measures. During the divided-attention task (but not during the threat cue only condition) individuals receiving a moderately high dose of alcohol had both attenuated P3 responses and attenuated fear indices relative to the no-alcohol condition and impairments in cognitive processes seemed to account for reductions in fear responses and behavioral inhibition.

General Findings of Alcohol Effects on Emotions

Extensive research on alcohol/affect relationships has yielded numerous findings. Although there are a number of consistencies in the literature (described below), there are also numerous inconsistencies. Many of these inconsistencies are undoubtedly attributable to the myriad methodological issues surveyed previously. Others are likely due to specific aspects of experimental protocols and measures of emotion. As noted by Lang, Patrick, and Stritzke (1999), the overwhelming majority of research on alcohol and affect focuses on negative emotions (especially anxiety), in large part because many of these studies were originally motivated by the tension-reduction hypothesis. Moreover, until relatively recently, there were few standardized protocols for assessing positive emotions. Despite seeming variability in findings noted by many reviewers (e.g., Greeley & Oei, 1999; Lang et al., 1999; Sayette, 1993a; Sher, 1987; Steele & Josephs, 1990; Stritzke et al., 1996), several general conclusions can be put forward. First, the effects of alcohol on negative emotions are most clearly demonstrated when a specific, discrete stimulus is used to induce a negative emotional state (e.g., threat of harm) and when intoxicating doses of alcohol are administered. Moreover, and consistent with cognitive theories, alcohol's effects on negative emotions appear to be somewhat context dependent, at least at lower doses. (Presumably at high doses, the direct pharmacological effects are prepotent and less likely to be moderated by environmental factors.) It is also important to note that alcohol-induced attenuation of negative emotions has been observed across multiple response domains (e.g., self-report, autonomic reactivity, facial expressions, and behavioral avoidance) (Greeley & Oei, 1999; Sher, 1987). (Although existing studies of alcohol effects on affect-modulated startle have yielded negative findings [Curtin, Lang, Patrick, & Stritzke, 1998; Stritzke, Patrick, & Lange, 1995], these studies have employed lower doses of alcohol than those associated with robust effects.) Finally, it bears reemphasizing that there are large individual differences in alcohol effects and that some of this variability appears related to risk for developing alcoholism (Newlin & Thomson, 1990; Sher, 1991; Sher & Wood, 2005), perhaps because alcohol is a more effective response modulator for some.

ALCOHOL CAN (AND PROBABLY DOES) CAUSE EMOTIONAL DYSREGULATION

A growing body of evidence suggests that alcohol use can increase underlying affective disturbance and disrupt cognitive functions important in emotional self-regulation. Support for this proposition comes from studies that find associations between alcohol use and both short- and long-term emotional change. Although the research literature tends to focus on affective changes that occur as a function of neuroadaptation to alcohol (e.g., see discussion of allostasis below), the recursive model described by Gross and Thompson (this volume) suggests that the consequences of intoxication can have profound effects on emotion. That is, intoxication-related behavioral acts can elicit negative reactions from others as well as from the self (e.g., regret over violating self-standards or embarrassment or shame over a public transgression), leading to negative affective consequences.

Short-Term Affective Dysregulation

Although alcohol consumption is presumably motivated by the acute positively and negatively reinforcing effects of alcohol, indulgence can also lead to punishment in the form of hangover. Hangover is an acute condition marked by dysphoria, including anxiety, depression, and a range of somatic symptoms (headache, fatigue, sleep disturbance, etc.; Slutske, Piasecki, & Hunt-Carter, 2003). Hangover is a well-known state to many drinkers and represents short-term perturbations in affective state that often follow alcohol consumption. These short-term changes may have important consequences for the drinker. Indeed, it is assumed that postconsumption dysphoria can motivate relief drinking (i.e., "hair of the dog") and that such a process can be significant in the etiology of alcohol use disorders (Piasecki, Sher, Slutske, & Jackson, 2005).

Long-Term Affective Dysregulation

Although short-term rebound effects from drinking, such as hangover, may be common, they are often isolated incidents in social drinkers. In contrast, heavy, chronic drinkers often experience a range of persistent changes relevant to emotional functioning. First, alcohol withdrawal symptoms are strongly associated with affective disturbance, primarily anxiety (e.g., Sellers, Sullivan, Somer, & Sykora, 1991) potentially setting up a vicious cycle whereby chronic, heavy alcohol use leads to affective disturbance which then motivates further drinking. Second, some forms of anxiety and mood disorders appear to be "alcohol induced" and differential diagnosis of substance-induced mood disorders is considered critical for nosology and treatment (American Psychiatric Association, 1994, 2000; Schuckit, 1994). Anxiety and mood disorders that remit spontaneously after a short period (less than a month) of abstinence and that only appear in the context of ongoing substance use should be considered substance induced and not "independent." Third, even ostensible "independent" anxiety and mood disorders often appear to temporally follow the occurrence of an alcohol use disorder (and this is especially true in the case of depression, Kessler et al., 1997). For example, in a multinational pool of five epidemiological studies (Merikangas et al., 1996), it was found that among those with co-occurring alcohol dependence and depression, 20% reported that the onset of the disorders occurred together, 38% reported that depression came first, and 42% reported that alcohol dependence came first (the study did not compare order of onset for anxiety disorders and alcohol dependence).

Notably, these epidemiological studies assume the accuracy of retrospective symptom reporting when trying to sequence disorders that may have been experienced decades earlier. Moreover, there can be co-occurrence between alcohol consumption and minor symptomatology prior to any formal symptom onset and many symptoms (e.g., tolerance to alcohol and worry) can have insidious onsets and be difficult to date. Unfortunately, few prospective studies of alcohol use disorder (AUD) comorbidity exist to help unravel the direction of effect. Those studies that do exist typically cover early periods of development (e.g., Costello, Erkanli, Federman, & Angold, 1999), when AUD symptomatology has not yet occurred, or begin later in development (e.g., Kushner, Sher, & Erickson, 1999) when extensive symptomatology is already in place. Moreover, Costello et al. (1999) found that comorbidity processes can begin in childhood, further highlighting the difficulty of disentangling cause and effect using retrospective reports in adults. Nevertheless, existing data do suggest that a prior diagnosis of alcohol dependence predicts both onset and persistence of anxiety disorders (Kushner et al., 1999). However, even well-conducted prospective studies beginning early in development are not capable of disentangling the direction of effect between alcohol involvement and psychiatric symptomatology as it is possible that third variables such as a common genetic diathesis influence both alcohol involvement and comorbid anxiety and mood disorders.

Putative Mechanisms of Alcohol-Induced Chronic Affective Changes

Several alternative mechanisms can be used to explain alcohol-related changes in emotional functioning. Chronic adaptation to alcohol can result in neuropharmacological changes associated with anxiety and depression. Typically, these chronic effects are the opposite of acute effects. For example, acute effects of ethanol are associated with increased GABA-ergic activity and anxiety reduction while chronic effects are associated with decreased GABA-ergic activity and heightened anxiety. In addition, acute alcohol effects are associated with increased dopaminergic and opioid activity and associated heightened reward while chronic effects are associated with decreased dopaminergic and opioid activity and associated dysphoria and/or anhedonia (see Fromme & D'Amico, 1999).

A general perspective on changes associated with the chronic use of various drugs of abuse is termed "allostasis." Allostasis refers to adaptive homeostatic changes that occur in response to repeated drug challenges (e.g., Koob & LeMoal, 2001). According to this theory, an organism responds to drug challenges by producing counter-directional (i.e., homeostatic) responses that increase over time. Allostasis explains the phenomenon of acquired tolerance, the tendency for a given dose of a drug to elicit progressively less response over time as proposed by Solomon and Corbit (1974) in their opponent-process theory and Siegel and colleagues (e.g., Siegel, Baptista, Kim, McDonald, & Weise-Kelly, 2000) in their Pavlovian account of tolerance development. However, the allostatic perspective goes further than opponent process and Pavlovian perspectives on tolerance that appear to assume a homeostatic or hedonic setpoint that the organism maintains over time, only intermittently perturbed by acute alcohol consumption. Specifically, the allostatic perspective posits that repeated homeostatic challenges present an adaptive burden and result in a shift of "setpoint" in the direction of the opponent process. Theoretically, such a process could explain intermediate- to long-term deviations in tonic mood, resulting in a more depressed and/or anxious alcohol-dependent person. Such a perspective is also consistent with the general principle that acute and chronic effects of alcohol are opposite in direction with respect to both neuropharmacological effects and their behavioral correlates.

An alternative, but not necessarily contradictory, approach describes the toxic effects of alcohol on neurocognitive functions important for self-regulation. Although alcohol-induced cognitive deficits are most associated with severe alcohol dependence, it has become increasingly clear that there is a monotonic dose–response relation between alcohol intake and neurocognitive functioning (Parsons, 1998) that can be observed at alcohol doses of 21 or more drinks per week (on average). Moreover, recent clinical data from humans and experimental data from rodents suggest that adolescence is a period of exquisite sensitivity to alcohol's effect on the brain (Monti et al., 2005). The importance of such neurocognitive compromise in emotion regulation is not yet clear. However, some types of deficits observed in humans (e.g., verbal, problem solving, and semantic memory skills) may be important in emotional self-regulation to the extent they relate to appraisal processes and other cognitive regulatory strategies.

A developmental perspective on adolescent alcohol use disorders suggests yet another, more speculative, possibility: that heavy alcohol involvement during this period of life preempts the developmental opportunities for learning various, affect-regulating, emotional-cognitive strategies. For example, alcohol consumption motivated by an acute interpersonal challenge can serve to reduce distress but can preclude the learning of more adaptive emotional regulation strategies. Such a perspective is consistent with the one proposed by Baumrind and Moselle (1985) for understanding the social–developmental consequences of adolescent substance use.

In summary, existing theories of the effects of alcohol on emotions typically view alcohol consumption as an emotional regulation strategy that serves to bring about a desired emotional state. At the same time, however, heavy alcohol consumption has chronic effects on affect and cognition that could, paradoxically, create more emotional dysregulation. Indeed, this may represent a core, pathological process in the development of severe alcohol dependence. Although these emotional changes induced by chronic consumption are presumably due to neuropharmacological changes in the brain, alcohol intoxication can lead to behavior culminating in a range of major life stressors. Such stressors (e.g., social rejection, job loss, legal problems, health problems, and humiliation) can also lead to affective disturbance. From a developmental perspective, preemption of normal social learning when alcohol is overused as an emotion regulation strategy is an additional mechanism to consider when considering the potential harm associated with heavy alcohol involvement in adolescence.

THE EFFECT OF EMOTIONAL STATES ON DRINKING

It is one thing to demonstrate that alcohol can alter emotions and other affective states. It is another to demonstrate that people (or animals) will use alcohol strategically to regulate emotions. To address this issue, we consider field surveys of alcohol and emotion, laboratory studies of stress-induced drinking, comorbidity between alcohol dependence and "emotional" disorders, studies examining the structure and correlates of alcohol outcome expectancies and "reasons for drinking," daily diary studies of mood and alcohol consumption, and studies of relapse in alcohol dependence.

Field Surveys of Drinking and Emotions

Field surveys of alcohol and emotions have produced mixed results. While some cross-sectional studies have found significant positive associations between various measures of "stress" and alcohol consumption and misuse (e.g., Aseltine & Gore, 2000; Cooper, Russell, Skinner, Frone, & Mudar, 1992), others have found small or nonexistent relationships (e.g., Rohsenow, 1982; Cahalan & Room, 1974). It is important to note that field studies are correlational in nature and therefore do not permit causal interpretations. For example, some research suggests that much of the alcohol/stressful event relationship can be attributed to aversive events that directly result from drinking (e.g., losing a job due to alcohol use; Hart & Fazaa, 2004). It should also be noted that several field studies have found relationships between stress and alcohol problems but not between stress and alcohol consumption (McCreary & Sadava, 2000), suggesting that tension-reduction drinking may be most relevant for pathological alcohol users. In addition, some research suggests that individual differences may mediate or moderate the stress/drinking relationship. For example, alcohol consumption appears to be more strongly related to stress among adolescents (e.g., Aseltine & Gore, 2000) than among older adults (e.g., Welte & Mirand).

Laboratory Studies of Emotion-Induced Drinking

Despite extensive experimental research on alcohol and emotion, few studies have examined the relationship between induced emotion and subsequent, ad lib drinking. In measuring *ad lib drinking*, one of two alternative contexts is typically used: (1) a totally unstructured drinking situation where participants have alcohol available to them if they wish to consume it, or (2) an unobtrusive "taste rating" task where participants are asked to rate a selection of different alcoholic beverages on various taste dimensions and consume as much as they need to in order to complete the task. Although somewhat constrained and artificial, studies of *ad lib* drinking can provide useful insights into the nature of different challenges that promote or inhibit alcohol consumption.

Most of the experimental research on affect-induced drinking suggests that individuals consume higher levels of alcohol when they anticipate a negative experience and when there are few alternative ways to cope with the experience. For example, Pelham et al. (1997) found that adult subjects who interacted with a deviant child confederate consumed significantly more alcohol than adult subjects who interacted with a non-deviant child confederate. Similarly, Kidorf and Lang (1999) found increases in alcohol consumption among undergraduate subjects who were asked to make videotaped speeches about their faults. This finding was especially strong for subjects high in trait anxiety and men who expected alcohol to increase social assertiveness. Other laboratory studies have found increases in alcohol consumption following such diverse stressors as difficult or unsolvable intellectual tasks, public speaking criticism, interpersonal evaluation, and failure feedback (Sher, 1987).

Although most laboratory research on stress-induced drinking assumes that drinking is motivated by the pharmacological properties of alcohol (sedative effects, etc.), other studies suggest that individuals drink before stressful tasks to create an excuse for potential failure, that is, for self-presentation reasons (i.e., self-handicapping; Jones & Berglas, 1978). For example, Tucker, Vuchinich, and Sobell (1981) administered either a solvable or an unsolvable test to college students who were then offered alcohol and told that they would be given a second test of equal or greater difficulty. Subjects who took the unsolvable test chose to drink more alcohol (i.e., to self-handicap) than subjects who took the solvable test, regardless of upcoming test difficulty. Notably, self-handicapping behavior decreased significantly when students were offered a performance-enhancing option (a study manual). Thus, it appears that participants chose to drink/self-handicap only when they did not have ways to improve future performance. From this perspective, alcohol consumption can represent either a cognitive strategy or a type of situational modification, where interpersonal expectations are altered by redefining the social context as more permissive than it otherwise might be.

As suggested earlier, the degree to which a stimulus will elicit drinking appears to be partially determined by the availability of alternative emotion regulation strategies. This finding may be particularly important in that alcohol consumption can lead to cognitive impairment and may disrupt attempts to cope effectively. The coping opportunities that might mitigate the occurrence of emotion-induced drinking are diverse, ranging from the opportunity to retaliate against an aggressor to reducing physiological arousal through relaxation to preparing oneself appropriately for the demands of a challenging task (Sher, 1987). That is, the "opportunity for coping" appears to be a general finding, replicable across experimental demands and types of coping/emotion-regulating activities. Thus, although individuals will use alcohol consumption as an emotion regulation strategy, other emotion regulation strategies (including other response-modulation strategies) may be preferred and used more often, even in those people who are willing to drink for emotion regulation reasons.

We note that there has been relatively little experimental research on the effects of positive emotions on alcohol consumption. This is unfortunate because individuals in our culture frequently report drinking for social and celebratory reasons. Notably, however, Gabel, Noel, Keane and Lisman (1980) found greater alcohol consumption following exposure to erotic, as opposed to neutral or negatively valenced, slides. In addition, two studies which found *decreased* drinking following social-evaluative stress (Holroyd, 1978; Pihl & Yankovsky, 1979) were based on comparisons to an esteem-enhancing (not neutral) control condition, suggesting that positive mood states may motivate drinking as much as negative mood states.

Comorbidity between Alcohol Dependence and Mood and Anxiety Disorders

It is widely believed that individuals with primary psychiatric disorders often drink to excess in order to cope with psychological distress, self-regulating their psychic suffering via alcohol (i.e., "self-medication"). Notably, several population-based, nationally representative studies support this hypothesis. For example, in the National Comorbidity Survey, Kessler et al. (1997) found that a prior lifetime anxiety or mood disorder substantially increased the likelihood of developing alcohol dependence, and this likelihood was greatly magnified for individuals with both anxiety and mood disorders. Specifically, for men/women, the odds ratio for developing alcohol dependence was 1.85/2.23 given a prior anxiety disorder alone, 1.83/2.72 given a prior mood disorder alone, 4.02/9.11 given a prior anxiety disorder + prior mood disorder, and 13.70/21.57 given a prior anxiety disorder + prior mood disorder + prior antisociality. Similarly, in the National Epidemiological Survey on Alcohol and Related Conditions (NESARC), Grant et al. (2004) found a moderate to strong association between alcohol dependence and affective disorders (odds ratios of 4.1 and 2.6 for "independent" [not alcohol-induced] mood and anxiety disorders, respectively) using past-year diagnoses. These data indicate that increasing levels of affective disturbance (especially when coupled with the high disinhibition associated with antisociality) are correlated with an increased likelihood of becoming alcohol dependent. Thus, mood and anxiety disorders may play an etiological role in the development of some forms of alcohol dependence.

Self-Reported Alcohol Motivations: Reasons for Drinking and Alcohol Outcome Expectancies

In contrast to psychiatric epidemiological studies that show robust associations between affective disorders and alcohol dependence, surveys of nonclinical samples typically show small, null, or negative correlations between drinking behavior and a range of trait and state markers of anxiety and depression (e.g., Greeley & Oei, 1999; Sher, 1987). This disjunction between clinical correlations (alcohol dependence with psychiatric disorders) and nonclinical correlations (drinking with anxiety, depression, neuroticism) suggests that affective disturbance needs to be extreme before it increases the risk of alcohol misuse (perhaps, so extreme as to overwhelm normal emotion regulation strategies). Despite this, it is clear that affect-based reasons for drinking are strongly associated with both alcohol consumption and alcohol problems in the general population (e.g., Cahalan, Cisin, & Crossley, 1969; Cooper, Frone, Russell, & Mudar, 1995). That is, individuals who report that they drink for emotional relief or to free themselves of their worries tend to consume alcohol heavily and to experience alcohol-related problems.

Reasons for drinking are clearly multidimensional. For example, Cooper (1994) found that a four-factor solution best described the structure of drinking motives with factors for (1) social reasons (e.g., "to be sociable"), (2) enhancement motives (e.g., "to get high," "because it's fun"), (3) coping motives (e.g., "to forget your worries," "because it helps when you feel depressed or nervous"), and (4) conformity motives (e.g., "to fit in"). Notably, enhancement and coping motives (but not social or conformity motives) were strongly associated with drinking, heavy drinking, and drinking problems. In a later study using population-based samples of adolescents and adults, Cooper et al. (1995) again found that the strongest predictors of drinking problems were enhancement and coping motives (although enhancement motives were more strongly associated with alcohol use). Notably, however, coping motives had a direct effect on alcohol problems, while the entire association between enhancement motives and drinking problems was mediated by alcohol use (i.e., there was no direct effect). These data suggest that drinking to regulate negative emotions is likely the strongest motivational correlate of problematic alcohol involvement.

A concept closely related to "reasons for drinking" is self-reported, alcohol outcome expectancies. Alcohol outcome expectancies can be defined as beliefs that people have about the affective, cognitive, and behavioral effects of drinking alcohol (Goldman, Brown, & Christiansen, 1987). Varying psychometric methods (e.g., exploratory and confirmatory factor analysis and multidimensional scaling) have been employed in the development of self-report expectancy measures designed to assess particular types of beliefs about drinking and to examine their relations with alcohol use and problems. Although the specific content of empirically derived factors varies across methods and measures, factors related to tension reduction, social and/or sexual facilitation, and enhanced cognitive or motor performance have been replicated across studies. Goldman, Del Boca, and Darkes (1999) suggest that outcome expectancies can be categorized along three basic dimensions: (1) positive versus negative expected outcomes (e.g., increased sociability vs. increased aggressiveness); (2) positive versus negative reinforcement (e.g., social facilitation vs. tension reduction); and (3) arousal versus sedation (e.g., stimulant vs. depressant effects).

Cross-sectional studies have consistently found associations between alcohol expectancies and both drinking behavior and drinking problems using diverse samples and methods. These studies suggest that drinking behavior is positively associated with positive outcome expectancies and negatively associated with negative outcome expectancies both cross-sectionally and prospectively. Moreover, these associations are robust across a variety of drinking patterns and remain significant (although weaker) after controlling for demographics and previous drinking behavior (Carey, 1995; Jones, Corbin, & Fromme, 2001). Outcome expectancies tend to develop in childhood (e.g., Anderson, Schweinsburg, Paulus, Brown, & Tapert, 2005), strengthen during adolescence (Smith, Goldman, Greenbaum, & Christiansen, 1995), and weaken during early adulthood (presumably, following extended experience with drinking; Sher, Wood, Wood, & Raskin, 1996).

While cross-sectional and longitudinal studies suggest expectancy/alcohol use associations, they do not imply causal relationships. Recent laboratory studies have addressed this issue by experimentally manipulating expectancies and observing subsequent changes in drinking behavior. For example, Roehrich and Goldman (1995) found that female undergraduates who had been primed with either alcohol-related words or an alcohol-related video drank significantly more beer in an ad lib "taste test" than undergraduates who were primed with neutral words or videos. Similarly, Carter, McNair, Corbin, and Black (1998) found that college students who were primed with positive, expectancy-related words (e.g., "confident" and "funny") drank significantly more than control subjects (primed with neutral words) while students who were primed with negative expectancy-related words (e.g., "sick" and "dizzy") drank significantly less than control subjects in a beer-tasting test. In a slightly different type of study, Sharkansky and Finn (1998) found that subjects who were told that alcohol would impair their performance on an impending cognitive task chose to drink less than subjects who believed that alcohol would not affect their performance. Other experimental studies have yielded similar results (e.g., Stein, Goldman, & Del Boca, 2000). Current research is increasingly focusing on the relation of expectancies to more distal risk factors such as genetics (Prescott, Cross, Kuhn, Horn, & Kendler, 2004; Slutske et al., 2002) and personality (Anderson et al., 2005; Finn, Bobova, Wehner, Fargo, & Rickert, 2005; Sher et al., 1991), based on the hypothesis that expectancies represent a common final pathway of diverse biopsychosocial influences on alcohol use and misuse (Goldman, Darkes, & Del Boca, 1999; Sher, 1991).

Daily Diary Studies

Most survey studies of alcohol and affective phenomena are cross-sectional and rely on retrospective reports of both affective states and drinking. These studies are problematic for several reasons. First, retrospective studies are subject to reporting biases that may be especially pronounced for events that occur under the influence of alcohol. Second, while cross-sectional studies correlate average levels of drinking with average levels of emotion, they do not address within-person, drinking/mood relationships. Thus, these studies cannot examine alcohol/emotion associations on an incident-by-incident basis or examine whether individuals drink more on days that they feel stress or sadness (Carney, Armeli, Tennen, Affleck, & O'Neil, 2000). Finally, cross-sectional studies do not address questions about the temporal order of cause-and-effect relationships. Specifically, it is unclear whether the emotion or other affect of interest precedes or follows alcohol consumption. Although prospective panel studies resolve this issue to some degree, they fail to address shorter-term, dynamic associations between drinking and emotion that may change over the course of minutes or hours

In contrast, daily diary and ecological momentary assessment (EMA) studies allow researchers to examine continually changing behaviors while using naturalistic conditions and minimizing retrospection bias. In daily diary studies, participants are instructed to record events or feelings that occurred during the day on structured nightly recording forms. In EMA studies, subjects are prompted several times per day to record feelings or behaviors (e.g., drinking or affect), in real time, on electronic devices, such as palmtop computers. To date, there have been relatively few daily diary/EMA studies of drinking and emotional regulation. Those studies that do exist suggest that alcohol consumption is associated with both positive and negative affective states (Swendsen et al., 2000; Hussong, Hicks, Levy, & Curran, 2001; Carney et al., 2000; Armeli, Tennen, Affleck, & Kranzler, 2000b; Steptoe & Wardle, 1999; Armeli, Carney, Tennen, Affleck, & O'Neill, 2000a; Mohr et al., 2001; Todd, Armeli, Tennen, Carney, & Affleck, 2003). In addition, these studies suggest that alcohol consumption tends to both precede and follow strong emotion (Swendsen et al., 2000; Hussong et al., 2001).

Critically, affect is not related to alcohol consumption in all individuals. For example, some studies have found that relationships between negative emotion and alcohol consumption are stronger for men than for women (Swendsen et al., 2000; Armeli et al., 2000a). Other studies suggest that both drinking context (Mohr et al., 2001; Armeli et al., 2003) and neuroticism moderate the affect/alcohol use relationship (Carney et al., 2000; Armeli et al., 2003). Unfortunately, these types of moderator studies are rare and their results tend to be contradictory. On the whole, however, diary studies indicate that some individuals use alcohol to regulate emotions but that this phenomenon is dependent on situational and dispositional factors. Several research teams are currently attempting to characterize the joint influence of emotional, situational, and individual difference variables that bound this phenomenon

Relapse, Cue Exposure, and Emotion

Research on emotional states and alcoholic relapse dates back to the seminal work of Marlatt and Gordon who, in the early 1970s, created a five-category typology of reasons for alcohol relapse based on responses from 65 alcoholic patients. Specifically, Marlatt and Gordon (1980) found that self-reported relapse was often attributed to (1) frustration, (2) social pressure, (3) intrapersonal temptation, (4) negative emotional states, or

(5) other miscellaneous triggers. Though not consistently replicated (Longabaugh, Rubin, Stout & Zywiak, 1997) Marlatt and Gordon's (1980) work was notable in that it highlighted the importance of situational and emotional factors in predicting relapse and helped broaden the field from one that was exclusively disease focused (i.e., relapse as a response to craving and physiological withdrawal) to one in which relapse was conceptualized as the result of psychological, environmental, and physiological factors and where emotions play a prominent role. Since Marlatt and Gordon's (1980) original publication, numerous prospective and retrospective studies have documented associations between psychological distress and alcoholic relapse (Curran, Kirchner, Worley, Rookey, & Booth, 2002; Flynn, Walton, Curran, Blow, & Knutzen, 2004; Cornelius et al., 2003; Miller, Westerberg, Harris, & Tonigan, 1996; Hodgins, el-Guebaly, & Armstrong, 1995). These studies have found associations between relapse and both pretreatment (Curran et al., 2002) and posttreatment (Curran & Booth, 1999; Flynn et al., 2004) psychological distress. For example, Curran et al. (2002) found that outpatient addictions clients with severe depressive symptomatology were significantly more likely to prematurely terminate treatment than were outpatient addictions clients without depressive symptomatology. Moreover, other studies have found positive associations between emotional distress and temptation to drink (Velasquez, Carbonari, & DiClemente, 1999). In addition, recent data suggest that reductions in psychological distress during treatment predict better posttreatment substance use outcomes (Long, Williams, Midgley, & Hollin, 2000).

Laboratory studies of cue exposure have also found associations between negative mood induction and desire to drink. For example, Litt, Cooney, Kadden, and Guapp (1990) induced both negative and neutral moods in alcoholic inpatients over a period of 4 days using a hypnotic mood-induction technique. Results showed that "desire to drink" ratings were higher following negative, as opposed to neutral, moods. Other studies have yielded similar findings among inpatient alcoholics (Cooney, Litt, Morse, Bauer, & Guapp, 1997; Payne et al., 1992) and nonalcoholic heavy drinkers (Zack, Poulos, Fragopoulos, & MacLeod, 2003).

Another body of literature suggests that various affective states may interact with alcohol cues to increase risk for relapse. For example, Greeley, Swift, and Heather (1992) found that scores on the Depression Adjective Checklist predicted desire to drink in the presence of alcohol cues (exposure to an alcoholic drink) but not in the presence of neutral cues (exposure to a nonalcoholic drink). Similarly, Rubonis et al. (1994) found that desire to drink in response to alcohol cues was exacerbated by negative mood induction among male and female alcoholics. Using a somewhat different methodology, Zack, Toneatto, and MacLeod (1999) found that negative affective cues primed alcohol concepts in a lexical decision task more strongly in problem drinkers with high, as opposed to low, levels of distress. Other studies, however, have failed to find interactive effects of psychological distress and alcohol cues in the prediction of drinking and more focused research is needed to clarify the relationships between negative mood, alcohol exposure, and relapse (Cooney et al., 1997; Payne et al., 1992).

SUMMARY AND CONCLUSIONS

Throughout recorded history, alcohol has been recognized as a transformative substance that can produce profound emotional effects. In addition, modern research has shown that alcohol can affect brain systems that regulate cognition and emotion. Notably, alcohol's effects on emotion are strongly conditioned on dose, time course of intoxication, situational factors, underlying affective state, and individual differences associated with both constitutional variables and acquired experience. As a result, simple generalizations concerning alcohol/emotion relations are not possible. However, under conducive circumstances, alcohol can strongly reduce negative emotions and increase positive emotions. Unfortunately, these benefits are often accompanied by considerable costs such as short-term negative emotional consequences. In addition, chronic, heavy alcohol use often leads to tonic changes in emotional state that may further motivate drinking. From this perspective, alcohol dependence may be considered, in part, a disorder of emotional regulation.

There has been little research on the determinants of emotion-related drinking in everyday life. Many of the research strategies used in the past, especially survey studies of drinkers and psychiatric epidemiological studies of alcohol-related comorbidity, fail to resolve the temporal dynamics of emotions and drinking. This situation is rapidly changing with the emergence of EMA studies, although even these have not yet provided sufficiently detailed assessments to fully contextualize the instigation of a drinking episode, its course, and its emotional consequences. The use of palmtop computers has revolutionized our ability to study emotion and drinking relations in the field and with the addition of emerging technologies (e.g., transdermal alcohol sensors and unobtrusive real-time recording of physiological activity), we should be able to transfer some of the measurement sophistication of the laboratory to the field.

Finally, while our review focused exclusively on alcohol and emotions, it is clear that many individuals use other psychoactive substances, both licit and illicit, for emotion regulation. The preferential choice of the use of one substance over another is undoubtedly attributable to myriad influences concerning personal experience (e.g., Khantzian, 1990), personality (e.g., Sher et al., 1999), accessibility, and cultural and subcultural norms of use. There are clearly many similarities in both the effects of and motivations for using different substances, but one must be careful not to overgeneralize from one substance to another. Drugs differ not only in terms of their psychological effects (and underlying neuropharmacology) but, importantly, to the extent they interfere with important life tasks, their potential for acute harm versus more chronic health problems, and the degree to which they preempt alternative emotion regulation strategies both situationally and developmentally. We believe, however, the focus on alcohol is instructive because it is a substance that is used by a large proportion of individuals in diverse cultures worldwide (unlike many illicit substances), because it can have profound effects on emotions and cognition (unlike nicotine), and because there are complex interactions between drinking, intoxication, and social context.

ACKNOWLEDGMENTS

Preparation of this chapter was supported by National Institute on Alcohol Abuse and Alcoholism Grant Nos. R37AA7231 and T32AA13526 to Kenneth J. Sher and Grant No. P50 AA11990 to Andrew C. Heath.

REFERENCES

American Psychiatric Association. (1994). *Diagnostic and statistical manual of mental disorders* (4th ed.). Washington DC: Author.

American Psychiatric Association. (2000). *Diagnostic and Statistical manual of mental disorders* (4th ed., text rev.). Washington, DC: Author.

Anderson, K. G., Schweinsburg, A., Paulus, M. P., Brown, S. A., & Tapert, S. (2005). Examining person-ality and alcohol expectancies using functional magnetic resonance imaging (fMRI) with adoles-cents. *Journal of Studies on Alcohol, 66,* 323–331.

Armeli, S., Carney, M. A., Tennen, H., Affleck, G., & O'Neil, T. P. (2000a). Stress and alcohol use: A daily process examination of the stressor-vulnerability model. *Journal of Personality and Social Psy-chology, 78,* 979–994.

Armeli, S., Tennen, H., Affleck, G., & Kranzler, H. R. (2000b). Does affect mediate the association between daily events and alcohol use? *Journal of Studies on Alcohol, 61,* 862–871.

Armeli, S., Tennen, H., Todd, M., Carney, M. A., Mohr, C., Affleck, G., et al. (2003). A daily process examination of the stress-response dampening effects of alcohol consumption. *Psychology of Addic-tive Behaviors, 17*(4), 266–276.

Aseltine, R. H., & Gore, S. L. (2000). The variable effects of stress on alcohol use from adolescence to early adulthood. *Substance Use and Misuse, 35,* 643–668.

Bandura, A. (1969). Social learning of moral judgments. *Journal of Personality and Social Psychology, 11*(3), 275–279.

Baumrind, D., & Moselle, K. A. (1985). A developmental perspective on adolescent drug abuse. *Advances in Alcohol and Substance Abuse, 4,* 41–67.

Cahalan, D., Cisin, I. H., & Crossley, H. M. (1969). American drinking practices: A national study of drinking behavior and attitudes. *Monographs of the Rutgers Center of Alcohol Studies, 6,* 260.

Cahalan, D., & Room, R. (1974). *Problem drinking among American men.* New Brunswick, NJ: Rutgers Center on Alcohol Studies.

Carey, K. B. (1995). Alcohol-related expectancies predict quantity and frequency of heavy drinking among college students. *Psychology of Addictive Behaviors, 9,* 236–241.

Carney, M. A., Armeli, S., Tennen, H., Affleck, G., & O'Neil, T. P. (2000). Positive and negative daily events, perceived stress and alcohol use: A diary study. *Journal of Counseling and Clinical Psychology, 68,* 788–798.

Carter, J. A., McNair, L. D., Corbin, W. R., & Black, D. H. (1998). Effects of priming positive and nega-tive outcomes on drinking responses. *Experimental and Clinical Psychopharmacology, 6,* 399–405.

Conger, J. J. (1956). Alcoholism: Theory, problem and challenge. II. Reinforcement theory and the dynamics of alcoholism. *Quarterly Journal of Studies on Alcohol, 17*(2), 296–305.

Cooney, N. L., Litt, M. D., Morse, P. A., Bauer, L. O., & Gaupp, L. (1997). Alcohol cue reactivity, negative-mood reactivity, and relapse in treated alcoholic men. *Journal of Abnormal Psychology, 106,* 243–250.

Cooper, M. L. (1994). Motivations for alcohol use among adolescents: Development and validation of a four-factor model. *Psychological Assessment, 6,* 117–128.

Cooper, M. L., Frone, M. R., Russell, M., & Mudar, P. (1995). Drinking to regulate positive and negative emotions: A motivational model of alcohol use. *Journal of Personality and Social Psychology, 69,* 990–1005.

Cooper, M. L., Russell, M., Skinner, J. B., Frone, M. R., & Mudar, P. (1992). Stress and alcohol use: Mod-erating effects of gender, coping and alcohol expectancies. *Journal of Abnormal Psychology, 101,* 139–152.

Cornelius, J. R., Maisto, S. A., Pollock, N. K., Martin, C. S., Salloum, I. M., Lynch, K. G., et al. (2003). Rapid relapse generally follows treatment for substance use disorders among adolescents. *Addic-tive Behaviors, 28,* 381–386.

Costello, E. J., Erkanli, A., Federman, E., & Angold, A. (1999). Development of psychiatric comorbidity with substance abuse in adolescents: Effects of timing and sex. *Journal of Clinical Child Psychology, 28,* 298–311.

Curran, G. M., & Booth, B. M. (1999). Longitudinal changes in predictor profiles of abstinence from alcohol use among male veterans. *Alcoholism: Clinical and Experimental Research, 23,* 141–143.

Curran, G. M., Kirchner, J. E., Worley, M., Rookey, C., & Booth, B. M. (2002). Depressive symptomatol-ogy and early attrition from intensive outpatient substance use treatment. *Journal of Behavioral Health Services and Research, 29,* 138–143.

Curtin, J. J., Lang, A. R., Patrick, C. J., & Stritzke, W. G. K. (1998). Alcohol and fear-potentiated startle: The role of competing cognitive demands in the stress-reducing effects of intoxication. *Journal of Abnormal Psychology, 107,* 547–557.

Curtin, J. J., Patrick, C. J., Lang, A. R., Cacioppo, J. T., & Birbaumer, N. (2001). Alcohol affects emotion through cognition. *Psychological Science, 12*(6), 527–531.

Di Chiara, G. (1997). Alcohol and dopamine. *Alcohol, Health and Research World, 21*, 108–114

Doty, P., & de Wit, H. (1995). Effect of setting on the reinforcing and subjective effects of ethanol in social drinkers. *Psychopharmacology, 118*(1), 19–27.

Finn, P. R., Bobova, L., Wehner, E., Fargo, S., & Rickert, M. E. (2005). Alcohol expectancies, conduct disorder and early-onset alcoholism: Negative alcohol expectancies are associated with less drinking in non-impulsive versus impulsive subjects. *Addiction, 100*, 953–962.

Flynn, H. A., Walton, M. A., Curran, G. M., Blow, F. C., & Knutzen, S. (2004). Psychological distress and return to substance use two years following treatment. *Substance Use and Misuse, 6*, 885–910.

Froehlich, J. C. (1997). Opioid peptides. *Alcohol, Health and Research World, 21*, 132–136.

Fromme, K., & D'Amico, E. J. (1999). Neurobiological bases of alcohol's psychological effects. In K. E. Leonard & H. T. Blane (Eds.), *Psychological theories of drinking and alcoholism* (pp. 422–455). New York: Guilford Press.

Gabel, P. C., Noel, N. E., Keane, T. M., & Lisman, S. A. (1980). Effects of sexual versus fear arousal on alcohol consumption in college males. *Behavior Research and Therapy, 18*, 519–526.

Goldman, M. S., Brown, S. A., & Christiansen, B. A. (1987). Expectancy theory: Thinking about drinking. In K. E. Leonard & H. T. Blane (Eds.), *Psychological theories of drinking and alcoholism* (pp. 272–304). New York: Guilford Press.

Goldman, M. S., Darkes, J., & Del Boca, F. K. (1999). Expectancy mediation of biopsychosocial risk for alcohol use and alcoholism. In I. Kirsch (Ed.), *How expectancies shape experience* (pp. 233–262). Washington, DC: American Psychological. Association.

Goldman, M. S., Del Boca, F. K., & Darkes, J. (1999). Alcohol expectancy theory: The application of cognitive neuroscience. In K. E. Leonard & H. T. Blane (Eds.), *Psychological theories of drinking and alcoholism* (2nd ed., pp. 203–246). New York: Guilford Press.

Grant, B. F., Stinson, F. S., Dawson, D. A., Chou, S. P., Dufour, M. C., Compton, W., et al. (2004). Prevalence and co-occurrence of substance use disorders and independent mood and anxiety disorders: Results from the national epidemiologic survey on alcohol and related conditions. *Archives of General Psychiatry, 61*(8), 807–816.

Greeley, J., & Oei, T. (1999). Alcohol and tension reduction. In K. E. Leonard, & H. T. Blane (Eds.), *Psychological theories of drinking and alcoholism* (2nd ed., pp. 14–53). New York: Guilford Press.

Greeley, J., Swift, W., & Heather, N. (1992). Depressed affect as a predictor of increased desire for alcohol in current drinkers of alcohol. *British Journal of Addiction, 87*, 1005–1112.

Gross, J. J., & Thompson, R. A. (2007). Emotion regulation: Conceptual foundations. In J. J. Gross (Ed.), *Handbook of emotion regulation* (pp. 3–24). New York: Guilford Press.

Hart, K. E., & Fazaa, N. (2004). Life stress events and alcohol misuse: Distinguishing contributing stress events from consequential stress events. *Substance Use and Misuse, 39*(9), 1319–1339.

Hodgins, D. C., el-Guebaly, N., & Armstrong, S. (1995). Prospective and retrospective reports of mood states before relapse to substance use. *Journal of Consulting and Clinical Psychology, 63*(3), 400–407.

Holdstock, L., & de Wit, H. (1998). Individual differences in the biphasic effects of ethanol. *Alcoholism: Clinical and Experimental Research, 22*(9), 1903–1911.

Holroyd, K. (1978). Effects of social anxiety and social evaluation on beer consumption and social interaction. *Journal of Studies on Alcoholism, 39*, 737–744.

Hull, J. G. (1981). A self-awareness model of the causes and effects of alcohol consumption. *Journal of Abnormal Psychology, 90*(6), 586–600.

Hull, J. G. (1987). Self-awareness model. In K. E. Leonard & H. T. Blane (Eds.), *Psychological theories of drinking and alcoholism* (pp. 272–304). New York: Guilford Press.

Hull, J. G., & Bond, C. F. (1986). Social and behavioral consequences of alcohol consumption and expectancy: A meta-analysis. *Psychological Bulletin, 99*(3), 347–360.

Hussong, A. M., Hicks, R. E., Levy, S. A., & Curran, P. J. (2001). Specifying the relations between affect and heavy alcohol use among young adults. *Journal of Abnormal Psychology, 110*, 449–461.

Jones, B. T., Corbin, W., & Fromme, K. (2001). A review of expectancy theory and alcohol consumption. *Addiction, 96*, 57–72.

Jones, E. E., & Berglas, S. (1978). Control of attributions about the self through self-handicapping strategies: The appeal of alcohol and the role of unachievement. *Personality and Social Psychology Bulletin, 4*, 200–206.

Kessler, R. C., Crum, R. M., Warner, L. A., Nelson, C. B., Schulenberg, J., & Anthony, J. C. (1997). Lifetime co-occurrence of DSM-III-R alcohol abuse and dependence with other psychiatric disorders in the National Comorbidity Survey. *Archives of General Psychiatry, 54*(4), 313–321.

Khantzian, E. J. (1990). Self-regulation and self-medication factors in alcoholism and the addictions: Similarities and differences. In M. Galanter (Ed.), *Recent developments in alcoholism* (Vol. 8, pp. 255–271). New York: Plenum Press.

Kidorf, M., & Lang, A. R. (1999). Effects of social anxiety and alcohol expectancies on stress-induced drinking. *Psychology of Addictive Behaviors, 13,* 134–142.

Koob, G. F., & LeMoal, M. (2001). Drug addiction, dysregulation of reward and allostasis. *Neuropsychopharmacology, 24,* 97–127.

Kranzler, H. R., & Anton, R. F. (1994). Implications of recent neuropsychopharmacologic research for understanding the etiology and development of alcoholism. *Journal of Consulting and Clinical Psychology, 62,* 1116–1126.

Kushner, M. G., Sher, K. J., & Erickson, D. J. (1999). Prospective analysis of the relation between DSM-III anxiety disorders and alcohol use disorders. *American Journal of Psychiatry, 156,* 723–732.

Lang, A., Patrick, C., & Stritzke, W. (1999). Alcohol and emotional response: A multidimensional–multilevel analysis. In K. E. Leonard & H. T. Blane (Eds.), *Psychological theories of drinking and alcoholism* (2nd ed., pp. 328–371). New York: Guilford Press.

Litt, M. D., Cooney, N. L., Kadden, R. M., & Guapp, L. (1990). Reactivity to alcohol cues and induced moods in alcoholics. *Addictive Behaviors, 15,* 137–146.

Long, C. G., Williams, M., Midgley, M., & Hollin, C. R. (2000). Within-program factors as predictors of drinking outcome following cognitive-behavioral treatment. *Addictive Behaviors, 25,* 573–578.

Longabaugh, R., Rubin, A., Stout, R. L., & Zywiak, W. H. (1997). Section IIA. Replication and extension of Marlatt's taxonomy: The reliability of Marlatt's taxonomy for classifying relapses. *Addiction, 91*(Suppl.), S73–S88.

Marlatt, G. A., Demming, B., & Reid, J. B. (1973). Loss of control drinking in alcoholics: An experimental analogue. *Journal of Abnormal Psychology, 81*(3), 233–241.

Marlatt, G. A., & Gordon, J. R. (1980). Determinants of relapse: Implications for the maintenance of behavior change. In P. O. Davidson & S. M. Davidson (Eds.), *Behavioral medicine: Changing health lifestyles* (pp. 410–452). New York: Brunner/Mazel.

Masserman, J. H., & Yum, K. S. (1946). Analysis of the influence of alcohol on experimental neuroses in cats. *Psychosomatic Medicine, 8,* 36–52.

McCreary, D. R., & Sadava, S. W. (2000). Stress, alcohol use and alcohol-related problems: The influence of negative and positive affect in two cohorts of young adults. *Journal of Studies on Alcohol, 61,* 466–474.

Merikangas, K. R., Whitaker, A., Angst, J., Eaton, W., Canino, G., Rubio-Stipec, M., et al. (1996). Comorbidity and boundaries of affective disorders with anxiety disorders and substance misuse: Results of an international task force. *British Journal of Psychiatry, 168*(Suppl. 30), 58–67.

Miller, W. R., Westerberg, V. S., Harris, R. J., & Tonigan, J. S. (1996). What predicts relapse?: Prospective testing of antecendent models. *Addiction, 91*(Suppl.), S155–S171.

Mohler, H., Fritschy, J. M., & Rudolph, U. (2002). A new benzodiazepine pharmacology. *Pharmacology and Experimental Therapeutics, 300,* 2–8.

Mohr, C. D., Armeli, S., Tennen, H., Carney, M. A., Affleck, G., & Hromi, A. (2001). Daily interpersonal experiences, context, and alcohol consumption: Crying in your beer and toasting good times. *Journal of Personality and Social Psychology, 80,* 489–500.

Monti, P. M., Miranda, R., Nixon, K., Sher, K. J., Swartzwelder, H. S., Tapert, S. F., et al. (2005). Adolescence: Booze, brains, and behavior. *Alcoholism: Clinical and Experimental Research, 29*(2), 207–220.

National Institute on Alcohol Abuse and Alcoholism. (1997). *Ninth special report to the U.S. Congress on alcohol and health from the secretary of health and human services.* Washington, DC: Author.

Nevo, I., & Hamon, M. (1995). Neurotransmitter and neuromodulatory mechanisms involved in alcohol abuse and alcoholism. *Neurochemistry International, 26*(4), 305–336.

Newlin, D. B., & Thomson, J. B. (1990). Alcohol challenge with sons of alcoholics: A critical review and analysis. *Psychological Bulletin, 108,* 383–402

Parsons, O. A. (1998). Neurocognitive deficits in alcoholics and social drinkers: A continuum? *Alcoholism: Clinical and Experimental Research, 22*(4), 954–961.

Payne, T. J., Rychtarik, R. G., Rappaport, N. B., Smith, P. O., Etscheidt, M., Brown, T. A., et al. (1992). Reactivity to alcohol-relevant beverage and imaginal cues in alcoholics. *Addictive Behaviors, 17,* 209–217.

Pelham, W. E., Lang, A. R., Atkeson, B., Murphy, D. A., Gnagy, E. M., Greiner, A. R., et al. (1997). Effects of deviant child behavior on parental distress and alcohol consumption in laboratory interactions. *Journal of Abnormal Child Psychology, 5,* 413–424.

Piasecki, T. M., Sher, K. J., Slutske, W. S., & Jackson, K. M. (2005). Hangover frequency and risk for alcohol use disorders: Evidence from a longitudinal high-risk study. *Journal of Abnormal Psychology, 114*(2), 223–234.

Pihl, R. O., & Yankofsky, L. (1979). Alcohol consumption in male social drinkers as a function of situationally induced depressive affect and anxiety. *Psychopharmacology, 65*, 251–257.

Pliner, P., & Cappell, H. (1974). Modification of affective consequences of alcohol: A comparison of social and solitary drinking. *Journal of Abnormal Psychology, 83*(4), 418–425.

Poznanski, A. (1959). Our drinking heritage. In R. G. McCarthy (Ed.), *Drinking and intoxication: Selected reading in social attitudes and controls.* New Haven, CT: College and University Press.

Prescott, C. A., Cross, R. J., Kuhn, J. W., Horn, J. L., & Kendler, K. S. (2004). Is risk for alcoholism mediated by individual differences in drinking motivations? *Alcoholism: Clinical and Experimental Research, 28*, 29–39.

Ramchandani, V. A., Bosron, W. F., & Li, T. K. (2001a). Research advances in ethanol metabolism. *Pathologie-Biologie, 49*, 676–682.

Ramchandani, V. A., Kwo, P. Y., & Li, T. K. (2001b). Effect of food and food composition on alcohol elimination rates in healthy men and women. *Journal of Clinical Pharmacology, 41*, 1345–1350.

Roehrich, L., & Goldman, M. S. (1995). Implicit priming of alcohol expectancy memory processes and subsequent drinking behavior. *Experimental and Clinical Psychopharmacology, 3*, 402–410.

Rohsenow, D. J. (1982). Social anxiety, daily moods, and alcohol use over time among heavy social drinking men. *Addictive Behaviors, 7*, 311–315.

Roueché, B. (1960). *The neutral spirit: A portrait of alcohol.* Boston: Little, Brown.

Rubonis, A. V., Colby, S. M., Monti, P. M., Rohsenow, D. J., Gulliver, S. B., & Sirota, A. D. (1994). Alcohol cue reactivity and mood induction in male and female alcoholics. *Journal of Studies on Alcohol, 55*, 487–494.

Sayette, M. A. (1993). An appraisal–disruption model of alcohol's effects on stress responses in social drinkers. *Psychological Bulletin, 114*(3), 459–476.

Sayette, M. A. (1999). Cognitive theory and research. In K. E. Leonard & H. T. Blane (Eds.), *Psychological theories of drinking and alcoholism* (2nd ed., pp. 247–291). New York: Guilford Press.

Sayette, M. A., Martin, C. S., Perrott, M. A., Wertz, J. M., & Hufford, M. R. (2001). A test of the appraisal disruption model of alcohol and stress. *Journal of Studies on Alcohol, 62*, 247–256.

Schuckit, M. A. (1994). *Substance-related disorders: DSM-IV sourcebook* (Vol. 1). Washington, DC: American Psychiatric Association.

Sellers, E. M., Sullivan, J. T., Somer, G., & Sykora, K. (1991). Characterization of DSM-III-R criteria for uncomplicated alcohol withdrawal provides an empirical basis for DSM-IV. *Archives of General Psychiatry, 48*, 442–447.

Sharkansky, E. J., & Finn, P. R. (1998). Effects of outcome expectancies and disinhibition on ad lib alcohol consumption. *Journal of Studies on Alcohol, 59*, 198–206.

Sher, K. J. (1985). Subjective effects of alcohol: the influence of setting and individual differences in alcohol expectancies. *Journal of Studies on Alcohol, 46*(2), 137–146.

Sher, K. J. (1987). Stress Response Dampening. In K. E. Leonard & H. T. Blane (Eds.), *Psychological theories of drinking and alcoholism* (pp. 272–304). New York: Guilford Press.

Sher, K. J. (1991). *Children of alcoholics: a critical appraisal of theory and research.* Chicago: University of Chicago Press.

Sher, K. J., Trull, T. J., Bartholow, B. D., & Vieth, A. (1999). Personality and alcoholism: Issues, methods, and etiological processes. In K. E. Leonard & H. T. Bland (Eds.), *Psychological theories of drinking and alcoholism* (2nd ed., pp. 54–105). New York: Guilford Press.

Sher, K. J., Walitzer, K. S., Wood, P. K., & Brent, E. E. (1991). Characteristics of children of alcoholics: Putative risk factors, substance use and abuse, and psychopathology. *Journal of Abnormal Psychology, 100*, 427–448.

Sher, K. J., & Wood, M. D. (2005). Subjective effects of alcohol II: Individual differences. In M. Earleywine (Ed.), *Mind-altering drugs: The science of subjective experience* (pp. 135–153). New York: Oxford University Press.

Sher, K. J., Wood, M. D., Richardson, A. E., & Jackson, K. M. (2005). Subjective effects of alcohol I: Effects of the drink and drinking context. In M. Earleywine (Ed.), *Mind-altering drugs: The science of subjective experience* (pp. 86–134). New York: Oxford University Press.

Sher, K. J., Wood, M. D., Wood, P. K., & Raskin, G. (1996). Alcohol outcome expectancies and alcohol use: A latent variable cross-lagged panel study. *Journal of Abnormal Psychology, 105*, 561–574.

Siegel, S., Baptista, M. A., Kim, J. A., McDonald, R. V., & Weise-Kelly, L. (2000). Pavlovian psychopharmacology: The associative basis of tolerance. *Experimental and Clinical Psychopharmacology, 8*(3), 276–293.

Slutske, W. S., Cronk, N. J., Sher, K. J., Madden, P. A. F., Bucholz, K. K., & Heath, A. C. (2002). Genes, environment and individual differences in alcohol expectancies among female adolescents and young adults. *Psychology of Addictive Behaviors, 16*, 308–317.

Slutske, W. S., Piasecki, T. M., & Hunt-Carter, E. E. (2003). Development and initial validation of the hangover symptoms scale: Prevalence and correlates of hangover symptoms in college students. *Alcoholism: Clinical and Experimental Research, 27*(9), 1442–1450.

Smith, G. T., Goldman, M. S., Greenbaum, P. E., & Christiansen, B. A. (1995). Expectancy for social facilitation from drinking: The divergent paths of high-expectancy and low expectancy adolescents. *Journal of Abnormal Psychology, 104*, 32–40.

Solomon, R. L., & Corbit, J. D. (1974). An opponent-process theory of motivation: I. Temporal dynamics of affect. *Psychological Review, 81*(2), 119–145.

Steele, C. M., & Josephs, R. A. (1988). Drinking your troubles away: II. An attention-allocation model of alcohol's effect on psychological stress. *Journal of Abnormal Psychology, 97*(2), 196–205.

Steele, C. M., & Josephs, R. A. (1990). Alcohol myopia: Its prized and dangerous effects. *American Psychologist, 45*(8), 921–933.

Steele, C. M., Southwick, L., & Pagano, R. (1986). Drinking your troubles away: The role of activity in mediating alcohol's reduction of psychological stress. *Journal of Abnormal Psychology, 95*(2), 173–180.

Stein, K. D., Goldman, M. S., & Del Boca, F. K. (2000). The influence of alcohol expectancy priming and mood manipulation on subsequent alcohol consumption. *Journal of Abnormal Psychology, 109*, 106–115.

Steptoe, A., & Wardle, J. (1999). Mood and drinking: A naturalistic study of alcohol, coffee and tea. *Psychopharmacology, 141*, 315–321.

Stritzke, W. G., Lang, A. R., & Patrick, C. J. (1996). Beyond stress and arousal: A reconceptualization of alcohol–emotion relations with reference to psychophysiological methods. *Psychological Bulletin, 120*, 376–395.

Stritzke, W. G. K., Patrick, C. J., & Lang, A. R. (1995). Alcohol and human emotion: A multidimensional analysis incorporating startle-probe methodology. *Journal of Abnormal Psychology, 104*, 114–122.

Swendsen, J. D., Tennen, H., Carney, M. A., Affleck, G., Willard, A., & Hromi, A. (2000). Mood and alcohol consumption: An experience sampling test of the self-medication hypothesis. *Journal of Abnormal Psychology, 109*, 198–204.

Todd, M., Armeli, S., Tennen, H., Carney, M. A., & Affleck, G. (2003). A daily diary validity test of drinking to cope measures. *Psychology of Addictive Behaviors, 17*, 303–311.

Tucker, J. A., Vuchinich, R. E., & Sobell, M. B. (1981). Alcohol consumption as a self-handicapping strategy. *Journal of Abnormal Psychology, 90*, 220–230.

Velasquez, M. M., Carbonari, J. P., & DiClemente. (1999). Psychiatric severity and behavior change in alcoholism: The relation of the transtheoretical model variables to psychiatric distress in dually diagnosed patients. *Addictive Behaviors, 24*, 481–496.

Warren, G. H., & Raynes, A. E. (1972). Mood changes during three conditions of alcohol intake. *Quarterly Journal of Studies on Alcohol, 33*(4-A), 979–989.

Weiss, F., & Koob, G. F. (1991). The neuropharmacology of ethanol self-administration. In R. E. Meyer, G. F. Koob, M. J. Lewis, & S. M. Paul (Eds.), *Neuropharmacology of ethanol* (pp. 125–162). Boston: Birkhauser.

Welte, J. W., & Mirand, A. L. (1995). Drinking, problem drinking and life stresses in the elderly general population. *Journal of Studies on Alcohol, 56*, 67–73.

Wood, M. D., Vinson, D. C., & Sher, K. J. (2001). Alcohol use and misuse. In A. Baum, T. Revenson, & J. Singer (Eds.), *Handbook of health psychology* (pp. 281–318). Hillsdale, NJ: Erlbaum.

Zack, M., Poulos, C. X., Fragopoulos, F., & MacLeod, C. M. (2003). Effects of negative and positive mood phrases on priming of alcohol words in young drinkers with high and low anxiety sensitivity. *Experimental and Clinical Psychopharmacology, 11*, 176–185.

Zack, M., Toneatto, T., & MacLeod, C. M. (1999). Implicit activation of alcohol concepts by negative affective cues distinguishes between problem drinkers with high and low psychiatric distress. *Journal of Abnormal Psychology, 108*, 518–531.

CHAPTER 29

Dialectical Behavior Therapy for Pervasive Emotion Dysregulation
THEORETICAL AND PRACTICAL UNDERPINNINGS

MARSHA M. LINEHAN
MARTIN BOHUS
THOMAS R. LYNCH

The aim of this chapter is to describe the application and the theoretical rationale of a set of emotion regulation skills developed within the context of dialectical behavior therapy (DBT; Linehan, 1993a, 1993b) DBT is a comprehensive cognitive-behavioral treatment developed originally for suicidal individuals meeting criteria for borderline personality disorder (BPD), expanded to treat patients with BPD more generally or with substance dependence and since expanded to treat other personality disorders as well as other mental disorders whose criterion behaviors are functionally related to problems in emotion regulation. The data for the efficacy of DBT in treating disorders characterized by pervasive and difficult-to-manage emotion dysregulation is extensive, including eight randomized clinical trials conducted across five independent research teams (Koons et al., 2001; Linehan, Armstrong, Suarez, Allmon, & Heard, 1991; Linehan et al., 1999; Linehan et al., 2002; Linehan et al., 2006; Lynch, Morse, Mendelson, & Robins, 2003; Verheul et al., 2003; Telch, Agras, & Linehan, 2001; Safer, Telch, & Agras, 2001; Lynch et al., in press; van den Bosch, Verheul, Schippers, & Van den Brink, 2002). In this chapter we give a description of how we define and teach the concepts of both emotion and emotion dysregulation. We then provide an overview of the relationship of BPD to emotion regulation and argue that the disorder can best be considered one of pervasive emotion dysregulation across both negative and positive emotions. Although we use BPD as an exemplar of severe emotion dysregulation, we believe the model we propose can be applied to other difficult-to-manage disorders of emotion regulation.

DBT is considered the front-line treatment for BPD and, thus, by extension can be considered a comprehensive treatment for emotion dysregulation. Training in skills to decrease emotional reactivity and to regulate emotional response is a primary focus of DBT. Each DBT skill set was derived either from more basic research on emotions and emotion regulation or from procedures used in clinical interventions already found efficacious in treating emotional disorders such as anxiety and fear, depression and grieving, and anger. We have no data at present, however, to say whether the combination of specific skills in DBT are a necessary or sufficient component of a treatment for pervasive emotion dysregulation. Component analyses are under way but not completed. We describe the research that we believe is needed now to evaluate these skills independent of their context within DBT.

EMOTION AND EMOTION DYSREGULATION

The Dialectical Behavior Therapy Model of Emotion

We are well aware that proposing any definition of the construct "emotion" is fraught with difficulty and even among emotion researchers, although there may be agreement on the fuzzy outlines of a definition, there is rarely agreement on any one concrete definition. That being said, teaching patients about emotions and emotion regulation, by necessity, requires some attempt at a description of emotions if not an exact definition. Drawing on many others, primarily Ekman (Ekman & Davidson, 1994), we view emotions as complex, brief, involuntary, patterned, full-system responses to internal and external stimuli. Similar to others, we emphasize the importance of the evolutionary adaptive value of emotions in understanding them today (Tooby & Cosmides, 1990, cited by Ekman, 1994). Although we view emotional responses as systemic, they can for the sake of discussion be viewed as consisting of a number of transacting components or subsystems. Admitting that there are any number of ways to divide up a complex system, we find the following five subsystems of practical use in both understanding and learning to regulate emotions: (1) emotional vulnerability to cues; (2) internal and/or external events that serve as emotional cues, including attention to and appraisals of the cues; (3) emotional responses, including physiological responses, cognitive processing, experiential responses and action urges; (4) nonverbal and verbal expressive responses and actions; and (5) aftereffects of the initial emotional "firing" including secondary emotions (see Figure 29.1). Similar to Scherers' (1994) conception of emotion, emotions are viewed as "a sequence of interrelated, synchronized changes in the states of all organismic subsystems (information processing/cognition, support/ANS, execution/motivation, action/SNS, monitoring/subjective feeling)" (Scherer, 1994, p. 27). Although one might ordinarily think of emotions as responses to internal and/or external events (i.e., as events separate from the events that prepare and cue the individual to respond emotionally), our view is that it is useful to consider emotional cues and the state of the individual (both biological and psychological) as occurring as part of a discrete emotional system across segments of time. From this dialectical point of view, emotions are transactional events where both context and response are integral parts of the emotional system; that is, the emotional response of the person is not separated from the emotionally evocative cue of the context and both are seen to reciprocally influence each other. (See Mesquita & Albert, this volume, for similar discussion.) Similarly, we find it useful to consider the patterned actions associated with emotional responses to be part and parcel of the emotional response rather than consequences of

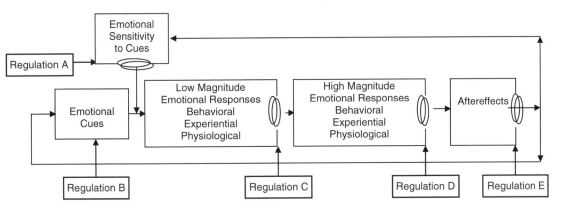

FIGURE 29.1. Model of emotion generation and points of regulation. Adapted from Gross (1998b). Copyright 1998 by the American Psychological Association. Adapted by permission.

the emotion. By combining all these elements into one transactional system we emphasize that modifying any component of the emotional system is likely to change the functioning of the entire system. In short, if one wants to change one's own emotions, it can be done by modifying any part of the system. Like Davidson and colleagues (Davidson, 1998) we contend that emotion regulation can be both automatic as well as consciously controlled and that emotion-regulatory processes are an integral part of emotional responding. In DBT, our focus is on (1) increasing conscious control and (2) eliciting sufficient practice to overlearn skills such that ultimately the regulation becomes automatic.

Pervasive Emotion Dysregulation

Emotion dysregulation is the inability, even when one's best efforts are applied, to change or regulate emotional cues, experiences, actions, verbal responses, and/or nonverbal expressions under normative conditions. Pervasive emotion dysregulation is when the inability to regulate emotions occurs across a wide range of emotions, adaptation problems, and situational contexts. Pervasive emotion dysregulation is conceptualized as due to an increased vulnerability to high emotionality combined with an inability to regulate intense emotion-linked responses. Emotion vulnerability, from this theoretical position, is defined as heightened sensitivity to emotional stimuli, intense reactions to such stimuli, and a slow, delayed return to an emotional baseline. Characteristics of pervasive emotion dysregulation include an excess of aversive emotional experiences, an inability to regulate intense physiological arousal, problems turning attention away from emotional stimuli, cognitive distortions and failures in information processing, insufficient control of impulsive behaviors related to strong positive and negative affects, difficulties organizing and coordinating activities to achieve non-mood-dependent goals when emotionally aroused and a tendency to "freeze" or dissociate under very high stress (see Figure 29.2). (See Ochsner & Gross, this volume, and Campbell-Sills & Barlow, this volume, for further discussion.) Pervasive dysregulation occurs across the entire emotional system, including the behavioral, physiological, cognitive, and experiential subsystems of emotional responding.

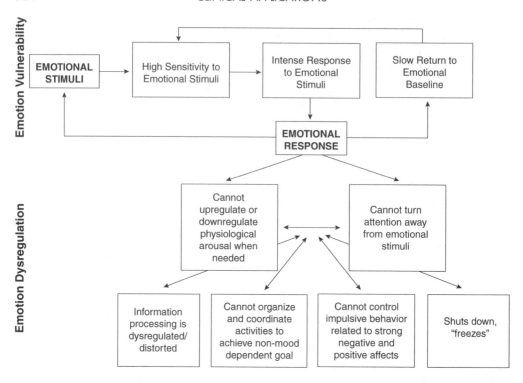

FIGURE 29.2. Pervasive emotion dysregulation schematic.

BORDERLINE PERSONALITY DISORDER: A MODEL OF PERVASIVE EMOTION DYSREGULATION

The Disorder

BPD is a severe mental disorder with a serious dysregulation of the affective system at its core. Patients show a characteristic pattern of instability in affect regulation, impulse control, interpersonal relationship, and self-image. The often severe functional impairment leads to substantial treatment utilization and a mortality rate by suicide of almost 10%, which is 50% higher than the rate in the general population (American Psychiatric Association, 2001). BPD affects approximately 1–2% of the general population, up to 10% of outpatients treated for mental disorders, and up to 20% of inpatients (Torgersen, Kringlen, & Cramer, 2001). Because of the severity of the disturbance and the intensive treatment use, patients with BPD constitute a disproportionately large subset of psychiatric inpatients and outpatients, consuming considerably more mental health resources than most other psychiatric groups (Bender et al., 2001; Zanarini, Frankenburg, Khera, & Bleichmar, 2001)

Affective dysregulation in BPD is viewed as a consequence of an interplay between genetic vulnerability and sociobiographical experience, resulting in enhanced sensitivity to emotional stimuli and inability to effectively modulate emotional responses and response tendencies. Specifically, most DSM-IV BPD criterion behaviors can be defined either as a direct consequence of emotion dysregulation or as responses that function to modulate the aversive emotional states. (Linehan, 1993a; McMain, Korman, & Dimeff, 2001). In a vicious cycle, this dysfunctional modulation of aversive emotions then serves as negative reinforcement for the criterion behaviors.

Enhanced Sensitivity

According to Linehan's theory, emotion dysregulation in BPD is hypothesized to consist of greater emotional sensitivity (low threshold for recognition of or response to emotional stimuli), greater emotional reactivity (high amplitude of emotional responses), and a slower return to baseline arousal (long duration of emotional responses) (Linehan, 1993a). To date, there have been relatively few studies examining the first component of Linehan's emotion dysregulation theory in BPD: "*high sensitivity to emotional stimuli.*" Wagner and Linehan (1999) compared recognition of facial emotional expressions between women diagnosed with BPD: non-BPD women who reported a history of sexual abuse, and normal controls. They found that BPD patients were primarily accurate perceivers of others' emotions and showed a tendency toward a heightened recognition of fear. In contrast, Levine, Marziali, and Hood (1997) reported that 30 male and female BPD patients were *less accurate* compared to 40 gender-balanced non-BPD controls at recognizing facial expressions of anger, fear, and disgust. Both of these studies used facial affect stimuli at 100% expression. Using morphing technology that allows examination of accurate perception at lower levels of intensity, Lynch et al. (2005) demonstrated that as facial expressions morphed from neutral to full intensity, participants with BPD correctly identified facial affect at an earlier stage than healthy controls. Participants with BPD were more sensitive than healthy controls at identifying emotional expressions in general, including both negative (i.e., anger) and positive (i.e., happiness) emotional expressions. These findings could not be explained by participants with BPD responding faster with more errors, supporting contentions that heightened emotional sensitivity is a core feature of BPD (Lynch et al., 2005).

Enhanced Reactivity

Emotional reactivity has been measured by both self-reports of emotional intensity and by measures of brain activity during presentation of emotional stimuli. A number of experimental and ambulatory monitoring field studies indicate that individuals with BPD report intense emotional experiences (Ebner-Priemera et al., in press; Levine et al., 1997; Stein, 1996; Stiglmayr et al., 2001). Cowdry et al. (1991) analyzed 14 days of morning and evening mood self-ratings in 16 subjects with BPD and showed a high degree of mood variability in comparison to other psychiatric groups.

Emotional challenge paradigms have been applied in neuroimaging studies to investigate neural correlates of affect processing. The materials used have been both standardized (e.g., emotional slides) and personalized (e.g., autobiographic scripts). Using standardized negative emotional material from the International Affective Picture System (IAPS) Herpertz et al. (2001) found increased activity in the amygdala of six patients with BPD and without comorbid psychiatric disorders compared to healthy controls. Donegan et al. (2003) examined neural responses to neutral, sad, fearful, and happy facial expressions (Ekman & Friesen, 1979, series) in 15 BPD and 15 control subjects. BPD patients showed greater left amygdala activation to all facial expressions regardless of valence (i.e., sadness, fear, and happiness) but also to neutral faces, compared with controls. The lack of differentiation between the four expressions raises questions regarding stimulus specificity of the left amygdala response. However, results also appear to extend findings by Lynch et al. (2005) and contentions by Linehan that BPD is an exemplar of pervasive dysregulation across both negative and positive emotions.

Using the method of script-driven imagery, Schmahl, Vermetten, Elzinga, and Bremner (2004) used autobiographical scripts to investigate processing of stressful memories in patients with BPD. Exposed to memories of traumatic life events, women with BPD failed to show increased blood flow in the anterior cingulate cortex (ACC), the orbitofrontal cortex (OFC), and the dorsolateral prefrontal gyrus, as did women without BPD. In addition, regional blood flow was investigated during imagination of situations of abandonment (Schmahl et al., 2004); significant decreases in the ACC and medial prefrontal cortex in women with BPD were found in this study. Taken together, structural and functional neuroimaging studies in patients with BPD have revealed a dysfunctional network of brain regions that mediate emotion regulation. The medial prefrontal cortex (mPFC) including ACC is involved in determination of stress, sense of controllability and emotion activation (Lane et al., 1997; Reiman, 1997) The mPFC has also inhibitory connections to the amygdala (Devinsky, Morrell, & Vogt, 1995; Vogt, Finch, & Olson, 1992). And plays a major role in downregulation of activated amygdala. Thus, the recent studies support the hypothesis of a dual brain pathology including frontal and limbic circuits causing enhanced reactivity and prolonged activation of aversive emotions. (See Beer & Lombardo, this volume, and Hariri & Forbes, this volume, for further discussion of brain functioning and emotion.)

Prolonged Activation

There is an almost absolute dearth of published studies examining the third component of the Linehan emotion dysregulation schematic, "*slow return to emotional baseline*" Linehan (1993a) suggests that problems with recovery from peak emotional intensity makes individuals with BPD more vulnerable to other triggers in their environment that might refire or exacerbate reactive emotional responding. Thus, patients with BPD may have special difficulties "turning off" the processing of either emotionally negative information, specifically, or emotionally arousing material in general. That said, to our knowledge, only one study has found support for the third component of Linehan's theory. Stiglymayr and his associates (Stiglmayr, Shapiro, Stieglitz, Limberger, & Bohus, 2001; Stiglmayr, Grathwol, Linehan, Fahrenberg, & Bohus, 2005) compared subjectively perceived states of aversive tension between female patients with BPD with normal controls. Highly significant differences were found regarding the duration and intensity of subjectively perceived states of aversive tension in the group with BPD.

DIALECTICAL BEHAVIOR THERAPY EMOTION REGULATION SKILLS

Overview

Emotion regulation skills in DBT are taught in the context of mindfulness skills, which are viewed as central in DBT and are thus labeled the "core" skills. These skills represent a behavioral translation of Zen meditation and practice and include observing, describing, spontaneous participating, nonjudgmentalness, focused awareness in the present moment, and focusing on effectiveness (rather than being "right"). Unlike standard behavior and cognitive therapies which ordinarily focus on changing distressing emotions and events, a major emphasis of mindfulness, and, thus, DBT, is on learning to bear emotional pain skillfully. Representing a natural progression from mindfulness skills, distress tolerance skills encompass the ability to experience and observe emotions without evaluation and without necessarily attempting to change or control emotional experiencing, arousal, or distress. In essence, distress tolerance skills target reducing maladaptive behavioral reactivity (e.g., impulsive acts and secondary negative emotions) to emotional responses without changing the distressing emotional response itself. Emotion regulation skills, in contrast, target the reduction of emotional distress through exposure to the primary emotion in a nonjudgmental atmosphere and application of set of specific skills. Whereas distress tolerance skills focus on *tolerating* distressing emotions, emotion regulation skills focus on *changing* distressing emotions.

All the skills in DBT target emotion regulation in one way or another. Our approach to developing the skills was to combine an approach that focused on targeting specific emotion components with a simultaneous emphasis on targeting specific time points in the emotion-generative process. Our model of emotional processes is very similar to that developed by Gross (1998a). He distinguished two points of emotion regulation. The first is at the point of the emotion cue where regulatory processes of situation selection, situation modification, attention deployment, and cognitive change are important and the second is at the point of the emotional response tendencies where processes of response modulation are important. As can be seen in Figure 29.1, DBT added three additional time points. First DBT adds a focus on vulnerability to emotional arousal. (See Davidson, Fox, & Kalin, this volume, and Peterson & Park, this volume, for similar discussions.) The idea here is that individuals will vary over time in their vulnerability to the same emotional cues. One can increase vulnerability to positive emotional cues and decrease vulnerability to negative emotional cues. Second, although we agree that there is a need to reduce emotional response tendencies once they have been initiated (i.e., the tendency to over- or underrespond or escalate or suppress an emotional response), there is also a need for emotion regulation once an emotional response is full blown (i.e., well past the point of initiation). Regulatory processes that may have been effective in the initial stages of an emotional response with low intensity emotions may be much less effective under condition of highly intense emotional arousal. Third, emotions have aftereffects that can serve as new emotional cues, refiring the same emotion again or precipitating a secondary emotion. In some respects, one can say emotions are self-organizing attractors and a major task in modulating emotions already fired is to stop refiring the emotion.

In addition to the five sets of emotion-regulatory processes proposed by Gross (Gross & Thompson, this volume), DBT targets five additional processes: biological change and context change (at the point of vulnerability to emotion cues), consequence expectancy change and response appraisal change (at the point of low intensity emotional response tendencies), and emotion reactivity change (at the point of emotional aftereffects). We moved the emotion-modulation process described by Gross as operating at the point of emotional response tendencies to more clearly focus at the point of high intensity emotional responding. The point of emotional response is the culminating point of emotional response tendencies combined with emotion-regulating processes. In the case of the pervasively dysregulated individual, this point is likely to be a point of extreme and intense emotions due to in adequate or misapplied regulation strategies. As will be seen, there is an extensive overlap of the skills prescribed in DBT and the emotion regulation procedures proposed by Gross.

Thus, we articulate two distinct types of emotional responses. Low-magnitude emotional response tendencies that include relatively low to moderate intensity responses and high-magnitude emotional responses that reflect responses of high intensity that are also products of emotion regulation processes occurring at the response tendency level. Thus, as in the Gross model (Gross, 1998b, 1999) our model describes emotional responses as sharing many qualities of emotional response tendencies and also reflecting the influence of emotion regulation or lack thereof on these tendencies. Our model focuses on both *intensity* and *timing* of responses. Emotion regulation strategies that work well when deployed in advance of a stressful experience may fail to help one regulate emotions already evoked. In addition, emotion regulation strategies that work well at relatively low emotion intensity may not work well at high intensity. In general, intensity and temporal issues have rarely been explored in studies of emotion regulation.

In what follows, we describe the specific skills taught in DBT. (See Table 29.1 for an outline of emotion regulation tasks and corresponding DBT skills.) The names of many of the skills are arbitrary and were developed by extensive pilot testing to do two things: entice clients into trying the skills and aid them in remembering the core idea of often complex sets of skills. Although we have organized the skills according to the regulation process they are most centrally related to, it should be clear that the functions of each set of skills can apply across many of the regulation processes. Our categorization, therefore, is somewhat arbitrary but, nonetheless helpful in understanding the skills. This is particularly the case for mindfulness skills which in one way or another can be viewed as critical at every juncture in the emotion regulation process.

TABLE 29.1. Emotion Regulation Tasks and Corresponding DBT Skills

Time point	Regulation process	DBT skills
A. Emotional Vulnerability	a_i Biological Change	Change Biological Sensitivity (PLEASE Skills) [Mindfulness Skills]
	a_{ii} Context Change	**A**ccumulate Positives **B**uild Mastery [Mindfulness Skills]
B. Emotional Cue	b_i Situation Selection/ Modification	Problem Solving Interpersonal Effectiveness Skills **C**ope Ahead by Covert Rehearsal [Mindfulness Skills]
	b_{ii} Attention Deployment	Distract Crisis Survival Skills [Mindfulness Skills]
	b_{iii} Situation Appraisal Change	Check the Facts [Mindfulness Skills]
C. Low Magnitude Emotional Responses Tendencies	c_i Consequences Expectancies Change	Pros and Cons (Crisis Survival Skill) [Mindfulness Skills]
	c_{ii} Response Appraisal Change	Reality Acceptance [Mindfulness]
D. High Magnitude Emotional Responses	d_i Physiological Response Modulation	Change Physiology (TIP skills)
	d_i Behavioral Response Modulation	Opposite Action [Mindfulness Skills]
E. Emotional Aftereffects	e_i Reactivity to Emotions Change	Identify and Label Emotions [Mindfulness Skills]

Note. See text for explanation of acronyms.

Changing Vulnerability to Emotional Cues

Emotional disorder, particularly when characterized by pervasive emotional dysregulation, is most often characterized by an imbalance of high negative emotionality with low positive emotionality although highly activated positive emotion, as in the case of mania, would also constitute disorder. An important task in learning to downregulate negative emotions is to decrease vulnerability to negative or distressing emotions and increase the probability of positive events and emotions, the latter to both increase happiness and increase resilience in stressful situations. By vulnerability we mean both sensitivity to and intensity of reactions to emotional cues. Changing emotion vulnerability changes the "establishing operation" or reinforcing effects of particular events and the subsequent behavior of the individual (Michael, 1993). For example, food deprivation is an establishing operation that momentarily increases the salience of food as a form of reinforcement. Two sets of processes are needed here: biological change and context change.

Biological change refers to reducing biological vulnerability to negative emotional cues. The data are clear that there are broad individual variations in physiological reactivity to emotional stimuli (Boyce & Ellis, 2005). Even when some components of this variability may be due to immutable genetic dispositions and early developmental experiences, most components can come under the control of the individual. Accordingly, DBT skills were designed to target behaviors that contribute to biological homeostasis and the reinforcing effects of various stimuli known to influence emotional reactivity. The DBT "**PLEASE**" skills target treating *P*hysical i*L*lness (Anderson, Hackett, & House, 2004), balancing nutrition and *E*ating (Smith, Williamson, Bray, & Ryan, 1999; Green, Rogers, Elliman, & Gatenby, 1994), staying off nonprescribed mood-*A*ltering drugs, getting sufficient but not too much *S*leep (Brendel et al., 1990), and getting adequate *E*xercise (Stella et al., 2005).

Context change refers to creating both psychological and environmental contexts conducive to emotional resiliency (i.e., the ability to minimize negative effects and maximize positive effects of exposure to emotional cues). Although emotional reactivity may move from relatively greater plasticity to progressively lower plasticity over time (Turkheimer & Gottesman, 1991; Waddington, 1966) one can influence vulnerability to emotional arousal by modifying the context in which emotional cues occur. DBT targets external context by teaching skills for accumulating positive life events and targets psychological context by teaching skills for building a sense of generalized mastery.

Although individuals do at times report both positive and negative emotional experiences contemporaneously (Ebner-Priemera et al., 2005) the building of a life with a sufficient number of positive events, particularly when those events are important to the individual, will increase the individual's resilience in the face of negative events. Increasing the number of pleasurable events in one's life is one approach to increasing positive emotions. In the short term, this involves increasing daily positive experiences. In the long term, it means making life changes and working on goals related to important life values so that pleasant events will occur more often. Building a general sense of mastery is done by engaging in activities that build a sense of competence and self-efficacy. Both skills have been shown to predict decreased vulnerability to negative emotional states (Rosenbaum, Lewinsohn, & Gotlib, 1996; Joiner, Lewinsohn, & Seeley, 2002; de Beurs et al., 2005; Bengtsson-Tops, 2004). The focus on mastery is very similar to activity and mastery scheduling in cognitive therapy for depression which has been shown to reduce depression even when the active focus on cognitive change is removed from the treatment (Jacobson et al., 1996; Dimidjian et al., in press).

Changing Emotional Cues

Situation Selection/Modification

One way to regulate emotions is to regulate situations that increase unwanted emotions (e.g., stimulus control). This can be done by either avoiding or modifying situations that generate the unwanted emotions. DBT teaches a simple set of *problem-solving* skills aimed at changing or developing strategies for eliminating, reducing, or avoiding emotionally problematic situations. The focus here is on defining those situations that cue unwanted emotions and then applying standard problems-solving steps such as those outline by D'Zurilla and Nezu (1999) and others. Because many problems are interpersonal and even if not may require interpersonal interactions to solve, DBT also includes a set of *interpersonal effectiveness skills* for asking for what one needs and saying no to unwanted requests. These skills focus on how to obtain a wanted objective while simultaneously maintaining both the interpersonal relationship as well as one's own self-respect, and doing so alters the emotional cues. However, problem solving, particularly interpersonal problem solving, often requires one to come into contact with emotional cues. Consequent high emotional arousal can interfere with the requisite coping necessary to solve the problem. With highly emotionally sensitive individuals, coping ahead with emotional situations via covert rehearsal of problem solving can be helpful in building the coping skills necessary for problem solving (Fourkas, Avenanti, Urgesi, & Aglioti, 2006; Barkley, 2001). *Coping ahead* may also work by increasing the individual's appraisal of his or her own ability to cope with the challenges of the emotional event, effectively increasing a sense of mastery and self-efficacy.

Attentional Deployment

There is consensus that cognitive processes play an important role in eliciting and regulating emotions. Many of these cognitive processes are implicit and automatic in nature (Ohman & Soares, 1993). At the input level, situations, whether external or internal stimuli, are appraised as either emotionally significant or emotionally insignificant. This appraisal process is operated by a range of cognitive processes relying on various levels of automaticity, voluntariness, and complexity (Smith & Kirby, 2000). At the output level, emotional states prime or facilitate specific cognitive modes. Christianson (1992) has shown that negative emotions bias attention toward the focal aspects of the situation that are emotionally relevant. Such focal attention might feed back in continuous appraisal, biasing the evaluation of the situation toward the activated emotion (McNally, 1995). Thus, from a regulation perspective, emotions might be modulated at different stages through cognitive processes: through appraisal that gives emotional meaning to a situation and through the cognitive processing mode that is elicited by the emotional state. Philippot, Baeyens, Douilliez, and Francart (2004) suggested that this process should result in an attentional bias for "schema-relevant" stimuli. Therefore, one important therapeutic approach involves training people to redirect their attention toward elements that are incongruent with their negative interpretation in order to develop a more balanced and objective view of the situation (Philippot et al., 2004).

Situation Appraisal Change

DBT focuses on analyzing and correcting situation appraisals by teaching a set of skills collected under the general rubric of *checking the facts*. These skills focus on discriminating assumptions, interpretations, ruminative thoughts, and worries from the actual observed facts of situations. Support for this model of emotion regulation has been demonstrated in a number of studies comparing different reappraisal strategies, including nonappraisal control conditions, following presentation of emotional cues (Lazarus & Abramovitz, 1962; Speisman, Lazarus, Mordkoff, & Davison, 1964). The mechanisms by which appraisal change works, however, are not clear. In an elegant set of cross-sectional studies, Sheppard and Teasdale (2000, 2004) measured changes in two aspects of affective information processing in response to pharmacotherapy: (1) "schema access" and (2) "metacognitive monitoring." Schema access is similar to the directing of attention to a negative thought or stimulus, whereas metacognitive monitoring can be thought of as mapping onto concepts of attentional disengagement (e.g., intentionally or nonconsiously turning away from negative stimuli or thoughts about the self). Sheppard and Teasdale found that currently depressed subjects differed significantly from controls on both tasks, whereas partially remitted individuals displayed an intermediate pattern of results. Specifically, their metacognitive monitoring resembled that of controls, while schema access was indistinguishable from fully symptomatic subjects. Their results suggest that remission was not the result of changes in depressive schemata but instead was a consequence of improvements in metacognitive skills similar to those taught in mindfulness. In other words, patients in remission still produced dysfunctional cognitions, but they showed improved abilities to recognize those thoughts as dysfunctional and changed their response to the negative cognition (i.e., see a thought as a thought, not literally true) instead of changing the content of the thought (i.e., reappraisal). Considering this, it is evident that further research must be conducted before conclusions regarding the mechanisms behind cognitive change can be firmly established.

Changing Emotional Response Tendencies

The regulation of action tendencies associated with emotions is an important step in regulating dysfunctional emotions. For example, cue exposure in the treatment of anxiety necessarily requires preventing of cognitive, emotional, and behavioral avoidance of the cue. Indeed, evidence has accumulated that, at least in the case of anxiety (especially social phobia), any lessening of the strength of anxiety stimuli, for example, by including safety cues, will reduce the effectiveness of interventions (Otto, Smits, & Reese, 2005). While many treatment manuals seem to assume that clients can easily prevent dysfunctional responses, DBT makes no such assumptions as the population that DBT was designed for has great difficulty inhibiting emotion-based responses. Thus, DBT provides a range of distress tolerance skills aimed at inhibiting impulsive emotional responses that interfere with long-term emotion regulation.

Consequence Expectancies Change

Changing emotional behaviors can be extremely difficult when they are followed by reinforcing consequences; thus, identifying the functions and reinforcers for particular emotional behaviors can be useful. Generally, emotions function to communicate to others and/or to motivate one's own behavior (Blair, 2003; Horstmann, 2003). Emotional behaviors can also have two other important functions. The first, related to the communication function, is to influence and control other people's behaviors; the second is to validate one's own perceptions and interpretations of events (i.e.,"if I feel it, it must be true"). The function of the latter can be seen as stabilizing the individuals concepts of self (Izard, Libero, Putnam, & Haynes, 1993). The key idea here is that all components of emotions may come under the control of operant conditioning. For example, across studies, displays of embarrassment (vs. nondisplay) following a transgression resulted in higher liking, greater forgiveness, and increased willingness to provide aid (see Keltner & Anderson, 2000, for review). Distressed behavior prompts both negative and solicitous emotions but deters hostile reactions (Biglan, Rothlind, Hops, & Sherman, 1989), and descriptions of how a person might feel in hypothetical depressive situations can be conditioned using social reinforcement (Lam, Marra, & Salzinger, 2005). Thus, changing consequence expectancies changes the probability of a response, including emotional responses. In DBT, the skill taught is evaluation of pros and cons of specific emotional reactions. The goal is to bring into present awareness both short- and long-term negative consequences of problem emotions and likely positive consequences of either changing negative emotions or enhancing positive emotions. Research has shown that asking normal controls to consider pros and cons on a task related to handling an interpersonal problem leads to the development of a "deliberative mind-set" in a subsequent task, compared to people asked to consider an action-oriented approach to the interpersonal problem (Gollwitzer, Heckhausen, & Steller, 1990). In addition, poor rational problem-solving skills (i.e., defining and formulating the problem and generating alternative solutions) was an important predictor variable of suicidality, hopelessness, and depression in a suicidal psychiatric sample and moderately predictive of the same variables in a college student sample (D'Zurilla, Chang, Nottingham, & Faccini, 1998).

Response Appraisal Change

Response appraisal change refers to changing one's appraisal of a negative emotion from appraising the experience as one that cannot be tolerated and experienced willingly and, therefore, must be avoided or changed. The principal DBT skills here are those of reality acceptance. Emotion acceptance has been shown when compared to emotion suppression or a neutral control to result in less subjective anxiety or avoidance in panic patients undergoing a carbon dioxide challenge (Levitt, Brown, Orsillo, & Barlow, 2004). In addition, coaching in an acceptance mind-set when compared to coaching of a control-your-emotions mindset or a placebo significantly increased the amount of time a subject was willing to spend in a cold pressor task (Hayes et al., 1999). With respect to emotions, DBT reality acceptance skills ("turning-the-mind" toward acceptance, radical acceptance, and willingness) focus on radical (meaning complete) acceptance of the current emotion and willingness to experience even aversive emotions.

Changing Emotional Responses

Physiological Response Modulation

DBT provides a set of skills designed specifically to downregulate the extreme physiological arousal that often accompanies intense emotions. These skills as a group are called the TIP skills referring to changing body **T**emperature, **I**ntense Exercise, and **P**rogressive relaxation. The function of these skills is to impact high arousal quickly with skills that do not require a correspondingly high level of cognitive processing to complete. The first skill has to do with using cold, icy water on the face, a method derived from research on the human dive reflex which is elicited by a combination of breath holding and face immersion with cold water. The dive reflex is thought to be a physiologically protective oxygen mechanism whereby the subject is kept alive during submergence. The physiological response involves both branches of the autonomic nervous system: parasympathetic activation (bradycardia) and concurrent sympathetic activation (vasoconstriction) (Hurwitz & Furedy, 1986). Acute bouts of intense exercise are also recommended if arousal is very high. Most important here is that the intensity of the exercise. Cox, Thomas, Hinton, and Donahue (2004) compared intensity of exercise (60% VO2max, 80% VO2 max, and a no-exercise control) and found that while intensity of exercise conditions did not differ in state anxiety immediately after exercise, a significant difference favoring the 80% VO2max condition over the control condition emerged at 30 minute postexercise. Progressive relaxation, one of the most commonly used methods of relaxation, consists of first tensing an entire limb, holding it for a brief moment, and then relaxing it. This procedure, with sufficient practice, can become a rapid method of reducing generalized physical tension (Pawlow & Jones, 2002).

Behavioral Response Modulation: Opposite Action All the Way

One strategy to change or regulate an emotion is to change its behavioral–expressive component by not only preventing emotional actions but also acting in a way that opposes or is inconsistent with the emotion. The DBT skill of *opposite action* is based on the idea that, as Barlow (1988) noted, the "essential step in the modification of emotional disorders is the direct alteration of associated action tendencies" (p. 313). Others have made this same point. Izard stated that treatment for anxiety disorders involves "the individual learn[ing] to act his way into a new feeling" (cited in Barlow, 1988, p. 410).

Cognitive-behavioral interventions for anxiety or fear disorders all include this one common element: Individuals have to approach the object/situation that is fearful, thus acting counter to (and inhibiting) their prominent urges to avoid. Effective treatments for anger also require the individual to act counter to the urges associated with anger (attack physically or verbally) by leaving the situation. Anger interventions also focus on opposite perspective taking: shifting from aggression and blame to gentleness and forgiveness (e.g., Tafrate, Kassinove, & Dundin, 2002). A number of researchers have observed that effective therapies for depression (sadness) all share a common thread: they activate behavior. For example, successful treatments for depression, such as cognitive therapy (Beck, Rush, Shaw, & Emery, 1979) and behavioral activation (BA; Martell, Addis, & Jacobson, 2001), require that the individual galvanize him- or herself to engage in activities that give a sense of mastery or pleasure. This engagement runs counter to the urges associated with depression, such as withdrawal, fatigue, and shutting down.

Opposite Action "all the way" targets changing the entire range of physical responses that accompany action, including visceral responses, body postures, and facial expression as well as movements. A large literature has demonstrated that the activation of a specific physical state activates the other facets of the corresponding emotion responses, be it via the face (Matsumoto, 1987), posture (Stepper & Strack, 1993), or respiration. Vice versa, there is ample empirical evidence that modulating one's physical state alters one's emotional state (Philippot et al., 2004). Also targeted in "all the way" opposite action are emotion-linked thought patterns and verbal responses.

It is very important to note that the idea here is to act contrary to an emotion, not to mask or hide emotions (Gross & Levenson, 1993).

In part, opposite action is hypothesized to work by influencing classically conditioned emotional responses (Lynch et al., in press). Opposite action may also create sensory feedback from facial muscles and skin that can be transformed directly into emotional experience without cognitive mediation (Izard, 1977; Tomkins, 1962). Overall, these studies indicate that facial expression can be sufficient (but not necessary) to elicit an emotional experience, and the intensity of facial expression is positively correlated with the subjective experience of emotion (e.g., Duclos & Laird, 2001; Hess, Kappas, McHugo, Lanzetta, & Kleck, 1992; Matsumoto, 1987; Soussignan, 2002; Strack, Stepper, & Martin, 1988; Tourangeau & Ellsworth, 1979). Finally, self-perception of expressive behavior and appraisals regarding proprioceptive sensations has been proposed to influence subjective emotional experience (Laird, 1974, 1984). Opposite action may influence emotion by changing the perception of the emotional event. Thus, by behaving opposite to the automatic response or action urge of an emotion the meaning of the emotional event may be altered automatically and without conscious effort (Lynch et al., 2005). In essence, the individual concludes that he or she is feeling safe because she is "acting as if" all is safe.

Changing Emotional Aftereffects: Reactivity to Emotions Change

Aftereffects of emotions on attention, memory, and reasoning are fairly well established (see Dolan, 2002, for a review). As noted previously, these aftereffects can increase the probability of a refiring of the same or similar emotion. Interrupting the cycle can be enhanced if the individual actually notices and identifies a current ongoing emotion which can then guide application of change strategies applicable to specific emotions or emotion groups. There is emerging evidence that low emotional awareness and problems identifying and describing one's own emotions are linked to a variety of emotional disorders (Subic-Wrana, Bruder, Thomas, Lane, & Kohle, 2005; Taylor, 1984; Bydlowski et al., 2005). For example, these characteristics are important components of alexithymia (Lane et al., 1996), a condition characterized by widespread difficulties in experiencing and processing emotions. (See Stegge & Meerum Terwogt, this volume, for further discussion of these points.)

As noted previously, emotions are complex behavioral responses. Their identification often requires the ability not only to observe one's own responses but also to describe accurately the context in which the emotion occurs. Thus, learning to identify an emotional response is aided enormously if one can observe and describe (1) the event prompting the emotion; (2) the interpretations or appraisal of the event that prompt the emotion; (3) the phenomenological experience, including the physical sensations, associated with the emotion; (4) the expressions and actions associated with the emotion; and (5) the aftereffects of the emotion on other types of functioning. Instructions for identifying emotions are given in the DBT *Observe and Describe Emotions Skills*. This skill is based on the research showing that processing emotional experience with greater specificity has advantages for improved emotion regulation over emotional processing that is overgeneral or nonspecific (e.g., Williams, 1996; Williams, Stiles, & Shapiro, 1999; Borkovec, Ray, & Stober, 1998). Indeed recent research has demonstrated that priming individuals with overgeneral emotional memories results in more intense emotional experience compared to priming specific emotional memories or a control condition (Schaefer et al., 2003). In addition, experimentally manipulated anxiety regarding public speaking has been shown to be reduced by observing and describing specifically the fear-producing cues, in contrast to general impressions regarding cues that resulted in higher fear (Philippot, Burgos, Verhasselt, & Baeyens, 2002). Drawing from the work of both Shaver (Shaver, Schwartz, Kirson, & O'Connor, 1987) and Hupka (Hupka, Lenton, & Hutchinson, 1999). Linehan developed a taxonomy of 10 basic emotions (anger, disgust, envy, fear, jealousy, joy, love, sadness, shame, and guilt), listing for each emotion (1) the family of emotion names associated with the basic emotion, and typical (2) prompting events, (3) interpretations or appraisals, (4) biological changes and experiences, (5) expressions and actions, (6) aftereffects, and (7) secondary emotions associated with each family of emotions. Using the taxonomy, clients are coached in learning to observe and describe both their primary and their secondary emotions to various events.

DIALECTICAL BEHAVIOR THERAPY CORE MINDFULNESS SKILLS: THEIR ROLE IN EMOTION REGULATION

Mindfulness is the "core" skill in DBT and when used with respect to current emotions means observing, describing, and "allowing" emotions without judging them or trying to inhibit them, block them, or distract from them. It is hypothesized to operate on a number of emotion-regulatory processes simultaneously. Consequently, we review this skill separately and the impact it is hypothesized to have on each component of the DBT emotion regulation model.

Changing Vulnerability to Emotional Cues

Biological Change

Mindfulness is hypothesized to reduce biological vulnerability to negative emotional cues. Indeed, research has demonstrated that for those with experience in mediation, a meditative state was associated with increased prefrontal and basal ganglia activation, as well as decreased activation in anterior cingulate and gyrus occipitalis, electroencephalogram (EEG) patterns consistent with improved capability in moderating the intensity of emotional arousal, and increased left anterior EEG activation (also associated with positive affect) (Aftanas & Golosheykin, 2005; Davidson et al., 2003; Ritskes, Ritskes-Hoitinga, Stodkilde-Jorgensen, Baerentsen, & Hartman, 2003).

Context Change

Mindfulness is hypothesized to create an *internal context* that functions as an *extinction reminder*. Prior research has demonstrated that the extinction of classically conditioned responses is context dependent (Bouton & Brooks, 1993; Bouton, 1993, 2002). Indeed, Bouton (1993) has argued that renewal effects (i.e., a reemergence of the originally conditioned response due to a change in context following extinction) may be due to a failure to retrieve a memory of extinction. An extinction reminder is a cue that is paired with an extinction response and when re-presented upon return to the original conditioning environment functions to reduce renewal effects (Bouton & Brooks, 1993). It is hypothesized that new associations to previously avoided (or pursued) conditional stimuli (CS) become increasingly dominant via repeated practice of mindfulness. The extinction reminder is activated simply by engaging in the act of mindful awareness (i.e., re-presents the cue) whenever the previously avoided CS appears.

Changing Emotional Cues

Situation Selection/Modification

Mindfulness may influence situation selection by nonjudgmentally expanding awareness regarding situations that in the past have evoked emotional experience. This awareness is hypothesized to increase sensitivity to the current contingencies in the environment allowing the opportunity for new learning. Thus, by seeing reality "as it is" (i.e., being in the present moment without historical filters), mindfulness may enhance the ability of an individual to make decisions regarding what situations to avoid, attempt to problem-solve, or cope ahead with.

Attentional Deployment

Mindfulness may influence emotion via attentional control. Mindfulness involves learning to *control the focus of attention,* not the object being attended to (e.g., observing a thought as a thought or emotion as emotion, without an attempt to change the thought or emotion). Being able to disengage from emotional stimuli may reduce the tendency to experience negative affect (Ellenbogen, Schwartzman, Stewart, & Walker, 2002), and redeploying attention has been postulated to lead to a "flexibility of attention" that may free up cognitive resources (Jerslid, 1927; Posner, 1980; Teasdale, Segal, & Williams, 1995). Thus, mindfulness may help modulate emotional experience by enhancing the practitioners' ability to turn their attention from that which is not useful (or effective) and attend to what is (Lynch et al., 2005; Lynch & Bronner, 2006).

Situation Appraisal Change

Mindfulness may alter situation appraisal by reducing literal belief in emotional appraisals. Mindfulness teaches individuals to observe appraisals as only thoughts that are not necessarily literally true. This is hypothesized to increase sensitivity to the current contingencies in the environment, allowing the opportunity for new learning. In this context, mindfulness in DBT would *not* be predicted to reduce the frequency of distressing thoughts but instead to decrease the influence these thoughts have on subsequent behavior and emotions (see more on this in the section "Response Appraisal Change").

Changing Emotional Response Tendencies

Consequence Expectancies Change

Mindfulness involves focusing on effectiveness (rather than being "right") and evokes concepts related to wisdom. Research has demonstrated that people with higher wisdom-related knowledge have higher affective involvement (e.g., interest and attentiveness) but lower affective arousal (Kunzmann & Baltes, 2003) and greater preference for the use of cooperative skills during conflict (Kunzmann & Baltes, 2003). Thus, mindfulness may lead to consequences that reinforce adaptive behavior, particularly in the interpersonal realm.

Response Appraisal Change

Mindfulness is hypothesized to influence the habitual or automatic response to emotional behaviors and any associated appraisals (Lynch et al., in press). A number of theoretical accounts of emotion have described emotions as *response tendencies* (e.g., Gross, 1998a) that have evolved over millennia to serve humans in their quest for survival (LeDoux, 2002). Mindfulness may alter automatic response tendencies by altering the response from habitual avoidance (or habitual approach) to that of "observe" (Lynch, Chapman, Rosenthal, Kuo, & Linehan, 2006). Indeed, by engaging in a response that is incompatible with an emotion (e.g., *observing* a defensive emotion rather than automatically *avoiding* it), the practice of mindfulness may parallel reciprocal inhibition research showing that changing the behavioral response also alters the meaning of the cues eliciting the emotion (e.g., Wolpe, 1954). Thus, without deliberately trying to change what is observed, mindful *observation itself* may alter emotional experience.

Changing Emotional Responses: Opposite Action

Mindfulness may alter rigid or habitualized attempts to overcontrol private experiences (e.g., emotions, cognitions, and sensations). By accepting or observing aversive experience rather than automatically attempting to change experience, mindfulness may function as *nonreinforced exposure* to previously avoided emotions, thoughts, and sensations. Thus, mindfulness can be conceptualized as consistent with interoceptive exposure (Craske, Barlow, & Meadows, 2000). By not avoiding, changing, judging, or attempting to escape interoceptive experience, the mindful practitioner develops new associations to previously avoided CSs (Lynch et al., 2006).

Changing Emotional Aftereffects: Reactivity to Emotions Change

Mindfulness to current emotions requires experiencing emotions without judging them or trying to inhibit them, block them, or distract from them. The basic idea here is that exposure to painful or distressing emotions, without association to negative consequences, will extinguish their ability to stimulate secondary negative emotions. The natural consequences of a person's judging negative emotions as "bad" are feelings of guilt, anger, and/or anxiety whenever feeling emotionally distressed. The addition of these secondary feelings to an already negative situation simply makes the distress more intense and tolerance more difficult. Thus, mindfulness is hypothesized to maximize a quick return to emotional baseline.

DIRECTIONS FOR FUTURE RESEARCH

Psychopathology Research

Construct Validity of Emotion Dysregulation

We proposed the construct of emotion dysregulation (Figure 29.2) and described the characteristics as including an excess of aversive emotional experiences, an inability to regulate intense physiological arousal, problems turning attention away from emotional stimuli, emotion-linked cognitive distortions, failures in information processing under high emotional arousal, insufficient control of impulsive behaviors related to strong positive and negative affects, difficulties organizing and coordinating activities to achieve non-mood-dependent goals when emotionally aroused, and a tendency to "freeze" or dissociate under very high stress. Although each of these is a known characteristic associated with high emotional arousal, we do not know how they go together or whether there are one or more "tipping" points that differentiate normative difficulties regulating extreme emotional arousal versus nonnormative difficulties that predict serious emotional disturbance.

Construct Validity of Pervasive Emotion Dysregulation

We proposed the construct of pervasive emotion dysregulation and conceptualized it as a combination of a tendency to high emotionality across a wide array of both positive and negative emotions together with an inability to regulate intense emotion-linked responses. The validity of this construct has not been evaluated, nor are there measures of the construct. The high incidence of comorbidity across emotional disorders suggests that the construct may be a useful one. Research is needed to both validate and identify the parameters of the construct. We further proposed BPD as a model of pervasive emotion dysregulation. Research designed specifically to evaluate this contention, particularly research comparing BPD to other emotional disorders, is needed.

Construct Validity of Emotion Vulnerability

We have defined emotion vulnerability as sensitivity to emotional stimuli, intense reactions to such stimuli, and a slow, delayed return to an emotional baseline. Once again, BPD is presented as a model of emotion vulnerability. First, the complexity of the constructs being examined highlights the importance of recognizing and measuring emotion vulnerabilty as a multidimensional construct (Campbell & Fiske, 1959). Second, although it appears evident that the intensity of all emotions is enhanced in BPD, the empirical evidence that patients with BPD are generally hypersensitive to emotion-eliciting cues and/or have prolonged return to emotional baselines when aroused are promising but not strong. For example, with respect to sensitivity to emotional cues, it is not clear whether such sensitivity is specific to emotional cues or, in contrast, is a generalized response to all new stimuli. Nor is it clear whether mode of stimulation (visual, auditory, somatic, etc.) makes a difference. Finally, although hypothesized as a trait, it is not clear how problems associated with heightened emotion vulnerability are influenced by current affect or cognitive load.

Neurobiology of Emotion Dysregulation

There is clear evidence for both structural and functional alterations in the fronto-limbic circuits within patients with BPD. However, it remains unclear whether these findings are specific for patients with BPD or are characteristic of individuals with emotion regulation difficulties in general. It is also unclear what and where neurobiological alterations are associated with pervasive emotion dysregulation: within the amygdala, the prefrontal–amygdaloid interaction, the hippocampus–amygdala interplay. There is only beginning research on restitution of these neurobiological alterations after successful treatment. Research on the neurobiology of social emotions such as shame or guilt is in its infancy. (See Beer & Lombardo, this volume, and Hariri & Forbes, this volume, for further discussion.)

Intervention Research

As noted previously, there are substantial data indicating that comprehensive DBT, including individual therapy, skills training, skills coaching, and team meetings for therapists, is effective for individuals with BPD and for other emotional disorders. What is not known is whether the skills taught in DBT are an important component of the treatment's effectiveness. A previous pilot study by Linehan and colleagues (described in Linehan, 1993a) found that DBT group skills training in the absence of a DBT individual therapist was not effective with women meeting criteria for BPD. This is not a complete surprise because the role of the DBT skills trainer is skills acquisition whereas the role of the DBT individual therapist is skills utilization. A larger study of the efficacy of DBT skills training alone versus individual therapy alone versus comprehensive DBT is currently ongoing. There are, however, some data that skills utilization is positively correlated to treatment outcome (Bohus, Limberger, Kleindienst, & Schmahl, 2006) and weekly DBT skills training alone with half-hour telephone coaching is effective in treating chronic depression (Lynch et al., 2003).

We do not know whether some DBT skills are more useful than others, nor are there data regarding the role of competence of skills application (i.e., whether application of the "right skill at the right time" is important). It is also not clear which skills are the right skills for various situations. (See Loewenstein, this volume, and Wranik, Barrett, & Salovey, this volume, for discussion of similar points.) Given the propensity for emotional avoidance among many emotionally disturbed individuals, it is extremely important to find out when to teach patients to distract from unwanted emotions and emotional stimuli and when to expose them to emotions and emotional stimuli. In DBT we make a distinction between moderate versus extreme emotional responses. Extreme emotional responses are defined as those accompanied by cognitive processing so compromised that skills requiring high use of cognitive resources (e.g., problem solving and checking the facts) are unlikely to be successful. With extreme responses, skills more directly affecting somatic arousal (e.g., deep breathing and applying ice water to the face) or attention (e.g., distraction) are recommended. Data verifying the wisdom of these recommendations are sorely lacking. This is particularly important in light of the increasing use of mindfulness-based treatment interventions that teach individuals to notice and accept ongoing emotional responses. The question might be reframed as follows: When is mindfulness of current emotions (a DBT skill) more or less important?

Although there is a fair amount of evidence for most of the specific skills taught in DBT when tested in experimental conditions, there is little evidence that they are effective as treatment interventions, particularly for those with serious emotion regulation disorders. The systematic examination of the DBT skills, both individually and in combination, is an essential first step in improving treatment for deregulated individuals. This is particularly important for the skill of opposite action. Linehan has suggested that opposite action will be effective across a wide range of both dysfunctional positive and negative emotions. Even the experimental literature is meager here and much more research is needed on opposite action as a clinical intervention. For example, a recent study by Rizvi and Linehan (2006) found promising results for opposite action with shame, but other emotions have not been studied explicitly. Thus, although thoroughly evaluated in efficacy studies, there has been substantially less emphasis on the processes by which treatments produce change and future research must work to narrow this gap.

REFERENCES

Aftanas, L., & Golosheykin, S. (2005). Impact of regular meditation practice on EEG activity at rest and during evoked negative emotions. *International Journal of Neuroscience, 115,* 893–909.

American Psychiatric Association. (2001). Practice guideline for the treatment of patients with border-line personality disorder—Introduction. *American Journal of Psychiatry, 158.*

Anderson, C. S., Hackett, M. L., & House, A. O. (2004). Interventions for preventing depression after stroke. *Cochrane Database Systems Review,* CD003689.

Barkley, R. A. (2001). The executive functions and self-regulation: An evolutionary neuropsychological perspective. *Neuropsychological Review, 11,* 1–29.

Barlow, D. H. (1988). *Anxiety and its disorders: The nature and treatment of anxiety and panic.* New York: Guilford Press.

Beck, A. T., Rush, A. J., Shaw, B. F., & Emery, G. (1979). *Cognitive therapy of depression.* New York: Guilford Press.

Beer, J. S., & Lombardo, M. V. (2007). Insights into emotion regulation from neuropsychology. In J. J. Gross (Ed.), *Handbook of emotion regulation* (pp. 69-86). New York: Guilford Press.

Bender, D. S., Dolan, R. T., Skodol, A. E., Sanislow, C. A., Dyck, I. R., McGlashan, T. H., et al. (2001). Treatment utilization by patients with personality disorders. *American Journal of Psychiatry, 158,* 295–302.

Bengtsson-Tops, A. (2004). Mastery in patients with schizophrenia living in the community: Relation-ship to sociodemographic and clinical characteristics, needs for care and support, and social net-work. *Journal of Psychiatric and Mental Health Nursing, 11,* 298–304.

Biglan, A., Rothlind, J., Hops, H., & Sherman, L. (1989). Impact of distressed and aggressive behavior. *Journal of Abnormal Psychology, 98,* 218–228.

Blair, R. J. (2003). Facial expressions, their communicatory functions and neuro-cognitive substrates. *Philosohphical Transactions of the Royal Society of London, B, Biological Sciences, 358,* 561–572.

Bohus, M., Limberger, M., Kleindienst, N., & Schmahl, C. (2006). *Long term follow up of DBT inpatient treatment.* Unpublished manuscript.

Borkovec, T. D., Ray, W. J., & Stober, J. (1998). Worry: A cognitive phenomenon intimately linked to affective, physiological, and interpersonal behavioral processes. *Cognitive Therapy and Research, 22,* 561–576.

Bouton, M. E. (1993). Context, time, and memory retrieval in the interference paradigms of pavlovian learning. *Psychological Bulletin, 114,* 80–99.

Bouton, M. E. (2002). Context, ambiguity, and unlearning: Sources of relapse after behavioral extinc-tion. *Biological Psychiatry, 52,* 976–986.

Bouton, M. E., & Brooks, D. C. (1993). Time and context effects on performance in a Pavlovian dis-crimination reversal. *Journal of Experimental Psychology: Animal Behavior Processes, 19,* 165–179.

Boyce, W. T., & Ellis, B. J. (2005). Biological sensitivity to context: I. An evolutionary–developmental the-ory of the origins and functions of stress reactivity. *Development and Psychopathology, 17,* 271–301.

Brendel, D. H., Reynolds, C. F., III, Jennings, J. R., Hoch, C. C., Monk, T. H., Berman, S. R., et al. (1990). Sleep stage physiology, mood, and vigilance responses to total sleep deprivation in healthy 80-year-olds and 20-year-olds. *Psychophysiology, 27,* 677–685.

Bydlowski, S., Corcos, M., Jeammet, P., Paterniti, S., Berthoz, S., Laurier, C., et al. (2005). Emotion-processing deficits in eating disorders. *International Journal of Eating Disorders, 37,* 321–329.

Campbell, D. T., & Fiske, D. W. (1959). Convergent and discriminanat validation by the multitrait–multimethod matrix. *Psychological Bulletin, 56,* 81–105.

Campbell-Sills, L., & Barlow, D. H. (2007). Incorporating emotion regulation into conceptualizations and treatments of anxiety and mood disorders. In J. J. Gross (Ed.), *Handbook of emotion regulation* (pp. 542–559). New York: Guilford Press.

Christianson, S. A. (1992). Emotional stress and eyewitness memory: A critical review. *Psychological Bul-letin, 112,* 284–309.

Cowdry, R. W., Gardner, D. L., O'Leary, K. M., Leibenluft, E., & Rubinow, D. R. (1991). Mood variabil-ity: A study of four groups. *American Journal of Psychiatry, 148,* 1505–1511.

Cox, R. H., Thomas, T. R., Hinton, P. S., & Donahue, O. M. (2004). Effects of acute 60 and 80% VO2max bouts of aerobic exercise on state anxiety of women of different age groups across time. *Research Quarterly for Exercise and Sport, 75,* 165–175.

Craske, M. G., Barlow, D. H., & Meadows, E. (2000). *Mastery of your anxiety and panic–3rd edition (MAP-3): Therapist guide for anxiety, panic, and agoraphobia*. San Antonio, TX: Graywind Publications/Psychological Corporation.

Davidson, R. J. (1998). Anterior electrophysiological asymmetries, emotion, and depression: Conceptual and methodological conundrums. *Psychophysiology, 35*, 607–614.

Davidson, R. J., Fox, A., & Kalin, N. H. (2007). Neural bases of emotion regulation in nonhuman primates and humans. In J. J. Gross (Ed.), *Handbook of emotion regulation* (pp. 47–68). New York: Guilford Press.

Davidson, R. J., Kabat-Zinn, J., Schumacher, J., Rosenkranz, M., Muller, D., Santorelli, S. F., et al. (2003). Alterations in brain and immune function produced by mindfulness meditation. *Psychosomatic Medicine, 65*, 564–570.

de Beurs, E., Comijs, H., Twisk, J. W., Sonnenberg, C., Beekman, A. T., & Deeg, D. (2005). Stability and change of emotional functioning in late life: Modelling of vulnerability profiles. *Journal of Affective Disorders, 84*, 53–62.

Devinsky, O., Morrell, M. J., & Vogt, B. A. (1995). Contributions of anterior cingulate cortex to behaviour. *Brain, 118*(Pt. 1), 279–306.

Dimidjian, S., Hollon, S., Dobson, D., Schmaling, K., Kohlenberg, B. S., Addis, M., et al. (in press). Randomized trial of behavioral activation, cognitive therapy, and antidepressant medication in the acute treatment of adults with major depression. *Journal of Consulting and Clinical Psychology*.

Dolan, R. J. (2002). Emotion, cognition, and behavior. *Science, 298*, 1191–1194.

Donegan, N. H., Sanislow, C. A., Blumberg, H. P., Fulbright, R. K., Lacadie, C., Skudlarski, P., et al. (2003). Amygdala hyperreactivity in borderline personality disorder: implications for emotional dysregulation. *Biological Psychiatry, 54*, 1284–1293.

Duclos, S. E., & Laird, J. D. (2001). The deliberate control of emotional experience through control of expressions. *Cognition and Emotion, 15*, 27–56.

D'Zurilla, T. J., Chang, E. C., Nottingham, E. J., & Faccini, L. (1998). Social problem-solving deficits and hopelessness, depression, and suicidal risk in college students and psychiatric inpatients. *Journal of Clinical Psychology, 54*, 1091–1107.

D'Zurilla, T. J., & Nezu, A. M. (1999). *Problem-solving therapy: A social competence approach to clinical intervention* (2nd ed.). New York: Springer.

Ebner-Priemera, U. W., Shaw-Welch, S., Grossman, P., Reisch, T., Linehan, M. M., & Bohus, M. (in press). Psychophysiological ambulatory assessment of affective dysregulation in borderline personality disorder. *Psychiatry Research*.

Ekman, P. (1994). All emotions are basic. In P. Ekman, & R. J. Davidson (Eds.), *The nature of emotion* (pp. 15–19). New York: Oxford University Press.

Ekman, P., & Davidson, R. J. (1994). *The nature of emotion: Fundamental questions*. New York: Oxford University Press.

Ekman, P., & Friesen, W. (1978). *Pictures of facial affect*. Palo Alto, CA: Consulting Psychologists Press.

Ellenbogen, M. A., Schwartzman, A. E., Stewart, J., & Walker, C. D. (2002). Stress and selective attention: The interplay of mood, cortisol levels, and emotional information processing. *Psychophysiology, 39*, 723–732.

Fourkas, A. D., Avenanti, A., Urgesi, C., & Aglioti, S. M. (2005). Corticospinal facilitation during first and third person imagery. *Experimental Brain Research, 168*, 143–151.

Gollwitzer, P. M., Heckhausen, H., & Steller, B. (1990). Deliverate vs. implemental mind-sets: Cognitive tuning toward congruous thoughts and information. *Journal of Personality and Social Psychology, 59*, 1119–1127.

Green, M. W., Rogers, P. J., Elliman, N. A., & Gatenby, S. J. (1994). Impairment of cognitive performance associated with dieting and high levels of dietary restraint. *Physiological Behaviour, 55*, 447–452.

Gross, J. J. (1998a). Antecedent- and response-focused emotion regulation: Divergent consequences for experience, expression, and physiology. *Journal of Personality and Social Psychology, 74*, 224–237.

Gross, J. J. (1998b). The emerging field of emotion regulation: An integrative review. *Review of General Psychology, 2*, 271–299.

Gross, J. J. (1999). Emotion and emotion regulation. In L. A. Pervin & O. P. John (Eds.), *Handbook of personality: Theory and research* (2nd ed., pp. 525–552). New York: Guilford Press.

Gross, J. J., & Levenson, R. W. (1993). Emotional suppression: Physiology, self-report, and expressive behavior. *Journal of Personality and Social Psychology, 64*, 970–986.

Gross, J. J., & Thompson, R. A. (2007). Emotion regulation: Conceptual foundations. In J. J. Gross (Ed.), *Handbook of emotion regulation* (pp. 3–24). New York: Guilford Press.

Hariri, A. R., & Forbes, E. E. (2007). Genetics of emotion regulation. In J. J. Gross (Ed.), *Handbook of emotion regulation* (pp. 110–132). New York: Guilford Press.

Hayes, S. C., Bissett, R. T., Korn, Z., Zettle, R. D., Rosenfarb, I. S., Cooper, L. D., et al. (1999). The impact of acceptance versus control rationales on pain tolerance. *Psychological Reports, 49,* 33–47.

Herpertz, S. C., Dietrich, T. M., Wenning, B., Krings, T., Erberich, S. G., Willmes, K., et al. (2001). Evidence of abnormal amygdala functioning in borderline personality disorder: A functional MRI study. *Biological Psychiatry, 50,* 292–298.

Hess, U., Kappas, A., McHugo, G. J., Lanzetta, J. T., & Kleck, R. E. (1992). The facilitative effect of facial expression on the self-generation of emotion. *International Journal of Psychophysiology, 12,* 251–265.

Horstmann, G. (2003). What do facial expressions convey: Feeling states, behavioral intentions, or action requests? *Emotion, 3,* 150–166.

Hupka, R. B., Lenton, A. P., & Hutchinson, K. A. (1999). Universal development of emotion categories in natural language. *Journal of Personality and Social Psychology, 77,* 247–278.

Hurwitz, B. E., & Furedy, J. J. (1986). The human dive reflex—An experimental, topographical and physiological analysis. *Physiology and Behavior, 36,* 287–294.

Izard, C. E. (1977). Distress—anguish, grief, and depression. In C. Izard (Ed.), *Human emotions* (pp. 285–288). New York: Plenum Press.

Izard, C. E., Libero, D. Z., Putnam, P., & Haynes, O. M. (1993). Stability of emotion experiences and their relations to traits of personality. *Journal of Personality and Social Psychology, 64,* 847–860.

Jacobson, N. S., Dobson, K. S., Truax, P. A., Addis, M. E., Koerner, K., Gollan, J. K., et al. (1996). A component analysis of cognitive-behavioral treatment for depression. *Journal of Consulting and Clinical Psychology, 64,* 295–304.

Jerslid, A. T. (1927). Mental set and shift. *Archives of Psychology, 14*(89), 81.

Joiner, T. E., Jr., Lewinsohn, P. M., & Seeley, J. R. (2002). The core of loneliness: Lack of pleasurable engagement—more so than painful disconnection—predicts social impairment, depression onset, and recovery from depressive disorders among adolescents. *Journal of Personality Assessment, 79,* 472–491.

Keltner, D., & Anderson, C. L. (2000). Saving face for Darwin: The functions and uses of embarrassment. *Current Directions in Psychological Science, 9,* 192.

Koons, C. R., Robins, C. J., Tweed, J. L., Lynch, T. R., Gonzalez, A. M., Morse, J. Q., et al. (2001). Efficacy of dialectical behavior therapy in women veterans with borderline personality disorder. *Behavior Therapy, 32,* 371–390.

Kunzmann, U., & Baltes, P. B. (2003). Wisdom-related knowledge: Affective, motivational, and interpersonal correlates. *Personality and Social Psychology Bulletin, 29,* 1104–1119.

Laird, J. D. (1974). Self-attribution of emotion: The effects of expressive behavior on the quality of emotional experience. *Journal of Personality and Social Psychology, 29,* 475–486.

Laird, J. D. (1984). The real role of facial response in the experience of emotion: A reply to Tourangeau and Ellsworth, and others. *Journal of Personality and Social Psychology, 47,* 909–917.

Lam, K., Marra, C., & Salzinger, K. (2005). Social reinforcement of somatic versus psychological description of depressive events. *Behaviour Research and Therapy, 43,* 1203–1218.

Lane, R. D., Reiman, E. M., Bradley, M. M., Lang, P. J., Ahern, G. L., & Davidson, R. J. (1997). Neuroanatomical correlates of pleasant and unpleasant emotion. *Neuropsychologica, 35,* 1437–1444.

Lane, R. D., Sechrest, L., Reidel, R., Weldon, V., Kaszniak, A., & Schwartz, G. E. (1996). Impaired verbal and nonverbal emotion recognition in alexithymia. *Psychosomatic Medicine, 58,* 203–210.

Lazarus, A. A., & Abramovitz, A. (1962). The use of "emotive imagery" in the treatment of children's phobias. *Journal of Mental Science, 108,* 191–195.

LeDoux, J. (2002). *Synaptic self.* New York: Viking/Penguin.

Levine, D., Marziali, E., & Hood, J. (1997). Emotion processing in borderline personality disorders. *Journal of Nervous and Mental Disease, 185,* 240–246.

Levitt, J. T., Brown, T. A., Orsillo, S. M., & Barlow, D. H. (2004). The effects of acceptance versus suppression of emotion on subjective and psychophysiological response to carbon dioxide challenge in patients with panic disorder. *Behavior Therapy, 25,* 747–766.

Linehan, M. M. (1993a). *Cognitive-behavioral treatment of borderline personality disorder.* New York: Guilford Press.

Linehan, M. M. (1993b). *Skills training manual for treating borderline personality disorder.* New York: Guilford Press.

Linehan, M. M., Armstrong, H. E., Suarez, A., Allmon, D., & Heard, H. L. (1991). Cognitive-behavioral treatment of chronically parasuicidal borderline patients. *Archives of General Psychiatry, 48*, 1060–1064.

Linehan, M. M., Comtois, K. A., Murray, A., Brown, M. Z., Gallop, R. J., Heard, H. L., et al. (2006). Two-year randomized trial + follow-up of dialectical behavior therapy vs. therapy by experts for suicidal behaviors and borderline personality disorder. *Archives of General Psychiatry, 63*, 757–766.

Linehan, M. M., Dimeff, L. A., Reynolds, S. K., Comtois, K., Shaw-Welch, S., Heagerty, P., et al. (2002). Dialectical behavior therapy versus comprehensive validation plus 12 step for the treatment of opioid dependent women meeting criteria for borderline personality disorder. *Drug and Alcohol Dependence, 67*, 13–26.

Linehan, M. M., Schmidt, H., III, Dimeff, L. A., Craft, J. C., Kanter, J., & Comtois, K. A. (1999). Dialectical behavior therapy for patients with borderline personality disorder and drug-dependence. *American Journal of Addiction, 8*, 279–292.

Loewenstein, G. (2007). Affective regulation and affective forecasting. In J. J. Gross (Ed.), *Handbook of emotion regulation* (pp. 180–203). New York: Guilford Press.

Lynch, T. R., & Bronner, L. L. (2006). Mindfulness and dialectical behavior therapy: Application with depressed older adults with personality disorders. In R. A. Baer (Ed.), *Mindfulness-based approaches: A clinician's guide.* New York: Elsevier.

Lynch, T. R., Chapman, A. L., Rosenthal, M. Z., Kuo, J. R., & Linehan, M. M. (2006) Mechanisms of change in dialectical behavior therapy: Theoretical and empirical observations. *Journal of Clinical Psychology, 62*, 459–480.

Lynch, T. R., Cheavens, J., Cukrowicz, K. C., Thorp, S., Bronner, L., & Beyer, J. (in press). Treatment of older adults with co-morbid personality disorder and depression: A dialectical behavior therapy approach. *International Journal of Geriatric Psychiatry.*

Lynch, T. R., Morse, J. Q., Mendelson, T., & Robins, C. J. (2003). Dialectical behavior therapy for depressed older adults: A randomized pilot study. *American Journal of Geriatric Psychiatry, 11*, 33–45.

Lynch, T. R., Rosenthal, M. Z., Kosson, D., Cheavens, J., Lejuez, C. W., & Blair, R. J. (2005). *Heightened sensitivity to facial expressions of emotion in borderline personality disorder.* Manuscript submitted for publication.

Martell, C. R., Addis, M., & Jacobson, N. S. (2001). *Depression in context: Strategies for guided action.* New York: Norton.

Matsumoto, D. (1987). The role of facial response in the experience of emotion: More methodological problems and a meta-analysis. *Journal of Personality and Social Psychology, 52*, 769–774.

McMain, S., Korman, L. M., & Dimeff, L. A. (2001). Dialectical behavior therapy and the treatment of emotion dysregulation. *In Session: Psychotherapy in Practice, 57*, 183–196.

McNally, R. J. (1995). Automaticity and the anxiety disorders. *Behavior Research and Therapy, 33*, 747–754.

Mesquita, B., & Albert, D. (2007). The cultural regulation of emotions. In J. J. Gross (Ed.), *Handbook of emotion regulation* (pp. 486–503). New York: Guilford Press.

Michael, J. (1993). Establishing operations. *The Behavior Analyst, 16*, 206.

Ochsner, K. N., & Gross, J. J. (2007). The neural architecture of emotion regulation. In J. J. Gross (Ed.), *Handbook of emotion regulation* (pp. 87–109). New York: Guilford Press.

Ohman, A., & Soares, J. J. (1993). On the automatic nature of phobic fear: Conditioned electrodermal responses to masked fear-relevant stimuli. *Journal of Abnormal Psychology, 102*, 121–132.

Otto, M. W., Smits, J. A. J., & Reese, H. E. (2005). Combined psychotherapy and pharmacotherapy for mood and anxiety disorders in adults. *Clinical Psychology: Science and Practice, 12*(1), 87–91.

Pawlow, L. A., & Jones, G. E. (2002). The impact of abbreviated progressive muscle relaxation on salivary control. *Biological Psychology, 60*, 1–16.

Peterson, C., & Park, N. (2007). Explanatory style and emotion regulation. In J. J. Gross (Ed.), *Handbook of emotion regulation* (pp. 159–179). New York: Guilford Press.

Philippot, P., Baeyens, C., Douilliez, C., & Francart, B. (2004). Cognitive regulation of emotion: Application to clinical disorders. In P. Philippot & R. S. Feldman (Eds.), *The regulation of emotion* (pp. 71–100). New York: Erlbaum.

Philippot, P., Burgos, A. I., Verhasselt, S., & Baeyens, C. (2002). *Specifying emotional information: Modulation of emotional intensity via executive processes.* Paper presented at the 2002 International Society for Research on Emotion Conference, La Cuenca, Spain.

Posner, M. I. (1980). Orienting of attention. *Quarterly Journal of Experimental Psychology, 32*, 3–25.

Reiman, E. M. (1997). The application of positron emission tomography to the study of normal and pathologic emotions. *Journal of Clinical Psychiatry, 58*(Suppl. 16), 4–12.

Ritskes, R., Ritskes-Hoitinga, M., Stodkilde-Jorgensen, H., Baerentsen, K., & Hartman, T. (2003). MRI scanning during Zen meditation: The picture of enlightenment? *Constructivism in the Human Sciences, 8*, 85–90.

Rizvi, S. L., & Linehan, M. M. (2006). The treatment of maladaptive shame in borderline personality disorder: A pilot study of "opposite action." *Cognitive and Behavioral Practice, 12*, 437–447.

Rosenbaum, M., Lewinsohn, P. M., & Gotlib, I. H. (1996). Distinguishing between state-dependent and non-state-dependent depression-related psychosocial variables. *British Journal of Clinical Psychology, 35*(Pt. 3), 341–358.

Safer, D. L., Telch, C. F., & Agras, W. S. (2001). Dialectical behavior therapy for bulimia nervosa. *American Journal of Psychiatry, 158*, 632–634.

Schaefer, A., Collette, F., Philippot, P., van der, L. M., Laureys, S., Delfiore, G., et al. (2003). Neural correlates of "hot" and "cold" emotional processing: A multilevel approach to the functional anatomy of emotion. *NeuroImage, 18*, 938–949.

Scherer, K. (1994). Toward a concept of "model emotions." In P. Ekman & R. J. Davidson (Eds.), *The nature of emotion* (pp. 25–31). New York: Oxford University Press.

Schmahl, C. G., Vermetten, E., Elzinga, B. M., & Bremner, J. D. (2004). A PET study of memories of childhood abuse in borderline personality disorder. *Biological Psychiatry, 55*, 759–765.

Shaver, P., Schwartz, J., Kirson, D., & O'Connor, C. (1987). Emotion knowledge: Further exploration of a prototype approach. *Journal of Personality and Social Psychology, 52*, 1061–1086.

Sheppard, L. C., & Teasdale, J. D. (2000). Dysfunctional thinking in major depressive disorder: A deficit in metacognitive monitoring? *Journal of Abnormal Psychology, 109*, 768–776.

Sheppard, L. C., & Teasdale, J. D. (2004). How does dysfunctional thinking decrease during recovery from major depression? *Journal of Abnormal Psychology, 113*, 64–71.

Smith, C. A., & Kirby, L. D. (2000). Consequences requires antecedents: Towards a process model of emotional elicitation. In J. D. Forgas (Ed.), *Feeling and thinking: The role of affect in social cognition* (pp. 83–106). New York: Cambridge University Press.

Smith, C. F., Williamson, D. A., Bray, G. A., & Ryan, D. H. (1999). Flexible vs. Rigid dieting strategies: Relationship with adverse behavioral outcomes. *Appetite, 32*, 295–305.

Soussignan, R. (2002). Duchenne smile, emotional experience, and autonomic reactivity: A test of the facical feedback hypothesis. *Emotion, 2*, 52–74.

Speisman, J. C., Lazarus, R. S., Mordkoff, A., & Davison, L. (1964). Experimental reduction of stress based on ego-defense theory. *Journal of Abnormal Psychology, 68*, 367–380.

Stegge, H., & Meerum Terwogt, M. (2007). Awareness and regulation of emotion in typical and atypical development. In J. J. Gross (Ed.), *Handbook of emotion regulation* (pp. 269–286). New York: Guilford Press.

Stein, K. F. (1996). Affect instability in adults with a borderline personality disorder. *Archives of Psychiatric Nursing, 10*, 32–40.

Stella, S. G., Vilar, A. P., Lacroix, C., Fisberg, M., Santos, R. F., Mello, M. T., et al. (2005). Effects of type of physical exercise and leisure activities on the depression scores of obese Brazilian adolescent girls. *Brazilian Journal of Medical and Biological Research, 38*, 1683–1689.

Stepper, S., & Strack, F. (1993). Proprioceptive determinants of emotional and nonemotional feelings. *Journal of Personality and Social Psychology, 64*, 211–220.

Stiglmayr, C., Grathwol, T., & Bohus, M. (2001). *States of aversive tension in patients with borderline personality disorder: A controlled field study in progress in ambulatory assessment.* Seattle: Hogrefe and Huber.

Stiglmayr, C., Grathwol, T., Linehan, M., Fahrenberg, J., & Bohus, M. (2005). Aversive tension in patients with borderline personality disorder: A computer-based controlled field study. *Acta Psychiatrica Scandinavica, 111*, 379.

Stiglmayr, C. E., Shapiro, D. A., Stieglitz, R. D., Limberger, M. F., & Bohus, M. (2001). Experience of aversive tension and dissociation in female patients with borderline personality disorder—A controlled study. *Journal Psychiatric Research, 35*, 111–118.

Strack, F., Stepper, S., & Martin, L. L. (1988). Inhibiting and facilitating conditions of the human smile: A nonobtrusive test of the facial feedback hypothesis. *Journal of Personality and Social Psychology, 54*, 768–777.

Subic-Wrana, C., Bruder, S., Thomas, W., Lane, R. D., & Kohle, K. (2005). Emotional awareness deficits in inpatients of a psychosomatic ward: A comparison of two different measures of alexithymia. *Psychosomatic Medicine, 67*, 483–489.

Tafrate, R. C., Kassinove, H., & Dundin, L. (2002). Anger episodes in high- and low-trait-anger community adults. *Journal of Clinical Psychology, 58*, 1573–1590.

Taylor, G. J. (1984). Alexithymia: Concept, measurement, and implications for treatment. *American Journal of Psychiatry, 141*, 725–732.

Teasdale, J. D., Segal, Z., & Williams, J. M. (1995). How does cognitive therapy prevent depressive relapse and why should attentional control (mindfulness) training help? *Behaviour Research and Therapy, 33*, 25–39.

Telch, C. F., Agras, W. S., & Linehan, M. M. (2001). Dialectical behavior therapy for binge eating disorder: A promising new treatment. *Journal of Consulting and Clinical Psychology, 69*, 1061–1065.

Tomkins, S. S. (1962). *Affect, imagery, consciousness* (Vol. 1). New York: Springer.

Tooby, J., & Cosmides, L. (1990). The past explains the present: Emotional adaptations and the structure of ancestral environment. *Ethology and Sociobiology, 11*, 375–424.

Torgersen, S., Kringlen, E., & Cramer, V. (2001). The prevalence of personality disorders in a community sample. *Archives of General Psychiatry, 58*, 590–596.

Tourangeau, R., & Ellsworth, P. C. (1979). The role of facial response in the experience of emotion. *Journal of Personality and Social Psychology, 37*, 1519–1531.

Turkheimer, E., & Gottesman, I. I. (1991). Individual differences and the canalization of human behavior. *Developmental Psychology, 27*, 18–22.

van den Bosch, L. M. C., Verheul, R., Schippers, G. M., & Van den Brink, W. (2002). Dialectical behavior therapy of borderline patients with and without substance use problems: Implementation and long-term effects. *Addictive Behaviors, 27*, 911–923.

Verheul, R., van den Bosch, L. M. C., Koeter, M. W. J., de Ridder, M. A. J., Stijnen, T., & van den, B. W. (2003). Dialectical behaviour therapy for women with borderline personality disorder: 12-month, randomised clinical trial in The Netherlands. *British Journal of Psychiatry, 182*, 135–140.

Vogt, B. A., Finch, D. M., & Olson, C. R. (1992). Functional heterogeneity in cingulate cortex: The anterior executive and posterior evaluative regions. *Cerebral Cortex, 2*, 435–443.

Waddington, C. H. (1966). *Principles of development and differentiation*. New York: Macmillan.

Wagner, A. W., & Linehan, M. M. (1999). Facial expression recognition ability among women with borderline personality disorder: Implications for emotion regulation? *Journal of Personality Disorders, 13*, 329–344.

Williams, J. B. W., Stiles, W. B., & Shapiro, D. A. (1999). Cognitive mechanisms in the avoidance of painful and dangerous thoughts: Elaborating the assimilation model. *Cognitive Therapy and Research, 23*, 285–306.

Williams, J. M. G. (1996). Cognitive mechanisms in the avoidance of painful and dangerous thoughts: Elaborating the assimilation model. *Cognitive Therapy and Research, 23*, 285–306.

Wolpe, J. (1954). Reciprocal inhibition as the main basis of psychotherapeutic effects. *Archives of Neurology and Psychiatry, 72*, 205–276.

Wranik, T., Barrett, L. F., & Salovey, P. (2007). Intelligent emotion regulation: Is knowledge power? In J. J. Gross (Ed.), *Handbook of emotion regulation* (pp. 393–407). New York: Guilford Press.

Zanarini, M. C., Frankenburg, F. R., Khera, G. S., & Bleichmar, J. (2001). Treatment histories of borderline inpatients. *Comprehensive Psychiatry, 42*, 144–150.

CHAPTER 30

Stress, Stress-Related Disease, and Emotional Regulation

ROBERT M. SAPOLSKY

The study of stress is now close to a century old, having been spawned by the work and insights of Walter Cannon and Hans Selye. In the initial years of the field, the subject was entirely the purview of biologically oriented scientists, and it was not until some decades later that the transition began to the present point, where the subject is as much the domain of psychologists. This shift, long resisted by the founding biologists, has allowed the field to mature to a dramatic extent. Moreover, as an ironic point that is reviewed, the introduction of a psychological orientation to the field has helped explain the origins of stress-related disease far better than could ever have been done with the purely biologically based approach.

This chapter reviews how the original biologically dominated view of stress and health came to accommodate an enormous input from psychologists. This is not meant to be mere historicism. Instead, it paves the way for appreciating the five main points of this piece:

1. In the face of an acute physical challenge, the body mobilizes the stress response, which is central to surviving that challenge.
2. In contrast, chronic mobilization of the stress response carries a wide array of pathophysiological risks.
3. Overwhelmingly, it is psychological, rather than physiological stress, which activates the stress response chronically enough to have disease consequences.
4. The power of purely psychological states to alter stress-related physiology implies that thought and emotion can make us sick. As such, the regulation of both becomes critical to health.
5. The appropriate regulation of thoughts and emotions not only decreases the likelihood of pathogenic activation of the stress response due to psychological factors but also increases the likelihood that the behavioral responses to psychological stressors that are chosen are adaptive ones.

THE PHYSIOLOGICAL STRESS RESPONSE

It was Cannon who formalized long-standing ideas regarding physiological regulation with the term "homeostasis." This was the idea that all physiological endpoints have an ideal level (an ideal body temperature, level of glucose in the bloodstream, heart rate, etc.), that the purpose of physiological regulation is to achieve a state of homeostasis (or "homeostatic balance"), in which as many of those endpoints are optimized as possible. While the classic homeostatic concept has been updated in recent years, as discussed later, the concept is the central dogma of physiology.

For the founding generation of stress researchers, anchored in the homeostasis concept, a "stressor" was defined as anything that perturbs homeostatic balance, while the "stress response" was defined as the neural and endocrine adaptations that, collectively, reestablish homeostasis (e.g., Cannon, 1936). Thus, a stressor can be something that induces a temperature extreme; blood loss; sharp pain; the need for a sudden, explosive expenditure of energy; and so on. And as was shown in rich detail, the stress response is ideally evolved for solving such acute challenges to homeostasis.

The first component of the stress response to be defined was the secretion of adrenaline (or, as known in the United States, epinephrine), along with the secretion of the related norepinephrine. Such secretion is under the control of the sympathetic nervous system (one branch of the larger autonomic nervous system) and was identified around 1914 by Cannon, who coined the term the "fight-or-flight response." It was in the 1930s that another key endocrine branch of the stress response was identified by the other founding father of the field, Hans Selye. Selye was the first to delineate the stress-induced secretion by adrenal glands of a class of steroid hormones called glucocorticoids (such as cortisol, also known as hydrocortisone). Glucocorticoids, along with the sympathetic hormones (i.e., epinephrine RT al., and norepinephrine), form the backbone of the stress response (Selye, 1936a, 1936b).

Other endocrine secretions were soon linked to the stress response. As with glucocorticoids and the sympathetic hormones, a typical stressor causes increased secretion of hormones that include beta-endorphin, prolactin, vasopressin, and glucagon. In addition, the stress response involves decreased secretion of other hormones, such as those of the reproductive system (e.g., estrogens and androgens), growth (such as the somatomedins), and energy storage (such as insulin), along with inhibition of the parasympathetic branch of the autonomic nervous system. While the exact orchestration of these various neural and hormonal changes varies to some extent, depending on the particular stressor (a phenomenon now called a stress signature), this is the basic stress response (Sapolsky, Romero, & Munck, 2000).

Collectively, these adaptations are critical to surviving the sort of short-term physical stressor that concerned the first generations in the field. Energy storage is curtailed and energy is mobilized from storage sites throughout the body, such as fat cells, for delivery to exercising muscle. Cardiovascular tone is increased to enhance the delivery of such energy; specifically, blood pressure and heart rate are elevated, blood flow to unessential regions (such as the intestines) is inhibited, and blood flow to exercising muscle is increased. Long-term processes such as growth, digestion, tissue repair, and reproduction are inhibited until more auspicious times. Immune defenses are enhanced, pain perception is blunted, and certain aspects of cognition are enhanced (Munck, Guyre, & Holbrook, 1984; Sapolsky et al., 2000). The critical role played by these adaptations can be appreciated in considering sufferers of diseases in which the

608 CLINICAL APPLICATIONS

stress response fails due to impaired secretion of glucocorticoids (as in Addison's disease), or of catecholamines (as in Shy–Drager syndrome). In these disorders, the loss of homeostasis caused by an infection, injury, surgical procedure, or even an outburst of energy expenditure can be life-threatening (Raison & Miller, 2003).

Therefore, as originally conceptualized, the purpose of the stress response was to reestablish homeostasis. It was not until the 1980s that it was widely accepted that part of the endocrine stress response, involving some of the slower-acting hormones, also brings about recovery from the primary stress response. For example, the energy-mobilizing effects of the primary stress response are eventually counterbalanced by hormones that stimulate appetite and promote energy storage in adipose tissue. Or, as another example, the immune-stimulating effects of the primary stress response are eventually countered by hormones that inhibit immunity. This delayed inhibition is thought to prevent the immune system from becoming so activated as to erroneously respond to normal constituents of the body as if they are invasive pathogens (i.e., an autoimmune disease) (Munck et al., 1984).

Thus, in the contemporary version of the Cannon school, the stress response can be viewed as a set of rapid adaptations designed to deal with an acute challenge to homeostasis with an explosive expenditure of energy, a curtailment of physiological unessentials, and the laying of the groundwork for recovering from this dramatic physiological shift. In an important modification in recent years, Taylor et al. (2000) have argued that the fight-or-flight response to homeostatic challenge tends to be an attribute of males, and that the disproportionate reliance on male subjects in stress research has erroneously produced the impression that this is "the" standard stress response. Instead, they argue, quite validly, that females of many social species respond to challenges to homeostasis with affiliative and nurturing behaviors (what they have termed the "tend and befriend" response), and that this profile depends on stress-responsive hormones generally ignored by the Cannon school, namely, vasopressin and oxytocin.

This classic Cannon model of thinking about stress was recognized to include a scenario in which the outcome is death rather than adaptation. This is one in which the physiological stressor is so severe as to overwhelm the adaptive capacity of the stress response. Consider an animal mildly injured while evading a predator. The stress response, in this instance, is highly adaptive, including local vasoconstriction and platelet aggregation to staunch the flow of blood at the site of injury, water retention to counter the hypotensive effects of the blood loss, stress-induced analgesia to block the pain of the injury, and so on. However, if the wounding is sufficiently severe, the stress response becomes insufficient and death ensues. Or, consider the scenario of a prey species running to evade a predator. Acutely, sufficient energy might be diverted from storage sites to muscle in order to power successful evasion; however, should the crisis be prolonged, energy stores become depleted, resulting in death. Thus, in these scenarios, it is not that the stress response is maladaptive (i.e., injurious on its own) but is simply insufficient. A very contrasting scenario will soon be discussed.

Over the subsequent decades, physiologists added nuances to this picture. The stress response, for example, was shown to be sensitive in a dose-response manner to the extent of homeostatic imbalance. For example, there is a fairly linear relationship (within a survivable range) between the extent of blood loss induced in an experimental hemorrhage in a laboratory animal and the magnitude of glucocorticoid secretion (Gann, Cryer, & Pirkle, 1977). In another realm, cell biologists were delineating how epinephrine, for example, triggers the breakdown of molecules of energy storage in fat cells, while molecular biologists uncovered, for example, different genetic versions of genes coding for glucocorticoid receptors.

Thus, the stress response is highly adaptive, being capable of buffering the body from all but the most extreme of homeostatic challenges. This essentially optimistic view was championed by Cannon, best captured in the title of one of his books, *The Wisdom of the Body* (Cannon, 1932/1963). It was not until the work of Selye, beginning a decade later, that this was shown to be only half of the story.

CHRONIC ACTIVATION OF THE STRESS RESPONSE, AND THE EMERGENCE OF STRESS-RELATED DISEASE

Selye, in challenging homeostasis in his study subjects, introduced an element under-explored by Cannon and colleagues, namely, *chronic* exposure to stressors. And under those circumstances, Selye observed a very different picture than the view of the stress response as being purely adaptive and beneficial. Instead, Selye observed pathology, specifically a triad of disorders that became the cornerstone of the field, namely, the emergence of peptic ulcers, enlargement of the adrenal glands, and atrophy of immune organs (such as the thymus) (Selye, 1936a, 1936b). We now recognize this to have been the first evidence of stress-related disease.

Selye's most creative contribution was to show that a remarkably diverse array of stressors could all cause the same triad of pathologies. What he soon appreciated was that the key commonality of these stressors was their chronicity.

In trying to explain why chronic stressors could prove pathogenic, Selye speculated that a prolonged physiological stressor triggered a state of endocrine "exhaustion" in the organism (Selye, 1979). For example, in that view, the relevant glands become depleted of the hormones that mobilize energy, that increase water retention, that accelerate heart rate, and so on. In effect, the stress response fails, leaving the organism undefended against the stressor. However, virtually no evidence has emerged support-ing the notion of an exhaustion stage, the idea that the stress response can become depleted as a result of chronic stressors. Instead, in the face of prolonged stressors, the stress response continues to be mobilized robustly and, over time, *the stress response itself becomes damaging*. In many ways, this is the most important concept of the field (Munck et al., 1984).

This consequence is readily appreciated when considering what occurs when the various facets of the stress response are prolonged. Mobilization of energy from storage sites throughout the body, when prolonged, will lead to atrophy of muscle, fatigue, and increased risk of adult-onset diabetes. Moreover, chronic activation of the counter-regulatory features of the metabolic stress response will lead to obesity. Next, while acute increases in cardiovascular tone can be highly adaptive, chronic increases will raise the risk of cardiovascular and cerebrovascular disease. Chronic inhibition of diges-tion increases the risk of an array of malabsorption disorders. Prolonged inhibition of growth in developing organisms can seriously impair normal maturation; at an extreme are syndromes of arrested growth for reasons of stress (i.e., stress dwarfism). Chronic deferring of tissue repair, will compromise wound healing; as one special domain of this, impairing the capacity to repair early-stage erosions in stomach walls (typically caused by the bacteria *Helicobacter pylori*) increases the risk of ulcers. Continuing this theme, while transient inhibition of reproductive physiology may be of no patho-physiological consequences, prolonged inhibition will impair fertility in both sexes. Next, while the delayed inhibition of immune function during a transient stressor may help to avoid the sort of overactivation of the immune system that biases toward autoimmunity, prolonged inhibition can result in frank immune suppression and increased risk of infectious disease. Finally, the same hormones that, acutely, can sharpen aspects of cognition during stress, can have a wide array of deleterious effects in the nervous system, including impairment of synaptic plasticity atrophy of dendritic process, and inhibition of neurogenesis (Sapolsky et al., 2000).

(This overview should make clear the basis of the original triad of pathologies reported by Selye, namely the increased risk of ulcers, the hypertrophied adrenal glands [due to increased demand for glucocorticoid synthesis and secretion], and the atrophy of immune tissues.)

Thus the work of Cannon showed that in the face of an acute stressor, the stress response is vital to successful adaptation to the challenge. However, as shown in the work of Selye, in the face of chronic stressors, the stress response itself can become pathogenic across a wide array of organ systems. What we think of as "stress-related diseases" are not the direct consequences of an overabundance of stressors, or of a failure of the stress response .but instead, are the result of overactivation of the stress response.

This raised a critical conundrum, one not appreciated for decades by the stress physiologists: Most physiological stressors, if severe enough to activate the stress response to a magnitude that would prove damaging if prolonged, would kill the organism long before the stress response itself would become damaging. Moreover, no degree of homeostatic imbalance, no matter how severe, can give rise to the broad and varied collection of slowly emerging pathologies. For example, a severe hemorrhage kills within minutes to hours; there are no pathophysiological routes by which, instead, it causes hypertension, impaired resistance to rhinoviruses (the cause of the common cold), or anovulatory reproductive cycles.

Thus, when could stress (outside the artificial context of the laboratory) ever be prolonged enough to cause the slow emergence of these stress-related diseases, rather than relatively rapid death? And the answer, which ushered in a psychological perspective in the field, is now clear—the prolonged stressors that produce disease through chronic activation of the stress response are those that are overwhelmingly psychological rather than physical in nature.

PSYCHOLOGICAL MODIFIERS OF PHYSIOLOGICAL STRESSORS

The importance of psychological factors in stress-related disease became clear by the late 1950s, beginning with the work of John Mason, and carried on by his intellectual descendents, such as Seymour Levine, Martin Seligman, and Jay Weiss (Mason, 1968). The clarity and elegance of this approach could be shown with a single example of the sorts of studies carried out. Consider a rat being exposed, intermittently and unpredictably, to an electric shock. As would be expected, the stress response would be mobilized; this should be viewed as adaptive, insofar as most organisms (i.e., those not in cages) would respond to such pain with the muscular expenditure of fleeing.

Now, a variable is added to this paradigm. As one example, 10 seconds before each shock, a warning bell would sound, thereby converting an unpredictable stressor into a predictable one. And, remarkably, less of a stress response would occur (e.g., less secretion of glucocorticoids) (Seligman & Meyer, 1970; Weiss et al., 1971a, 1971b, 1971c; Davis & Levine, 1982). Such predictability is generally interpreted as protecting for two reasons: (1) by signaling the impending nature of the stressor, predictability aids the planning of coping strategies during the stressor; and (2) when accurate, predictive information also signals when one is safe (for at least 10 seconds) (Seligman, 1975).

This genre of research demonstrates the importance of a second variable, in this case a sense of control. For the same external physiological stressor (e.g., shocks), less of a stress response will be activated in a rat that believes that, by lever pressing, it is avoiding getting an even larger number of shocks (Houston, 1972). Similar findings apply to humans. This has been demonstrated in experiments (with designs remarkably similar to the shock/lever press design in rodents) (Brier et al., 1987), as well as in the work force, where low-demand/low-control occupations produce more stress-related disease than do high-demand/high-control occupations (Lundberg & Frankenhaeuser, 1978; Karasek & Theorell, 1990).

Another variable uncovered concerns the perception of whether things are worsening or improving, amid the identical external physiological stressor. Thus, for example, a stress-response is triggered in a baboon who, as a result of tense, competitive interactions with a rival, is declining in the dominance hierarchy, but not in a baboon experiencing the same rate of those interactions with a rival where, as a result, his rank is rising (Sapolsky, 1992).

Collectively, these studies show that psychological context can modulate the linkage between a physiological stressor and the magnitude of the subsequent stress-response.

Such findings raised the issue of whether psychological context could modify the primary response of the body to a physiological stressor (i.e., to alter the extent to which homeostasis was lost). In other words, when an optimal psychological context reduced the stress response caused by a physical stressor, would that be because the stressor was now less of a challenge to homeostasis, or, for the same extent of loss of homeostasis, because less of a stress response would be mobilized? For example, for the identical physical fight with a rival baboon, would a salutary psychological context (i.e., it becoming clear that the fight would result in a rise in rank) mean that muscles required less energy to be mobilized than if it became clear that the result would be a drop in rank? For the same fight, would a salutary outcome produce less blood loss following a canine slash than that produced by an adverse psychological outcome?

There is little evidence that psychological context could make a physical stressor less homeostatically challenging. This is seen in a recent study examining the neural processing of pain, and of the psychological context in which pain occurs. A painful stimulus to a finger activates a certain number of pain receptors beneath the skin. This leads to activation of spinal pain pathways that, among other consequences, activate an array of brain regions. Functional brain imaging allows one to roughly dichotomize the areas activated into somatosensory regions processing the primary pain signal, and higher-order, more interpretive brain regions that assign meaning to the primary sensory information (such as the anterior cingulate). One can then generate the pain signal in a different psychological context. Specifically, an inert cream, that the subject has been told has analgesic properties, is applied prior to the painful stimulus. In this situation, subjective pain perception is blunted (i.e., the cream works as a placebo). And on a neurobiological level, the primary sensory processing regions of the brain are activated as before (reflecting activation of the same number of local pain receptors in the skin in response to the homeostatic imbalance of the injury), while there is blunted activation of the upstream interpretive parts of the brain (Wager et al., 2004).

Subsequent studies have expanded on the idea that psychological context can modulate the stress response. Some demonstrate the importance of factors such as novelty or discrepancy from expectation, showing their partial similarity to variables such as control and predictability (Haidt & Rodin, 1999).

Collectively, these findings represented landmark challenges to the purely physiological school of thinking about stress and health (and findings that were strongly resisted by physiologists, most notably Selye himself). These also paved the way for studies that were even more troubling to the physiologists.

PSYCHOLOGICAL INITIATORS OF THE STRESS RESPONSE

The studies just described demonstrate that psychological context can modify the connection between the extent of homeostatic imbalance and the magnitude of the stress response mobilized. Studies done during the Mason era also showed that the stress response can be initiated by certain psychological contexts, even in the absence of any physiological stressor.

The clearest demonstration of this is shown in an elegant, subtle style of study. In it, a rat is placed daily in a cage capable of delivering shocks and has been trained to lever-press in order to minimize such shocks. Placement of the rat in the cage with the lever removed causes a substantial stress response, even in the absence of any shocks (Coover, Ursin, & Levine, 1973). In other words, loss of senses of control and predictability, in the absence of loss of physiological homeostasis, can activate the stress response. This approach even allowed for the same sort of quantitative precision shown earlier in stress physiology. For example, increasing gradations of a sense of unpredictability causes increasing magnitudes of a stress response, independent of any actual physical stressor (Levine, Weiner, & Coe, 1989).

The activation of the stress response in the absence of any physical challenge to homeostasis was profoundly bewildering to stress physiologists (Selye, 1975). This bewilderment was made even stronger by Mason's (1975a, 1975b) that physical stressors activate the stress response only insofar as they induce a sense of loss of control, predictability, and so on.

As emphasized by Selye, this extreme view could not be the case; this is because a robust stress response is activated by a surgical incision in anesthetized individuals (i.e., with no capacity to experience psychological distress) (Selye, 1975a, 1975b). Nonetheless, the findings generated by the Mason school decisively made the idea that stress and health can be understood in purely physiological terms untenable.

Thus, psychological context can alter the linkage between a physiological stressor and the stress response. Moreover, psychological stressors can initiate the stress response in the absence of a physiological stressor. Furthermore, psychological stress is at the core of understanding why chronic stress is pathogenic. As such, the regulation of thought and emotion is of great relevance to health. How such regulation occurs is, of course, the focus of the rest of this book.

ALLOSTASIS AND EMOTION REGULATION

The issue of regulation of emotion and thought in the context of stress and disease becomes relevant in an additional realm. To appreciate this, one must consider a recent trend in physiology, namely, the new concept of "allostasis." As introduced by the physiologists Sterling and Eyer (1988; Sterling, 2003), and championed by the neurobiologist McEwen (e.g., McEwen, 2004), this neologism represents a more modern and expansive version of the homeostasis concept. One difference between homeostasis and allostasis concerns setpoints. The homeostatic realm of thinking focuses on the idea that there exist single optimal setpoints for each measure (e.g., an ideal blood pressure, or level of circulating glucose, or body temperature). Allostatic thinking, in contrast, emphasizes that an optimal setpoint for any physiological measure can differ dramatically by circumstance (what has been termed "constancy through change").

It is the second difference between the two—homeostasis and allostasis—that is most pertinent. In the concept of homeostasis, homeostatic imbalance is solved locally; in contrast, allostatic imbalance is viewed as being solved with more global responses. This can be illustrated with a metaphor. Suppose a period of drought in California brings about the challenge of a water shortage. A local, "homeostatic" solution might be to mandate that all new shower heads must be low-flow. In contrast, an allostatic solution might involve that change, but along with it, convincing people to conserve water, rethinking the irrigation of semiarid California farmland in order to grow rice, acting to slow down global warming, and so on. In the same way, consider a water shortage in the body. A purely homeostatic solution would be for the kidneys to increase water retention in response to a local signal of dehydration. In the more accurate allostatic scenario, the detection of dehydration is signaled to the brain. This triggers an array of adaptations, including water retention in the kidneys, withdrawal of water from places in the body where it readily evaporates (skin, mouth, and nose), and adaptations that can consist of behavior (such as developing a sense of thirst and drinking).

The allostatic concept is powerful, insofar as it is a more accurate description of physiology than is the homeostatic concept. For our purposes, the most important feature of allostasis is recognizing that the solution to a physiological challenge, in some circumstances, can involve behavior.

This raises an important problem. Specifically, it is difficult to fix one aspect of physiology without potentially having adverse effects in some other domain of balance, and the more far-flung and varied the allostatic compensations, the more likely it is that something else will be impaired in the process (Sterling, 2003). This represents the drawbacks of bodies evolving to, in effect, detect locally and fix globally. And within the context of physiological regulation, behavioral means of correction can be among the most far-flung.

This fact becomes relevant in considering stress and health. Allostasis teaches that sometimes a stressor, including a psychological stressor, can be dealt with by behavioral means. And in some circumstances, that behavior can prove more damaging than the stressor itself. The habitual consumption of alcohol to solve the psychological stressor of anxiety illustrates this point. It may provide a local solution (i.e., decreasing the immediate state of anxiety). However, it may have more serious adverse global consequences (e.g., cirrhosis of the liver). Moreover, it may ultimately worsen the primary source of loss of homeostasis, namely the anxiety. This might be through local means, such as the fact that while alcohol is anxiolytic when blood alcohol levels are rising, it is anxiogenic when levels are falling. In addition, the worsening might occur through more indirect means, such as increased anxiety about job stability due to alcohol-induced absenteeism.

As another example, consider the tendency of individuals who are anxious, fearful, or frustrated to act aggressively toward another individual (this is shown with the increases in child and spousal abuse that occur during times of economic stress). While displacement aggression may temporarily quell a stress response (Virgin & Sapolsky, 1997), its long-term social consequences are often maladaptive.

This leads to a key point, namely, that the behavioral coping responses that are the least adaptive in the long run are often the easiest and most tempting in the short run.

This underlines the importance of this volume: the appropriate regulation of thoughts and emotions not only decreases the likelihood of pathogenic activation of the stress response due to psychological factors but also increases the likelihood that the behavioral responses to psychological stressors that are chosen are adaptive ones.

This point incorporates the world of addiction, of self-defeating behaviors and self-fulfilling prophesies, of winning battles and losing wars. Most important, it tells us much about the tendency of the members of so many social species, including our own, to resort to the most damaging of all behavioral coping outlets for stress. Meyer Friedman was the pioneering cardiologist who became a founding parent of behavioral medicine by being the first to describe the Type A personality. In discussing the adverse consequences of that behavioral profile, he would emphasize what he considered to be the most malign consequence of being Type A, and it was an opinion that often surprised colleagues. It was that, thanks to their particular style of behavioral coping, Type A individuals consistently displace aggression on to those around them; as he would state, the prime purpose of his research was not to reduce the incidence of heart disease, but to make people kinder to each other (personal communication). Within the realm of stress and health, the greatest challenge of emotional regulation is to resist the temptation of avoiding ulcers by giving them to others.

ACKNOWLEDGMENTS

Manuscript assistance and advice was provided by Alan Basbaum, James Gross, Brian Knutson, and Jon Levine.

REFERENCES

Brier, A., Albus, M., Pickar, D., Zahn, T. P., Wolkowitz, O., & Paul, S.. (1987). Controllable and uncontrollable stress in humans: Alterations in mood and neuroendocrine and psychophysiological function. *American Journal of Psychiatry, 144,* 1419

Cannon, W. (1914). The interrelations of emotions as suggested by recent physiological researches. *American Journal of Psychology, 25,* 256.

Cannon, W. (1932/1963). *The wisdom of the body.* New York: Peter Smith.

Cannon, W. (1936, May). The role of emotion in disease. *Annals of Internal Medicine, 9.*

Coover, G., Ursin, H., & Levine, S. (1973). Plasma corticosterone levels during active avoidance learning in rats. *Journal of Comparative Physiology and Psychology, 82,* 170–174.

Davis, H., & Levine, S. (1982). Predictability, control, and the pituitary–adrenal response in rats. *Journal of Comparative Physiology and Psychology, 96,* 393–404.

Gann, D., Cryer, G., & Pirkle, J. (1977). Physiological inhibition and facilitation of the adrenocortical response to hemorrhage. *American Journal of Physiology, 232,* R5–R9.

Haidt, J., & Rodin, J. (1999). Control and efficacy as interdisciplinary bridges. *Review of General Psychology, 3,* 317.

Houston, B. (1972). Control over stress, locus of control, and response to stress. *Journal of Personality and Social Psychology, 21,* 249.

Karasek, R., & Theorell, T. (1990). *Health work, stress, productivity, and the reconstruction of working life.* New York: Basic Books.

Levine, S., Wiener, S., & Coe, C. (1989). The psychoneuroendocrinology of stress: A psychobiological perspective. In S. Levine & F. Brush (Eds.), *Psychoendocrinology* (pp. 1–21). San Diego, CA: Academic Press.

Lundberg, U., & Frankenhaeuser, M. (1978). Psychophysiological reactions to noise as modified by personal control over noise intensity. *Biological Psychology, 6,* 51–59.

Mason, J. (1968). A review of psychoendocrine research on the pituitary–adrenal cortical system. *Psychosomatic Medicine, 30*, 576.

Mason, J. (1975a). A historical view of the stress field: Part II. *Journal of Human Stress, 1*, 6.

Mason, J. (1975b). A historical view of the stress field: Part I. *Journal of Human Stress, 1*, 22.

McEwen, B. (2004). Protection and damage from acute and chronic stress: Allostasis and allostatic overload and relevance to the pathophysiology of psychiatric disorders. *Annals of the New York Academy of Science, 1032*, 1.

Munck, A., Guyre, P., & Holbrook, N. (1984). Physiological functions of glucocorticoids during stress and their relation to pharmacological actions. *Endocrinology Review, 5*, 25–44.

Raison, C., & Miller, A. (2003). When not enough is too much: The role of insufficient glucocorticoid signaling in the pathophysiology of stress-related disorders. *American Journal of Psychiatry, 160*, 1554–1565.

Sapolsky, R. (1992). Cortisol concentrations and the social significance of rank instability among wild baboons. *Psychoneuroendocrinology, 17*, 701.

Sapolsky, R., Romero, M., & Munck, A. (2000). How do glucocorticoids influence the stress-response?: Integrating permissive, suppressive, stimulatory, and preparative actions. *Endocrinology Review, 21*, 55–89.

Seligman, M. (1975). *Helplessness: On depression, development and death.* San Francisco: Freeman.

Seligman, M., & Meyer, B. (1970). Chronic fear and ulcers with rats as a function of the unpredictability of safety. *Journal of Comparative Physiology and Psychiatry, 73*, 202.

Selye, H. (1936a). A syndrome produced by diverse nocuous agents. *Nature, 138*, 32.

Selye, H. (1936b). Thymus and adrenals in response of the organism to injuries and intoxications. *British Journal of Experimental Pathology, 17*, 234.

Selye, H. (1975). Confusion and controversy in the stress field. *Journal of Human Stress, 1*, 37–44.

Selye, H. (1979). *The stress of my life.* New York: Van Nostrand.

Sterling, P. (2003). Principles of allostasis: Optimal design, predictive regulation, pathophysiology and rational therapeutics. In J. Schulkin (Ed.), *Allostasis, homeostasis, and the costs of adaptation* (pp. 56–85). Cambridge, MA: MIT Press,

Sterling, P., & Eyer, J. (1988). Allostasis: A new paradigm to explain arousal pathology. In S. Fisher & J. Reason (Eds.), *Handbook of life stress, cognition, and health* (pp. 629–649). New York: Wiley.

Taylor, S., Klein, L., Lewis, B., Gruenewald, T., & Gurung, R., Updegraff, J. (2000). Biobehavioral responses to stress in females: Tend-and-befriend, not fight-or-flight. *Psychological Review, 107*, 411–429.

Virgin, C., & Sapolsky, R. (1997). Styles of male social behavior and their endocrine correlates among low-ranking baboons. American *Journal of Primates, 42*, 25–39.

Wager, T., Rilling, J., Smith, E., Sokolik, A., Casey, K., Davidson, R., et al. (2004). Placebo-induced changes in fMRI in the anticipation and experience of pain. *Science, 303*, 1162–1167.

Weiss, J. (1971a). Effects of coping behavior in different warning signal conditions on stress pathology in rats. *Journal of Comparative Physiology and Psychology, 77*, 1.

Weiss, J. (1971b). Effects of punishing the coping response (conflict) on stress pathology in rats. *Journal of Comparative Physiology and Psychology, 77*, 14.

Weiss, J. (1971c). Effects of coping behavior with and without a feedback signal on stress pathology in rats. *Journal of Comparative Physiology and Psychology, 77*, 22.

Author Index

Ersland, S., 467
Esaki, T., 124, 125
Eslinger, P. J., 71, 76, 78
Espinet, S. D., 150, 151
Essex, M. J., 297, 298
Etscheidt, M., 574
Eugene, F., 50, 51
Evans, D., 332, 336, 341
Everitt, B. J., 144
Everly, G. S., 470
Evers, C., 8, 370, 440
Exline, J. J., 513
Eyer, J., 612

Faber, R. J., 409
Fabes, R. A., 229, 231, 256, 257, 291, 294, 295–296, 296, 297, 298, 299, 300, 301, 339, 525, 531
Facchin, P., 96
Faccini, L., 592
Fadiga, L., 431
Fahrenberg, J., 586
Fairburn, C. G., 536
Fales, C. L., 207
Fallgatter, A., 121
Falls, W. A., 30
Fan, J., 337, 338
Fanselow, M. S., 28, 29, 35, 55
Farah, M. J., 71, 75, 76, 77, 99, 141, 145, 218
Fargo, S., 572
Farrell, J., 275, 276
Faw, B., 397
Fazaa, N., 569
Fazio, R. H., 433
Federman, E., 567
Feeney, J. A., 454, 455
Fehr, B., 398
Fehr, E., 212
Fein, S., 437
Feinman, S., 482
Feinstein, J. S., 340
Feit, A., 385, 386
Feldman Barrett, L., 92, 271
Feldman, L. A., 394
Feldman, R., 239, 254
Fellows, L. K., 71, 75, 76, 77, 99, 145
Fera, F., 119, 120, 122, 123, 124, 126
Ferenz-Gillies, R., 451, 452, 453, 458
Ferguson, E. D., 7
Ferguson, M. J., 401, 430
Ferguson, T. J., 276
Fernandez, G., 174
Ferrari, J. R., 411
Ferrell, R. E., 113, 114, 117, 125
Ferry, A. T., 31
Festinger, L., 418
Feuk, L., 112
Fiedler, K., 7
Field, D., 317
Field, T., 255
Fiez, J. A., 214

Fig, L. M., 38
Finch, D. M., 586
Findler, L., 457
Fine, S. E., 296
Fingerman, K. L., 310, 315
Finkenauer, C., 468, 469, 475, 476, 478
Finn, P. R., 572
Finucane, M. L., 382
Fisberg, M., 589
Fischer, K. W., 448
Fischl, B., 31, 38, 39
Fischle, M., 383
Fischman, A. J., 104
Fisher, P., 291, 336, 338
Fiske, D. W., 598
Fiske, S. T., 207, 432
Fissell, C., 214
Fissell, K., 219
Fitzsimons, G. J., 437, 440
Fitzsimons, G. M., 136, 430, 431, 432
Fivush, R., 260, 482
Flanagan, K. D., 279
Flavell, E., 273
Flavell, J. H., 273
Fleming, W. S., 451, 452, 453, 458
Fletcher, C. W., 172
Fletcher, G. J. O., 174
Flett, G. L., 411
Flint, J., 114, 118
Floden, D., 145
Flombaum, J. I., 338
Flood, M. F., 256
Florian, V., 452, 453, 454, 455, 457
Flory, J. D., 113, 114
Floyd, N. S., 32
Flugge, G., 58–59
Flynn, H. A., 574
Foa, E. B., 548
Fockenberg, D. A., 435
Fogassi, L., 431
Folkman, S., 278, 310, 322, 358, 359, 397, 449
Fonagy, P., 375, 451
Fong, C., 437
Fong, G. W., 96, 97, 209, 214
Foot, P., 208
Forbes, E. E., 8, 110, 598
Forgas, J. P., 434–435
Forman, E. M., 258
Fourkas, A. D., 590
Fowler, C., 374, 377
Fox, A., 8, 18, 74, 81, 87, 253, 292, 311, 535
Fox, A. S., 61, 62, 207
Fox, M. D., 340
Fox, N., 290, 291
Fox, N. A., 12, 60, 229, 231, 232, 234, 235, 238, 240, 241, 242, 253, 334
Frackowiak, R. S., 141
Fragopoulos, F., 574
Fraley, R. C., 362, 446, 447, 452, 456

Francart, B., 399, 590
Francis, D., 239
Francis, D. D., 239
Frank, M. J., 219
Frank, R. H., 78, 181
Frankel, A. N., 549
Frankel, C. B., 18, 270, 490
Frankel, M., 71, 74
Frankenburg, F. R., 584
Frankenhaeuser, M., 611
Frankenstein, U. N., 95
Franz, C. E., 169
Frattaroli, J., 470
Frederick, S., 187, 188, 213
Fredman, D., 112
Fredrickson, B. F., 320
Fredrickson, B. L., 175, 314, 417, 550
Fredrikson, M., 119
Freimer, N. B., 114, 115, 118
Fresco, D. M., 175, 542, 549
Freud, A., 182, 374, 377
Freud, S., 7, 374, 380
Frey, K. A., 35
Frick, P. J., 531, 532–533
Friedman, N. P., 20
Friedman, R. J., 493
Friesen, W., 585
Friesen, W. V., 309, 313, 394
Frijda, N., 206, 270, 271, 472, 473
Frijda, N. H., 5, 7, 18, 160, 171, 394, 396, 397, 448, 489, 495, 496, 497, 498, 499
Friston, K., 214
Frith, C. D., 92, 150, 431
Frith, U., 150
Fritschy, J. M., 564
Froehlich, J. C., 563
Fromm, E., 515
Fromme, K., 563, 564, 567, 572
Frone, M. R., 569, 571
Frosch, C., 233, 241
Frosch, C. A., 262
Frost, R. O., 414
Fry, P. S., 409
Frye, D., 136, 137, 138
Frysztak, R. J., 36
Fuchs, E., 58–59
Fukui, K., 119
Fulbright, R. K., 585
Funder, D., 379
Fung, H., 260, 315, 316
Fung, H. H., 314, 486
Furedy, J. J., 593
Furmark, T., 121
Fuster, J., 31, 144

Gabel, P. C., 570
Gable, S. L., 468
Gabrieli, J. D. E., 18, 50, 51, 89, 93, 94, 98, 104, 338, 341, 343, 381, 387, 432, 535
Gado, M. H., 57
Gage, F. H., 58
Galaburda, A. M., 78

Subject Index

inhibition of emotional
experience and, 451–452
jealousy and, 459
overview, 461–462
Awareness of an emotion
atypical development, 278–281
external versus internal cues,
273–278
overview, 271, 282–283

Balancing, response, 323–324
Basal amygdala, 29–30
Basal ganglia
emotional regulation and, 72t
integrating top-down with
bottom-up approaches, 89–90,
91f, 92–93, 92f
mindfulness skills and, 595–596
Basal nuclei, 36–37
Basolateral complex (BLA), 31
Behavior
caregiver influences and, 241–
243
core features of emotions and,
5
cultural regulation of, 497–499
intuitiveness and, 200n
moral aspects of anger and,
515–516
religious practice and, 509–511
response modulation and, 15
socioemotional selectivity
theory, 322
treatment of anxiety and mood
disorders and, 553–555
Behavior, antisocial. See also
Externalizing disorders
arousal and, 533
attention-deficit/hyperactivity
disorder (ADHD), 529
emotion regulation and, 531–
534
patterns of, 527
Behavior genetics, 111–115
Behavioral activation, 594–595
Behavioral association studies, 115
Behavioral Inhibition System, 334–
335
Behavioral responses to emotions,
5
Behavioral therapy, 39–40
Beliefs
affective forecasting and, 197
Carnegie Mellon University
study on intuitions and
beliefs, 188–191, 191t, 192t,
193–196, 193t, 194t, 195t
emotional awareness and, 274–
275
emotional climate of family life
and, 258–259
religious, 506–509
"Big Five" personality domains,
354–363, 355t, 360t
Binge eating, 414–415

Biological basis. See also
Physiological basis
caregiver influences and, 238–
241
inhibition, 27–28
mindfulness skills and, 595–596
temperament and, 331–332
Blood alcohol concentration
(BAC), 561
Borderline personality disorder,
584–586. See also
Psychopathology
Bottom-up approach
cognitive control of emotion
model, 100–102, 101f, 102f
implications of, 102–105
integrating with top-down
approaches, 89–90, 91f, 92–
93, 92f
overview, 88–89
Boundary issues, 12–13
Brain bases of emotion and
emotion regulation, 310–311.
See Neural bases of emotion
and emotion regulation
Brain damage, 73–77
Brain-derived neurotrophic factor
(BDNF), 116–117
Broaden-and-build theory, 175
Buddhism. See also Religion, role of
in emotional regulation
anger and, 514
meditation and, 511

Candidate gene association
approach, 112–113
Cardiovascular functioning
lifespan development and, 311–
312
stress response and, 607–608,
609–610
Caregiver influences. See also
Parenting
attachment and, 236–238
cultural models of self and
relating and, 494–495
development of emotion
regulation and, 235–236,
238–243
overview, 229–234, 243–244
Caregiving quality, 301–302
Carnegie Mellon University study
on intuitions and beliefs
overview, 188–191, 191t, 192t,
193–196, 193t, 194t, 195t
scenarios from, 197–199
Catastrophizing, 174
Catecho-O-methyltransferase
(COMT)
imaging genetics, 116–117
personality and, 113–114
Caudate, 72t
CAVE (Content Analysis of
Verbatim Explanations), 167,
173

Central effects of an emotional
experience
overview, 473
social sharing of emotions and,
480
Central physiology, 5
Change, cognitive. See also
Rationalization; Reappraisal
anxiety and mood disorders
and, 550–551
"Big Five" personality domains,
355t
cognitive control of emotion
model, 100–102, 101f, 102f
coping styles and, 360t
extraversion and, 356
overview, 14–15, 96–100, 181–
182, 351–352, 352f
social–cognitive constructs and,
365t
treatment of anxiety and mood
disorders and, 552–553
Childhood. See also Developmental
processes
attentional deployment and, 13–
14
cognitive change and, 14–15
development of emotion
regulation skills during, 231
spatial processing systems, 338
temperament and, 335–336
training of executive attention
and, 343–344
Children's Behavior Questionnaire
(CBQ), 338
Choice, intertemporal, 213–215,
214f, 215f
Christianity. See also Religion, role
of in emotional regulation
anger and, 514, 516–518
changing concepts of, 505–506
guilt and, 512–513
meditation and, 511
Cingulate control systems
cognitive change and, 96–100
genetics of emotion regulation
and, 121–123
intertemporal choice and, 214–
215, 214f
placebo affect and, 98
regulation of attention via
emotion and, 340
Clarity
emotional intelligence and, 364–
366, 365t
social sharing of emotions and,
476t
Classification of affect regulation
strategies, 181–182, 374f
Clinical–empirical model of
emotion regulation
conflict, defense and
compromise, 377–380
coping and decision making,
380–383